D1333459

K07778

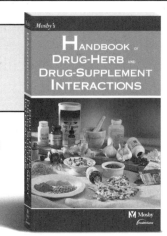
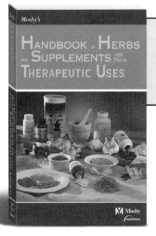
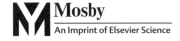

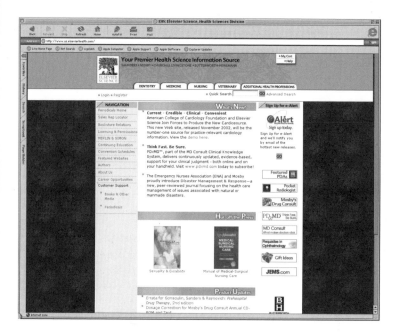

Clinical Guide to
Nutrition and Dietary Supplements
in
Disease Management

Clinical Guide to
Nutrition and Dietary Supplements
in
Disease Management

Jennifer R. Jamison, MBBCh, PhD, EdD,
FACNEM, Grad Dip Human Nutr
Professor of Diagnostic Sciences
Department of Complementary Medicine
RMIT University
Bundoora Campus
Victoria, Australia

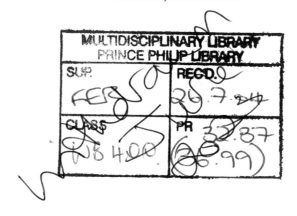
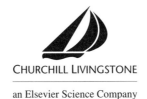
CHURCHILL LIVINGSTONE

an Elsevier Science Company

CHURCHILL LIVINGSTONE
an Elsevier Science Company

Notice

Complementary and alternative medicine is an ever-changing field. Standard safety precautions must be followed, but as new research and clinical experience broaden our knowledge, changes in treatment and drug therapy may become necessary or appropriate. Readers are advised to check the most current product information provided by the manufacturer of each drug to be administered to verify the recommended dose, the method and duration of administration, and contraindications. It is the responsibility of the licensed prescriber, relying on experience and knowledge of the patient, to determine dosages and the best treatment for each individual patient. Neither the publisher nor the editors assume any liability for any injury and/or damage to persons or property arising from this publication.

Publishing Director: Linda Duncan

Publishing Manager: Inta Ozols

Associate Developmental Editor: Melissa Kuster Deutsch

Project Manager: Peggy Fagen

Designer: Mark Bernard

Library of Congress Cataloging-in-Publication Data

Jamison, Jennifer R.
  Clinical guide to nutrition and dietary supplements in disease management / Jennifer R. Jamison.
    p. cm.
Includes bibliographical references and index.
ISBN 0-443-07193-4 (alk. paper)
  1. Dietary supplements. 2. Diet therapy. 3. Nutrition. I. Title

RM258.5.J35 2003
615.8′54–dc21

                                                                                    2003048515

Preface

Nutritional medicine is gaining popularity as health professionals become more aware of scientifically proven links between diet and disease and laypersons find it increasingly agreeable to self-medicate using natural remedies. The mushrooming interest in herbs and supplements has recently resulted in the publication of a plethora of texts in this area. The texts tend to fall into two distinct categories: either they are well referenced, detailed, and tending to the esoteric, offering little practical advice to the generalist, or they are full of handy hints but lack any evidence of being based on scientifically validated information. It is hoped that this text will provide scientifically sound information while providing useful clinical guidance to those embarking on a pathway that boldly traverses conventional and alternative health care.

Part One focuses on a number of important principles in the use of diet, nutrient, and herbal supplements. Part Two discusses certain disorders that are prevalent and/or particularly amenable to nutrient or herbal intervention. No attempt has been made to provide a comprehensive list of anecdotally useful interventions. Instead, the attempt has been to identify at least one probable mechanism involved in the pathogenesis of each listed condition and to demonstrate how selection of particular foods, nutrients, and/or herbs can offer biologically plausible intervention. Part Three provides additional details on popular nutrients, herbs, and functional foods. Rather than attempting to list all the active constituents in herbs, only major physiologically active constituents are noted. When exploring the potential clinical usefulness of dietary supplements, I have made an attempt to provide an overview of current scientific thinking. In clinically effective doses, herbs and nutrient supplements constitute drug therapy; accordingly safe clinical care in nutritional medicine requires careful attention to dose, side effects, and interactions. Pregnant and breastfeeding women should be particularly cautious.

Nutritional medicine is a rapidly advancing area that holds enormous promise. It is hoped that this text will be a useful aid in an exciting but often confusing area of health care.

Jennifer R. Jamison

Contributors

Colm Benson, ND, BHSc
Health Services Manager
Analytical Reference Laboratories
Victoria, Australia

Ian Brighthope, MBBS, Dip Agr Sc, MATA, FACNEM
President
Australasian College of Nutritional and Environmental Medicine
Victoria, Australia

Paul Holman, MA, MB, Bchir, MRCPsych
Consultant Psychiatrist
Victoria, Australia

Toni Jordan, BSc, Grad Cert BA, AACNEM
National Sales & Marketing Manager
Nutrition Care Pharmaceuticals
Victoria, Australia

Contents

Foreword

The question of what to eat has been around since the dawn of humanity. Eating is fundamental to survival. The content of foods not only influences our short-term feelings of well being and satiety but also a profoundly affects our long-term health, longevity, and risk of developing both acute and chronic diseases.

Although it is becoming increasingly acknowledged that diet is one of the most important factors in determining our health, there are many factors that can be considered when determining our food choices. These include social factors such as tradition, culture, religion, social status, fashion, branding, societal norms, media exposure, education, mass-marketing, peer pressures, and commercial interests; pragmatic factors such as availability, location, production methods, distribution and storage, time of day, affordability, and cooking methods; and individual factors such as time pressures, impulses, instant versus delayed gratification, physical activity, boredom, hunger, personal taste, education, past exposure, weight considerations, ethical beliefs, environmental concerns, desired health status, and specific medical conditions. It is important not only that we consider all of these factors but also that we understanding how these factors interact.

In addition to making choices about what to eat, we must also contend with an expanding range of options for supplementing our diets. A visit to any health store or pharmacy will attest to the vast number of products available, including products containing vitamins, trace elements, and minerals; fish and plant oils; probiotics; amino acid and protein combinations; herbal and plant products, including teas, tinctures, extracts, powders, tablets, and whole plant extracts; and a vast array of combination products that include many of these ingredients in various formulations and potencies.

The scientific study of nutrition aims to determine how different nutritional substances interact with life processes and contribute to healthy functioning and to determine how they may be manipulated to help prevent and treat disease. Nutritional medicine is based on evidence accumulated from a variety of different sources, including basic biochemical investigations and in vitro studies looking at fundamental biologicalprocesses; animal studies looking at dietary manipulations in specific diseases and deficiency states; and human trials that range from randomized, double-blind, placebo-controlled studies of specific interventions for specific diseases, to case-control studies, cohort studies, and individual case series, to epidemiological studies looking at patterns of nutrition and disease in large populations.

Evaluating the available evidence can be very confusing, because it is often difficult to understand how in vitro or biochemical studies are relevant to clinical use. In addition, research results are not always clear-cut, as evidenced by the often-conflicting results and ongoing controversies among experts. Furthermore, it may be difficult to determine the independence of the information because many powerful forces behind the scenes control what studies are done and how information is presented.

Given the vast array of food choices, the many possibilities for supplementation, and the numerous studies on different nutrients and diseases, it is easy to become overwhelmed by the complexity of it all. This complexity is further increased when we consider the possible interactions that nutritional factors may have with pharmaceutical interventions and the highly individual physiological, psychological, and social factors that contribute to our overall health status.

Despite the difficulties involved, the use of any therapy should be based on the best available evidence and informed decision making on behalf of both practitioners and patients. Such decision making is both a subtle art and an inexact science, and it is up to individual practitioners and patients to seek the necessary information upon which to base their decisions.

This book attempts to help guide us through this maze of information. The author has a long history of teaching and performing research in nutritional medicine and provides a well-referenced, evidence-based account of the clinical use of nutritional interventions in the treatment of specific diseases. This book should make the task of finding relevant information easier and therefore go along way toward helping us make informed decisions that contribute to the prevention and alleviation of human disease.

Marc Cohen, MBBS (Hons) PhD, BMed Sc (Hons), FAMAS
President, Australasian Integrative Medicine Association (AIMA)
Head of Department,
Department of Complementary Medicine,
Faculty of Life Sciences
RMIT University

PART ONE

PRINCIPLES OF NUTRITIONAL MEDICINE

■ CHAPTER 1 ■

THE SCIENCE OF NUTRITIONAL MEDICINE

> The science of nutritional medicine identifies dietary choices and supplements likely to benefit most people: it uses evidence-based medicine to cate to the norm.

Nutritional medicine holds enormous promise for health care in the new millennium. New insights are anticipated to emerge from the often disagreeable discourse between conventional and alternative health professionals. Instead of a conceptual gulf caused by adherence to discrepant practice paradigms, practitioners of conventional and alternative medicine are likely to join forces in delivering a humanized yet scientific form of health care. Increasing acceptance of natural medicine and enhanced criticism of the mechanistic nature of conventional practice have fostered a transformation in health care. Conventional health care is undergoing an overhaul. The reductionist approach characteristic of the biomedical model is increasingly being modified to embrace the more holistic interactive approach captured by the infomedical model. Table 1-1 compares the biomedical and infomedical models. The system proposed within the infomedical model is one of continual interaction between and within mind and body.[1] The clinical repercussions of this changed perception include recognition of a consciously active role for the patient, acceptance of clinical uncertainty as an inevitable component of care, and a renewed appreciation of the complexity of those processes that influence the balance between health and disease.

The paradigm shift in contemporary health care is characterized by a profound change in how the relationships between physician and patient, mind and body, and cause and effect are viewed. Instead of conforming to a dominant-submissive relationship, patients are emerging as partners in health care. Instead of viewing mind and body as separate, patients and physicians are recognizing psyche and soma as inseparable. Health and disease triggers are no longer viewed as being limited to physical, chemical, or microbial factors; psychosocial stimuli are also perceived to advance wellness or disease. In contrast to the belief that individual disease triggers have a unilinear cause-effect relationship, multiple causes are perceived to

TABLE 1-1 ■ Paradigms and Nutritional Research

MODEL	BIOMODEL	INFOMEDICAL
Stimulus-response relationship	Unidirectional cause-effect	Circular self-organizing interaction
Meaningful outcome	Statistical significance	Substantive improvement
Meaningful information	Objectively measured	Subjective and objective data
Strongest research design	Double-blind, placebo-controlled clinical trial	Case study series
Clinical benefit	Universally applicable knowledge	Local knowledge and patient-focused care

mutually influence health status. The interplay of somatic and extrasomatic factors is envisaged in the initiation and progression of disease. The recognition of the many factors that determine clinical outcomes has provided impetus to the need to revisit the causative role of foods, herbs, and nutrients in the promotion of health and the management of disease.

Interaction of various biologic systems makes it difficult to predict the clinical repercussions of particular interventions.

STRATEGIES FOR ESTABLISHING CAUSE-EFFECT RELATIONSHIPS

When the reductionist approach is applied in clinical research, the gold standard is a randomized, double-blind, placebo-controlled clinical trial. The strength of this research design lies in its ability to most clearly link cause and effect. Establishing a causal relationship provides valuable insight into both pathogenesis and clinical intervention. The reductionist approach, with its emphasis on linking specific causes with particular outcomes, favors a single-nutrient approach. It is particularly useful for evaluating nutrients as drug substitutes. However, this approach is problematic on at least two fronts. On the one hand, the research methodology of blinded placebo-controlled trials is subject to ethical constraints. On the other hand, the appropriateness and validity of the single-nutrient approach are being questioned. The growing conviction that plant biologic activity confers benefit when plants are consumed by humans challenges the use of single-nutrient therapy.[2] An inverse relationship between the risk of death from coronary heart disease and vitamin E intake from food has been detected,[3] yet this inverse association is not associated with vitamin E supplements. Disjunction between this relationship is even more puzzling when it is recalled that higher doses of vitamin E than those achievable by diet alone are needed to protect low-density lipoprotein from oxidation. Oxidized low-density lipoprotein is a major risk factor for coronary heart disease.

The fundamental virtue of the reductionist approach is that it tends to clarify cause-effect relationships. It can be used to detect factors that predispose to disease and to identify interventions that alter the course of disease. Although randomized, double-blind, placebo-controlled clinical trials are the most scientifically sound approach to establishing cause-effect relationships, other research designs can be used to ascertain the likelihood of such a relationship. Although the probability of a cause-effect relationship is greatest when substantiating evidence can be obtained from studies in humans, other strategies that identify a correlation between dietary choices and wellness or disease have been developed. Animal studies and other laboratory investigations meet a number of the criteria required to establish a cause-effect relationship.

Biologic plausibility is an important criterion that should be met in any postulated cause-effect relationship. The biologic plausibility of using nutrients to influence pathophysiologic processes is well established. The role of nutrients in diverse biochemical pathways is well documented in numerous laboratory studies. A logical extrapolation of the proven ability of nutrients to affect biologic processes in the test tube is to postulate their use in clinical care. However, laboratory evidence does not constitute proof that nutrient intervention is effective in clinical practice. For example, genistein inhibits thrombin formation and platelet activation in vitro, yet dietary supplementation with soy protein isolates rich in isoflavones has no significant effect in vivo.[4,5] Reductionist science works well at the level of the basic sciences. It is more problematic when intact organisms are studied. Animal experiments lend themselves to mechanistic exploration, and analogous situations can be identified but are seriously limited by questions about cross-species validity. This latter dilemma is addressed by epidemiologic studies.

Epidemiologic studies have species relevance but are quasi-experimental and rely on statistical methods for control. Because each approach has its own limitations, epidemiologic studies rely on a variety of research methods. In this way the possibility of a cause-effect relationship is increased. Criteria used to establish a cause-effect relationship that may be tested by means of epidemiologic studies include the following: consistency between different studies supporting a relationship between intervention and outcome, an appropriate temporal relationship (i.e., cause precedes effect), and a strong and dose-responsive relationship between intervention and outcome. Data to meet these criteria can be collected from analytic epidemiologic trials in which cohort or prospective longitudinal studies are done; from descriptive studies based on prevalence, survey, or cross-sectional studies; and from case studies and case reports, the weakest source of evidence (see Box 1-1). Analytic epidemiology provides good descriptions and suggests useful diet-disease inferences. Case-control studies provide useful clues but low-level exposures, confounding and methodologic errors can cause researchers to overlook both protective and harmful repercussions of nutritional intervention. Contradictions become apparent when data from different research methods are compared. For example, animal studies

■ Box 1-1 ■

RESEARCH STANDARDS WITHIN THE BIOMEDICAL MODEL

Acceptable data gathering methods

Three research designs providing adequately strong evidence for ascertaining effectiveness are:

1. Randomized, controlled trials. These experimental studies are ideally:
   - Placebo-controlled (i.e., the outcome of an inert intervention is compared with the test remedy)
   - Double-blinded (i.e., neither the patient/subject nor the clinician/researcher knows who is in which group)
   - Randomized to avoid subject selection bias
   - Prospective
2. Cohort studies are analytic observational studies. They attempt to correct for known confounding variables, but selection bias is a problem. Cohort studies follow persons:
   - Who have been exposed to risk factors and control subjects who have no known exposure
   - Longitudinally over time (i.e., are prospective)
3. Case-control studies are descriptive observational studies. Observer recall and selection bias are problems. Case control studies:
   - Are retrospective in design
   - Involve cases that are selected on the basis of having the disease

Ranking of evidence*

Ranking of sources of evidence according to likelihood that the research design or information gathered is capable of providing acceptable evidence for effectiveness is based on the system used by the Canadian and US Preventive Taskforces in which evidence was categorized as follows:

Category I: Evidence obtained from at least one properly randomized trial

Category II-1: Evidence obtained from well-designed controlled trial without randomization

Category II-2: Evidence from well-designed cohort or case-control studies (i.e., analytical epidemiologic)

Category II-3: Evidence from multiple time series (i.e., comparisons between times and places with or without intervention) and dramatic results of uncontrolled experiments

Category II-4: Evidence from animal experiments

Category III-Evidence from the following:
- Opinions of respected authorities based on clinical experience
- Descriptive studies or case reports
- Reports of expert committees

---

* Canadian Task Force: The periodic health examination, *Can Med Assoc J* 121:1193-254, 1979.
US Preventive Services Task Force: *Guide to clinical preventive services: report of the U.S. preventive services task force,* ed 2, Baltimore, 1996, Lippincott Williams & Wilkins.

suggest fat restriction decreases breast cancer; descriptive epidemiologic studies support an inverse relationship, but case-control studies show little effect and cohort studies show few associations.[6]

Establishing clinical reality is fraught with difficulty despite clear guidelines within the biomedical model. An eclectic approach is often used to enhance the reliability and validity of conclusions. For example, in the case of functional foods, it has been suggested that before particular benefits are claimed, evidence should be obtained from diverse sources and weighted as follows: epidemiologic studies (25%), intervention studies (35%), animal models (25%), and mechanism of action (15%).[7] Gathering data from diverse study modes goes some way toward accommodating the multiple health and disease triggers that continually interact to determine clinical outcome.

In contrast to the biomedical model, which supposes that outcomes are predictable, the holistic infomedical model accepts that clinical outcomes are unpredictable and that uncertainty is the rule rather than the exception. The infomedical model accepts discrepancies explaining the inexplicable as an inherent feature of the circular cybernetic of interacting information systems characteristic of living organisms. The infomedical model seemingly provides a framework in which dietary choices and the interaction between nutrition and health or disease triggers can be better accommodated. However, the infomedical model has yet to clarify the rules of a research design for investigating nutritional medicine. A template that accommodates the diverse and interacting influences of behavioral choices and dietary complexity, while permitting objective measurement of clinical outcomes, is needed.

The biomedical model abhors uncertainty and seeks to limit clinical unpredictability by withholding unproven therapy. The infomedical model advocates interventions that have yet to achieve scientific validation. Such discrepancies in the use of nutritional information have resulted in two schools of nutritional "medicine."

> Within the infomedical model, clinical evaluation and confirmation of biologically plausible interventions is necessary, because outcomes are inherently unpredictable.

THE DILEMMA OF LINKING DIET AND DISEASE

The conservative school enjoys scientific respectability at the expense of patients who may be deprived of the benefits of nutritional therapy, albeit this is inadequately proven. The alternative school, consistent with its focus on maximizing wellness in individual patients, may serve as a source of nutritional misinformation.

When faced with conflicting results, the conservative school withholds potentially beneficial therapy until it meets rigorous scientific standards.

Delays in therapeutic management are a direct consequence of relying on the gold standard of a randomized, placebo-controlled clinical trial. In the absence of such trials, postulates supported by biologically plausible mechanisms need to be treated with skepticism. This is done because conventional nutritional medicine recognizes that the side effects of a therapy with uncertain efficacy approximate infinity. However, such a stance is fraught with contradictions. Although the medical profession hesitates to advocate routine nutritional supplementation for patients, one study showed that half the female physicians surveyed in the United States took a multivitamin-mineral supplement.[8]

Nonetheless, as demonstrated by epidemiologic studies involving diet and colon cancer, hesitation in providing unproven dietary advice is not without justification.[9] Results of case-control studies suggest that an increased energy intake increases the risk of colon cancer. Descriptive studies suggest that fat is associated with an increased risk for this disease. A high-fat diet is inevitably a high-energy diet. However, a meta-analysis that included 13 case-control studies suggested that total energy intake, rather than the intake of fat, correlated with the risk of colon cancer. On the other hand, case-control studies suggest that animal, but not vegetable, fat correlates positively with colon cancer. To complicate matters, cohort studies, after controlling for energy, showed no association with fat but suggested that red meat, especially beef, was associated with a risk for colon cancer. Animal experimentation has added a further dimension, suggesting that genetically distinct colon cancers respond discretely to nutritional intervention. High consumption of monounsaturated fats, mostly derived from olive oil, was associated with a statistically significant decrease in the risk of cancer with wild-type Ki-ras genotype but not in the risk of Ki-ras–mutated cancers.[10] To further confuse matters, a high calcium intake was found to be associated with a decreased risk of Ki-ras–mutated tumors but not wild-type tumors. A major source of calcium for humans is milk, a rich source of animal fat! Contradictory findings do not lend themselves to confident clinical intervention. Although it is desirable to provide unambiguous dietary advice, it is even more important to justify prescription of nutritional supplements. Appropriate dietary advice and nutrient prescriptions are most likely to arise when cause-effect or food/nutrient-health relationships are established.

Difficulties associated with identifying causal associations between diet and disease make safe, effective, and timely nutritional intervention problematic. Variables making intervention equivocal for conventional practitioners of nutritional medicine include the following.[11,12]

- Metabolic uniqueness: This ensures that a correlation between dietary intake and pathogenesis enjoys a degree of individual variation. This uniqueness is of sufficient significance for authorities to maintain that although it is possible to enunciate recommended daily allowances to prevent nutrient deficiencies, it precludes community prescription of optimal intake levels. A further repercussion of metabolic individuality is the indeterminate relationship of blood nutrient levels to dietary intake because of the complexity of metabolic interactions.

- Inappropriate merging of data: Data from nonidentical diseases may be inadvertently merged. Colorectal cancer represents three diseases: cancer of the proximal colon, the distal colon, and the rectum.[11] Epidemiologic evidence suggests that cancer of the distal colon is linked to fat, whereas cancer of the rectum is more closely associated with alcohol consumption.

- Dietary complexity: It is likely that the diet of free living individuals contains a number of compounds, generally assumed to be innocuous, that have unrecognized biologic effects. Results from epidemiologic studies, active pharmacologic principles identified in traditional plants, and the role of natural antioxidants in maintaining food quality would seem to support this construct.[13] Dietary studies are based on responses to whole foods. Attempts to adopt a reductionist approach in nutritional epidemiology are clouded both by the propensity for individual micronutrients to be present in numerous food sources and the impact of the physical characteristics of a food on physiologic responses. Nutrient interactions and the diversity of nutrients in any one food make it difficult to predict the effect of supplementation with single nutrients. Data from two cohort studies, one in males older than 10 years and one in females older than 12 years, suggested that several carotenoids may reduce the risk of lung cancer.[14] Because carotenes are a group of compounds with different potencies, such findings do not provide adequate evidence for recommending single-nutrient supplementation. Mechanistic explanations do not help to clarify the situation. Supplementation with lycopene, the most powerful carotenoid antioxidant, may be advisable if the protection afforded is the result of singlet oxygen quenching. However, if the benefit results from the propensity of vitamin A and retinenes to regulate epithelial cell differentiation and maintenance, then lycopene supplementation is a poor choice. Lycopene, unlike the other carotenes, appears devoid of provitamin A activity.

- Nutrient bioavailability: Depending on its exact chemical nature, the bioavailability of a nutrient varies. The availability and absorption of carotenes are influenced by food preparation. Lycopene is best absorbed from heated tomatoes consumed in oil.[15] The two major soy isoflavones, genistein and daidzein, differ in bioavailability, with daidzein being more readily excreted in urine.[16] Similar statements apply to carotenoids and tocopheryl. Nutrient interaction may also influence bioavailability as demonstrated by feeding tocopherol with and without vitamin A.[17] Components of plants, which are themselves not active, may improve the stability, solubility, bioavailability, or half-life of physiologically active chemicals. Synergy is a particularly important concept with respect to herbal pharmacology.

- Pitfalls associated with dietary analysis in free living population groups: Errors in judging portion size, problems of recall, dietary variability over time, and food table inaccuracies confound study outcomes. Furthermore, it is recognized that overweight and obese persons increasingly underreport their total energy intake and, presumably, their total fat consumption. Concerns about the accuracy of dietary self-reporting caused by measurement error biases have even led to the suggestion that current reporting instruments may be inadequate for analytic epidemiologic studies of dietary fat and disease risk.[11]

- Time lapse between dietary exposure and disease: A decade or more may pass between the initiation of carcinogenesis and the overt development of cancer.[18]
- Difficulties associated with human trials: Human trials raise ethical questions and require substantial financial and manpower resources.

In contrast to conventional reductionist thinking, alternative medicine practitioners work within a holisitic model that accepts uncertainty as inevitable. Rather than finding virtue in delaying the use of potentially useful therapy until scientifically sound advice can be given, alternative medicine practitioners may require only that a therapeutic regimen be biologically plausible and supported by personal clinical experience accumulated from individual case studies. Attribution of a particular outcome to a natural intervention based on its likely impact on pathophysiologic processes is potentially fraught with danger. Individual behavioral differences can distort biochemical, not to mention clinical, outcomes. Daily oral supplementation with 30 mg of beta-carotene significantly raises serum beta-carotene levels. Daily supplementation with 30 mg of beta-carotene successfully prevents the serum-depleting effect of steroid contraceptive use but fails to prevent serum depletion of beta-carotene induced by cigarette smoking.[19] Biologic plausibility is not synonymous with clinical validity. Pathophysiologic reality cannot be assumed in the clinical context, and it certainly cannot alone be anticipated to confer clinical effectiveness.

> Thus biologic plausibility is a desirable but inadequate justification for intervention.

A multitude of variables may confound the extrapolation of in vitro findings to in vivo situations. Flavonoids such as quercetin are an example. Some, but not all, prospective epidemiologic studies have shown that the intake of flavonols (e.g., quercetin) and flavones is inversely associated with subsequent coronary heart disease.[20] Possible explanations for these discrepancies include the nature, concentration, and ratio of the members of the flavonoid group ingested, the whole-food environment of the relevant flavonoid glycoside, the efficacy of the intestinal flora at splitting the flavonoid ring, and the relative concentration and nature of other nutrients including antioxidants in the host. Quercetin, like other flavonoids, has been shown in vitro and in animal studies to modify eicosanoid biosynthesis, protect low-density lipoprotein from oxidation, inhibit platelet aggregation, and promote relaxation of cardiovascular smooth muscle.[21] Direct translation of these in vitro effects into clinical care would result in quercetin-dampening inflammation, prevention of atherosclerotic plaque formation, inhibition of thrombosis, prevention of arrhythmia, and reduction of hypertension. Although quercetin has yet to demonstrate this potential in in vivo studies, it is a strong antioxidant and is believed to offer effective protection against lipid oxidation in the cell membrane.[22] One mechanism of action may be through protection of ascorbate. However, concurrent pulse-radiolytic generation has shown that dihydroquercetin, but not quercetin, is capable of reducing the ascorbyl radical.[23] Another interesting finding is that ascorbic acid in elderberry juice protects the anthocyanins, but not quercetin, against oxidative degradation.[24] The interaction between vitamin C and quercetin in vivo is open to speculation. It remains unclear whether quercetin acts as an antioxidant in vivo.[25] One simplistic explanation for discrepancies between in vivo and in vitro findings may be failure to absorb nutrients. In fact, flavonoids in foods are largely considered nonabsorbable because they are bound to sugars and only become available after removal of the glycoside by bacteria in the colon. However, a recent study showed that humans absorb the quercetin glycosides from onions (52%) far better than those from pure aglycone (24%).[26] Because human subjects can absorb significant amounts of bioavailable quercetin, it is unlikely that this theory can explain the quercetin paradox.

SCIENCE AND CLINICAL REALITY

With so many variables confusing clear scientific understanding, it is not altogether surprising to find that some old wives tales may be emerging as scientifically sound. The current status of garlic as therapy and nutritional intervention for the common cold deserves special mention.

Garlic: A Popular Panacea

Garlic has long been touted as health-promoting. Increasing evidence indicates that garlic has antimicrobial, antithrombotic, antitumor, hypolipidemic, antiarthritic, and hypoglycemic activity.[27-29] Epidemiologic, animal, and in vitro studies have provided evidence for an anticarcinogenic effect of active ingredients in garlic. Although garlic is clearly not a panacea for cancer, its broad range of beneficial effects are today deemed worthy of serious consideration in clinical trials for the prevention and treatment of cancer. Garlic is reported to stimulate immunity. It enhances the activity of various cells, such as macrophages and natural killer cells, and increases the production of cytokines. Garlic is associated with the beneficial T_H1 antitumor response characteristic of effective cancer immunotherapies.[30] In a meta-analyses of the epidemiologic literature on the association between garlic consumption and risk of various cancers, investigators concluded that a high intake of both raw and cooked may be associated with a protective effect against stomach and colorectal cancers.[31] However, heterogeneity of effect estimates, differences in dose estimation, publication bias, and the possibility that results were confounded by total vegetable consumption do preclude definitive conclusions.

Similarly, garlic has potential as an agent for prevention and treatment of atherosclerosis and atherosclerosis-related diseases.[32] In animal models, garlic may prevent and achieve regression of atherosclerosis in the artery wall. It has been postulated that garlic indirectly affects atherosclerosis by reduction of hyperlipidemia and hypertension. It may also reduce the risk of a critical occlusion by preventing thrombus formation. The observed effects in animal studies could be explained as garlic reducing the lipid content in arterial cells. By preventing intracellular lipid accumulation, a trigger for atherosclerotic cell proliferation and extracellular matrix synthesis is neutralized. In a meta-analysis of randomized, double-blind, placebo-controlled trials, Stevinson et al[33] concluded that garlic is superior to placebo in reducing total cholesterol levels. However, because the size of the effect was modest, these authors questioned the usefulness of garlic for treating hypercholesterolemia; whereas other investigators concluded that, on the basis of a number of new rigorously designed controlled studies, there is increasingly less evidence for lipid-lowering properties of garlic preparations.[34] Despite encouraging results from early studies, there is growing pessimism that garlic could ever be regarded as an antihyperlipidemic agent. However, this does not preclude garlic as a useful option for enhancing cardiovascular health. Marginal reduction of blood cholesterol levels is only one of garlic's potential effects on coronary artery disease. The direct effects of garlic on aortic elasticity, its antioxidant properties, and antiplatelet aggregation effects need evaluation before judgment on the impact of garlic on cardiovascular health can be made. Modest changes to the pathogenesis of coronary heart disease at diverse levels may well combine to provide a meaningful clinical outcome. Use of garlic may not be clinically justified according to a reductionist approach in which each of its effects is individually evaluated. However, it may be regarded as a valuable health adjunct when the totality of its clinical impact is appreciated. Although garlic is regarded as one of the potentially safe herbs,[35] garlic supplementation does affect warfarin activity.[36]

Within the framework of the biomedical model, when the efficacy of an intervention is uncertain and side effects are present, risk is considered to approximate infinity. Such reservations are consistent with the universal applicability outcome criterion of the biomedical model. Within the framework of the infomedical model, any intervention that achieves a health gain without untoward effects is deemed clinically worthwhile. When the focus is on the individual and subjective data are considered, garlic can be an important intervention option in the treatment of a patient seeking a "natural" approach.

The Dilemma of the Common Cold

Nutritional controversy not only surrounds the use of particular nutrients and herbs, it also besets the prevention and management of prevalent ailments somewhat resistant to conventional medication. With an annual cost exceeding $3.5 billion in the United States alone, coryza, or the common cold, has long been a condition of general interest. Despite widespread lay belief, the medical profession generally regards prevention of colds by vitamin C as a myth.[37] Dr. Linus Pauling's conclusion in the 1970s that vitamin C had physiologic effects on the common cold was of major importance, because it conflicted with the prevailing consensus that the only physiologic effect of vitamin C on human beings was prevention of scurvy.[38] Pauling, in a single placebo-controlled trial conducted with schoolchildren in a Swiss skiing camp, found a significant decrease in the incidence and duration of the common cold in the group taking 1 g of vitamin C daily. Pauling's extrapolation of this finding to the general population was in error as to the magnitude of the effect, but its general thrust has not been invalidated. A recent American survey indicated that two of three patients believed that vitamin C reduced cold symptoms.[39] Further recent scientific results support the patients' perspective. A clinical trial demonstrated an 85% decrease in flu and cold symptoms in the test group, compared with the control group.[40] The test group in this study, on reporting symptoms, was treated with 1000 mg of vitamin C per hour for the first 6 hours, followed by 1000 mg every 8 hours thereafter. In one review 23 studies were analyzed, and the authors concluded that vitamin C in daily doses of 2 g or greater was most effective in managing the common cold.[41] In another study 30 randomized and nonrandomized trials were reviewed, and the authors concluded that long-term daily supplementation with vitamin C in large doses did not appear to prevent colds, although they did concede that the duration of cold symptoms was moderately reduced by relatively high doses.[42]

Although vitamin C enjoys more popular acclaim, it is not the only nutrient that may affect the common cold. Trials of zinc supplementation for colds have been ongoing for more than a decade, with contradictory results.[43] Formulation of the zinc medication may contribute to such contradictions: addition of citric or tartaric acid, sorbitol, or mannitol may reduce zinc availability in the supplement. Furthermore, not only may the medium in which the active principle is delivered affect outcome, variations in the pathogenesis of the condition may modify therapeutic efficacy. In one trial it was reported that zinc acetate had no effect but that zinc gluconate may reduce the average duration of symptoms by 1 day, from 3.5 to 2.5 days.[44] This benefit was only detected with experimentally induced colds, and not in cases of natural infection. Echinacea is another increasingly popular but unproven cold remedy.[45]

Numerous explanations are possible for the conflicting results of nutritional interventions to manage the common cold. The dose of the nutrient used, the frequency and duration of administration, and the form or chemical environment of the supplement all influence outcome. The stage of the infection at which therapy is initiated and the extent to which the supplement is absorbed affect efficacy. The patient's nutritional and immune status, any associated disorders, and other medications also have an impact.

A PRAGMATIC APPROACH WITH HEALTH THE OBJECTIVE

Increasingly, the sound science offered by a reductionist approach is being applied to nutritional medicine with encouraging results. A systematic review of current thinking in nutritional medicine is being undertaken; the objective is to determine how food, herbs, and nutrients may promote health and prevent disease.

Although superficially the framework of the drug-paradigm testing model provides a gold standard for evaluating nutritional intervention, perfunctory implementation of this framework invites erroneous conclusions. Results from clinical trials are poor or largely fail to support epidemiologic findings that suggest antioxidants reduce the risk of cardiovascular disease and cancer.[46,47] Several explanations for such discrepancies, which cast serious doubt on the validity of clinical trials, can be offered. These include failure to recognize that nutrients achieve their outcome as a result of synergistic metabolic interrelationships, that stereochemistry influences efficacy, and that it is simplistic to presume a direct dose-response relationship in a cybernetic system.[47] Furthermore, within the reductionist drug paradigm, when the magnitude of the outcome of a nutritional intervention fails to achieve a statistically significant effect, rejection of the remedy tends to follow. In contrast, the ability of an intervention to achieve discernible improvement in the individual patient demands recognition within the infomedical model.

When certain individuals respond to a nutritional intervention, the framework of the infomedical model leads the investigator to consider the reason for such discrepancies. Issues ranging from biologic individuality to age-specific responses need to be addressed. The possibility that subclinical depletion of one or more nutrients may distinguish responders from nonresponders needs to be explored. Failure to have prescribed an effective clinical dose and the prospect of having unbalanced nutrient-nutrient interactions also need to be considered. Within the infomedical framework, a marginal but statistically insignificant improvement triggers a search for reasons that some patients respond when others do not. Instead of encouraging rejection of the intervention, such a marginal improvement serves as an impetus for further investigation to achieve better understanding. On the other hand, an unproven therapy may do more harm than good.

Reliable information about the efficacy, safety, and cost of nutrient and herbal interventions is a prerequisite for cost-effective care. Such data are not always available, and concern has been expressed that control of nutritional and herbal products by licensing of remedies with equivocal benefits and few risks, as evidenced by a long history of safe use, may increase societal health care costs.[48] It is along this tightrope that nutritional medicine must progress. The dilemma is well demonstrated by vitamin E. In view of the very low risk of reasonable supplementation and the difficulty in obtaining more than about 30 IU/day from a balanced diet, Pryor[49] advocates vitamin E supplementation. However, a calculation based on observational data suggests that 170 to 250 persons would need to take vitamin E for 10 years to prevent one myocardial infarction or stroke.[50] Furthermore, Pearce et al[50] remind readers that, although observational data suggest a cardiovascular benefit from vitamin E supplementation, the results of controlled clinical trials are inconsistent regarding the effect on nonfatal myocardial infarction. A protective effect of vitamin E against fatal myocardial infarction has not been demonstrated.[50] On the other hand, a survey of 180 American cardiologists indicated that about half took vitamin E prophylactically.[51] The issue is to agree on a point at which the weight of the scientific evidence is to be judged adequate.

Nutrient intervention need not be delayed until absolute proof of its efficacy has been documented; therapy may be initiated when the weight of the scientific evidence is judged to be adequate

SCIENCE ADAPTING TO CLINICAL REALITY

Science is never "complete," and the infomedical model recognizes that outcomes are indeterminate. It is possible, or even probable, that each condition for which a nutrient provides benefit will have a unique dose-effect curve. Furthermore, different nutrients may be anticipated to interact (e.g., antioxidants appear to act synergistically), so supplementation with one might be more effective if it is combined with another. Because of the great amount of time required, conduction of trials that adequately probe the dose-effect curve for promising nutrients for each condition they might affect or studies of all the possible combinations of other micronutrients that might act to enhance effectiveness is an insurmountable task.

The situation with herbal medicine is no less problematic. Herbs contain numerous interacting constituents. It has even been suggested that a new paradigm needs to be used whereby the pharmacologic effects of traditional herbs such as ginseng can be understood in the light of their polyvalent actions as demonstrated by ginseng saponins with their positive antimutagenic, anticancer, antiinflammatory, antidiabetes, and neurovascular effects.[52]

Recent recognition that two different kinds of clinical investigations, explanatory and pragmatic trials, are scientifically valid suggests an opportunity for substantial progress.[53] Pragmatic trials do not require that the patient or the therapist be unaware of the treatment being given and can even be designed to take patient preferences into account. This approach is not free of pitfalls. In fact, for most psychiatric disorders, a given treatment is not considered effective without a placebo control. The placebo response rate in psychiatric conditions varies widely across patient groups; it may be as high as 65% in a group of patients with major depression.[54] Even triangulation of results derived from diverse studies, while providing a useful template for determining the interface between exploration and therapy, cannot eliminate this problem. For example, it is difficult to judge how much of the clinical improvement is due to the treatment in open studies in which a treatment is given to a group of patients and their response is hypothetically contrasted to the treatment outcome with a known drug. A second type of investigation compares the experimental treatment with a drug of established efficacy. Even if an experimental treatment appears comparable to a standard drug in terms of response, it may be that a placebo would have done as well as either treatment over the course of the study. Investigations in which a treatment is compared with placebo, sometimes with the use of a standard drug as a third arm of the study, therefore remain an important dimension in therapeutic validation. Such methodological modifications are making it increasingly appropriate and feasible to evaluate alternative medicine by means of scientifically accepted methodology.

The infomedical model accepts that intervention in the face of uncertainty is normal. The biomedical model provides a research methodology for minimizing such uncertainty. It provides a system for incrementally increasing understanding and reducing, but not eliminating, uncertainty. Modern nutritional science and herbal medicine need to continue to build on an eclectic science. Increasingly, clinical trials are showing statistically significant benefits. Within an eclectic science, clinical trials that show benefit but not statistical significance are also recognized as contributing to knowledge. Although review of these trials should be rigorously undertaken to identify methodological flaws such as an inappropriate combination of nutrients, failure to use a pharmacologically active dose, and inadequate attention to individual biologic variation, contributions from these studies should not be automatically discarded. The clinical reality of nutritional medicine is that it is the response of each individual, and not the population norm, that matters. Ultimately, patients remain the best index of therapeutic efficacy (see Case Study). Claims that a protocol lacks adequate scientific validation should serve to trigger further clinical investigation; even flawed trials may alert investigators to particular subgroups. Evidence accumulated from the clinical experience of practitioners can no longer be ignored.

It is the task of future studies to identify populations that can benefit from nutritional and herbal supplementation, to define doses and treatment duration, to recognize drug interactions, and in the case of nutrients, to clarify whether mixtures, rather than single nutrients, are more advantageous. The infomedical model ensures a patient-centered focus, and the biomedical model seeks to balance the benefits and risks of intervention. Models are

CASE STUDY

Ian Brighthope

One of the most severe causes of acute viral infection that I have encountered was that of Ms. M, a 19-year-old who presented with adult chicken pox (varicella). The treatment program can be applied to any acute viral infection including influenza, infectious mononucleosis (glandular fever), and the common cold. Ms. M had a massive outbreak of vesicles on her trunk, limbs, and face; but the most serious were those in her nasopharynx extending to the laryngopharynx and esophagus. She was in severe pain, with cough and total dysphagia. It was midnight when she called, and I began making preparations for immediate admission to the infectious diseases hospital. Adult chicken pox can be rapidly fatal.

At the time of presentation, I gave Ms. M an intravenous infusion of fluids and most importantly, the following:

- Intravenous sodium ascorbate equivalent to 30 g of vitamin C over 30 minutes
- Intravenous zinc (30 mg of elemental zinc)
- Intramuscular high-potency B vitamins, including 15 mg of folic acid and 50 to 100 mg of the other B vitamins

She left the clinic that night. The next morning she rang to make an appointment. She had gone home the previous night with the intention of going to the hospital after collecting some belongings. She felt so much better and was able to speak and drink water within 2 hours of receiving the injections that she decided not to go until morning.

When I saw her the next morning, she was feeling much better and smiling. The discharging lesions had mostly crusted over. She had no more cough and was asking whether it were really necessary to be hospitalized. I had never seen such a dramatic change in a patient's condition, although I had witnessed thousands of cases that had improved with the use of megadose intravenous vitamin C. I decided to wait for the results of a complete blood count and chest x-ray before deciding on admission. The complete blood count confirmed an acute viral infection with an increased erythrocyte sedimentation rate and lymphocytes, and the chest x-ray was essentially clear. I gave her repeat treatments of the intravenous therapy for 2 days, at the end of which she had only four to five lesions remaining. I added some Echinacea, 1500 mg administered twice daily, to an oral regimen of vitamins, antioxidants, and 8 to 10 g of vitamin C daily. She remains well and takes supplements on a regular basis. She has not had a cold or the flu for 10 years despite a stressful, busy lifestyle.

This protocol can be used for any acute viral infection (e.g., severe glandular fever, influenza, or chicken pox).

merely frameworks for viewing the world. The real world does not conform to any one model, but rather exhibits characteristics described in both the biomedical and infomedical models. The findings of the "old science" provide a good foundation for future developments. Studies in which well-established research methods are used are demonstrating a scientific basis for nutritional remedies long considered folklore by conservative medicine.

Herein lies the fascination and frustration of nutritional medicine. Establishing common ground between conservative and alternative nutritional medicine is likely to emerge as nutritional medicine draws from both models. The final result will inevitably need to be a blend of science and art.

REFERENCES

1. Foss L: The challenge to biomedicine: a foundations perspective, *J Med Philos* 14:165-91, 1989.
2. Cordain L: Cereal grain: humanity's double-edged sword, *World Rev Nutr Diet* 84:19-73, 1999.
3. Ascherio A: Antioxidants and stroke, *Am J Clin Nutr* 72:337-8, 2000.
4. Wilcox JN, Blumenthal BF: Thrombotic mechanisms in atherosclerosis: potential impact of soy proteins, *J Nutr* 125(suppl 3):631S-8S, 1995.
5. Gooderham MH, Adlercreutz H, Ojala ST, et al: A soy protein isolate rich in genistein and daidzein and its effects on plasma isoflavone concentrations, platelet aggregation, blood lipids in normal men, *J Nutr* 126:2000-6, 1996.
6. Dwyer JT: Human studies on the effects of fatty acids on cancer: summary, gaps, and future research, *Am J Clin Nutr* 66(suppl 6):1581S-6S, 1997.
7. Milner JA: Functional foods: the US perspective, *Am J Clin Nutr* 71(suppl 6):1654S-9S, 2000.
8. Frank E, Bendich A, Denniston M: Use of vitamin-mineral supplements by female physicians in the United States, *Am J Clin Nutr* 72:969-75, 2000.
9. Giovannucci E, Goldin B: The role of fat, fatty acids, and total energy intake in the etiology of human colon cancer, *Am J Clin Nutr* 66 (suppl 6):1564S-71S, 1997.
10. Bautista D, Obrador A, Moreno V, et al: Ki-ras mutation modifies the protective effect of dietary monounsaturated fat and calcium on sporadic colorectal cancer, *Cancer Epidemiol Biomarkers Prev* 6:57-61, 1997.
11. Weisburger JH: Dietary fat and risk of chronic disease: mechanistic insights from experimental studies, *J Am Diet Assoc* 97(suppl 7):S16-23, 1997.
12. Wynder EL, Weisburger JH, Ng SK: Nutrition: the need to define "optimal" intake as a basis for public policy decisions, *Am J Public Health* 82:346-50, 1992.
13. Chesson A, Collins A: Assessment of the role of diet in cancer prevention, *Cancer Lett* 114:237-45, 1997.
14. Michaud DS, Feskanich D, Rimm EB, et al: Intake of specific carotenoids and risk of lung cancer in 2 prospective US cohorts, *Am J Clin Nutr* 72:990-7, 2000.
15. Arab L, Steck S: Lycopene and cardiovascular disease, *Am J Clin Nutr* 71(suppl 6):1691S-5S, 2000.
16. Hendrich S, Lee KW, Xu X, et al: Defining food components as new nutrients, *J Nutr* 124(suppl 9):1789S-92S, 1994.
17. Eicher SD, Morrill JL, Velazco J: Bioavailability of alpha-tocopherol fed with retinol and relative bioavailability of D-alpha-tocopherol or DL-alpha-tocopherol acetate, *J Dairy Sci* 80:393-9, 1997.
18. Bertram JS, Kolonel LN, Meyskens FL: Rationale and strategies for chemoprevention of cancer in humans, *Cancer Res* 47:3012-31, 1987.
19. Palan PR, Chang CJ, Mikhail MS, et al: Plasma concentrations of micronutrients during a nine-month clinical trial of beta-carotene in women with precursor cervical cancer lesions, *Nutr Cancer* 30:46-52, 1998.

20. Hollman PC, Katan MB: Health effects and bioavailability of dietary flavonols, *Free Radic Res* 31(suppl):S75-80, 1999.
21. Formica JV, Regelson W: Review of the biology of Quercetin and related bioflavonoids, *Food Chem Toxicol* 33:1061-80, 1995.
22. Chen ZY, Chan PT, Ho KY, et al: Antioxidant activity of natural flavonoids is governed by number and location of their aromatic hydroxyl groups, *Chem Phys Lipids* 79:157-63, 1996.
23. Bors W, Michel C, Schikora S: Interaction of flavonoids with ascorbate and determination of their univalent redox potentials: a pulse radiolysis study, *Free Radic Biol Med* 19:45-52, 1995.
24. Kaack K, Austed T: Interaction of vitamin C and flavonoids in elderberry (Sambucus nigra L.) during juice processing, *Plant Foods Hum Nutr* 52:187-98, 1998.
25. Wiseman H: The bioavailability of non-nutrient plant factors: dietary flavonoids and phyto-oestrogens, *Proc Nutr Soc* 58:139-46, 1999.
26. Hollman PC, Katan MB: Absorption, metabolism and health effects of dietary flavonoids in man, *Biomed Pharmacother* 51:305-10, 1997.
27. Sato T, Miyata G: The nutraceutical benefit: part iv: garlic, *Nutrition* 16:787-8, 2000.
28. Agarwal KC: Therapeutic actions of garlic constituents, *Med Res Rev* 16:111-24, 1996.
29. Ali M, Thomson M, Afzal M: Garlic and onions: their effect on eicosanoid metabolism and its clinical relevance, *Prostaglandins Leukot Essent Fatty Acids* 62:55-73, 2000.
30. Lamm DL, Riggs DR: The potential application of Allium sativum (garlic) for the treatment of bladder cancer, *Urol Clin North Am* 27:157-62, xi, 2000.
31. Fleischauer AT, Poole C, Arab L: Garlic consumption and cancer prevention: meta-analyses of colorectal and stomach cancers, *Am J Clin Nutr* 72:1047-52, 2000.
32. Orekhov AN, Grunwald J: Effects of garlic on atherosclerosis, *Nutrition* 13:656-63, 1997.
33. Stevinson C, Pittler MH, Ernst E: Garlic for treating hypercholesterolemia. A meta-analysis of randomized clinical trials, *Ann Intern Med* 133:420-9, 2000.
34. Berthold HK, Sudhop T: Garlic preparations for prevention of atherosclerosis, *Curr Opin Lipidol* 9:565-9, 1998.
35. Klepser TB, Klepser ME: Unsafe and potentially safe herbal therapies, *Am J Health Syst Pharm* 56:125-38, 1999.
36. Evans V: Herbs and the brain: friend or foe? The effects of ginkgo and garlic on warfarin use, *J Neurosci Nurs* 32:229-32, 2000.
37. Truswell AS: Nutrition—the myths, *Royal Prince Alfred Mag* 82:13, 1984.
38. Hemila H: Vitamin C supplementation and the common cold—was Linus Pauling right or wrong? *Int J Vitam Nutr Res* 67:329-35, 1997.
39. Braun BL, Fowles JB, Solberg L, et al: Patient beliefs about the characteristics, causes, and care of the common cold: an update, *J Fam Pract* 49:153-6, 2000.
40. Gorton HC, Jarvis K: The effectiveness of vitamin C in preventing and relieving the symptoms of virus-induced respiratory infections, *J Manipulative Physiol Ther* 22:530-3, 1999.
41. Hemila H: Vitamin C supplementation and common cold symptoms: factors affecting the magnitude of the benefit, *Med Hypotheses* 52:171-8, 1999.

42. Douglas RM, Chalker EB, Treacy B: Vitamin C for preventing and treating the common cold, *Cochrane Database Syst Rev* 2000;(2):CD000980.
43. Marshall I: Zinc for the common cold, *Cochrane Database Syst Rev* 2000;(2):CD001364.
44. Turner RB, Cetnarowski WE: Effect of treatment with zinc gluconate or zinc acetate on experimental and natural colds, *Clin Infect Dis* 31:1202-8, 2000.
45. Giles JT, Palat CT, Chien SH, et al: Evaluation of echinacea for treatment of the common cold, *Pharmacotherapy* 20:690-7, 2000.
46. Tran TL: Antioxidant supplements to prevent heart disease: real hope or empty hype? *Postgrad Med* 109:109-114, 2001.
47. Wheatley C: Vitamin trials and cancer: what went wrong? *J Nutr Env Med* 8:277-288, 1998.
48. Ashcroft DM, Po AL: Herbal remedies: issues in licensing and economic evaluation, *Pharmacoeconomics* 16:321-8, 1999.
49. Pryor WA: Vitamin E and heart disease: basic science to clinical intervention trials, *Free Radic Biol Med* 28:141-64, 2000.
50. Pearce KA, Boosalis MG, Yeager B: Update on vitamin supplements for the prevention of coronary disease and stroke, *Am Fam Physician* 62:1359-66, 2000.
51. Mehta J: Intake of antioxidants among American cardiologists, *Am J Cardiol* 79:1558-60, 1997.
52. Ong YC, Yong EL: Panax (ginseng)—panacea or placebo? Molecular and cellular basis of its pharmacological activity, *Ann Acad Med Singapore* 29:42-6, 2000.
53. Walker LG, Anderson J: Testing complementary and alternative therapies within a research protocol, *Eur J Cancer* 35:1614-8, 1999.
54. Quitkin FM: Placebos, drug effects, and study design: a clinician's guide, *Am J Psychiatry* 156:829-36, 1999.

▪ CHAPTER 2 ▪

THE ART OF NUTRITIONAL MEDICINE: PATIENT-CENTERED CARE

PAUL HOLMAN

"Facts are fine, but the accumulation of facts does not necessarily give rise to wisdom, or even foster good judgement."[1]

At the very end of the 19th century, Dr. Max Bircher-Benner opened a small sanatorium in Zurich. At this clinic, patients with largely chronic, intractable conditions were treated with a partially raw vegetarian diet, hydrotherapy, and psychotherapy. As Bircher-Benner's experience grew, so did the comprehensiveness of this "holistic" regimen, which seems so similar to the approaches that we recognize today as intrinsic to integrative medicine.

One hundred years later, we can acknowledge the genius of this pioneer and affirm, albeit in slightly different language, a set of principles that guided his practical, everyday dealings with patients.

The first principle states that the generality of conventional medical diagnosis needs to be complemented by the clinical reality of the unique individual.

The complexity of the individual in his or her environment necessitates quite radical departures from our over-focused compartmentalized ways of thinking. An organism is in a constantly shifting balance with its environment, and breakdown in an organism's integrity arises when its adaptational capacity has been exceeded in a particular environmental setting. Bircher-Benner and other early theorists noted two general sets of factors that predispose to such adaptational failure:

- Toxemia—the result of environmental challenges in forms such as infections, toxins, (including foods), allergens, and psychosocial stress
- Enervation—deficiency and depletion of both physical and psychologic nutrients and the state of exhaustion that results from prolonged, excessive challenge

The second principle embodies the concept of self-regulation.

Holistic practitioners have faith in the organism's ability to know what it needs, given the opportunity. The valuing, facilitation, and maintenance of this faculty constitutes an individual's best hope for enduring vitality and recovery from illness. These principles are treated in greater detail in the following sections.

APPROACHING THE UNIQUE INDIVIDUAL

Our first task in approaching a new patient is to undertake a preliminary assessment. The importance of taking a broad look at the assessment process in medicine is expressed well in the truism that we see what we expect to see. This is as true, unfortunately, in science and medicine as it is in everyday life. We wear perceptual and conceptual blinkers derived from our experience, training, and the built-in biases in our nervous systems. Consequently, we tend to make only those observations that are accommodated by conditioned ways of seeing and thinking. It is one of the great dilemmas of life that we need frameworks to interpret our experience, but to be truly alive and creative, we must not be bound by them.

Naturally enough, I was introduced to the assessment process in my first week at medical school. A comprehensive medical history scheme was contained in a handy blue book. After a brief introduction to this important document, we students were dispatched to the wards to try out the history-taking process. My colleague and I found ourselves on a surgical ward with a man in his late 60s who was recovering from an inguinal hernia operation. My companion, being of a more confident nature, plunged into the process and left no stone unturned. My mind wandered until I heard him asking the poor fellow about his sex life, and in particular, the frequency with which he indulged in solitary sexual pleasure. I tried to mentally disassociate myself from the proceedings but much later realized that I had already learned valuable lessons about being sensitive and selective. My colleague went on to become an anesthetist, and I, a psychiatrist—physicians supposedly at opposite ends of the communication spectrum in medicine. It is possible that, unknown to ourselves, we both made important decisions about our future careers on that first day of history-taking. *Chacun à son gout.*

The "blue book" method of categorical diagnosis has of course been spectacularly successful in many respects. Its purpose is to provide comprehensive description, means for assessing progress and planning treatment, and avenues for research in etiology. These goals have often been met in areas of medicine in which disease is acute, anatomically localized, and/or related to identifiable environmental agents (e.g., microorganisms) or insult (e.g., trauma). It has been less useful in dealing with problems that are chronic, multisystemic, and not so obviously related to identifiable environmental factors.

The greatest success of the blue book method has been in the establishment of uniform medical practice and standards. In looking back at my training, I can see now that one of the great imperatives of medical education is to minimize dangerous mistakes. Such is the obvious merit of this approach and the rigorous efficiency with which it is inculcated that few seem to notice that the scientific method as applied to individual medical practice is completely ignored. The idea that a physician would make original observations, form hypotheses, and test these hypotheses in the treatment process is anathema. Not only are physicians conditioned to rigidly follow the protocols of their training, but it is now (probably correctly) assumed that physicians are not equipped to evaluate the results of ongoing medical research, either by virtue of their limited time or insufficient expertise. Consequently, medical truths must be filtered through a prevailing orthodoxy of evidence-based medicine and its supporting medical establishment. Thus we are left with practitioners who are basically technicians following diagnostic and therapeutic decision trees that would often be more effectively implemented by a computer or an individual with less extensive training. Openness, imagination, questioning, and original observations have become fringe activities in medicine long overdue for revival.

All this is hardly surprising when one considers that contemporary medicine has no encompassing philosophy of health or disease. It has simply become a patchwork of disparate and often unrelated approaches driven by largely pragmatic concerns. Attempts to find unifying theories are often regarded as naïve and fruitless and ultimately not helpful in the search for new therapeutic avenues.

The situation should be different in psychiatry in which problems *are* complex, pervasive, and often chronic and involve the person within his or her social and work contexts. Psychiatrists certainly pay lip service to the biopsychosocial model and are trained to formulate cases with these interacting strands in mind. In practice, clinicians and researchers alike still cling to an outdated Linnean nosology, exemplified by the *Diagnostic and Statistical Manual*, with which to provide the central plank of diagnosis.

Cloninger[3] has been critical of mainstream psychiatric nosology on a number of grounds, pointing out the following.

- There is extensive descriptive, prognostic, and even etiologic heterogeneity within *Diagnostic and Statistical Manual* categories.
- There is considerable overlap between categories.
- The current system does not have a model of health (and therefore of disease), and as a consequence, cannot address the concerns of individuals or society about achieving and maintaining health, happiness, and community.

Although his comments are directed at the discipline of psychiatry, there is much here that applies to medicine as a whole.

It is worth spending some time considering Cloninger's model of assessment because it represents a fundamental shift in the medical paradigm that is of far-reaching importance for all the healing disciplines. Its relevance lies in the fact that it is a dimensional and not a categorical model and examines the functional interaction between regulatory systems in the brain. Functional capacity and interaction are key concepts in the establishment of new approaches to understanding biologic complexity. Cloninger takes as his starting point the conception of temperament and character as the most obvious manifestations of the whole person in his or her physical and social environments. He sees temperament as resulting from inherited biases in central nervous system (CNS) processing and learning, and extensive research has revealed four independently inherited dimensions of temperament related to four dissociable brain systems.[3] This is already an important step, making a linkage between observable, heritable, temperamental characteristics and brain systems that mediate certain fundamental aspects of organismic regulation, learning, and behavior. Cloninger's four dimensions of temperament are harm avoidance (anxiety proneness versus risk taking), novelty seeking (impulsiveness versus rigidity), reward dependence (approval seeking versus aloofness), and persistence (determination versus fickleness). The organization of these variables is essentially the same in other mammals.

Character, the result of social learning about the self in relation to others, is seen as having three dimensions—self-directedness, cooperativeness, and self-transcendence (the ability to experience oneself as part of a greater whole).

Although Cloninger's system is still just a model, it is far more encompassing than the current nosologic methods for a number of reasons.

- It starts with a consideration of the whole person from both biologic and social standpoints and defines measurable dimensions of observable behavior and subjective experience.
- It is part of a model of healthy functioning and the maturational process in humans.
- The dimensions of temperament have a wide range of measurable, and therefore researchable, physical (e.g., genetic, neurochemical, hormonal) and psychologic (e.g., behavioral, social) correlates. This facilitates research across disciplinary boundaries and makes recognition of complex psychobiologic patterns easier. For example, the dimension of harm avoidance is related to activity in serotonergic brain systems. A significant score on this dimension shows a predisposition to anxiety and mood disturbances. Individuals with high scores in the dimension of harm avoidance tend to have low energy, require more rest, and seem to recover more slowly from illnesses.[4] Here is a useful set of observations in unraveling some of the complexities of chronic fatigue syndrome and its relation to stress and mood disturbance.
- Cloninger's model recognizes that the systems and processes underlying the temperament and character dimensions interact with one another and the environment to produce a picture of multidimensional complexity. The unique patterns of individual behavior, as well as abnormalities of behavior and experience, emerge as a result of interactions among multiple diathetic and stress-related factors. Apparently similar pathologic outcomes may therefore arise from variable origins. Thus although the trait of harm avoidance, for example, may predispose

to depression, higher scores in the dimensions of self-directedness and cooperativeness mitigate this predisposition.
- For the purposes of this chapter, the Cloninger paradigm forms a connection between contemporary psychobiology and largely ignored bodies of information concerning constitution.

A large body of research now supports the utility of this approach. However, it is still in its infancy, and only time will tell whether other fledgling disciplines such as psychoneuroimmunology will take up the Cloninger model either as a suitable structure around which information can be organized or as an appropriate model on which to base their own paradigm shifts.

There is a close parallel between Cloninger's work and that of early constitutional theorists such as William Herbert Sheldon, a physician and psychologist who attempted to correlate body type with personality. These pioneering endeavors still have practical relevance today and deserve more than the often cursory consideration that they often receive.

Constitution

Constitution may be defined as the total biologic makeup of an individual as a manifestation of the way in which hereditary factors have interacted with the environment from gamete formation through to adult life. Constitution manifests most obviously through physique (somatotype) and temperament, and these two areas have been most studied by constitutional theorists and practitioners.

Somatotype. In the Western tradition, reference to body type goes back to Hippocrates (5th century BC), who observed that people with long thin bodies (habitus phthisicus) were susceptible to tuberculosis, whereas individuals with short thick bodies (habitus apoplecticus) were prone to vascular disease and apoplexy. Typologies that followed this early Greek lead persisted into the 19th century, but serious scientific study began only after the introduction of systematic anthropometry by di Giovanni at the University of Padua in the late 1800s. Early in the 20th century, biologists and anthropologists sought to refine discrete typologies that were often tripartite or quadripartite in nature. An example is that formulated by Ernst Kretschmer, who divided physiques into the well-known athletic, pyknic, asthenic, and dysplastic types.[5]

A significant advance was made in the 1940s when Sheldon introduced the somatotype concept of continuous variation along three dimensions of physique, which he described as endomorphic, mesomorphic, and ectomorphic.[6] Sheldon's work deserves detailed examination because it forms the foundation for most subsequent somatotyping investigation.

According to Sheldon, each of the three dimensions of physique derives from one of the three basic embryonic germ layers—endoderm, mesoderm, and ectoderm. Thus in the endomorph, tissues derived from the endoderm (i.e., the gastrointestinal tract and associated organs) come to dominate the physique. Sheldon lists endomorphic characteristics as roundness and softness of body, central concentration of mass, predominance of abdominal and thoracic volume over the extremities, predominance of proximal segments of limbs over distal segments, large head, short neck, no muscle relief, and smoothness of contours throughout. In contrast, the second constitutional type, the mesomorph, has a squareness and hardness of body, rugged prominent muscling, large prominent bones, sharp muscle relief, and a large trunk without central concentration of mass. The third type, the ectomorph, is linear and fragile and has a delicate body. The bones are small, and the muscles are slight and "thready." Shoulder drop is a constant feature, the trunk is relatively short, and the limbs are relatively long. In contrast to mesomorphy, the facial mass is small compared with the cranial mass.

The importance of Sheldon's work lies in the fact that he defined clear criteria for the three components and then applied a detailed and painstaking scaling technique in the analysis of photographs of 4000 individuals. For the purposes of anthropometric analysis, the body was divided into five regions, each of which was subjected to a number of specific measurements. On the basis of these measurements and with the use of a seven-point rating scale for each component, a constitutional profile was established for each individual. Thus an athletic muscular mesomorph with very little fat might be described with the profile 161.

Sheldon was interested in the relationships between the somatotype, physical disease, and temperament. For example, with regard to illness predisposition, he noted a clear relationship between mesoendomorphy and cardiovascular disease, between mesoendomorphic endomorphy and gall bladder disease, and between duodenal ulcers and a low endomorphy component. It would have been fascinating if Sheldon's pioneering work had been developed in a systematic way; unfortunately, interest in somatotyping waned in the 1950s and 1960s, and research was patchy and inconclusive.

Carter and Heath[7] attempted to overcome some of the flaws in Sheldon's work by developing a system that was much more objective and reproducible. They simplified the basic definitions as follows: endomorphy, relative fatness; mesomorphy, musculoskeletal robustness related to stature; and ectomorphy, relative linearity. Using only a modest number of physical measurements supplemented by a photoscopic examination, investigators can reliably rate a somatotype on three scales, which, although theoretically open, in practice span the following ranges: endomorphy, ½ to 16; mesomorphy, ½ to 12; and ectomorphy, ½ to 9. Ratings greater than 7 are regarded as extremely high.

The Heath-Carter somatotype method is now widely accepted as valid and reliable, and this tool has been used in extensive research. Unfortunately, it has largely been confined to the fields of sports education and anthropology, since there is little current interest in somatotype correlation with physical or psychologic health. Nonetheless, the earlier observations on mesoendomorphy and predisposition to cardiovascular disease and type 2 diabetes have been repeatedly confirmed and many other (weaker) correlations have been found between somatotype dimensions and a number of physical and physiologic variables. Similarly, it is now clear that the heritability of the components varies and that the effects of environment are significant for endomorphy, minor for mesomorphy, and not significant for ectomorphy. The correlation between childhood and young adult somatotype is poor. Overall, the Heath-Carter endeavor has provided us with a brief and precise way of describing physique (i.e, with an anthropological identification tag).

The clinical significance of the somatotype rating resides in a number of areas.

- It has some predictive value in estimating predisposition to physical and psychologic disease.
- It systematically connects us with a rich descriptive medical literature, both ancient and contemporary.
- It is a tool for further research into constitutional types.

The second point merits further consideration.

Medical writing has traditionally concerned itself with comprehensive description. Thus in Western medical literature, particularly in the last 200 years, we have a wealth of clinical information cast in the form of vivid medical portraits of individuals and their conditions. Over the last 50 years or so, the individual person has been lost or obscured, first by a greater emphasis on accuracy and conformity in the description of symptoms and later by the methodology of medical trials. The somatotype method allows us to reintroduce the physical reality of patients into the medical history and also gives us a firm reference point with which to correlate our observations with those of other physicians, past and present. The value of constitutional description as a factor linking clinical descriptions from different sources is illustrated in various works.[8,9]

In an article on the hypoadrenocortical state and its management, Tintera[8] describes a constitutional type prone to low adrenocortical function that falls short of overt Addison's disease. In a series of 200 cases, a particular physique was identified, characterized by asthenic habitus, thin and dry skin, scanty perspiration, sparse body hair, cervical lymphadenitis, postural hypotension, and cold extremities. Such patients tended to exhibit a positive Rogoff sign (tenderness in the vertebrocostal angle), and on laboratory investigation, to show low urinary 17-ketosteroid levels, eosinophilia, and a flat glucose tolerance test result. Patients in this series tended to experience fatigue, anxiety, depression, faintness, insomnia, allergies, dermatoses, and a variety of symptoms related to autonomic imbalance.

Tintera believed that these individuals were particularly prone to "adrenal exhaustion" under stress and that therapy should aim at resting and supporting the adrenal glands and stabilizing blood sugar levels. Consequently, he recommended a high-protein, low–refined-carbohydrate diet with supplements of vitamins B and C. He placed particular emphasis on vitamins B_6

and B$_{12}$. A crucial part of the therapy, however, was the administration of intravenous or intramuscular adrenocortical extract over variable periods to "rest" the adrenal glands.

In contrast, Bieler's[9] main distinction lay between individuals who had either a dominant thyroid gland or a dominant adrenal gland. The "thyroid type" was described as slender, fine-boned, and long-limbed; and the "adrenal type" closely resembled Sheldon's mesomorph. Bieler's work has been extended by Abravanel[10] into a four-part typology. Table 2-1 outlines a number of key features of the Bieler thyroid type and compares it with Tintera's description of the hypoadrenal type, Sheldon's description of the ectomorph, and the traditional Ayurvedic Vata type.[11]

The remarkable similarity in these descriptions strongly suggests that a very real clinical entity is being described, but from differing viewpoints. Each approach adds valuable information that can be used in understanding etiology and in implementing appropriate treatment. The connecting thread is the description of the physical reality of the constitutional type. A similar exercise can be done with the other types.

Temperament.   Sheldon was particularly interested in the connection between physical constitution and temperament, although he did not hold any simplistic view as to the relationship between the two. He saw personality as a product of "the play of a complex pattern of environmental pressures upon a living organism that carries an innately determined constitutional patterning."[6] He used the terms *viscerotonia, somatotonia,* and *cerebrotonia* to describe the temperaments often found in association with the three constitutional types. The viscerotonic individual is described as a relaxed, comfortable person who participates easily in social gatherings and who shows a warm interest in and tolerance of the human race. A person of this type enjoys food and easily expresses his or her emotions. The person with a somatotonic temperament is extremely active and energetic with a tendency to self-assertion and even aggression. Such an individual is extroverted in action but not in affect. The extreme cerebrotonic individual is an introvert and thus under strong inhibitory control with regard to feelings and socialization. He or she is easily overstimulated and tends to withdraw from social gatherings.

Although subsequent research has shown that there is an element of constitutional or predictable behavior associated with particular somatotypes, the majority of investigative efforts have been confused by the variety of somatotyping methods and the problems inherent in psychologic inventories. Most of the psychologic tools used for assessing personality and behavior fail to distinguish between temperament (inherited) and character (acquired traits). The most significant correlations will obviously arise only between somatotype and temperament variables.

Cloninger's *Temperament and Character Inventory* seems to offer a way out of the confusion.[4] Research with twins has now clearly demonstrated that the heritability of each of the four temperament traits is substantial in both

TABLE 2-1 ■ Comparison of Four Systems of Constitutional Classification

PHYSIQUE	SHELDON ECTOMORPH	TINTERA ASTHENIC HABITUS	BIELER-ABRAVANAL LONG, THIN, DELICATE	AYURVEDA SLIM, THIN BONES
Teeth	Crowded	Crowded lower incisors	Crooked	Crooked
Hair	Fine	Sparse	Fine, thinly distributed	Sparse
Skin	Pale, dry	Thin, dry	Fine	Thin/dry
Sweat	—	Scanty	Variable	Little
Temperature	Gets cold easily	Cold extremities	Cold extremities	Prefers hot weather
Energy	Prone to fatigue	Prone to fatigue	Tires easily	Low stamina
Immune	Prone to allergies	Prone to allergies	Allergies and infections	—
Digestion	Less suited to vegetarian diet	Frequent GI problems	Poor	Irregular
Food	Needs more calories and protein	More protein, less carbohydrate	More protein, less carbohydrate	More flesh food than other types
Endocrine	—	Hypoadrenocorticism	Dominant thyroid	—
Sleep	Poor	Poor	Poor	Light
Temperament	Sensitive, anxious	Nervous, irritable	Anxious	Anxious, insecure, changeable
Explanatory hypothesis	Dominance of tissues derived from ectoderm (CNS, skin)	Low adrenal cortex function	Dominant thyroid	Dominant vata (movement, homeostasis, communication)

CNS, Central nervous system; *GI,* gastrointestinal.

sexes and that the traits are homogeneous and independent. In contrast, alternative models, measured by such tools as the Eysenck Personality Questionnaire, are genetically heterogeneous. We can expect that research that examines correlations between somatotype and these four temperament variables might show definite relationships, and in fact, it is tempting to speculate with Arraj[12] that there would be correlations between harm avoidance and ectomorphy, novelty seeking and mesomorphy, and reward dependence and endomorphy. My own clinical observations leave me in no doubt that there is a significant correlation between ectomorphy and harm avoidance and that this combination of characteristics predisposes the ectomorphic group to a higher incidence of anxiety and chronic fatigue syndrome.[13]

We would also expect, of course, that an individual's somatotype might affect his or her character development. However, research in this area is complicated by the fact that there are only poor correlations between the somatotype of the child and the adult. Long-term follow-up research may partially answer the question.[14] Kagan[14] has noted that his cohort of shy children tend to be ectomorphic and fair-complexioned. Tracking these children into adult life will provide some clues about the complex interactions of somatotype, temperament, and character.

Genetic and Metabolic Profiling.   At the biochemical level, the enormous complexity of cellular activity makes individuality more difficult to characterize. Roger Williams, way ahead of his time, demonstrated a wide variation in animal nutrient requirement and showed that human differences in biochemical parameters were much greater than differences in physical appearance.[15]

Our understanding of biochemical individuality will no doubt be greatly enhanced by the mapping of the human genome and complementary DNA microarray technology (gene chips). However, we should not underestimate the challenges that will arise in interpreting the vast complexity so revealed, and more will be said on this point in the following section on models of health and disease.

Francis S. Collins, Director of the National Human Genome Research Institute in the United States, has contextualized the likely changes that will come in the wake of this technology by making the following predictions.[16]

- By 2010, predictive genetic tests for a dozen conditions will be available.
- By 2020, cancer treatments will be targeted to gene fingerprints of tumors, and customized pharmacotherapy will be in use.
- By 2030, comprehensive genetic health care will be available, and there will be serious debate over the desirability of "designer babies."

Ground-breaking work in the area of genetics as it applies to nutritional and environmental medicine has been accomplished by Reading[17] who sees most disease as arising from food sensitivities (especially grain and milk products) with secondary impairment of nutrient absorption. The family tree may be especially useful in determining which foods are likely causes of disease. Thus grain or milk sensitivity may be suggested by information from the following areas:

- Diagnosed illnesses such as celiac disease, cancer of the bowel, or autoimmune syndromes such as systemic lupus erythematosus
- Recurrent undiagnosed symptoms such as chronic gastrointestinal problems, tiredness, headaches, or depression

The secret of this approach is to be very familiar with the protean manifestations of food and environmental sensitivities and to recognize patterns as they recur through generations. For example, the index of suspicion for gluten sensitivity in an autistic child would be raised if the mother was experiencing irritable bowel syndrome and a grandparent had been given diagnoses of systemic lupus erythematosus and depression.

While the exciting prospects offered by genetic research play themselves out in the many and diverse fields of biology and medicine, we are left with the task of making clinically useful decisions about individual biochemical differences and needs. Measures of nutrient status provide some help but are accompanied by the many problems outlined in Chapter 6. This and other factors have led to the search for a metabolic typology that would guide dietary nutrient prescription. Attempts at metabolic typing have not been overwhelmingly successful, although the approaches of two pioneers, George Watson and William Donald Kelley, deserve consideration from both historical and clinical points of view.

Watson[18] found that nutrients had differential effects on individuals, especially with respect to psychologic state, and he developed a theory based on cellular oxidation to explain his findings. In this scheme there are two basic metabolic types—fast oxidizers and slow oxidizers. Fast oxidizers show a disproportionately fast oxidation of carbohydrates and glucogenic amino acids together with slow but still more rapid than normal oxidation of fats and ketogenic amino acids. Such individuals will tend to have higher blood carbon dioxide levels and lower pH values. In contrast, slow oxidizers show a slow oxidation of carbohydrates and glucogenic amino acids with a slow but preferential utilization of fats and ketogenic amino acids. Such individuals will tend to have lower carbon dioxide levels in a generally more alkaline biochemical environment. The aim of therapy is to provide macronutrients and micronutrients that will assist the more inefficient aspects of metabolism. Thus the slow oxidizer needs to consume less fat and more complex carbohydrates, together with cofactors that would assist in carbohydrate metabolism. The opposite is true of the fast oxidizer who needs to rely less on carbohydrates and more on the metabolic effects of protein and fat.

A detailed discussion of this process is beyond the scope of this chapter, but Table 2-2 provides an overall summary of the strategies. Watson did not provide us with any descriptive correlations between his concept of metabolic type and somatotype. Despite the lack of scientific validation of these concepts, this work continues.[19]

TABLE 2-2 ■ Metabolic Typing Systems of Watson and Kelley

WATSON FAST OXIDIZER	SLOW OXIDIZER
Needs	Needs
Vitamins B_3 (amide), B_5, B_{12}	Vitamins B_1, B_2, B_3, B_6, folate
Vitamins A, E	PABA, biotin
Choline, inositol	Vitamins A, C, D
Calcium, phosphorus, iodine, zinc	Potassium, magnesium, iron, copper, manganese, chromium
↑ Protein ↓ carbohydrate	↓ Fat ↑ carbohydrate

KELLEY PARASYMPATHETIC	SYMPATHETIC
Appearance	Appearance
Flabby, stocky, poor muscle tone, lethargic	Tall, slim, well-developed muscles, hyperactive
Needs	Needs
Vitamins B_3 (amide), B_5, B_{12}	Vitamins B_1, B_2, B_3, B_6, folate
Choline, inositol	PABA, biotin
Vitamins C, E	Vitamins C, D, K
Calcium, phosphorus, zinc	Potassium, magnesium, zinc, chromium
Meat in diet	HCl, pancreatic enzymes
	Vegetarian diet

HCl, hydrochloric acid; PABA, para-aminobenzoic acid.

Kelley's story is an interesting one.[20] In the mid 1960s, he developed inoperable pancreatic cancer, and in the face of a very poor prognosis, he accepted the advice of his mother that he radically change his diet to a whole-food one consisting of fruits, vegetables, and whole grains. Over subsequent months, he found his condition improving, and, with the judicious use of pancreatic enzyme supplements and various detoxification procedures, he was eventually cured. He published his account of this process in 1974.[21] His book is full of the evangelical zeal that one frequently finds in literature written by early converts to whole-food and natural diets. Kelley was subsequently disappointed to find that his regimen did not work for his wife who had become severely ill with a fatigue syndrome after exposure to paint fumes. In contrast, her recovery was eventually effected by adding substantial quantities of meat to her diet; this stimulated Kelley's interest in exploring individual differences and the concept of metabolic type. Elaborating on earlier work that examined the effects of nutrients on the autonomic nervous system,[22,23] he formulated a model in which he made a distinction between sympathetic and parasympathetic metabolic types. Some of the major characteristics of these two types are shown in Table 2-2, although over time his approach became quite elaborate.[24,25]

Table 2-2 makes it apparent that there is a remarkable similarity in the descriptions of Watson and Kelley, with almost identical therapeutic recommendations despite an apparent theoretical contradiction (one might expect fast oxidizer to be sympathetically dominated). As far as we know, Watson and Kelley were not influenced by one another, making their data all the more intriguing. The simplest explanation is that both investigators were identifying a spectrum of differing protein and carbohydrate needs. It would also explain the different supplement recommendations; meat eaters, for example, would require more calcium and lipotropic factors, whereas vegetarians would require more B vitamins. Clinical experience indicates that the protein/carbohydrate ratio is probably the most important thing to get right in a person's overall dietary plan. A questionnaire for assessment of this ratio is available.[20] The results of the questionnaire can form the basis for a preliminary diet that is higher in protein, higher in carbohydrates, or intermediate. The dietary proportions are then adjusted according to the individual's response over subsequent weeks. Woolcott's[20] system is a good example of the use of "enlightened experimentation," and the reader is advised to study this material as a matter of priority.

The other metabolic typing system that has received a lot of recent attention is the blood group method.[26] D'Adamo's[26] basic message is that dietary lectins interact with blood group antigens to cause disease. Freed,[27] an authority on lectins, acknowledges that although lectins can cause disease, he does not believe that they do so necessarily in the blood group classification proposed by D'Adamo. However, it is not surprising that this scheme works for many people. Individuals with the most common blood group (O) are put on a "Stone Age" diet. In my experience, such a diet suits a majority of people, and so there will be many satisfied customers on this basis alone.

FINDING A USEFUL MODEL OF HEALTH AND DISEASE

We may never arrive at a grand unified theory in biology or medicine, but this does not mean that we cannot consider what the requirements of such a theory would be. Even in our present state of pervasive ignorance, we can guess that a grand unified theory in medicine would have some of the following characteristics:

- It would involve systemic thinking (i.e., that in a system, the whole is greater than the sum of the parts, and the parts are defined in relation to the whole and to one another). Such thinking applies not only to the internal functioning of the individual but also to the organism in its social, environmental, and planetary contexts. Thus systems thinking encompasses a range from intracellular dynamics to global ecology.
- Any new model must involve thinking in terms of information—how it is encoded, transmitted, transduced, and interpreted. Unifying theories in physics are turning to information theory to bridge the gaps between quantum and Newtonian physics and to explain the anomalies of the quantum model.[28] A model of information processing complements

systems theory very well in biology. Rossi[29] has dealt at some length with the ways in which information is transduced between the multiple hierarchical levels of biologic organization, how it changes form between levels, and how constant feedback processing is essential to maintain form and behavior within acceptable limits. Just as communities, societies, and organizations inevitably break down when communication and free flow of information are restricted, so do organisms.

- Systems are about relationships. Relationships involve constant communication and reciprocity (feedback). Without communication and information flow, there can be no relationship and no system.
- New models in biology must accommodate theories of complexity and the theoretic subset known as *chaos theory*. It seems as if many, if not all, biologic systems behave in ways reminiscent of chaotic systems. Rossi[29] has reviewed the subject and has drawn attention to the fact that rhythmicity is a powerful organizing force in complex systems and that the study of chronobiology provides new insights into the ways that multiple complex systems can coordinate with one another. Chaos theory has many important lessons for biology, not the least of which is that wide-ranging effects spring from small changes in initial conditions ("butterfly effect").
- New models must take into account the mysterious qualities of self-organization and self-regulation to be found in biologic systems. Self-regulation implies that an organism will tend to "know" what it needs to correct its own imbalances and that self-healing is the rule rather than the exception. The concept of *vis mediatrix naturae* is an acknowledgment of this fact and is easily forgotten in this age of "the high-tech fix."

Some of these requirements can be encompassed in the very simple model represented in Figure 2-1. In this model, information flows between the organism and the environment, is distributed as widely and democratically as possible within the organism, and is processed at many different levels. The CNS acts as an information-rich area, mediating activity at the organism-environment interface; and DNA, the other principal information-rich domain (ubiquitously distributed throughout the organism), sets the limits on biologic structure and function. It is tempting to see the CNS and DNA as control centers for the organism. However, this would be misleading because we could equally say that the environment is ultimately in control. Control, in fact, does not reside at any particular location; there is only constant adaptation to the demands of the organism-environment interface. It would be equally untrue to say that there is "top-down" organization from the CNS intersecting with "bottom-up" organization from DNA. The only true statement that we can make is that organization resides with the organism as a whole in its environment and that we have very little knowledge of this organism as a whole, although we are constantly tempted to hack the poor long-suffering thing apart in our efforts to "shoe-horn" it into the shape of machines or computers or other products of our limited imagination.

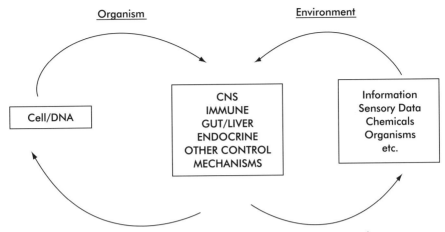

FIG. 2-1 Möbius loop of information transduction and exchange. *CNS,* Central nervous system.

The preliminary mapping of the human genome has raised enormous expectations that this knowledge will unlock the secrets of health and disease. No doubt it will contribute greatly to this process, but it will also open up new realms of complexity. How does a relatively modest complement of 30,000 or so genes express itself to generate and maintain an organism? How is the activity of the genes coordinated? How do they interact and how is this complex melody modified by environmental factors? To answer these questions one needs completely new ways of handling information, and the emerging science of bioinformatics will rely heavily on computer programs that can sift the burgeoning literature, recognize patterns in data, and make connections between disparate areas of research.[30]

The most sanguine of the medical crystal ball gazers promises us all a gene chip on our desks within 10 years. Such an idea gives us pause for thought. Chapter 6 examines the problem of coordinating the modest amount of information that we already collect. Suffice it to say that at this stage, data on the expression of several thousand genes will require a very intelligent program to make sense of such a wealth of information in the context of the clinical presentation and the plethora of other data (biochemical and otherwise) that we are now capable of assembling. At the end of the day, we will probably be left with the same paradox that we face now: the more we know of the microscopic, the more we need to know of the macroscopic (i.e., the organism in its environment) to make sense of that information. Thus the need for systems thinking will become increasingly important.

Consider the issue of disease. In the previously described model of the organism in its environment, health might be defined in a general way as the maintenance of a dynamic stability at the organism-environment boundary with free flow of information across this boundary. We might then define disease as arising when the adaptational capacities of the organism have been exceeded in a particular environmental setting, producing dysfunction or disharmony at the organism-environment boundary (see Figure 2-2). Such disharmonies will be marked with changes in the flow of information at the disturbed boundary, and consequently, throughout the organism.

It is likely that the challenge to adaptation presented by psychosocial stimuli (e.g., work stress) is as significant as the challenges posed by physical stimuli (e.g., toxins, microorganisms). Both classes of stimuli can be regarded as types of information that need to be processed by the organism.

This simple model can be elaborated in various ways. The environmental medicine movement has long used the analogy of a container (representing the adaptational capacities of the organism) being filled from various sources of environmental challenge. Symptoms and disease arise when the container overflows.

As already mentioned, the naturopathic tradition uses the twin concepts of toxemia and enervation, which interact in mutually reinforcing ways. As a refinement of these models, we can now summarize the main components of the environmental challenge and the competence of organismic response in the following way:

Environmental Challenge

- Social relationships
- Trauma—physical and psychosocial
- Foods, chemicals, supplements, medications, microorganisms, inhalants, weather, light, and other factors
- The ecology of the gut

Organismic Response

- Genes/constitutional factors
- The mediating informational network—mechanisms of control and adaptation that facilitate self-regulation (includes chaotobiologic and chronobiologic considerations)

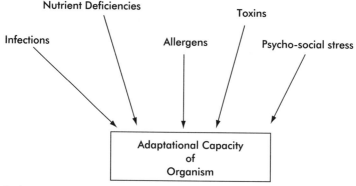

FIG. 2-2 The container model of adaptational capacity.

- Organismic needs that support self-regulation—this usually means what is deficient, for example, rest or nutrients (physical, psychologic, and social)

This list provides a good guide to the areas that should be addressed in the assessment process. By evaluating each of these areas, we can begin to form a picture of how adaptation might have broken down in any one individual. We do not have the advantage of an overriding schema that would easily make sense of disparate findings. Part of the attraction of a medical system such as Ayurveda is that its detailed and elaborate structure rests on the foundation of simple principles—namely the three gunas (Rajas/active principle, Tamas/limiting principle, and Sattwa/balancing principle) and the five elements. Since these principles are universal, they operate across the boundaries of self/world and body/mind/spirit and form links that make tracing the roots of disharmony both logical and comprehensive. For example, with a vata (ether/air) imbalance, the physician can look to those environmental influences such as the weather, season, and diet that have those elemental qualities and that may be manifesting in the patient's life in an excessive way. Thus a vata excess might be the result of irregularity of habits, excess coffee, or cold food.

The yin/yang principle also has enormous descriptive and explanatory utility, eloquent testimony to which can be found in its common use in Western culture. It may yet show its usefulness in tracking the dynamic interplay of complex systems. In fact, an example from biochemistry is supplied by Dolittle[31] in which he describes the step-by-step process of blood clotting in terms of the play of action/reaction, yang and yin.

There is certainly a need for explanatory principles as we slowly drown in our current tidal wave of often isolated "facts." It is possible that traditional wisdom holds some keys that with appropriate polishing will unlock the doors to the sort of synthesis that we are seeking.

HELPING SELF-REGULATION

The concept of self-regulation has always been dangerous and controversial. At its core, self-regulation is about the individual's ability and right to determine what is best for him or her and to do so if necessary in the face of authority and authoritative opinion. This is the core of the liberal democratic tradition and should equally be at the heart of medicine.

The practice of self-regulation is based on self-observation, which, if practiced conscientiously, leads an individual to understand what his or her needs are and how to satisfy them. However, an important starting point is to make observations, and we physicians must be able to cultivate this seldom taught process before we can help our patients to cultivate greater powers of self-observation for themselves. We must begin by admitting that our meager knowledge concerning the human being is vastly outweighed by our ignorance.

It is humbling to imagine what doctors in 200 years would make of our ramblings today, and we should therefore open ourselves to "not knowing" and to the benefits of direct knowledge through unprejudiced observation. We may realize in this process that we have completely lost the ability to see anything that we are not expecting to see. Or if we do see something new, we tend to forget about it; a veil is drawn across our minds. We need practice. Spending time with someone who looks at things differently from us, (e.g., a body worker or a practitioner of traditional Chinese medicine) can be helpful. There is no better way of acquiring a new behavior or modus operandi than immersing oneself in the company of an expert who is actively engaged in his or her specialty. We are programmed to learn by modeling in such situations—a fact enshrined in the apprentice system of skills acquisition. Such an experience of full participation can provide a jolt to the perceptual processes and allow us to actually see facets of an individual that we would not have thought possible.

Having made our observations, we can then function as scientists, forming hypotheses and organizing appropriate experiments. The word *experiment*, of course, tends to send shivers down the spine in the helping professions. In this context, however, I am referring to a process of enlightened experimentation in which physician and patient participate in a process of trying safe interventions and carefully monitoring the results. Such trial-and-error methods are the norm in medicine anyway, except that physicians are not usually forthcoming about the fact. The critical difference in enlightened experimentation is that the patients are educated about the process and know that they bear some responsibility for active participation, monitoring, and decision making.

Perhaps the most fundamental point about observation and experimentation was passed on to me by Dr. Eric Lederman, a physician, psychiatrist, homeopath, and naturopath who introduced me to the subject of nutrition when I was probably too young to appreciate it fully. I remember very clearly his advice that to understand dietary treatment, one had to experiment on oneself. My experience over the subsequent 25 years has borne this out fully. Self-observation and self-knowledge derived from trial-and-error experimentation with oneself are absolutely essential to get the feel of the far-reaching effects of dietary change, supplementation, and all the other aspects of lifestyle manipulation.

Through such observation, one is easily convinced that the essential aspect of self-regulation is the body's ability to register what it needs. Normally, this expresses itself only in very obvious ways (e.g., resting when tired, eating when hungry). For example, we know that the body can be quite subtle in its appreciation of nutritional deficiencies. Some women get marked cravings for meat in the face of a falling iron level, and pregnancy seems to be a time when cravings and aversions reflect organismic needs to nurture and protect the fetus. Surprisingly, we pay little attention to this ability, which is often overridden or obscured by habits and expectations. The epidemic of weight problems (overweight and underweight) in our culture is eloquent testimony to the fact that even the simpler aspects of dietary self-regulation are a challenge to many.

It is easy for the physician to take over the body's authority and impose his or her ideas of what is right for the person. This may be acceptable as a temporary expedient, but it keeps the patient powerless and dependent. The healer's role is in fact to help patients reestablish their organismic sensitivity and to learn what they in their uniqueness require and when they require it. This is the most important part of enlightened experimentation.

Self-regulation also means that the organism can set its own priorities (i.e., it can know in what order the different facets of a problem should be addressed). Actually, people often know what they require, but they may not have the words to express what is needed or believe that they do not have permission to speak. Often psychologic methods, such as Gendlin's[32] focusing or guided imagery, can help increase sensitivity to the body's signals and the interpretation of these signals.

Information flow is vital to the process of self-regulation. The practitioner provides feedback to the client at many levels, and the client receives feedback at many levels from the process of enlightened experimentation. The keys are client willingness, active participation, and intelligent appreciation of the process. The practitioner must complement these qualities in an equal partnership with the patient and always be willing to admit ignorance. This produces a special sort of relationship in which mutual feedback is food for the treatment process. Self-regulation also ensures that the body is very "forgiving" of treatment mistakes and excesses. Thus the body detoxifies therapeutic poisons, rids itself of excesses, and may not immediately protest when we are on some new yet unproductive treatment path.

REFERENCES

1. Kunz-Bircher R: *The Bircher-Benner health guide*, St. Leonards, 1981, Allen & Unwin.
2. Callaway E: Two modest proposals, *Biol Psychiatry* 22:665-6, 1987.
3. Cloninger CR: A new conceptual paradigm from genetics and psychobiology for the science of mental health, *Aust N Z J Psychiatry* 33:174-86, 1999.
4. Cloninger CR: *The temperament and character inventory: a guide to its development and use*, St. Louis, 1994, Center for Psychobiology of Personality, Washington University.
5. Kretschmer E: *Köperbau und charakter*, Berlin, 1921, Springer-Verlag.
6. Sheldon WH: *The varieties of human physique*, New York, 1940, Harper and Brothers.
7. Carter JEL, Heath BH: *Somatotyping development and applications*, Cambridge, 1990, Cambridge University Press.
8. Tintera J: The hypoadrenorortical state and its management, *New York State Journal of Medicine* 35(13), 1955. Reproduced in Light MH, editor: *Hypoadrenocorticism* 1-14, 1974, Adrenal Metabolic Research Society.
9. Bieler H: *Food is your best medicine*, New York, 1968, Ballantine Books.

10. Abravanel ED: *Dr. Abravanel's body type diet*, New York, 1983, Bantam.
11. Svoboda R: *Prakruti: your ayurvedic constitution*, Twin Lakes, Wis, 1989, Lotus Press.
12. Arraj J: *Tracking the elusive human: an advanced guide to the typological worlds of C. G. Jung, vol 2*, Chiloquin, Ore, 1990, Inner Growth Books.
13. Holman CP: Treating the ectomorphic constitution, *J Nutr Env Med* 6:359-70, 1996.
14. Kagan J: Born to be shy? In Conlon R, editor: *States of mind*, New York, 1999, John Wiley & Sons.
15. Williams RJ, Kalita NK: *A physician's handbook on orthomolecular medicine*, New York, 1977, Pergamon Press. New York.
16. Coghlan A, Marchant J: Secrets of the genome, *New Sci* 2278:5, 2001.
17. Reading CM, Meillon RA: *Your family tree connection*, Chicago, 1988, Keats Publishing.
18. Watson G: *Nutrition and your mind*, New York, 1972, Harper & Row.
19. Wiley R: *Biobalance*, Orem, Utah, 1989, Essential Science Publishing.
20. Woolcott W: *The metabolic typing diet*, New York, 2000, Doubleday.
21. Kelley WD: *One answer to cancer*, 1974, Kelley Foundation.
22. Lee R: *Protomorphology: the principle of cell autoregulation*, 1947, Lee Foundation.
23. Pottinger FM: *Symptoms of visceral disease*, St. Louis, 1919, Mosby.
24. Kelley WD: *The metabolic type*, 1976, Kelley Foundation.
25. Valentine T, Valentine C: *Medicine's missing link*, London, 1989, Thorsons.
26. D'Adamo P: *The eat right diet*, London, 1998, Century.
27. Freed DLJ: Book review, *J Nutr Envir Med* 9:168-9, 1999.
28. Von Baeyer HC: In the beginning was the bit, *New Sci* 2278:26-33, 2001.
29. Rossi EL: *The symptom path to enlightenment*, Los Angeles, 1996, Palisades Gateway Publishing.
30. Cohen D: Machine head, *New Sci* 2279:26-9, 2001.
31. Doolittle J: The evolution of vertebrate blood coagulation, *Thromb Haemost* 70:24-8, 1993.
32. Gendlin ET: *Focusing*, 1978, Everest House.

■ CHAPTER 3 ■

SELF-REGULATION: PATHOPHYSIOLOGIC MECHANISMS INFLUENCING HEALTH AND DISEASE

> The healing relationship is best conceived of as a form of "dialogue" — not only between patient and practitioner but also between nutrient triggers and self-regulating systems.

Health is the result of balanced interchange between mutually interacting physiologic processes: a change in one system affects the function of the entire organism.[1] Imbalance in one system may modify the function of other organ systems; similarly, imbalance in one system may be minimized by changes in interacting systems.

Homeostatic mechanisms interact to maintain bodily functions within viable limits. Negative feedback systems tend to minimize fluctuations and restore the status quo. Positive feedback systems prime the organism to cope with untoward events.

Homeostasis depends on successful communication. Messages are transmitted by means of one of two distinct systems. The nervous system transmits messages as electrical impulses along neural pathways, and the endocrine system conveys chemical information in the blood and interstitial fluid. Three prerequisites to a homeostatic system are a receptor, a control center, and an effector. The receptor receives information from the environment in the form of stimuli. Stimuli may be physical, chemical, microbial, or psychosocial in nature. The control center determines the set point at which a process is to be maintained. The effector provides an afferent pathway that feeds information back to influence the stimulus. Consistent with the infomedical model, the flow of information in a homeostatic feedback system is circular, rather than linear. Multiple triggers, interacting at the level of diverse organ systems, converge and diverge at various interfaces to determine health or disease, wellness or dysfunction. Nutrition is one factor that contributes to the cybernetic circularity of mutual causality.

This chapter explores how diet, herbs, and supplements can modify physiologic and pathologic mechanisms. It demonstrates how biologic plausibility provides a sound basis for guiding investigation into nutritional management and shows how the complex interactions involved in homeostasis make it difficult to accurately predict clinical outcome despite sound pathophysiologic principles.

NEGATIVE FEEDBACK SYSTEM OF GLUCOSE HOMEOSTASIS

Negative feedback systems prevent extreme change. They continually adjust the system to maintain function within an acceptable range. A negative feedback system is one in which the afferent pathway depresses the control mechanism and seeks to neutralize the input. It keeps a balance between input and output. Most homeostatic systems depend on negative feedback. Examples include control of blood glucose levels, blood pressure, heart rate, and respiratory rate.

> A negative feedback system dampens biologic responses, keeping them within an acceptable physiologic range.

Adenosine Triphosphate: The Currency of Cellular Energy

Complete catabolism of glucose produces energy (adenosine triphosphate [ATP]), water, carbon dioxide, and heat. Glucose is the major source of fuel for all cells; it is immediately available from the blood, and the levels are replenished as required. The gastrointestinal tract extracts simple sugars from foods and absorbs monosaccharides into the bloodstream, elevating the blood sugar level. As organs extract glucose from the bloodstream to meet their particular metabolic requirements, blood glucose levels start to fall. Glycogen, the storage form of carbohydrate in animals, is then converted to glucose. Glycogen, the human equivalent of starch in plants, is produced and stored in the liver and skeletal muscle. The liver stores about 100 g of glycogen and provides an immediately available reserve of glucose (see Figure 3-1). When energy is required, glycogen is broken down to glucose, which is further catabolized to pyruvate with the generation of two molecules of ATP. Under aerobic conditions, pyruvate enters the tricarboxylic acid cycle and generates reduced nicotinamide adenine dinucleotide and the reduced form of flavin adenine dinucleotide, which produce cellular energy via the electron transport chain. Hepatic glycogen can maintain blood glucose levels for about 4 hours after absorption. Glucose released from muscle glycogen is used to fuel skeletal muscle.

Glycogen from skeletal muscles may indirectly contribute to restoration of blood glucose levels by release of metabolic intermediates such as pyruvic acid or lactic acid. Only glucose derived from liver glycogen directly restores blood glucose levels. As glycogen is depleted, new sources of glucose are sought. Gluconeogenesis is the process whereby noncarbohydrate sources of energy are recruited. Glucogenic amino acids and glycerol can be

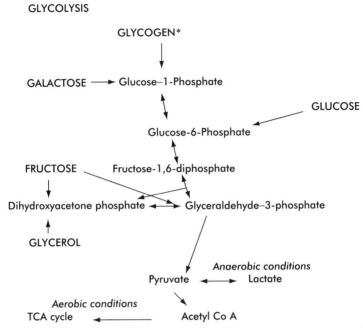

FIG. 3-1 Carbohydrates as a source of energy. *Liver glycogen serves as a store to regulate blood glucose levels between meals; muscle glycogen cannot release glucose into the blood.

used to restore blood glucose levels and, in conjunction with fatty acids, boost energy reserves. With prolonged fasting, the body adapts by relying more on fat and protein as its energy sources. All tissues, except the brain, increasingly use fatty acids as their dominant energy source. If fasting continues for longer than 5 days, the brain starts to supplement its use of glucose with ketone bodies as its fuel source (see Figure 3-2). When glucose is plentiful and intracellular ATP levels are high, further glucose breakdown is inhibited. Glucose is then converted to the energy storage forms of glycogen or fat. Fat is the major form of stored energy.

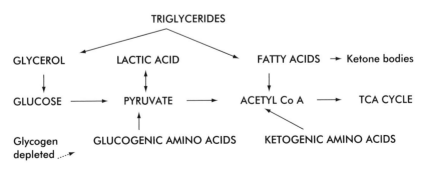

TCA cycle - Tricarboxylic acid cycle (Krebs)

FIG. 3-2 Energy sources.

> Liver glycogen is depleted after 12 to 15 hours of fasting; muscle glycogen is depleted by prolonged strenuous exercise.

A Finely Poised Negative Feedback System

Voluntary triggers, such as exercise intensity and dietary selection, affect blood glucose levels, which can be maintained between 4.5 and 7.5 mmol/L. The blood glucose level is the result of the interaction of multiple systems that combine to stabilize blood glucose levels within a defined range (see Figure 3-3). After ingestion of a high-carbohydrate meal, glucose is absorbed directly into the bloodstream, and blood glucose levels peak. When blood glucose levels are high, the liver converts glucose to glycogen for short-term storage and to fat for long-term storage, reducing blood glucose levels. Hormones secreted in response to rising blood glucose levels assist the liver in reducing blood glucose levels. Thyroxin increases cellular uptake and uti-

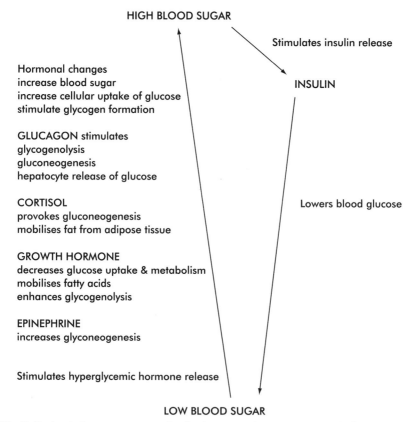

FIG. 3-3 Blood glucose—a negative feedback system. Gluconeogenesis is the formation of glucose from noncarbohydrate sources (i.e., fat and protein). Glycogenolysis is the breakdown of glycogen to glucose.

lization of glucose for energy, while insulin binds to membrane receptors of target cells and facilitates the entry of glucose. Within minutes of its release, insulin increases the cellular uptake of glucose some 20-fold. Only brain cells can actively take up glucose in the absence of insulin.

Insulin reduces blood glucose levels by stimulating utilization of glucose for energy, stimulating glucose uptake by cells, and enhancing synthesis of glycogen (glycogenesis) and by inhibiting production of glucose (gluconeogenesis). This endocrine-mediated, homeostatic, negative feedback system seeks to restore blood glucose levels to within a physiologically acceptable range.

Hours after the last meal, blood glucose levels are maintained above 4 or 5 mmol/L by the liver, which makes glucose available through glycolysis. When hepatic glycogen stores are depleted and blood glucose requires replenishing, the liver converts amino acids and glycerol to glucose. The increase in blood glucose levels is achieved by increased gluconeogenesis with the help of glucagon, epinephrine, cortisol, and growth hormones and by glycogenolysis with the aid of glucagon and epinephrine.

The liver, along with various hormones, plays a particularly important role in blood glucose homeostasis (see Figure 3-3). The endocrine system secretes hormones that elevate or depress blood glucose levels as required.

> Blood glucose levels trigger release of hormones that increase or decrease utilization or production of glucose as needed.

Disorders of Blood Glucose

Given all the variables that converge to influence blood glucose levels, it is scarcely surprising that blood glucose levels may deviate outside a physiologic range. When the blood glucose level rises, the condition is called *hyperglycemia*; when it falls, it is called *hypoglycemia*.

Hypoglycemia. Hypoglycemia may be triggered by extraneous administration of insulin, by fasting, or by alcohol abuse. Hypoglycemia occurs within 24 hours of a drinking binge unaccompanied by food. Symptomatic hypoglycemia appears to be related to the rate of decline in the blood glucose level, the actual blood glucose level, and the intensity of the homeostatic response attempting to normalize blood glucose levels.

When the blood glucose level drops to around 4 to 5 mmol/L, epinephrine and glucagon are secreted to increase blood glucose levels. Increased levels of catecholamine have a physical impact, and persons with hypoglycemia may experience headache, palpitations, sweating, tremors, and restlessness. At a level of 4 mmol/L, sophisticated tests can detect early cognitive changes. As the blood glucose level falls below 4 mmol/L, cognitive changes become more marked; at this level, neurogenic evidence of hypoglycemia appears. Neuroglycopenic symptoms range from confusion and impaired performance to behavioral changes, such as irrational anger and aggression. Visual disturbances such as diplopia may be experienced. When the blood glucose level falls below 3 mmol/L, neuroglycopenic symptoms predominate and drowsiness is noted; there is also a substantial risk for coma and seizures when the blood glucose level drops below 2.5 mmol/L.

> No single threshold at which the blood glucose level triggers symptoms of hypoglycemia has been established.

Fasting hypoglycemia is gradual in onset, and symptoms persist until fasting ceases. In contrast, functional or reactive hypoglycemia occurs suddenly, 2 to 5 hours after a meal, and symptoms are transient. Catecholamine-mediated symptoms include transient episodes of dizziness, weakness, poor concentration, anxiety, and depression. Characteristic neuroglycopenic symptoms are chronic or intermittent fatigue, episodic tiredness within 1 hour of eating, and sleep disturbance. Although the underlying mechanism remains disputed, fasting hypoglycemia has been hypothesized to be triggered by enhanced insulin sensitivity, impaired glucose homeostatic mechanisms, and food or chemical sensitivity. The condition is more often encountered in persons who consume large quantities of coffee, tea, alcohol, and tobacco and in those who have a sweet tooth.

Hyperglycemia.   Hyperglycemia may result from increased levels of cortisol, epinephrine, or glucagon; defective insulin release; or increased insulin resistance. It is estimated that around one in three persons in countries with a Western lifestyle have a degree of insulin resistance and the health consequences associated with this metabolic derangement.[2]

Blood glucose levels tend to rise because tissues are less responsive to the insulin-driven clearance of glucose from the bloodstream. A self-perpetuating, disturbed, positive-feedback, metabolic cycle may be established as persistent hyperglycemia further enhances insulin resistance.

Insulin resistance, also characterized by higher fasting and postglucose-loading insulin levels, seems to be a common feature and a possible contributing factor to various health problems including polycystic ovary disease, dyslipidemia, hypertension, cardiovascular disease, sleep apnea, certain hormone-sensitive cancers, obesity, and type 2 diabetes mellitus.[3]

> The ability of insulin to dispose of glucose in the liver, skeletal muscle, and other peripheral tissues is compromised in insulin resistance

Diabetes mellitus is a prevalent condition of aberrant carbohydrate and lipid metabolism characterized by increased blood glucose levels. Two variants of diabetes mellitus have been described. Lean patients with diabetes are usually insulin-deficient, whereas obese patients with diabetes are characteristically insulin-resistant and have a relative insulin deficiency. Insulin-dependent diabetes usually presents in young people who complain of weight loss, thirst, and frequent urination. Without insulin replacement, ketosis may develop and these patients may lose consciousness. In contrast, patients with noninsulin-dependent, or type 2, diabetes are usually older and obese, often have a family history of diabetes, and experience excessive fatigue. Insulin resistance or decreased tissue sensitivity to insulin is associated with an increased prevalence of abnormal blood lipids, hypertension, and a tendency for blood to clot.[4] In patients with type 2 diabetes, lifestyle and dietary management may be sufficient to control blood glucose levels. Lifestyle and nutritional management of diabetes mellitus are discussed in detail in Part II.

Natural Intervention Measures

An intact negative feedback system usually compensates for dietary and energy utilization fluctuations. In persons in whom this system is defective, lifestyle choices may exacerbate or minimize clinical repercussions.

> Pathophysiologic stress can be modulated by dietary choices.

Glycemic Index: A Useful Guide to Food Selection. The glycemic index is the degree to which a food raises blood glucose levels relative to the same amount of oral glucose. Sugar, fruit juice, white bread, and pasta have a high glycemic index. A meal rich in simple sugars taxes the system by suddenly delivering a large bolus of glucose to the pancreas. The blood glucose level determines the amount of insulin secreted by the pancreas. A large bolus of absorbed glucose stimulates release of a large amount of insulin. Because a diet of simple sugars is rapidly absorbed, the glucose substrate for insulin is rapidly exhausted, and the blood glucose level drops rapidly. On the other hand, a diet rich in complex carbohydrates results in slower absorption of glucose because digestive juices take longer to reach and break down the polysaccharides in whole foods. Prolonged slower absorption of glucose results in both a smaller amount of insulin being released and a more prolonged delivery of substrate. Foods with a low glycemic index (i.e., foods that cause a more controlled and moderate rise in the blood glucose level) include legumes, barley, oats, and rice. A high-fiber diet is reputed to reduce postprandial blood glucose levels, maintain a lower basal blood glucose concentration, and enhance sensitivity to insulin.[5]

> Control of the blood glucose level is enhanced by selecting foods with a low glycemic index.

The glycemic index of food is influenced by its texture and content (e.g., the physical state of fiber, the type of carbohydrate present, and the presence of fat).[6] Rice, for example, has a lower glycemic index than potatoes because rice has a branched chemical structure and potatoes have a linear chain chemical structure. White rice is preferred, because brown rice contains lectins to which the patient may be sensitive. Although the precise mechanisms that determine a food's glycemic index remain obscure, it has been noted that the quality of fiber is itself an important glycemic determinant. Like fat, viscous fiber may induce a smaller glycemic response because of its slower gastric emptying time. In addition to delaying gastric emptying, water-soluble fiber delays glucose absorption from the small intestine by creating an unstirred water barrier and reducing intestinal motility. In contrast, insoluble fiber retards glucose absorption by insulating starch from intestinal hydrolytic enzymes and accelerating intestinal transit. In any event, persons with reactive hypoglycemia benefit from dietary choices that result in a low-sugar, high–complex-carbohydrate diet. Frequent small meals may also be helpful.

Carbohydrates and Athletic Performance.   Knowledge of glucose homeostasis is useful to endurance athletes. High-carbohydrate diets can increase an athlete's endurance by increasing glycogen stores. Exercise depletes muscle glycogen. When muscle glycogen is depleted, muscles become fatigued. The complete breakdown of glycogen to glucose and energy can only occur in the presence of sufficient oxygen. During intense exercise, an oxygen debt can develop, and muscle glycogen is converted by means of pyruvic acid into lactic acid. Pain results when lactic acid accumulates in muscle faster than the circulation removes it. Lactic acid is converted to glucose in the liver.

The first 20 minutes of moderate exercise is fuelled mainly by glycogen. As muscle glycogen stores decrease, the blood glucose level rises as liver glycogen is broken down. With time, glycogen utilization and stores decrease, and fat becomes an important source of energy. Training increases the quantity of glycogen stored in muscle; it increases the muscle mitochondria, and therefore, the aerobic metabolism of muscle; and it increases lean body mass. An adequate protein intake is also necessary.

Glycogen stores can be increased by eating a diet rich in carbohydrates.

Athletes can use a diet high in carbohydrates to trigger increased glycogen storage. Athletes require a daily intake of 9 to 10 g of carbohydrates per kilogram body of weight, or 60% to 70% of their energy intake from carbohydrates, to maximize their potential. Glycogen repletion should be started as soon as possible after exercise. Consumption of about 0.7 g of carbohydrate per kilogram of body weight is recommended every 2 hours for the first 4 to 6 hours after exercise. Simple sugars are more effectively absorbed than starches, and liquid supplements are often the preferred option after exercise. Carbohydrate loading may be undertaken by either of the following:

- Reducing training efforts and increasing carbohydrate intake 48 to 72 hours before competition. Body weight should be increased by 1 to 2 kg. Associated with each gram of glycogen stored are 3 g of water.

- Reducing carbohydrate intake to 50% of total calories for the first half week before competition while gradually decreasing training intensity. During the second half of the week, training is further reduced, but carbohydrates are boosted to 70% of calories or 10 g/kg body weight. Meals should be eaten 3 to 6 hours before the event and should contain at least 100 g of carbohydrates or approximately 4.5 g/kg body weight. Carbohydrates should be avoided 30 to 45 minutes before competition.

Recent research suggests that a high-carbohydrate maintenance diet coupled with cutting down on training for one or more days before a major sporting event can result in equally high levels of muscle glycogen. This strategy prevents the side effects of extreme fatigue during the depletion phase and muscle soreness caused by water retention in muscle fibers during the glycogen repletion/high-carbohydrate intake stage.

During exercise, carbohydrates will improve performance if the exercise lasts for more than 1 hour. The optimal range of intake is 20 to 30 g of carbohydrate for each 30 minutes. After exhaustive exercise, it can take 24 hours to replenish glycogen muscle stores. Because the rate of glycogen synthesis is potentially 50% greater during the first 2 hours after exercise, optimal recovery after exercise can be achieved by the following:

- Consuming carbohydrate-rich foods and drinks as soon as possible after finishing exercise. High levels of glycogen synthetase are present, and muscle cell walls are highly permeable and sensitive to insulin immediately after exercise. Carbohydrates are most rapidly absorbed if no fat or protein is present. Fruit and fruit juices are ideal choices.
- Continuing to drink over the next few hours, even if not thirsty.
- Keeping alcohol, and to a lesser extent caffeine, consumption to a minimum.

Recent studies suggest that the glycemic index of foods is an important consideration in exercise. It appears that consumption of foods with a low glycemic index before prolonged exercise may provide a more slowly released source of glucose for exercising muscles and result in greater endurance. It has therefore been suggested that generous amounts of foods with a low glycemic index (apples, peaches, baked beans, lentils, bran cereals, milk, and yogurt) should be eaten before prolonged exercise. In contrast, during exercise, high–glycemic-index drinks are beneficial to prevent hypoglycemia and dehydration. After intense exercise, optimal recovery of muscle glycogen stores is achieved by consuming high–glycemic-index foods such as bread, pasta, corn flakes, potatoes, bananas, honey, fruit juice, and sports drinks.[7]

> The dominant effect of a negative feedback system is prevention of unacceptable fluctuations; it maintains biologic functions within a physiologically acceptable range.

POSITIVE FEEDBACK SYSTEM OF HEMOSTASIS

In contrast to the blood glucose level, hemostasis is largely controlled by a positive feedback system. A positive feedback system enhances the effect of the stimulus, and the control mechanism escalates the response. Positive feedback amplifies the repercussions of the initial stimulus. It sets off a series of events that may be self-perpetuating and cause the system to deviate further from its resting value. Labor in childbirth, complement activation, and the blood-clotting cascade all exemplify positive feedback systems.

> Homeostasis based on positive feedback systems often involves a balance between systems with opposing actions.

Blood serves as a liquid transport medium for nutrients, oxygen, and waste products. Blood retains its fluid state as long as it flows within an intact cardiovascular system. An intact endothelial lining protects against activation of coagulation, and swiftly flowing blood dilutes any activated clotting factors. Should the endothelial lining of the system be damaged, blood in the affected area is converted from a liquid to a solid in an effort to prevent uncontrolled blood loss. Hemostasis is the rapid, localized response to disruption of the endothelial lining of blood vessels, and it involves interaction of three processes: vascular spasm, platelet plug formation, and coagulation.

The process of converting blood from a liquid to a solid is coagulation; the process of preventing blood from solidifying in an intact vascular system is fibrinolysis. In health, there is a balance between coagulation and fibrinolysis. Coagulation and fibrinolysis interact, and each system is separately controlled by positive feedback. In contrast to negative feedback systems in which homeostatic balance is achieved within a single system, positive feedback systems require interaction between counterbalancing systems to achieve homeostasis.

> Hemostasis results from vascular spasm, platelet plug formation, and coagulation.

Vasospasm

Vascular constriction can significantly reduce blood loss for up to 30 minutes, during which time a platelet plug and then a clot are formed to seal the vessel. Vessels constrict in response to injury. Triggers for vasospasm include chemical stimulation by endothelial or platelet factors, direct physical injury to vascular smooth muscle cells, and reflex spasm after stimulation of local pain receptors.

> Vasospasm reduces blood flow to the area.

Platelet Plug Formation

Platelets play a vital role in hemostasis by forming a temporary seal and releasing factors that enhance coagulation. They become sticky when exposed to collagen, as in the case of vascular injury. Platelets attach to the damaged lining of the vessel wall, and degranulation is triggered. Platelets release various chemicals, including the following:

- Serotonin, a local vasoconstrictor
- Adenosine diphosphate, a chemical that attracts platelets and enhances platelet aggregation
- Thromboxane A_2 (TXA_2), a prostaglandin that intensifies platelet aggregation and vasoconstriction

A positive feedback cycle is established, resulting in the formation of a platelet plug that forms a template for coagulation. The same factors that damaged the blood vessel and released chemicals from damaged tissue initiate the coagulation cascade that ultimately results in clot formation (see Figure 3-4). Intact endothelial cells, which secrete prostacyclin (PGI_2), a prostaglandin that inhibits platelet aggregation, restricting platelet plug formation to areas of vascular damage.

> Platelets form a temporary vessel seal that reduces blood loss.

Coagulation

Conversion of blood from a liquid to a gel occurs through the phases of prothrombin activation, thrombin, and finally fibrin formation. Several of the clotting factors circulating in the plasma are synthesized in the liver. Vitamin K is required for the hepatic synthesis of factors II (prothrombin), VII, IX, and X.

Prothrombin may be activated by an intrinsic or extrinsic activation system. In both instances a number of clotting factors are sequentially activated to form a clotting cascade. Damage to the vascular endothelium with platelet adhesion to the disrupted endothelium triggers the intrinsic pathway. Tissue trauma with release of tissue thromboplastin triggers the shorter extrinsic pathway. Clot formation takes 3 to 6 minutes after activation of the intrinsic system, and it takes 15 seconds after activation of the extrinsic system following tissue damage. The final common pathway of both systems is activation of factor X, which forms a complex with factor V in the presence of calcium ions to form prothrombin activator. When activated, prothrombin, a plasma protein, produces an enzyme, thrombin. Thrombin converts fibrinogen, a plasma protein produced by the liver, to fibrin. Thrombin polymerizes

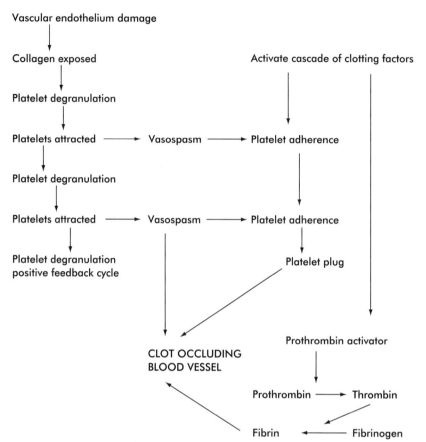

FIG. 3-4 Platelets in a positive feedback cycle.

fibrinogen, aligning its molecules and converting it into insoluble fibrin strands. Fibrin forms a gel-like substance and traps platelets; thus, the foundation of a clot is formed.

After activation by thrombin, fibrin-stabilizing factor acts as a cross-linking enzyme, binding fibrin strands and solidifying the clot. Within 30 to 60 minutes, platelet activity causes further clot retraction. Platelets contain contractile proteins that squeeze serum from the clot and plug damaged blood vessels. Other platelet constituents also contribute to vessel healing. Platelet-derived growth factor released from platelet granules stimulates division of smooth muscle cells and fibroblasts. Vessel healing results from the organization of the clot and regrowth of the vascular wall after cellular activation by platelet enzymes.

> The coagulation cascade changes blood from a liquid to a solid, forming a clot.

Fibrinolysis

Heparin is a natural anticoagulant normally found in small amounts in the plasma. Heparin, secreted by endothelial cells, inhibits the intrinsic pathway and prevents clot formation in healthy vessels. Even in traumatized vessels, coagulation is restricted to damaged areas.

Protein C and antithrombin III, produced in the liver, protect against inappropriate clot formation by inhibiting the activity of various intrinsic pathway coagulants. The behavior of thrombin, once activated, is carefully regulated. Activated thrombin is adsorbed onto fibrin and largely confined within the clot being formed. Furthermore, in the presence of calcium ions, thrombin simultaneously activates fibrin stabilizing factor (factor XIII) and catalyzes fibrinogen polymerization. Any thrombin that escapes into the circulation is inactivated by antithrombin III. The activity of antithrombin III is enhanced by heparin, released from the granules of platelets and mast cells.

> Interacting systems counterbalance coagulation, preventing widespread clotting.

In addition to providing safeguards that contain clot formation, the fibrinolytic system dissolves clots that have already formed. Fibrinolysis is the process that keeps blood as a liquid and prevents vascular occlusion. Plasminogen, an inactive plasma protein, is incorporated into clots. The presence of a clot stimulates vascular endothelial cells to secrete tissue plasminogen activator. Conversion of inactive plasminogen to plasmin results in dissolution of fibrin. Activated factor XII and thrombin also activate plasminogen. Fibrinolytic activity is largely confined to the clot. Fibrinolytic activity, initiated within 48 hours of coagulation, gradually declines until the clot is dissolved.

> Fibrinolysis increases vascular permeability and augments the inflammatory response.

The positive feedback systems in coagulation are countered by other positive feedback systems that impede clot formation. An imbalance of interacting positive feedback systems has serious consequences. A patient whose coagulation system evades normal control mechanisms starts bleeding. Disseminated intravascular coagulopathy results when clotting factors are depleted by disproportionate coagulation. Bleeding cannot be controlled because ineffective clots are formed in the presence of a hyperactive fibrinolytic system. Heparin is used to control bleeding in patients with disseminated intravascular coagulation. Less grave distortions of hemostasis can be mediated by dietary and nutrient measures.

> - Fibrinolysis counteracts coagulation, keeping the vascular system patent and preventing inappropriate clot formation; uncontrolled coagulation can lead to hemorrhage.
> - Interacting positive feedback systems are poised to prevent catastrophic exsanguination while maintaining tissue perfusion.
> - Dietary measures that modify platelet function can prevent vascular occlusion and reduce the risk of a heart attack.

Natural Intervention Measures

The vessel wall, coagulation, and fibrinolytic systems all influence hemostasis. Capillary fragility and disorders of platelets may result in easy bruising (see Figure 3-5). Suppression of platelet aggregation or adherence may prevent undesirable clot formation.

Dietary Choices and Platelet Function.   Dietary choices can inhibit platelet aggregation and prolong bleeding. Alcohol inhibits platelet aggregation, but wine may be more effective than ethanol alone. Wine and grape juice contain a wide variety of naturally occurring compounds, including fungicides, tannins, anthocyanins, and phenolic flavonoids (including flavonols and flavones). Phenolic flavonoids in wine are thought to exert their effects by reducing prostanoid synthesis from arachidonate- and nitric oxide–mediated platelet activity and by increasing vitamin E levels through decreasing the oxidative stress of platelets.[8] These compounds have demonstrated platelet inhibition in vitro and provide one explanation for the platelet-inhibitory properties of red wine and grape juice.[9] Animal experiments suggest that red wine and grape juice contain compounds absent from or present in lower concentrations in white wine. Persons at risk for thrombosis may benefit from regular consumption of red wine.

Omega-3 (ω-3) fatty acids, rich in deep sea cold water fish, are believed to be responsible for the prolonged bleeding tendency observed amongst Eskimos. Fish rich in ω-3 fatty acids include leather jacket, yellowfin tuna, blue grenadier, salmon, tuna, mackerel, herring, and mullet.[10] When buying fish, one should select specimens with clear, bright, bulging eyes; moist red gills; firm springy flesh; and a fresh, slightly briny smell. A diet that replaces meat and eggs with fish modifies the fatty acid composition of cell membranes. Increased consumption of fish and fish oils (eicosapentaenoic acid [EPA], docosahexaenoic acid) replaces ω-6 fatty acids, especially arachidonic acid (AA) in, among others, platelets and red blood cells.[11] The result is decreased production of TXA_2, a potent thromboxane, and increased production of TXA_3, a weak thromboxane. The net effect is less vasoconstriction and platelet aggregation. Increased production of the prostacyclins, PGI_3, and unchanged production of PGI_2 increases vasodilation and inhibits platelet aggregation.

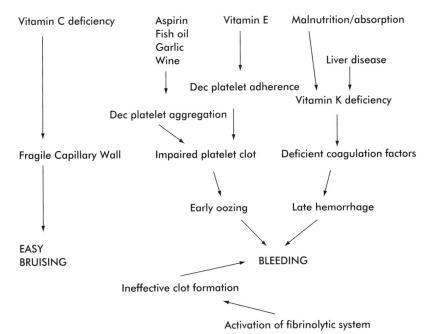

FIG. 3-5 Impaired hemostasis.

Persons taking anticoagulants may need to adjust their dose when converting to a diet rich in oily fish.

In addition to dietary choices, a lifestyle program to reduce the risk of clots may include adequate exercise and avoidance of stress. Although there is no clinical validation of the efficacy of stress management as an anticoagulant, there is evidence that mental stress enhances platelet aggregation.[12] However, because platelet function test results return to baseline values after about 30 minutes, the clinical validity of stress management as anticoagulant therapy is questionable.

Dietary Deficiency and Hemostasis. Just as increased consumption of certain foods may influence blood homeostasis, so may deficiency of certain nutrients affect hemostasis. Deficiency of vitamin C results in easy bruising caused by increased capillary fragility; deficiency of vitamin K results in prolonged bleeding caused by impaired hepatic synthesis of clotting factors. Eating fresh fruits and vegetables rich in vitamin C reduces the capillary fragility associated with scurvy. However, eating green leafy vegetables rich in vitamin K may not restore clotting factors. Synthesis of clotting factors requires normal liver function plus adequate vitamin K. In persons with normal liver function, impaired synthesis of clotting factors caused by vitamin K deficiency is usually attributable to malabsorption; in these patients, vitamin K injections may be necessary. Dietary deficiency of vitamin K is less likely to be clinically important, because bacteria present in the bowel normally produce vitamin K. Clinical reality is the result, not of a unilinear cause-effect relationship between vitamin K and the hepatic synthesis of clotting factors, but of the multisystem interaction of absorption and delivery of vitamin K to hepatocytes. Another clinical reality is that except in neonates, avoidance rather than prescription of vitamin K is likely. A diet rich in vitamin K is contraindicated in persons taking coumarin-based anticoagulants such as warfarin.

Nutrient Therapy. Lifestyle changes can modulate systems controlling hemostasis; however, larger intakes of nutrient can serve as more powerful triggers. Although correction of nutrient deficiency constitutes well-accepted clinical practice, prescription of nutrients in doses that exceed the recommended daily allowance requires more careful scrutiny of biologic mechanisms. Platelet adhesion and aggregation is an important early step in clot formation. Consequently, it is biologically plausible that natural interventions that reduce platelet stickiness would have an antithrombotic effect. A number of nutrients and herbs affect platelet adhesion.

Compared with control subjects, medical students who ate 10 g of raw garlic daily for 2 months demonstrated an increase in clotting time and fibrinolytic activity.[13] Garlic in doses of 800 mg has also been shown, in at least one double-blind, placebo-controlled trial, to decrease platelet aggregation and stickiness.[14] The ability of garlic to reduce the likelihood of thrombosis goes beyond basic science logic and has received a degree of clinical validation. In fact, consumption of garlic has even been cited as a risk factor for postoperative bleeding.[15]

Vitamin E in doses of 200 to 400 IU/day exerts an antithrombotic effect by inhibiting platelet adhesion. It has been suggested that after 2 weeks of supplementation, adhesion decreases by more than 75%.[16,17] Vitamin E interferes with platelet adhesion by inhibiting protein kinase C, resulting in decreased platelet pseudopodia formation. Vitamin E quinone, formed in vivo when vitamin E reacts with oxygen, is regarded as a potent anticoagulant. Although the results of clinical trials with vitamin E supplements are contradictory,[18] in view of its probable anticoagulant activity, vitamin E should not be taken for at least 48 hours before or after surgery.

Omega-3 fatty acids also reduce thrombosis by decreasing platelet aggregation, platelet TXA_2, and fibrinogen concentration and by increasing bleeding time and vascular prostacyclin (PGI_3).[19,20] Animal experimentation has confirmed multiple targeting of platelets and coagulation by fish oils. Researchers found that MaxEPA had an antithrombotic effect in arteries and, to a lesser extent, veins.[21] Dietary supplementation for 1 month with 2.28 g of ω-3 fatty acid ethyl esters twice daily resulted in impaired platelet aggregation that persisted for 8 weeks after the supplement was discontinued.[22]

Patients should be asked about consumption of garlic, vitamin E, and fish oil supplements; and use should be avoided before surgery to minimize the risk of untoward blood loss.

The physical state of blood is the result of multiple triggers for diverse, interacting feedback systems. Blood hemostasis exemplifies the complexity of biologic processes, as does acute inflammation.

ACUTE INFLAMMATION

Cause-effect outcomes are supported by a complex web of biologic interactions. Both positive and negative feedback systems are embedded in a lattice of interacting processes. Inflammation is a predictable and standard protective response to a noxious stimulus. It is one of a number of interlinking processes that serve to protect the individual and restore homeostasis. The inflammatory response is an integral component of nonspecific or innate immunity, because it provides the next level of protection when the superficial barrier has been breached. As part of the innate immune system, it provides immediate and general protection against the external environment; it also supplies a vital link to the specific immune system. Inflammatory cells process material used to prime the specific immune system, which then targets and attempts to eliminate designated foreign material.

Innate immunity provides immediate nonspecific protection, whereas specific immunity provides a slower, targeted protective response.

Superficial Barrier

Before the inflammatory response is triggered, the superficial barrier needs to be breached. The superficial barrier serves as a boundary between the individual and the external environment. It provides mechanical, chemical, and microbial protection. The skin and mucous membranes achieve mechanical protection. The mechanical barrier includes a respiratory escalator, a urinary lavage, and the physical impediment of an intact skin and mucosa. Organisms are flushed out of the respiratory tract by the cilia, which expel organisms trapped in a tenacious mucus blanket. Passing urine similarly expels organisms from the urinary tract through the urethra. The skin consists of a dry layer of keratinized cells that are regularly shed, along with any attached organisms. The gut lining is replenished every 48 to 72 hours. The chemical barrier includes stomach acid with its low pH, sebum with its rich fatty acids toxic to fungi, and lysozyme, a chemical found in saliva and tears, which lyses gram-positive bacteria. The mucosa of the gastrointestinal tract is initially protected against ingested microbes by the acid barrier of the stomach, whereas the large intestine houses commensal organisms. The microbial barrier of the intestine and vagina house commensal organisms that compete with potential pathogens for nutrients and create an environment hostile to a number of possible invaders.

The superficial barrier offers protection by mechanical, chemical, and microbial means.

Lifestyle choices can support or compromise the superficial barrier. Probiotics such as yogurt can replenish commensal gut bacteria, but cigarette smoking compromises the efficacy of the bronchial cilial escalator. Apparently, healthy foods may cause problems for susceptible persons. Lectins are molecules of nonimmunologic origin that bind to specific carbohydrate receptors, some of which line the gut wall. Lectins may provoke mast cells into releasing histamine. Histamine increases intestinal permeability, and the risk of absorbing allergens is increased. Persons susceptible to food allergy should avoid foods rich in lectins such as peanuts, beans, lentils, and wheat.

Nonspecific Immunity

Once the superficial barrier has been breached, the body mounts a cellular and humoral inflammatory response (see Figure 3-6). Phagocytosis and cytolytic elimination of foreign material are the primary activities of nonspecific immune cells.

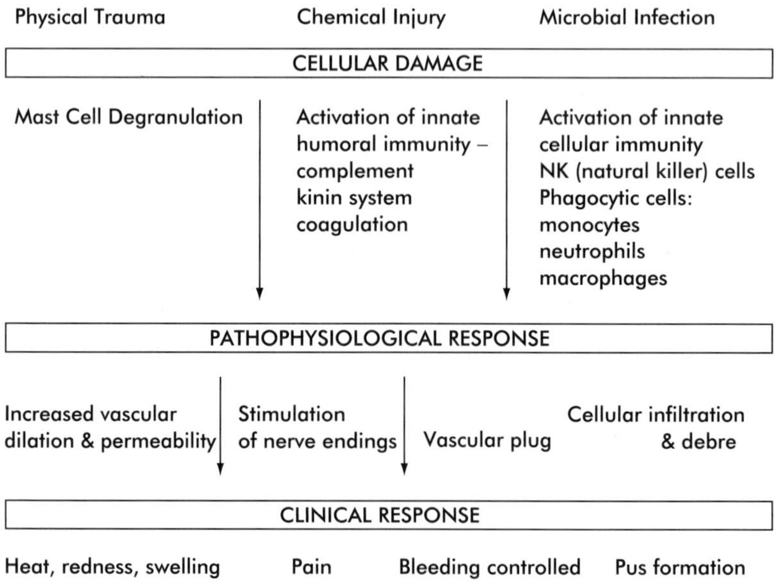

Physical Trauma	Chemical Injury	Microbial Infection
CELLULAR DAMAGE		
Mast Cell Degranulation	Activation of innate humoral immunity – complement kinin system coagulation	Activation of innate cellular immunity NK (natural killer) cells Phagocytic cells: monocytes neutrophils macrophages
PATHOPHYSIOLOGICAL RESPONSE		
Increased vascular dilation & permeability	Stimulation of nerve endings Vascular plug	Cellular infiltration & debre
CLINICAL RESPONSE		
Heat, redness, swelling	Pain Bleeding controlled	Pus formation

FIG. 3-6 Acute inflammation.

A positive feedback system is set up whereby cells, while responding to chemotactic factors released in the area of tissue injury, also contribute to the concentration of humoral factors in the inflammatory site. For example, platelet-activating factor (PAF)—a phospholipid found in neutrophils, macrophages, and platelets—stimulates aggregation and granule secretion by neutrophils and monocytes and enhances endothelial adhesion of leukocytes. It also attracts other neutrophils and monocytes to the area, thereby escalating the total response. PAF enhances platelet aggregation and encourages release of platelet contents. Platelets, in addition to being fundamental to hemostasis, contribute to the inflammatory response.

Cellular function influences diverse interacting systems: the positive feedback system that triggers platelets enhances the nonspecific inflammatory response and promotes blood coagulation.

Acute inflammation involves multiple cells secreting various chemicals that enhance the diverse aspects of the inflammatory process. Discrete triggers initiate similar processes. Diverse cells interact to achieve a common goal. Unilinear cause-effect relationships are submerged in a web of interacting processes. The more exaggerated the tissue response, the more severe are the redness, swelling, and pain. Fundamental to the clinical manifestations of acute inflammation is the need to trigger the vascular response.

Vascular Response. Mast cells serve as local activators of acute inflammation; they trigger the vascular response in acute inflammation. Mast cells release the chemical mediators of a local inflammatory response on exposure to physical trauma or chemical insult (e.g., toxins) or through an immunoglobulin E–mediated immunologic reaction. Chemicals immediately released on mast cell degranulation include the following:

- Histamine, which enhances vasodilation and aids perfusion of inflamed tissue
- Neutrophil chemotactic factor
- Eosinophil chemotactic factor

The immediate effect of mast cell degranulation is to increase blood flow and draw phagocytic cells to the local area. This vascular response is responsible for the heat, swelling, redness, and pain experienced early in inflammation. It is characterized by local redness and warmth caused by vascular dilation and swelling caused by fluid extravasation from affected vessels into the extracellular space.

As time passes, mast cells synthesize and secrete additional proinflammatory chemicals. Of the eicosanoid products of arachidonic acid (AA) metabolism, leukotrienes serve to further enhance vascular permeability and cellular chemotaxis. In contrast, although some of the prostaglandin products augment inflammation, some of the eicosanoid products of essential fatty acid metabolism tend to reduce inflammation. Dietary choices can affect this balance.

Mast cells play a fundamental role in inflammation, and lifestyle choices can influence mast cell function.

Cellular Response. Inflammation, in addition to a vascular response, involves a cellular response. The cellular response supports the vascular response and supplies building blocks necessary for nonspecific immunity, and later, specific immunity. The cellular response enhances the vascular response, removing debris and laying down connective tissue as part of the healing process. Both local (e.g., tissue) macrophages, mast cells, and endothelial cells and circulating cells are involved in inflammation.

Circulating cells drawn to the area include polymorphonuclear leukocytes, mononuclear phagocytic cells, and platelets. Polymorphonuclear leukocytes are produced in the bone marrow and circulate in the blood as neutrophils, basophils, and eosinophils. Neutrophils are highly effective phagocytes. They travel to sites of inflammation where they ingest foreign material. Eosinophils are not as efficient as killers but are more important in parasitic infections. Basophils contain granules of chemical factors that enhance inflammation; basophils are found in the blood and probably have a function similar to that of tissue-bound mast cells. The mononuclear phagocytic cells include monocytes and macrophages. In contrast to polymorphonuclear phagocytes, mononuclear phagocytes tend to remain confined to their local area. Macrophages process foreign material and present antigen to the specific immune system. They act as the link between innate and specific immunity.

Macrophages process antigens and provide a link between general and targeted immune responses.

Neutrophils, monocytes, and lymphocytes adhere to the vascular endothelium and migrate into the surrounding tissue. Interaction between leukocytes and the endothelial cells lining the blood vessels, leading to the migration of cells into damaged areas, involves the following:

- Tethering: Circulating cells are slowed. Tethering is mediated by selectins, which are lectin-like carbohydrate molecules. Selectins recognize specific carbohydrate sequences on either leukocytes or endothelial cells.
- Triggering: Factors present in the vessel are released, for example, cytokines and activated leukocyte adhesion molecules (e.g., integrins). Strong adhesion requires activation by interleukin 8 (IL-8) or PAF.
- Strong adhesion: Leukocytes are bound to the endothelium by means of integrin-mediated molecules.
- Motility: Adhered leukocytes migrate out of the blood vessel into the surrounding tissue. Local chemotactic factors direct this migra-

tion. Many of the cytokines that trigger adhesion also act as chemotactic factors.

Cells that dominate the early stages of the inflammatory response are the phagocytic and natural killer (NK) cells. NK cells are derived from a specific group of large granular lymphocytes, or null cells. These cells eliminate cancer- or virus-infected cells by nonspecifically targeting the cell membrane and releasing cytolytic enzymes. NK cells secrete chemicals that enhance the inflammatory response.

> Mononuclear and polymorphonuclear phagocytes participate in the inflammatory response, generating free radicals as they attempt to eliminate foreign or dead cells.

Phagocytic cells engulf and digest organisms and other foreign material. Triggers of phagocytosis are opsonized bacteria and diverse stimuli that activate cell membrane receptors (e.g., C5a). Enzymes in the primary granules of phagocytic cells such as proteases, lysozyme, and myeloperoxidase facilitate destruction of ingested material. Phagocytosis requires energy. Cellular energy (ATP) is generated through a process of oxidative phosphorylation, in which oxygen is converted to water through sequential steps that inevitably result in the generation of free radical by-products such as superoxide, hydrogen peroxide, and hydroxyl. Bacteria and viruses are destroyed by phagocytic cells with an oxidative burst that produces nitric oxide, superoxide, hydrogen peroxide, and halide anions (I^-, Cl^-, Br^-). Oxidants help fight infections. Hydrogen peroxide and superoxide are extremely toxic. Unless adequately contained, the cellular products that are toxic to bacteria can result in untoward cellular destruction. Reduced nicotinamide adenine dinucleotide phosphate oxidase reduces oxygen to superoxide. Superoxide dismutase rapidly converts superoxide to hydrogen peroxide, which is detoxified by catalase and oxidative reduction of glutathione (see Figure 3-7). Imprecise control of this and other physiologic processes that generate energy and render microbes innocuous can have pathologic consequences. Chronic infection and inflammation (i.e., chronic phagocytosis) have been associated with an increased risk of cancer. Chronic hepatitis carries an increased risk of liver cancer; schistosomiasis carries the risk of colon or bladder cancer, depending on the *Schistosoma* species responsible for the infection.

Although a positive feedback system is necessary to enhance the inflammatory response, an uncontrolled response can result in excess tissue damage. A second system is therefore required to counter the inflammatory response. Eosinophils carry chemicals that dampen the inflammatory response. Eosinophils contain enzymes that dampen the vascular effects of inflammatory response by various mechanisms including degradation of histamine and leukotrienes.

The inflammatory response has the potential to heal or harm.

Humoral Response. Inflammation is augmented by chemical mediators such as serotonin, histamine, kinins, eicosanoids, complement, and lymphokines. These chemicals enhance inflammation, aid phagocytosis, and interact with the specific immune system to achieve cytolysis. Inflammatory mediators may circulate, in an inactive form, in plasma or be produced by a diversity of cells. Interleukin-8 (IL-8) is produced by endothelial cells, fibroblasts, and macrophages. It is chemotactic for and activates neutrophils and nonhematopoeitic cells involved in wound healing. Platelets release histamine and PAF.

A number of chemicals in plasma, when activated, participate in the inflammatory process. Factor XII may activate coagulation and the kinin system. The kinin system generates bradykinin, which augments inflammation-enhancing vasodilation, vascular permeability, and pain. Coagulation, once activated by factor XII, generates fibrin and fibrinopeptides that are chemotactic and enhance vascular permeability. The fibrinolyic system activates factor XII, precipitating a cascade of interacting events including plasmin generation, complement C3 cleaving, and formation of fibrin split products. The complement system may be activated by the classical pathway involving an antibody-antigen (microbe) complex or by the alternate pathway after exposure to microbial polysaccharide. The consequences of complement activation are increased vascular permeability, neutrophil chemotaxis and activation, and opsonization of foreign cells followed by cytolysis. Complement is particularly effective in triggering elimination of bacteria.

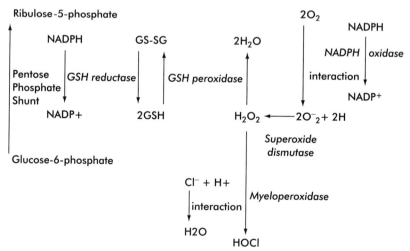

FIG. 3-7 Metabolic interactions. *GSH*, Reduced glutathione; *GSSG*, oxidized glutathione.

> Common triggers for diverse interacting positive or negative feedback systems can make clinical outcomes difficult to predict.

Inflammatory Response: A Fine Balance Between Healing and Harming

The body mounts an inflammatory response to tissue injury. The inflammatory process localizes cellular damage, removes cell debris and pathogens, and provides a framework for tissue repair and healing. Acute inflammation is dominated by a vascular response characterized by neutrophils and mast cells, whereas chronic inflammation is characterized by a proliferative response with macrophages and lymphocytes. When inflammation is exaggerated or prolonged, instead of healing, tissue destruction can result.

The mediators of the humoral response are potent chemicals. Although a humoral response is required to achieve local inflammation and healing, the chemical mediators of inflammation may have pathologic repercussions. Histamine provides a useful example. Histamine improves perfusion but also increases permeability of local capillaries and promotes exudation. Histamine is stored in an inactive bound form in mast cells, basophils, and platelets. The intestine, skin, and lungs are rich in histamine. Histamine is capable of activating cell membrane receptors in different organs. H_1 receptors are found mainly in smooth muscles and exocrine glands of the respiratory tract. H_2 receptors are found mainly in the parietal cells of the stomach. H_1 and H_2 receptors are also found in the brain and cardiac muscle. H_3 receptors inhibit the release of histamine in the central nervous system. The concentration and site of histamine release determine the repercussions of histamine release.

Activation of H_1 receptors increases the cellular level of cyclic guanosine monophosphate, which enhances contraction in smooth muscle and endothelial cells, chemotaxis in neutrophils, and prostaglandin synthesis in mast cells. Other cyclic guanosine monophosphate stimulants are biotin, ginseng, vitamin C in high doses, and leukotrienes. Histamine stimulation of H_1 receptors mediates the following:

- Muscle contraction of the bronchi, intestine, and uterus. Potential adverse consequences of smooth muscle contraction are bronchospasm, colic, and dysmenorrhea.
- Pulmonary vasoconstriction. Excess stimulation may precipitate pulmonary hypertension.
- Permeability of the postcapillary venules. One adverse effect of excess stimulation is edema. Increased vascular permeability enhances edema and pruritus. Other consequences are receptor stimulation (resulting in itching, pain, and sneezing), prostaglandin generation, and a positive chronotropic effect increasing heart rate.

H_1 receptors mediate the allergic response. In classic allergies, histamine and other mediators are released from mast cells after cross-linkage between two immunoglobulin E molecules on the mast cell membrane.

H_2 receptors stimulate mucus production in the bronchial tree and augment gastric acid production. Other consequences are increased production of cyclic adenosine monophosphate; inhibition of the release of lymphokines, basophil histamine, neutrophil enzymes, eosinophil migration; and T-lymphocyte–mediated cytotoxicity. Stimulation of H_2 receptors dampens lymphocyte, eosinophil, neutrophil, and mast cell activity.

> Lifestyle choices can modulate the balance between the interacting systems controlling the acute inflammatory response.

Dietary Modulation of Inflammation

The polyunsaturated fatty acids, linoleic (ω-6) and α-linolenic acid (ω-3), are essential for normal cellular function. They act as precursors for the synthesis of longer-chained polyunsaturated fatty acids such as AA, eicosapentaenoic acid (EPA), and docosahexaenoic acid (DHA), which have been shown to participate in numerous cellular functions affecting membrane fluidity, membrane enzyme activities, and eicosanoid synthesis (see Figure 3-8).

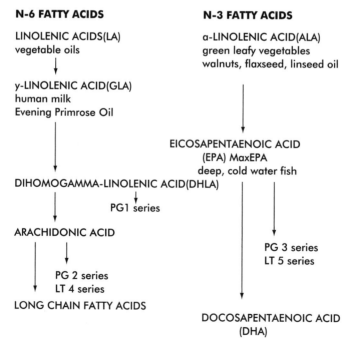

FIG. 3-8 Nutrient modulation of eicosanoid production.

Eicosanoids are involved in cell regulation; among their functions is modulation of inflammation. Two important groups of eicosanoids involved in inflammation are the leukotrienes and prostaglandins. The nature of the eicosanoid produced is influenced both by the unsaturated fatty acid substrate and the oxygenase enzyme system present. Although leukotrienes are more potent inflammatory mediators than prostaglandins,[11] the essential fatty acids from which the eicosanoid is generated determines its relative potency. Leukotrienes produced from the ω-6 series of fatty acids are 10 to 30 times more potent inflammatory agents than leukotrienes produced from the ω-3 fatty acids. Similarly, prostaglandin II, produced from AA (ω-6 intermediates), is clearly proinflammatory; whereas prostaglandins I and III, produced from dihommogammalinolenic acid (ω-6) and ω-3 fatty acids, do not or only marginally enhance inflammation.

Cyclooxygenase enzymes are necessary for prostaglandin production. Cyclooxygenase is found in all cells except red blood cells. Important eicosanoids produced by the action of cyclooxygenase on AA are prostaglandin E_2 (PGE_2), prostacyclin, and TXA_2 (see Figure 3-9). PGE_2 and prostacyclin mediate the vascular phase of inflammation, increasing vasodilation and microvascular permeability. They activate adenylate cyclase,

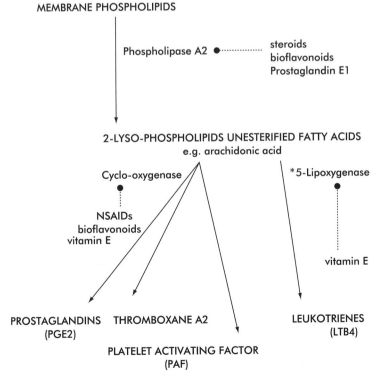

FIG. 3-9 Inflammation and arachidonic acid and metabolism. *5-Lipoxygenase detected in a limited number of cells (e.g., bone marrow–derived cells, synovial cells). Cyclooxygenase is virtually ubiquitous.

thereby increasing cellular levels of cyclic adenosine monophosphate, which modifies local immunity and reduces inflammation. Exercise and compounds in fruit and vegetables stimulate production of cyclic adenosine monophosphate.

TXA_2 is a powerful vasoconstrictor and enhances platelet aggregation; prostacyclin prevents platelet aggregation and with PGE_2 causes vasodilatation. In balance, the prostaglandin II series promotes inflammation. This is in contrast to the prostaglandin I and III series that arise from a different fatty acid substrate. Box 3-1 illustrates the protean effect of a single dietary change on the inflammatory process, and Box 3-2 shows how such dietary changes influence physiologic processes in other body systems.

The lipoxygenase enzymes are necessary for leukotriene production. This enzyme system is only encountered in inflammatory cells such as

---

■ Box 3-1 ■

WIDESPREAD IMPACT OF A SINGLE DIETARY CHANGE

An increased intake of fish oils results in changes to the following:
Macrophages
- Decreased adhesion to endothelial cells
- Decreased interleukin 1
- Decreased tissue necrosis factor
- Decreased platelet-activating factor

Neutrophils
- Reduced leukotriene B_4, a powerful inducer of leukocyte chemotaxis and adherence
- Increased leukotriene B_5, a weak inducer of inflammation and chemotatic agent
- Decreased superoxide

Vascular endothelium
- Decreased nitric acid
- Decreased platelet-derived growth factor
- Decreased ventricular arrhythmia
- Decreased endothelial stickiness

Platelets
- Reduced thromboxane A_2, a potent platelet aggregator and vasoconstrictor
- Increased thromboxane A_3, a weak platelet aggregator and vasoconstrictor
- Increased concentration of prostacyclin (PGI_3) with no decrease in PGI_2, resulting in an overall increase in prostacyclins that enhance vasodilation and inhibit platelet aggregation
- Decreased platelet aggregation and adhesiveness

```
■ Box 3-2 ■

SYSTEMIC EFFECT OF EICOSANOIDS

General functions of prostaglandins
  • Inhibition of gastric secretion
  • Stimulation of pancreatic and small intestine secretions
  • Induction of water and electrolyte flow into the intestinal lumen
  • Sensitization of nerve endings, causing pain
  • Maintenance of renal blood flow
  • Stimulation of release of anterior pituitary hormones

Increased prostglandin E₂
  • Relaxes bronchial smooth muscle
  • Increases mucus secretion
  • Decreases acid secretion in the stomach
  • Causes hyperalgesia
  • Contracts the myometrium
  • Stimulates renin release
  • Induces fever

Increased leukotriene C₄
  • Increases tracheal mucus production
  • Induces bronchoconstriction
  • Increases vascular permeability
  • Induces granulocyte accumulation
```

macrophages, mast cells, and all of the three polymorphonuclear leukocytes (neutrophils, basophils, and eosinophils). These cells dominate the cellular response to acute inflammation. Lipoxygenase produces leukotrienes (LT_4) and lipoxanes from AA in these inflammatory cells. Not surprisingly, this leukotriene series is unequivocally proinflammatory. Leukotriene B_4 attracts leukocytes, enhances their adhesion to endothelial cells, and activates them to secrete reactive oxygen species and degradation enzymes. Leukotrienes C_4, D_4, and E_4 stimulate smooth muscle contraction, which may result in vasoconstriction and bronchospasm. Vascular permeability and mucus production are also increased. Lipoxanes A and B inhibit human NK cell activity, stimulate smooth muscle causing arteriolar dilatation, stimulate chemotaxis and superoxide anion secretion, and activate protein kinase C. Excessive leukotriene formation has been linked to asthma, gout, atopic eczema, psoriasis, and ulcerative colitis.

Lipoxygenase is inhibited by vitamin E, quercetin, garlic, and curcumin.

The nature of the eicosanoids produced in inflammatory cells can be modified by diet. Tissue injury and phagocytosis trigger the release of phospholipids from cell membranes by phospholipase A_2. Persons with diets rich in meat and eggs have cell membranes rich in AA, an ω-6 fatty acid. Phospholipase A_2 releases AA from the cell membrane and initiates production of proinflammatory eicosanoids from the PGE_2 series and LT_4 series. Feeding linoleic acid to animals enhances PGE_2 production, induces IL-1 and IL-6 production in a positive curvilinear fashion, and increases leukotriene B_4 production in moderate doses and suppresses it in high doses.[23] In contrast, a diet rich in fish enhances eicosapentaenoic acid (EPA) deposition in cell membranes, and phospholipase A_2 is more likely to release and initiate production of noninflammatory products from the PGE_3 series and weakly inflammatory LT_5 series. Overall, eating fats rich in ω-6 fatty acids enhances IL-1 production and tissue responsiveness to cytokines; fats rich in ω-3 fatty acids have the opposite effect, because monounsaturated fatty acids decrease tissue responsiveness to cytokines, whereas IL-6 production is enhanced by the total unsaturated fatty acid intake.[23] The fatty acid precursor of the eicosanoids with the greatest proinflammatory impact in terms of quantity and quality is AA.

Decreased tissue stores of AA can be achieved by increased consumption of ω-3 fatty acids (see Figure 3-8). By replacing meat, meat products, eggs, and lard in the diet with fish, spinach, walnuts, soy products, canola oil, and linseed oil, the composition of cell membranes can be changed. Persons on a diet rich in these products have cell membranes rich in ω-3 fatty acids. Ingestion of dietary supplements of ω-3 fatty acids has been consistently shown to reduce both the number of tender joints on physical examination and the amount of morning stiffness in patients with rheumatoid arthritis.[24] The clinical benefits of the ω-3 fatty acids were not apparent until they had been consumed for at least 12 weeks. Furthermore, it appeared that to experience benefit, a minimum daily dose of 3 g of EPA and docosahexaenoic acid was necessary to achieve a significant reduction in the release of LTB_4 from stimulated neutrophils and of IL-1 from monocytes. An earlier randomized, controlled, double-blind study showed that patients with rheumatoid arthritis taking 10 g of fish oil per day reported a significantly decreased consumption of nonsteroidal anti-inflammatory drugs (NSAIDs) at 3 and 6 months.[25]

> Dietary fat selection can alter the eicosanoid environment of cell membranes to enhance or dampen the inflammatory response.

In addition to changing the fatty acid constitution of cells, nutritional measures can alter cellular enzyme activity. Certain flavonoids possess potent inhibitory activity against a wide array of enzymes including phospholipase A_2. Activated mast cells, basophils, neutrophils, eosinophils, macrophages, and platelets are susceptible to the modulating effects of flavonoids.[26] Bioflavonoids have an inhibitory effect on the release of AA from cell membranes, and consequently, can limit its availability as a substrate for cellular oxygenase enzymes. Quercetin and other flavonoids have been shown to modify eicosanoid biosynthesis, reducing prostanoid production and facilitating an anti-inflammatory response.[27] This outcome is not solely attributable to the effect of flavonoids on phospholipase A_2; flavonoids also have an inhibitory effect on cyclooxygenase. In addition to a membrane-stabilizing effect and their ability to inhibit oxygenase enzymes, flavonoids are free radical scavengers. Consequently, it is biologically plausible that they would be useful in cases of acute inflammation. Anecdotal evidence suggests that 400 mg of quercetin, taken 20 minutes before meals three times a day, is helpful in reducing acute inflammation. It is also reputed to reduce the swelling that results from hard contact sports when taken in doses of 0.6 to 1.8 g before participation.

Bioflavonoids are not the only nutrients believed to dampen inflammation. Vitamin C and curcumin, the active ingredient in turmeric, are also believed to modify cyclooxygenase enzyme activity. Vitamin E is believed to have an inhibitory effect on both cyclooxygenase and lipoxygenase activity. Quercetin, garlic, and chaparral are other lipoxygenase inhibitors.

Nitric oxide activates cyclooxygenase and lipoxygenase, leading to the production of physiologically relevant quantities of PGE_2 and leukotrienes.[28] Vitamin E, an antioxidant, can neutralize nitric oxide and other free radicals. Free radicals generated during inflammation create a self-propagating system in which they cause tissue damage, which in turn exacerbates cell damage. Vitamin E may interrupt this positive feedback cycle and prevent unquenched free radicals from damaging tissue. The dose of vitamin E may be crucial. The recommended daily intake of vitamin E is around 19 IU, although doses between 100 and 800 IU/day may be prescribed.[29] Vitamin E decreases platelet adhesion, and at levels greater than 400 IU/day, may increase clotting times.[30] Immune function in the elderly has been found to improve with a dose of vitamin E of 800 IU/day.[31] The cell membranes of immune cells have a high concentration of polyunsaturated fatty acids, and the rich supply of vitamin E in immune cells protects them against lipid oxidation. For persons with a high polyunsaturated fatty acid intake, it may be desirable to take vitamin E at doses of 400 to 800 IU/day to ensure an adequate vitamin E concentration. Absolute and relative vitamin E deficiencies impair the immune response at several levels.

> Fish, fish oil, vitamin E, bioflavonoids, and curcumin may dampen inflammation.

HOMEOSTASIS: BALANCE WITHIN A DYNAMIC INTERACTIVE SYSTEM

Homeostasis is achieved by the interaction of multiple systems. The impact of single-nutrient supplementation on homeostasis depends on the overall nutrient status. As an example, in the immune system, zinc deficiency results in increased susceptibility to infection and is associated with atrophy of the thymus and loss of T helper cell function. Correction of zinc deficiency enhances immune function; however, zinc excess, which can occur at doses of 150 mg daily, reduces chemotaxis, phagocytosis, and lymphocyte proliferation. Furthermore, zinc supplementation can cause copper deficiency, which impairs antibody production. Similarly, iron deficiency impairs T-cell activation and limits the ability of NK cells to stimulate interferon; on the other hand, iron excess enhances the growth of microorganisms and impairs immune function. Single nutrients do not act in isolation. A single nutrient can initiate various homeostatic responses by triggering any one of a number of interacting systems. Adaptation to change depends on the intensity and nature of each stimulus, the interaction between stimuli, the competence of each individual system, and the overall integrity of the interaction between systems. Food contains a multitude of nutrients, each of which may influence diverse physiologic processes. Table 3-1 lists some of the nutrients that interact to optimize mitochondrial oxidative phosphorylation.[32] A balanced food intake reduces the risk of creating a nutrient imbalance that stresses compensatory mechanisms. Furthermore, in herbal medicine, adaptogens such as *Astragalus* species and ginseng are recognized to provide a

TABLE 3-1 ■ Nutrients Contributing to Mitochondrial Oxidative Phosphorylation

NUTRIENT	POSTULATED DESIRABLE RANGE	EFFECT ON MITOCHONDRIAL FUNCTION
Glutathione	100-1000 mg	Antioxidant and phase 2 detoxification
N-acetyl-carnitine	50-200 mg	Fatty acid transport
N-acetyl cysteine	20-200 mg	Stimulates glutathione
Lipoic acid	50-1000 mg	Diverse protective effects
Catechin	50-1000 mg	HO and peroxynitrite quencher
Omega-3 fatty acids	500-2000 mg EPA	Membrane component, blocks cytokine activity
Selenium	100-500 μg	Activates GSH peroxidase
Manganese	2-5 mg	Component of superoxide dismutase
Zinc	10-50 mg	Component of superoxide dismutase
Copper	1-3 mg	Component of superoxide dismutase
Magnesium malate	50-1000 mg	Activates Krebs cycle
Sodium succinate	100-4000 mg	Activates Krebs cycle
Vitamin K	100-1000 μg	Protects electron chain transport
Co Q10	20-300 mg	Maintains electron pump
Vitamin E	100-1000 mg	Protects mitochondrial membrane
Riboflavin	10-200 mg	$FADH_2$ activator, Krebs cycle
Niacin	10-200 mg	NADH and NADPH production
Thiamine	10-200 mg	Transketolase activator

FADH$_2$, Reduced form of flavin adenine dinucleotide; *GSH,* reduced glutathione; *HO,* hyperbaric oxygen; *NADH,* reduced nicotinamide adenine dinucleotide; *NADPH,* reduced nicotinamide adenine dinucleotide phosphate.

measure of protection by maintaining homeostasis despite environmental stress.[33] The capacity of adaptogens to normalize the cellular environment makes them potentially useful prophylactic agents. The chemical complexity of herbs and whole foods provides a substrate with numerous and diverse triggers that may, assuming an appropriate combination, be conducive to wellness.

The diversity of stimuli that can trigger particular systems and the intricacy of physiologic interactions that seek to achieve homeostasis are the bane and boon of health care. The diversity of triggers that can be used to restore health provide a plethora of opportunities for intervention. The complexity of self-referent, mutually interactive systems makes selection of optimal intervention problematic and conclusive attribution of a clinical outcome to a particular intervention difficult.

REFERENCES

1. Cosford R: Insulin resistance, obesity and diabetes: the connection, *J Aust Coll Nutr Env Med* 18:3-10, 1999.
2. Grimm JJ: Interaction of physical activity and diet: implications for insulin-glucose dynamics, *Public Health Nutr* 2:363-8, 1999.
3. Kelly GS: Insulin resistance: lifestyle and nutritional interventions, *Altern Med Rev* 5:109-32, 2000.
4. Goldberg RB: Prevention of type 2 diabetes, *Med Clin North Am* 82:805-21, 1998.
5. Vinik AI, Jenkins DJ: Dietary fiber in management of diabetes, *Diabetes Care* 11:160-73, 1988.
6. Wood FC, Bierman EL: Is diet the cornerstone in management of diabetes? *New Engl J Med* 315:1224-7, 1986.
7. Thomas DE, Brotherhood JR, Brand JC: Carbohydrate feeding before exercise: effect of glycaemic index, *Int J Sports Med* 12:180-6, 1991.
8. Ruf JC: Wine and polyphenols related to platelet aggregation and atherothrombosis, *Drugs Exp Clin Res* 25:125-31, 1999.
9. Demrow HS, Slane PR, Folts JD: Administration of wine and grape juice inhibits in vivo platelet activity and thrombosis in stenosed canine coronary arteries, *Circulation* 91:1182-8, 1995.
10. Gibson RA: The effect of diets containing fish and fish oils on disease risk factors in humans, *Aust N Z J Med* 18:713-22, 1988.
11. Simopoulos AP: Omega-3 fatty acids in health and disease and in growth and development, *Am J Clin Nutr* 54:438-63, 1991.
12. Grignani G, Pacchiarini L, Zucchella M, et al: Effect of mental stress on platelet function in normal subjects and in patients with coronary artery disease, *Haemostasis* 22:138-46, 1992.
13. Gadkari JV, Joshi VD: Effect of ingestion of raw garlic on serum cholesterol level, clotting time and fibrinolytic activity in normal subjects, *J Postgrad Med* 37:128-31, 1991.
14. Kiesewetter H, Jung F, Jung EM, et al: Effect of garlic on platelet aggregation in patients with increased risk of juvenile ischaemic attack, *Eur J Clin Pharmacol* 45:333-6, 1993.

15. Burnham BE: Garlic as a possible risk for postoperative bleeding, *Plast Reconstr Surg* 95:213, 1995.
16. Jandak J, Steiner M, Richardson PD: Alpha-tocopherol, an effective inhibitor of platelet adhesion, *Blood* 73:141-9, 1989.
17. Steiner M: Vitamin E, a modifier of platelet function: rationale and use in cardiovascular and cerebrovascular disease, *Nutr Rev* 57:306-9, 1999.
18. Mensink RP, van Houwelingen AC, Kromhout D, Hornstra G: A vitamin E concentrate rich in tocotrienols had no effect on serum lipids, lipoproteins, or platelet function in men with mildly elevated serum lipid concentrations, *Am J Clin Nutr* 69:213-9, 1999.
19. Leaf A, Weber PC: Cardiovascular effects of n-3 fatty acids, *N Engl J Med* 318:549-57, 1988.
20. Saynor R, Gillott T: Changes in blood lipids and fibrinogen with a note on safety in a long term study on the effects of n-3 fatty acids in subjects receiving fish oil supplements and followed for seven years, *Lipids* 27:533-8, 1992.
21. Andriamampandry MD, Leray C, Freund M, et al: Antithrombotic effects of (n-3) polyunsaturated fatty acids in rat models of arterial and venous thrombosis, *Thromb Res* 93:9-16, 1999.
22. Cerbone AM, Cirillo F, Coppola A, et al: Persistent impairment of platelet aggregation following cessation of a short-course dietary supplementation of moderate amounts of N-3 fatty acid ethyl esters, *Thromb Haemost* 82:128-33, 1999.
23. Grimble RF, Tappia PS: Modulation of pro-inflammatory cytokine biology by unsaturated fatty acids, *Z Ernahrungswiss* 37(suppl 1):57-65, 1998.
24. Kremer JM: n-3 fatty acid supplements in rheumatoid arthritis, *Am J Clin Nutr* 71(suppl 1):349S-51S, 2000.
25. Skoldstam L, Borjesson O, Kjallman A, et al: Effect of six months of fish oil supplementation in stable rheumatoid arthritis. A double-blind, controlled study, *Scand J Rheumatol* 21:178-85, 1992.
26. Middleton E Jr: Effect of plant flavonoids on immune and inflammatory cell function, *Adv Exp Med Biol* 439:175-82, 1998.
27. Formica JV, Regelson W: Review of the biology of Quercetin and related bioflavonoids, *Food Chem Toxicol* 33:1061-80, 1995.
28. McCann SM, Licinio J, Wong ML, et al: The nitric oxide hypothesis of aging, *Exp Gerontol* 33:813-26, 1998.
29. Pearce KA, Boosalis MG, Yeager B: Update on vitamin supplements for the prevention of coronary disease and stroke, *Am Fam Physician* 62:1359-66, 2000.
30. Kim JM, White RH: Effect of vitamin E on the anticoagulant response of warfarin, *Am J Cardiol* 77:545-6, 1996.
31. Meydani M, Meisler J: A closer look at vitamin E: can this antioxidant prevent chronic disease, *Postgrad Med* 102:199-207, 1997.
32. Fluhrer J: Geriatrics. Presented at the ACNEM Primary Course, Melbourne, Australia, September 2000.
33. Wasaf T: Astragalus: spanning Eastern and Western medicine, *Am J Nat Med* 5:26-9, 1981.

CHAPTER 4

TOWARD NUTRITIONAL HEALTH: CHOOSING FOOD OR SUPPLEMENTS

> Hippocrates suggested some 2500 years ago: "Let food be thy medicine and medicine be thy food."[1]

In 1996, sales of dietary supplements increased 9% over the previous year and totaled $9.8 billion.[2] The community has long shown a predilection for taking dietary supplements, and health professionals are increasingly demonstrating a similar trend. Half of the 4501 female physicians aged 30 to 70 years who responded to an American survey took a multivitamin-mineral supplement; 35.5% of them did so regularly.[3] However, despite a vast array of options (see Table 4-1 and Part Three of this text), no more than 33% took any supplement other than calcium and less than 20% did so regularly. Given the array of nutritional supplements readily available, the issue has become one of prudent choice.

INDICATIONS FOR SUPPLEMENTATION

Dietary supplements include any substance consumed in addition to the regular diet. Dietary supplements must provide a nutrient that is either being undersupplied to cells or is capable of exerting a pharmacologic effect on cellular processes to be efficacious.[4] In other words, reasons for dietary supplementation range from an absolute or relatively inadequate dietary intake to use of nutrients and herbs as medications to correct cellular dysfunction. In the former, optimal function is achieved when a nutrient required by the organism reaches a specific concentration within the cell. Low-calorie diets may not deliver the quantity or variety of nutrients necessary for health unless nutrient-dense food is selected. However, during periods of increased physiologic demand (e.g., pregnancy and lactation), even normal diets may not supply the increased demand for particular nutrients such as iron or calcium. In the latter instance, when used as medication, the dietary supplement contains a constituent that is either not normally required by the cell or not required in the dose achieved by supplementation. In this case, the supplement may be perceived to act

TABLE 4-1 ■ Popular Community Remedies

SUPPLEMENT/CONSTITUENT	ACTION	POTENTIAL USE	SIDE EFFECTS
Green-lipped mussel	Prostaglandin inhibitor, anti-inflammatory effect	Rheumatoid arthritis	Flatulence, nausea; safe
Green tea/flavonoids, catechins	Antioxidant, cancer protective, antimicrobial	Reduces risk of cancer and cardiovascular disease	Aggravates bleeding tendency
Glucosamine/hexamine sugar	Used in synthesis of, e.g., glycoproteins, hyaluronic acid, glucosaminoglycan	Osteoarthritis	Constipation, diarrhea, drowsiness
Shark cartilage	Glycosaminoglycans, anti-angiogenesis factors	Osteoarthritis, adjunct cancer therapy	Gastrointestinal complaints, hepatitis
S-adenosylmethionine	Methyl donor	Depression, fibromyalgia osteoarthritis, cardiovascular disease	Nausea, dry mouth
Para-aminobenzoic acid	B vitamin group	Prevents sunburn	Rarely rash
Melatonin	Pineal hormone	Jet lag, insomnia	Nil of note, short-term use
Flaxseed oil/Lignans, α-linolenic acid (ω-3)	Phytoestrogenic effect, anti-inflammatory	?? Alternative to fish oil	Nil
Dehydroepiandrosterone (DHEA)	Adrenal hormone precursor of estrogen & androgens, stimulates insulin growth factor	Enhances immunity, well-being	Safe but could cause masculinization in females
Chitosan/polysaccharide	Binds fat molecules	Weight loss	Absorption of fat-soluble vitamins D, E, C in animals
Carnitine/amino acid derivative	Long-chain fatty acid transport across membranes, β-oxidation, transport of acyl coenzyme A	Adjunct treatment for diseases of atherosclerosis	Nausea, diarrhea, vomiting; L-carnitine less risk of toxicity than D-carnitine
α-Lipoic acid	Improves recycling of other antioxidants	Improves glucose utilization in diabetics	Occasional skin rash
Aloe vera	Hypoglycemia, hypolipidemia, antiinflammatory	Local application, moisturizer; orally, diabetes	Occasional allergy

as a drug. If nutritional supplements and herbs are deemed to be drugs, they will be subject to outcome claims and constraints not associated with foods.

LEGISLATIVE STANDARDS: STANDARDIZATION AND SAFETY

A major difference between supplements and drugs is in the legislative standards that must be met. In the case of drugs, issues such as administration of a safe, effective dose need to be meticulously addressed. Safe, effective drug therapy requires at least use of standardized drug formulas in previously determined doses. Although the importance of carefully scrutinizing the quality of supplements is recognized,[5] history suggests that standards need review. Herbal products are not regulated for purity and potency, and batch-to-batch variability is recognized to be associated with varying efficacy and side effects resulting from impurities.[6] Pharmacologic differences have been reported within a single species of herb (ginseng) cultivated in two different locations.[7] The variability of bioactive compounds present in different preparations makes it difficult to interpret the efficacy of herbs in analysis of clinical trials. Echinacea products can contain other plant extracts, can be derived from different plant species, can be obtained from different parts of the plant, and can be prepared in different ways (e.g., hydrophilic or lipophilic extraction).[8] Determining the efficacy of garlic from clinical trials has encountered a similar problem. In general, efforts to standardize herbal products are complicated by plant identification, genetic variation, agronomic factors, the part of the plant used, time and method of harvesting, postharvest handling, manufacturing technique, and stability.[9] Even the composition of tea leaves depends on the climate, season, horticultural practices, type, and age of the plant.[10] In addition to not getting the prescribed dose of an active principle, recipients may receive a toxic compound. In late 1989, an epidemic of eosinophilia-myalgia syndrome (several thousand cases) that resulted in 36 deaths in the United States was linked to contamination of a batch of tryptophan manufactured in Japan.[11] Nutrient supplement purity may vary with preparation procedures, and chemical variations in plant extracts may result from diverse agricultural practices. Although herbal preparations are more difficult to standardize, nutrients also have a record of not always meeting acceptable standards.

Therapeutic claims carry significant responsibility. If claims are to be made for nutrients and herbs as useful cancer chemotherapeutic agents, they will need to withstand scrutiny equivalent to the standards set for cytotoxic agents being developed for cancer chemoprevention.[12] The blueprint for chemotherapy evaluation passes through three phases of rigorous evaluation before registration; efficacy, dose toxicity, and long-term side effects are all assessed. The development, evaluation, manufacture, marketing, and prescription of drugs are rigorously regulated.

SUPPLEMENT CLAIMS

By definition, dietary supplements have not been designated drugs. In 1994, the Dietary Supplement Health and Education Act (DSHEA) set up a new framework for Food and Drug Administration (FDA) regulation in the United States.[13] The DSHEA defined dietary supplements as being neither a replacement for a conventional diet nor a drug. Unlike drugs, supplements are not intended to diagnose, treat, or prevent disease; also, they are not subject to clinical studies to establish their efficacy, safety, appropriate dosage, or potential interactions before marketing. In fact, supplements are considered safe until proven unsafe by the FDA. The DSHEA further broadened the definition for dietary supplements to include, with some exceptions, any product intended for ingestion as a supplement to the diet. Supplements include vitamins, minerals, herbs, botanicals, various other plant-derived substances, amino acids, concentrates, and metabolites.

> Vitamin, mineral, amino acid, herbal, and botanical supplements are assumed to be safe until proven unsafe by the FDA.

Supplement manufacturers are permitted to make certain types of claims in the United States. Nutrient-nutrient claims describe the concentration of nutrient in the food. Provided that the supplement contains an adequate concentration of the nutrient, disease-prevention claims are permitted if supplement-disease links have been established (e.g., "folic acid may prevent neural tube defects" or "calcium prevents osteoporosis"). Nutrition support claims can also be made. Since October 1999, foods containing at least 6.5 g of soy per serving that are low in fat, saturated fat, and cholesterol are permitted by the FDA to carry the following health claim: "Diets low in saturated fat and cholesterol that include 25 grams of soy protein may reduce the risk of heart disease."[14]

The agency reviewed results from 27 studies and concluded that soy protein had demonstrable value for lowering total cholesterol and low-density lipoprotein (LDL) cholesterol levels. Foods must contain (per serving) 6.25 g of soy protein, less than 3 g of fat, less than 1 g of saturated fat, less than 20 mg of cholesterol, and less than 480 mg of sodium in individual food items (less than 720 mg in a main dish and less than 960 mg in a meal) to qualify for the claim. Foods made with the whole soybean, such as tofu, may qualify for the claim if they have no fat other than that naturally present in the whole bean. When structure-function claims such as "fiber maintains bowel regularity" are made, a disclaimer stating that the supplement has not been evaluated by the FDA and is not intended to diagnose, treat, cure, or prevent disease must be inserted.

Since 1999, supplements in the United States have also been required to have a "Supplement Facts" label that includes the "reference daily intake" and a listing of other ingredients including binders, lubricants, coatings, colorings, and fillers.[15] Minerals must list their salt source, and herbs must list their common and Latin names. Such labeling reduces, but does not eliminate, the risk of inadvertent consumption of ingredients by sensitive individuals. It also provides useful health information for health-conscious consumers. Results of a cohort study suggest that food labels are useful for helping people reduce fat intake.[16]

> Regardless of whether the initial source is food or a supplement, it is the concentration and configuration of the active principle at the cellular site that determines the clinical response.

SUPPLEMENT OR FOOD

Regardless of nomenclature gymnastics, it is the performance of the active principle of the nutritional supplement or herb at the active site that determines efficacy. Both fish and fish oils are important sources of essential fatty acids. Essential fatty acids serve as dietary precursors for the formation of eicosanoids. Eicosanoids are powerful autocrine and paracrine regulators of cell and tissue functions ranging from inflammatory reactions, to blood pressure regulation, to bronchial and uterine muscle contraction. The risk of cardiovascular and other chronic diseases can be reduced by dietary choice, by supplementation, or by a combination of the two. Eating fish two to three times a week, taking 3 to 4 g of marine oil daily, or taking 1.2 g of long-chain polyunsaturated fat daily—representing 0.5% of total energy—may result in similar wellness outcomes.[17] However, the comparative efficacy of food versus supplementation is determined by diverse factors. Supplying equivalent concentrations of a nutrient in a food and a supplement does not necessarily or predictably translate into a similar clinical outcome.

Common Considerations

Variables that influence the clinical impact of food and supplements are the concentration, structure, and chemical environment of the nutrient or herb at the active cellular site. The clinical impact of discrepancies in the concentration of a nutrient in various supplements is but one consideration. Calcium carbonate contains around 40% of elemental calcium, and calcium lactate contains around 18%.[18] The elemental calcium in a 500-mg tablet of these two products is vastly different. Similarly, 100 mg of zinc gluconate contains 14 mg of zinc, whereas 100 mg of zinc oxide contains 80 mg. Filler adds substantially to the mass of a tablet. The supplement-matrix environment may have health repercussions. Sensitive individuals may fail to appreciate that corn protein may appear on labels as "natural vegetable coating." Even worse, certain unfortunate individuals may be allergic to the inert matrix used to bulk supplements. Even labeling supplements does not completely eliminate this hazard. The food-nutrient environment may encounter similar problems. Foods may contain substances to which individuals are allergic (e.g., the protein in cow's milk), or additives used in processing (e.g., monosodium glutamate) may create a risk for sensitive individuals. Before the active principle of a food or supplement can reach the operational site of a cell, it must be absorbed and transported. The concentration of a nutrient that reaches the cell from a meal is enormously influenced by its initial concentration, digestion, and absorption. This is true regardless of whether the source of the nutrient is food or a supplement.

Transformation of food during preparation, digestion, or metabolism may modify cellular activity and health risk. Food preparation procedures may prevent clinical toxicity. When cassava is soaked and boiled, hydrogen cyanide is leached out into the water and lost to the atmosphere during boiling. Peeling potatoes removes chlorogenic acid, an anticarcinogenic substance that binds benzo[a]pyrene, a potential carcinogen found in smoked or barbecued foods. Grilled potatoes should be eaten with their skins. Boiling potatoes causes nutrient losses: 50% of the vitamin C, 25% of the folate, and 40% of the potassium are forfeited. Microwaving and steaming are healthier options. The chemical state of a nutrient affects biologic availability. Lycopene is the fat-soluble pigment that gives tomatoes, guavas, and watermelon their color. Although these foods are rich in lycopene, food processing substantially alters the availability and absorption of this carotenoid. Lycopene from tomatoes appears more readily in the blood if the tomato is heated and eaten in a meal containing fat. Iron from meat is better absorbed than iron from vegetables. Vitamin C enhances the absorption of iron from vegetable sources, and phytates impair mineral absorption from the bowel.

As with food, the delivery system of nutritional supplements affects absorption. Absorption of calcium from a lactate matrix delivery system is greater than that from a carbonate one. Because the critical factor is the concentration of the nutrient that reaches the active site within the cell, consumption of an equivalent concentration of calcium from diverse sources may have dissimilar outcomes. Prudent nutritional supplement purchasing goes beyond noting the price. It involves reading the label, excluding the presence of allergens, calculating the actual concentration of the desired nutrient in each tablet, and noting associated elements that might influence absorption and metabolism. Although supplements may contain a known quantity and food, a less clearly established concentration of a nutrient, the dose of nutrient that reaches the cell is inevitably unknown. This is due partly to the medium in which the nutrient is ingested and partly to genetically determined physiologic differences between individuals.

Dietary and supplement choices, which result in unique nutrient combinations, further contribute to metabolic differences in cellular metabolism. The impact of diet and dietary supplements on drugs is well recognized. Patients taking monoamine oxidase inhibitors are advised to avoid aged cheeses and red wine. Patients taking oral contraceptives are prone to vitamin B_6 deficiency. Supplementation with vitamin B_6 may precipitate a relative vitamin B_2 deficiency. Similarly, increasing the amounts of particular herbs or foods also requires vigilance. Just as caution is advocated when ginkgo is recommended to patients taking anticoagulants,[19] so may wariness be necessary when a diet rich in cold water fish is advocated, because this may enhance bleeding time.[20]

Less well-described than the repercussions of food and supplement interactions with drugs are the more subtle interactions of diet with metabolic systems. The cytochrome P-450 enzymes are major catalysts involved in the biotransformation of xenobiotic chemicals and in the metabolism of endogenous substrates. P-450 enzymes may be induced or inhibited, and this influences the overall impact on xenobiotic chemicals such as drugs, carcinogens, and pesticides or endogenous chemicals such as steroids, fat-soluble vitamins, and eicosanoids. Food choices and food preparation procedures further affect the clinical outcome. Broccoli and cabbage induce certain P-450 enzymes. A key factor in the effectiveness of cruciferous vegetables in cancer prevention appears to be indole-3-carbinol induction of these cytochrome enzymes. Red wine and high-protein diets also enhance P-450 enzyme–catalyzed oxidation.[21] A high-protein diet may have clinical repercussion for asthmatic individuals taking theophylline, since protein has been shown to increase metabolism of this drug.

Charbroiled foods such as barbecued beef induce P-450 enzymes. In contrast, heterocyclic aromatic amines, formed by cooking meat at high temperatures, may inhibit P-450 enzymes. However, eating potato skins with the meat may reduce absorption of heterocyclic amines. Drinking grapefruit juice, an inhibitor of the intestinal cytochrome P-450 3A4 system, will also modify the overall effect.[22] Through the inhibition of an enzyme system responsible for the first-pass metabolism of many medications, grapefruit juice interacts with a variety of medications, leading to elevation of their serum concentrations. Grapefruit juice, through interaction with various members of the cytochrome P-450 enzyme subfamily in the intestinal mucosa, increases the bioavailability of caffeine, 17-β-estradiol and its metabolite estrone, and other substances.[23] Flavonoids, which are plentiful in plant foods, may directly stimulate or inhibit various P-450 enzyme reactions. A barbecue—in which meat and potatoes are cooked over the coals, accompanied by coleslaw and broccoli salad, and washed down with red wine and grapefruit juice—has diverse and complex affects on the P-450 enzyme system.

Genetic constitution provides the template on which metabolic reactions can be influenced by dietary selection or supplementation. Nutrients cause physiologic changes, whether they are consumed in the form of a food or a supplement. A randomized, double-blind, controlled trial demonstrated that administration of 20 mg of beta-carotene daily for 4 weeks significantly decreased the peroxidation products in the breath of smokers.[24] In this study no significant change in the breath peroxidation products of nonsmokers taking beta-carotene was noted. The clinical impact of supplementation in this study was influenced by more than just the quantity and quality of the supplement; it was also influenced by the internal environment of the recipient. Smokers have more oxidation products than nonsmokers, and beta-carotene only caused clinically measurable free radical quenching in persons with higher levels of peroxidation. The physiologic condition of the recipient is one variable that should never be overlooked when diet or supplementation is considered as a health-promoting or disease-preventing intervention.

The Case Against Use of Single Supplements

> In general, supplementation with a single nutrient carries a greater risk of metabolic imbalance than eating food, a complex nutrient system.

Foods alone and in combination have a profound effect on diverse pathophysiologic processes.[25] Apples, barley, blackberries, carrots, eggplant, oats, ginger, garlic, ginseng, mushrooms, onions, soybeans, and tea all have a lipid-lowering effect. Lemons, apples, cranberries, garlic, beets, cucumbers, squash, soybeans, cabbage, brussels sprouts, cauliflower, kale, broccoli, and spinach enhance drug detoxification. Licorice, oats, parsley, and ginseng have an anti-inflammatory effect; and garlic, onions, cranberries, and green tea have antimicrobial activity. Oranges, green tea, and garlic are antiproliferative; and anise, fennel, soybeans, and cabbage are antiestrogenic.

The variation and interactions of known and unrecognized nutrients in whole foods contribute to nutritional health in diverse, and sometimes unexpected, ways. This is one reason that "Dietary therapy may not be less costly than drug therapy, when calculated as dollars spent per mmol reduction in LDL, but it should have far-reaching benefits affecting known and suspected risk factors for cardiovascular benefits."[26] Nutrients modulate a number of physiologic processes; by providing whole groups of interacting nutrients, foods may achieve far-reaching health benefits.

Groups of antioxidants occur naturally in food. In fact, one explanation for the discrepancy between the health-promoting and protective effects of fruits and vegetables and the inconsistent outcomes of antioxidant supplements may be that benefits provided by whole foods result from the integrated reductive environment created by plant antioxidants of differing solubility in each of the tissue, cellular, and macromolecular phases.[27] Water-soluble ascorbate, glutathione, and urate act in concert with lipid-soluble tocopherols and carotenoids and intermediary soluble flavonoids and hydroxycinnamic acids. Dynamic interaction provides the optimal outcome. Evidence suggests the intake of certain fruits and vegetables can decrease oxidative DNA damage, whereas supplementation with ascorbate, vitamin E, or beta-carotene cannot.[28] Food may be more effective than supplements.

Although one explanation for the failure of individual nutrients to decrease oxidative DNA damage is loss of the additive effect of antioxidants interacting to maximize their clinical impact, another depends on the chemical structure of the nutrient. A large prospective cohort study of post-menopausal women showed that vitamin E, total vitamin A, and carotenoid intake did not appear to be associated with death from stroke. However, this study did identify an inverse association between death from stroke and intake of vitamin E–rich foods (e.g., mayonnaise, nuts, and margarine).[29] The authors concluded that their results suggested a protective effect from vitamin E–rich foods but did not support a protective role for supplemental vitamin E or other antioxidant vitamins. Similarly, although observational studies suggest that vitamin E from dietary sources may provide women with modest protection from breast cancer, there is no evidence that vitamin E supplements confer protection. The authors point out that studies have failed to show any consistent relationship between plasma and adipose tissue concentration of α-tocopherol and suggest the modest protection from breast cancer associated with dietary vitamin E may be due to effects of the other tocopherols and tocotrienols in the diet.[30] Nutrient heterogeneity provides a potential explanation for such discrepancies. Natural vitamin E (RRR-α-tocopherol) is distinct from the chemically synthesized supplement. Synthetic vitamin E (*dl-α*-tocopherol or all-*rac-α*-tocopherol) is a mixture of stereoisomers, of which *d-α*-tocopherol makes up 12.5%. The potency of the mixture is lower, with 1 mg of synthetic vitamin E being equivalent to 1.10 IU and 1 mg of natural vitamin E being equivalent to 1.49 IU.

Although dose requirements are changed by the stereochemistry of the nutrient mixture, efficacy may depend on the presence of the appropriate (i.e., functional) nutrient compound. In vitro studies of breast cancer cells indicate that α-, γ-, and δ-tocotrienol, and to a lesser extent, δ-tocopherol have potent antiproliferative and proapoptotic effects that would be expected to reduce the risk of breast cancer. In contrast to α-tocopherol, the most abundant form of vitamin E in supplements, γ-tocopherol, the most abundant form in the US diet, is a more effective trap for lipophilic electrophiles and inhibits prostaglandin E_2 synthesis in lipopolysaccharide-stimulated macrophages, interleukin 1β–activated epithelial cells, and cyclooxygenase-2 in intact cells.[31] It is possible that discrepant results are attributable to treatment with the wrong form of the supplement.

Use of carotenes may encounter a similar problem because, in nature, carotenes constitute a group of distinct compounds. A case-control study showed significantly inverse associations with prostate cancer with plasma concentrations of lycopene and zeaxanthin, borderline associations for lutein and β-cryptoxanthin, and no obvious associations for alpha- and beta-carotenes.[32] Nutrients classified within a single category may not provide an identical spectrum of functions, and even shared functions may be carried out with differing efficacy. Blood levels of carotene are inversely proportional to the number of deaths from ischemic heart disease.[33] Carotenes efficiently quench singlet oxygen. A human intervention trial to determine whether a moderately increased consumption of carotenoid-rich vegetables would influence antioxidant status was conducted in 23 healthy men.[34]

Consumption of carotenoid-rich vegetable products (carrot juice, spinach powder, and tomato juice) enhanced lipoprotein carotenoid concentrations, but only tomato juice (330 mL/day) reduced LDL oxidation. The antioxidant potency of carotenes is known to vary, being greatest for lycopene followed by alpha-carotene, beta-carotene, and lutein. However, because another study demonstrated that higher lycopene concentrations tend to be more protective against myocardial infarction in men who have never smoked,[35] it is possible that the cardiovascular benefits of lycopene may not be solely related to its antioxidant effect.

Lycopene may also inhibit cholesterol synthesis and enhance LDL degradation. When added to macrophage cell clones, lycopene decreased cholesterol synthesis and increased LDL receptors. A clinical investigation showed that administration of 60 mg of lycopene per day (equivalent to 1 kg of tomatoes) for 3 months resulted in a 14% decrease in LDL cholesterol with no change in high-density lipoprotein cholesterol.[36] Lycopene may prove particularly useful for cardiovascular health but may not be as effective as alpha-carotene against lung cancer. Lycopene, unlike many of the other carotenoids, has no vitamin A activity. There is strong evidence that beta-carotene has a protective effect against stroke,[37] but evidence to support a similar effect by other carotenoids is lacking. Nutrients grouped as a single category may have some, but not all, of their actions in common.

Assuming that the biologically active form is administered, nutrient supplements may be used to achieve somewhat predictable outcomes when provided in megadoses, if supplied as a group of metabolically interacting nutrients capable of achieving harmonious synergy at the cellular level. Beta-carotene is water-soluble and may be safely consumed in megadoses. Vitamin A is fat-soluble with a relatively narrow therapeutic window. In the presence of vitamin E, beta-carotene can be converted to vitamin A. Furthermore, vitamin A toxicity is not a concern because there is a threshold beyond which beta-carotene is not converted to vitamin A. Metabolic processes are interlinked by positive and negative feedback systems.

Consequently, supplementation may be safer and more effective if individual supplements are combined with other micronutrients. In view of the network of interactions between antioxidants, it has been suggested that it would be preferable to supplement with a group of antioxidants rather than with a single antioxidant.[38] For example, with respect to cardiovascular disease, vitamin E acts as a first risk discriminator, and vitamin C, as a second; and optimal health requires synchronous interaction of vitamins C, E, and A; carotenoids; and vegetable co-nutrients. Plasma values deemed desirable for primary prevention are equal to or greater than 30 μmol/L lipid-standardized vitamin E with an α-tocopherol/cholesterol ratio of 5.0 μmol/mmol, 50 μmol/L vitamin C with a targeted vitamin C/vitamin E ratio of 1.3 to 1.5, 0.4 μmol/L beta-carotene, or 0.5 μmol/L of an alpha- and beta-carotene combination.[39] This translates roughly into vitamin A, 1 mg; beta-carotene, 2 to 3.5 mg in nonsmokers and 7 to 12 mg in smokers; vitamin C, 70 to 145 mg in nonsmokers and 130 to 175 mg in smokers; and vitamin E, at least 67 mg daily. Furthermore, desirable ratios of these nutrients may be vitamin C/E greater than 1.3, carotene/vitamin E greater than 0.02, and vitamin C/carotene in excess of 100 or vitamin C/ beta-carotene in excess of 125. The risk of cancer and cardiovascular disease is postulated to double if values of these antioxidants drop 20% to 50% below these target thresholds.[39] Moreover, if beta-carotene is an essential antioxidant defense, its loading may promote cancer by creating imbalances in the antioxidant cascade. However, no increased risk of cancer is likely with beta-carotene levels below 3 μmol/L in nonsmokers.[39] Synergistic interactions are also well documented for constituents within a total extract of a single herb, as well as between different herbs in a formulation.[40] Furthermore, there is evidence that extracts of medicinal herbs, once isolated in their pure state, can produce pharmacologic effects that differ significantly from those produced by the whole herb.[41]

> "Although evidence of the efficacy of herbal preparations in treating various conditions is increasing, translating the results of efficacy studies into effective management in the clinical situation is hindered by the chemical complexity of the products, a lack of standardization of available preparations, and a paucity of well-controlled studies."[42]

In contrast to single nutrients synthesized in the laboratory, supplements extracted from herbs or plants provide groups of interacting compounds. Impurities and adulterants may be found in nutrient and herbal products. Because of a lack of stringent requirements for good manufacturing practices and the absence of standardization requirements, the active ingredient may be absent or highly variable among products from different manufacturers.[43] In time, such discrepancies may be controlled by better regulation. In the meantime, the plethora of interactions at the cellular level, uncertainty about optimal dose-response relationships, and the probability that some active principles are as yet unrecognized provide an argument for food as a preferred option to dietary supplements. Consistent with a holistic philosophy, food and herbs may achieve more than supplementation with its "parts."

FOOD AS THERAPY

Given the abundance of known nutrients and the probability that unrecognized compounds in food affect health and disease, cogent reasons for considering diet as a form of natural therapy remain. Food meets nutritional needs, promotes wellness, and reduces the risk of disease. Food modulates biologic functions, retarding or facilitating pathophysiologic processes.

Dietary Prevention of Disease

A prospective study in which men, aged 50 to 70 years, were followed up over 20 years demonstrated a correlation between dietary intake and all-cause mortality in different cultures.[44] Dietary habits have been reported to correlate with approximately 60% of cancers in women and 40% of cancers in men.[45] In another large prospective study of men, aged 40 to 75 years, with no diagnosed cardiovascular disease at baseline, the investigators concluded, after 8 years of follow-up, that major dietary patterns predicted the risk of coronary heart disease, independent of other lifestyle variables.[46] The prudent dietary pattern to emerge from this study was characterized by higher intake of vegetables, fruits, legumes, whole grains, fish, and poultry. This diet carried a lower risk than the Western pattern, characterized by a higher intake of red and processed meat, refined grains, sweets and dessert, French fries, and high-fat dairy products.

A prospective study of women showed that a dietary pattern characterized by consumption of foods recommended in current dietary guidelines was associated with decreased risk of mortality.[47] Another prospective epidemiologic study showed that the relative risk of mortality in men and women consuming two or fewer food groups was 1.5 and 1.4, respectively.[48] Diets that omitted several food groups were associated with an increased risk of mortality. Dietary diversity enhances the likelihood that all required nutrients will be available and that an adequate intake will be achieved. Very restrictive diets are more likely to be deficient in particular nutrients and to lack the diversity to compensate for marginal nutrient deficiency. The five food groups have long been advocated as a basic formula from which to select a balanced and diverse diet (see Table 4-2). Choosing most foods from grain products (6 to 11 servings), the vegetable group (3 to 5 servings), and the fruit group (2 to 4 servings), eating moderately from the dairy product group (2 to 3 servings) and meat/bean group (2 to 3 servings), and limiting fats to no more than 30 g/day constitute a sound fundamental approach. Although a healthy dietary pattern emphasizes certain food groups,[49] each food group makes a particular contribution (see Box 4-1).

TABLE 4-2 ■ The Five Food Groups

FOOD GROUP	MINIMUM INTAKE	MAXIMUM SERVINGS
Meat/legume/nut group	1 serving	Men, 4; women, 3
Bread/cereals	4 servings	Men, 8; women, 6
Vegetables/fruit	4 servings	Men, 8; women, 6
Milk/dairy products	1 serving	Men, 4; women, 3
Fat	15 g	30 g

The following represent one serving from the respective food groups: 15 to 30 g margarine (1 tablespoon or 20 g); 1 piece of fruit; 1/2 cup vegetables; 1 slice bread; 1/2 cup cereal; 1/2 cup pasta; 75 to 100 g meat; 3/4 cup cooked beans.

> The five food groups provide a rough guide, but health may be improved by improvising within defined boundaries such as increasing plant foods and reducing animal products.

Balancing the Five Food Groups

Although all food groups should be represented in the diet, there is a clear advantage associated with increasing the intake of certain food groups. Epidemiologic studies suggest that milk and milk products fit well into a healthy eating pattern emphasizing cereals and vegetables.

Many studies have linked increased consumption of milk and milk products with lower blood pressure and a reduced risk of hypertension. Calcium, bioactive peptides produced during digestion of milk proteins, and unidentified components in whole milk may protect against hypertension.[49] Folic acid, vitamins B_6 and B_{12}, and/or other unidentified components of skim milk may contribute to low homocysteine levels.[50] Lipid auto-oxidation in milk is affected by a complex interplay of pro-oxidants and antioxidants.[51] Antioxidative enzymes in milk include superoxide dismutase, which catalyzes the dismutation of the superoxide anion to hydrogen peroxide; catalase, which degrades hydrogen peroxide; and glutathione peroxidase, which degrades hydrogen and lipid peroxides. Lactoferrin may play an important role by binding pro-oxidative iron ions, and vitamin C interacts with iron and fat-soluble antioxidants. Vitamin E and carotenoids act as fat-soluble antioxidants in the milk fat globule. The concentrations of antioxidants in milk are affected by cow feeding rations and milk storage conditions.

In a 5-year prospective study of a large cohort of female health-care professionals with no history of cardiovascular disease or cancer, investigators

---

■ Box 4-1 ■

A HEALTHY DIETARY PATTERN

Lower total fat: Use monounsaturated fats and eat fish.

Avoid obesity: Adjust energy intake to need.

Increase cereal bran fiber foods: Eat a plant-based breakfast.

Eat a plant-rich diet: Have five or preferably 10 servings of vegetables, fruits, cooked tomato, and/or soy products daily.

Avoid pickles and smoked foods: Restrict salt intake to 5 g, and preferably 3 g, daily.

Limit fried and broiled foods: Eat fresh food or prepare food on grill or in microwave.

Increase calcium intake: Use only low-fat dairy products.

Avoid or limit alcohol: But drink 1 to 1.5 L of fluid each day.

Based on data from Weisburger JH: Approaches for chronic disease prevention based on current understanding of underlying mechanisms, *Am J Clin Nutr* 71(suppl 6):1710S-4S, 2000.

concluded that a higher intake of fruits and vegetables may be protective against cardiovascular disease.[52] The World Health Organization recommends a daily intake of more than 400 g of fruits and vegetables, but seven of the European Union Member States have a mean daily intake of less than 275 g.[53] According to the best current estimates of relative risk, more than 26,000 deaths before the age of 65 years would be prevented annually in the European Union if the intake of fresh plant produce was increased to equal the highest consumption levels. Although health benefits became evident with the consumption of at least three servings each day,[54] an increase from two fruits and three vegetables to two average-sized (120 to 150 g) pieces of fruit and five average-sized (60 to 90 g) servings of vegetables daily is recommended.[55] Careful selection of plant produce is also important, because plant foods do not have identical health effects. Red food, such as tomatoes rich in lycopene, may promote prostate health; and yellow-green vegetables, such as corn and leafy greens rich in lutein and zeaxanthin, may enhance retinal health. An improved health outcome is more likely if, instead of merely eating eight servings of fruits and vegetables daily, a color code is used. The objective becomes to eat a serving of each color of fruit or vegetable daily.[56] Red-purple foods (e.g., red apples, grapes, berries, and wine) contain anthocyanins, which are powerful antioxidants; orange foods (e.g., carrots, mangoes) contain beta-carotene; orange-yellow foods (e.g., oranges, lemons) contain citrus flavonoids; green foods (e.g., broccoli, brussels sprouts) contain glucosinolates; white-green foods (e.g., onion, garlic) contain allyl sulfides.[56] One serving of each of these colors meets the minimum recommendation of the National Cancer Institute and American Institute for Cancer Research guidelines to eat five to nine servings per day.

A survey of a cross-sectional sample of North Americans indicated that animal protein consumption was consistently higher in persons with higher cholesterol concentrations and consumption of plant proteins was consistently higher among persons with lower cholesterol concentrations.[57] More than two thirds of protein in the American diet is animal protein.[58] Meat, fish, and poultry protein contribute about twice as much as dairy protein. Dairy products in turn provide more dietary protein than grains, the major source of plant protein. Both the amount and the source of protein are important health-disease variables. Mediterranean diets are characterized by plentiful consumption of fruits, vegetables, and whole grains; moderate intake of alcohol; and limited consumption of animal products, saturated and hydrogenated fats, and refined carbohydrates.[59] A prospective cohort study, involving 141 Anglo-Celtic Australians and 189 Greek Australians aged 70 years or older indicated that a diet that adheres to the principles of the traditional Mediterranean diet is associated with longer survival among Australians, regardless of their Greek or Anglo-Celtic origins.[60] The increased availability of a variety of plant foods, the advent of nutrient-fortified plant foods or functional foods, and the use of vitamin and mineral supplements mean that convergence between the essential nutrient profiles of plant-only and plant-rich diets is possible.[61]

Omitting Animal Products

Although substantial health benefits can be achieved by merely limiting consumption of animal products, vegetarians go a step further and exclude them.

If the intake from a particular food group is to be increased, other foods must be restricted to retain overall energy balance. Although omission of particular food groups is not without its hazards,[62] careful food selection can result in dietary balance. Plant-based diets omit animal proteins. The spectrum of plant-based diets ranges from the plant-only diets of vegans and fruitarians to the plant-rich macrobiotic, lactovegetarian, semi-vegetarian, and meatless diets. Compared with nonvegetarians, Western vegetarians have a lower mean body mass index (BMI) (by about 1 kg/m^2); a lower mean plasma total cholesterol concentration (by about 0.5 mmol/L); a lower mortality from congestive heart disease (CHD) (by about 25%); and a lower risk for constipation, diverticular disease, gallstones, and appendicitis.[63] The benefits of a plant-based diet may be attributable to its inclusions, omissions, or both.

Plant protein sources in the vegetarian diet are largely legumes, nuts, and cereals. Foods in the vegetarian diet, if eaten alone, may provide an inadequate complement of amino acids. Complementary protein mixtures may be substituted to overcome such deficiencies and result in a diet that approximates the high biologic values of proteins found in animal products. Legumes are limited in their content of methionine and other sulfur-containing amino acids. Cereals lack lysine and threonine. Complementary protein meals combine legumes with cereals. Good complementary protein pairs include the following:

- Lentils with wheat or rice
- Soybeans with rice
- Peas with wheat
- Beans with corn

Regular consumption of nuts is associated with a one-third decrease in the risk of a major coronary event in adult women.[64] Eating 5 oz, compared with less than 1 oz, of nuts weekly reduces the relative risk of ischemic heart disease. Nuts are a rich source of L-arginine, and results of animal studies have indicated that this amino acid improves endothelial dilation and decreases platelet aggregation and monocyte adhesion.[65] The fatty acid profile of nuts is conducive to cardiovascular health. Nuts, because of their content of phytosterols, especially β-sitosterol, appear to offer some protection against colon, prostate, and breast cancer. Roasted peanuts contain 61 to 114 mg of phytosterols per 100 g, depending on the peanut variety, 78% to 83% of which is in the form of β-sitosterol.[66] Peanut butter, which represents 50% of the peanuts consumed in the United States, contains 144 to 157 mg of phytosterols per 100 g. Peanut flour, which results from partial removal of oil from peanuts, contains 55 to 60 mg of phytosterols per 100 g. Unrefined peanut oil with 207 mg of phytosterols per 100 g is a richer source of phytosterols than unrefined olive oil. Refining results in a reduction in phytosterol concentration, but hydrogenation after refining has a minimal effect on phytosterol content.

Of the legumes in the vegetarian diet, soybeans are a particularly interesting food source. Soybeans are a better source of minerals than other beans; and soybean-based foods are, for practical purposes, the only nutritionally relevant dietary sources of isoflavones.[67] Soybeans provide distinct dietary advantages. Inclusion of soybeans in a plant-based diet provides the following[68]:

- Protein of high biologic value. Soy protein is a complete protein equivalent to egg albumin. An average daily intake of 25 g of soy protein may be obtained from any combination of the following: 0.5 cup of soy flour (20 g of soy protein), 1 cup of soy milk (3 to 10 g of soy protein), 4 oz of tofu (5 to 13 g of soy protein), 0.5 cup of textured soy protein (6 to 11 g), or 3 tablespoons of soy protein isolate (22 g of soy protein). Substituting soy protein for high-fat animal protein diets has a beneficial effect on serum lipid levels. The beneficial cardiovascular effect is not only related to the type of protein ingested, it is also linked to the type of fat consumed.

- Polyunsaturated fat. Soybeans are rich sources of polyunsaturated fat (20%) compared with other beans (1%). The ratio of linoleic (ω-6) to α-linolenic acid (ω-3) is approximately 7:1.

- Fiber. One serving, 31 g or 1/6 cup, of uncooked soybeans provides 5.4 g of fiber, of which 2 g is soluble. Soybeans have a low glycemic index. Soy fiber supplements improve glucose tolerance and insulin response in subjects with glucose intolerance.[69] Other legumes are also good sources: a cup of cooked split peas provides 16 g of fiber, and the same amount of cooked kidney beans contains 12 g. An apple, an orange, or 10 dried apricot halves provide 3 g of fiber, as does a half cup of cooked oatmeal. Fiber is often found in the outer layer of foods. Eating whole foods provides a fiber advantage: a slice of whole-meal bread has 2 g of fiber, and a slice of white bread, 0.5 g.

- Minerals. Although availability varies depending on processing and phytate content, soybeans are a good vegetable source of minerals. The concentration of minerals are as follows: iron, around 16 mg/100 g dry weight; zinc, 4.8 mg/100 g dry weight; and calcium, 276 mg/100 g dry weight. Soybeans contain around 138 mg of calcium per 90-g serving (0.5 cup boiled soybeans), and bioavailability is largely equivalent to that in milk.[70]

- Oligosaccharides. Raffinose, stachyose, and verbascose serve as prebiotics and are fermented in the intestine to gas and short-chain fatty acids that may hinder hepatic cholesterol synthesis.

- Isoflavonoids. Flavonoids have antioxidant and estrogenic effects. At higher doses, flavonoids may act as mutagens, pro-oxidants that generate free radicals, and as inhibitors of key enzymes involved in hormone metabolism. Caution should be exercised in ingesting them at levels above that which would be obtained from a typical vegetarian diet.[71] Isoflavones are a subclass of flavonoids. The concentration of isoflavones is around 1 to 3 mg per gram of soy protein; one serving of traditional soy foods provides 25 to 40 mg of isoflavones.[72] Important soy isoflavone phytoestrogens are genistein and daidzein. Intestinal bacteria convert daidzein into several products, including equol; the amount and nature of products produced depends on the bowel microflora. In a randomized, crossover study, soy-enriched diets with low and high isoflavone content were compared; results indicated that consumption of soy that contained naturally occurring amounts of isoflavone phytoestrogens reduced lipid peroxidation in vivo and increased the resistance of LDL to oxidation.[67] This effect was dose-dependent. Equol is a particularly good inhibitor of LDL oxidation and membrane lipid peroxidation. In a study of 66 free living postmenopausal women, investigators concluded that soy with a higher isoflavone content is needed to protect against spinal bone loss compared with cardiovascular disease.[73] Isoflavones are weak estrogens; their biologic impact depends on the overall hormone environment. They are antiestrogenic in the high-estrogen environment of premenopausal women but become proestrogenic in the estrogen-depleted environment of menopause. Phyto-estrogens may affect the development of cancer.[74] They are also used as growth promoters in the animal feed industry.

A randomized trial demonstrated that a combination of vegetable protein (33 g of soy) and soluble fiber significantly improved the lipid-lowering effect of a low-saturated-fat diet.[75] Although these results support expanding the current dietary advice to emphasize particular foods, the potency of particular plant foods, such as those rich in phytochemicals, to cause harm from excessive consumption should not be ignored.[76] Nonetheless, it is only by targeting particular plant foods and/or the use of functional foods that the gap in effectiveness between a good diet and drug therapy may be reduced.

WHOLE VERSUS REFINED FOODS

The benefits of a plant-based diet are greatest when whole foods are consumed. For example, results of case-control studies suggest an inverse relationship between colon cancer and whole grain consumption.[77] The Adventist Health Study showed that a diet rich in nuts and whole-meal bread had a protective effect.[78] In fact, subjects in this study who consumed whole-meal bread rather than white bread experienced a cardiovascular advantage. The rationale for eating whole grains rather than refined starch includes preventing loss of the following[79]:

- Food structure. Preserving the structure of food influences the glycemic index of food. Intact whole grains of barley, rice, rye, oats, corn, buckwheat, and wheat have a glycemic index between 36 and 81. In contrast, the glycemic index of white bread and potatoes is greater than 90. Similarly, the plasma glucose response to an apple is lower than that to apple puree, which in turn is lower than that to apple juice. The starch in whole grains is more resistant to digestion than refined starch.
- Nutrients. Nutrients are concentrated in the outer portion of grains, and therefore refining reduces nutrient content. Vitamin E, removed during the refining process, protects polyunsaturated fatty acids in cell membranes from oxidative damage, inhibits nitrosamine formation, and keeps selenium in a reduced state. Selenium functions as a cofactor for glutathione peroxidase, an enzyme that protects against oxidative damage. It has been suggested that selenium prevents expression of neoplastic cells previously exposed to carcinogens. Selenium is lost in the refining process. Trace metals including copper, zinc, and magnesium are also more plentiful in whole grains. At levels of 20 to 35 g of fiber per day and three servings of whole grains per day, no adverse effects on minerals are noted.
- Fiber. Fiber influences bowel function. Course bran delays gastric emptying and accelerates small-bowel transit. Refining removes proportionally more insoluble than soluble fiber, and fermentation of insoluble fiber produces short-chain fatty acids. Fermentation of dietary fiber produces butyrate, a short-chain fatty acid shown to be antineoplastic.[80] Oats, rye, and barley are rich sources of soluble fiber. Oligosaccharides are prebiotics and create an environment conducive to the proliferation of beneficial intestinal bacteria.
- Phytonutrients. Phytochemicals are concentrated in the outer portion of grains. Phenolic acids are natural antioxidants and are believed to offer some protection against cancer. Their anticarcinogenic benefits involve induction of detoxification systems, particularly phase II conjugation reactions. Caffeic and ferulic acids are phenolic agents that prevent carcinogen formation from precursor molecules and block the reaction of carcinogens with critical cellular macromolecules. Wheat is a good source of ferulic acid, and wheat bran has the type of fiber that most consistently inhibits carcinogenesis.
- Phytic acid, a known antioxidant, forms chelates with various metals. Colonic bacteria produce oxygen radicals, and dietary phytic acid may suppress oxidant damage to the intestine by suppressing iron-catalyzed redox reactions.
- Lignans are hormonally active compounds found in whole grain wheat, oats, and rye meal. Plant lignans are converted by human gut bacteria into mammalian lignans, enterolactone and enterodiol. Lignans have a diphenolic structure similar to estrogenic compounds. Lignans are also found in seeds of flax, pumpkins, caraway, and sunflowers. Flaxseeds should not be heated but added to salads or foods after they are cooked.

Since they have a tough outer shell, soaking overnight in a little water will make them softer to eat. They can also be ground and added to baked goods. Flaxseed oil, although a good source of ω-3 fatty acids, is not a source of lignans because most of the lignan is found in the non-oil part of flaxseeds.

The advantages of whole foods are even more pronounced in organic foods produced through selective methods of cultivation and animal husbandry. Not only are organic crops free of pesticides, they appear to contain significantly more vitamin C, iron, magnesium, and phosphorus and significantly less nitrates than conventional crops.[81]

Whole foods are a healthier option than refined foods.

BEYOND THE FIVE FOOD GROUPS: FUNCTIONAL FOODS

The five food groups no longer provide a comprehensive overview of dietary options. Functional foods are whole foods or ingredients of whole foods that may provide a health benefit beyond that conferred by the nutrients the food contains.[82] They may either be consumed as part of or in addition to the regular diet. In the case of the former, prunes, because of their flavor and mild laxative effect, epitomize a functional food that may be consumed as a part of the regular diet.[83] In the case of the latter, dietary supplements, also variously termed *nutriceuticals*, *botanical supplements*, *herbals*, *ergogenic aids*, and *medical foods* (depending on the marketing strategy used), may be consumed. Functional foods may take many forms. They may be whole foods (e.g., prunes, cranberries), a macronutrient that achieves a specific physiologic function (e.g., resistant starch, ω-3 fatty acids), an essential micronutrient taken in quantities exceeding the recommended daily allowance (RDA), or a nonessential nutrient (e.g., oligosaccharide); or they may have no nutritive value (e.g., phytochemicals).[84]

The Federal Food, Drug, and Cosmetic Act does not provide a statutory definition of functional foods; consequently, the FDA has no authority to establish a formal regulatory category for such foods. Therefore existing food and drug regulations must suffice. In the United States, the FDA permits two types of labeling claims: those that are health claims and those pertaining to structure or function. Only health claims require pre-approval from the FDA. FDA-authorized health claims for the functional benefits of food include calcium for osteoporosis, folate for neural tube birth defects, fruits and vegetables for some cancers, and potassium for hypertension and stroke. For coronary heart disease, soy protein, plant sterol or plant stanol esters, fruits, vegetables, and grain products containing fiber, and soluble fiber as found in whole oats and psyllium seed husks are considered beneficial.[85] Other recognized health claims are based on a low content of "negative" nutrients such as sodium for hypertension, dietary saturated fat and cholesterol for coronary heart disease, and dietary fat for some types of cancer such as prostate, breast, and colon cancer. The primary determinant of the regulatory status of a food is its intended use as described by the label. A claim that cranberry juice helps maintain urinary tract health, provided it is not misleading, is an appropriate label for a functional food.[86] A claim that cranberry products prevent recurrence of urinary tract infections constitutes a drug claim and is not acceptable. Health claims must be supported by the scientific literature. Much current research on functional foods addresses the physiologic effects and health benefits of foods and food components, with the aim of authorizing specific health claims.[84]

Functional foods may be the result of selective breeding or enhancement of the plant substrate. Genetic engineering of plant foods to enhance concentrations of nutrients and other chemicals has become a viable option. However, although increased phytonutrient content through selective breeding or genetic improvement is possible, most, if not all, of the bioactive phytonutrients are bitter, acrid, or astringent.[87] Consumer tastes may provide functional food designers with a problem. Animal products may also be modified to assume the status of functional foods. Animal feeds rich in ω-6 fatty acids favor cell membranes rich in arachidonic acid, and animal feeds rich in ω-3 fatty acids increase the eicosapentaenoic acid (EPA) and docosahexaenoic acid (DHA) composition of cell membranes. Adding fish oils and vitamin E to the diet of hens has resulted in eggs with an appreciably decreased level of arachidonic acid and a dramatically increased concentration of ω-3 fatty acids, particularly EPA and DHA, in the yolk.[88] Yolk α-tocopherol levels increased linearly as dietary dl-α-tocopheryl acetate levels increased. Twenty-eight days of storage at room temperature (20° to 25° C) did not alter the yolk fatty acid profile, and moreover, the levels of vitamin E remained very close to those observed in fresh eggs. Experimental and epidemiologic studies, as well as randomized trials, have clearly demonstrated that ω-3 fatty acids reduce the risk of sudden cardiac death in patients with ischemic heart disease.[89] In view of these benefits, eggs may emerge as an important functional food for patients with heart disease. Foods with singular potential as functional foods because of their phytochemical content are soy and rice-bran products.[90]

Functional foods may result from manufacturing procedures.[25] A food product may be made functional by eliminating a component known to have an adverse health consequence (e.g., an allergen) or by increasing the concentration of a beneficial component (e.g., folic acid). Foods enriched with physiologic doses of vitamins and folate-supplemented breakfast cereal have been shown to correct abnormalities of folate in the elderly[91] and reverse elevated homocysteine levels.[92] Functional foods may be produced by adding a component not normally present (e.g., stanols) or by replacing a macronutrient (e.g., fat) with one that confers greater benefit. Carbohydrates such as dextrins, maltodextrins, modified food starches, polydextrose, and gums are well-known fat substitutes often used to add moisture to low-fat baked foods. Protein-based fat substitutes such as microparticulated protein products, egg white, and milk may be used to duplicate the texture of ice cream. Food processing can increase the bioavailability of or enhance the stability of compounds that confer a beneficial effect.

Functional foods appear to have a particularly promising impact on cardiovascular and gastrointestinal health. Many functional foods have been found to be beneficial in the prevention and treatment of cardiovascular disease.[93] Eating adequate amounts of soybeans, oats, psyllium, flaxseed, garlic, tea, fish, grapes, nuts, and/or stanol- and sterol-ester enhanced margarine on a consistent basis decreases the risk of cardiovascular disease. Resultant decreased blood lipid levels, improved arterial compliance, reduced LDL oxidation, decreased plaque formation, improved free radical scavenging, and inhibition of platelet aggregation promote cardiovascular health.

Gastrointestinal function may be enhanced by prebiotics and probiotics. Probiotic foods provide an adequate number of viable, functional bacteria with a good shelf life.[94] Among the variables to be considered are acid and bile stability and intestinal mucosal adhesion properties of the probiotic culture. The benefits of probiotic bacteria include improved digestion (e.g., modulation of lactose intolerance), enhanced production of organic acids potentially conferring some protection against colon cancer, reduced production of toxic metabolites (e.g., ammonia, phenols), restoration of gut flora after antibiotic therapy, breakdown of carcinogens, and vitamin synthesis (e.g., vitamins K and B_{12}, folic acid, and biotin). With the potential to enhance intestinal health through stimulation of immunity, competition for limited nutrients, inhibition of epithelial and mucosal adherence, inhibition of epithelial invasion, and production of antimicrobial substances, probiotics represent an exciting prophylactic and therapeutic advance.[95]

Prebiotics are nondigestible food ingredients that beneficially affect the host by selectively stimulating the growth and/or activity of a limited number of probiotic bacterial species (e.g., lactobacilli and bifidobacteria) resident in the colon.[96] In addition to providing a probiotic substrate, prebiotics stimulate absorption of several minerals and improve mineralization of bone.[97] Animal experiments showed that nondigestible oligosaccharides increased the availability of calcium, magnesium, zinc, and iron. Good plant sources of these oligosaccharides are onions, asparagus, wheat, and artichoke leaves.

Increased consumption of functional foods and their associated bioactive components provides a viable approach to optimizing nutrition.[25] Functional foods can enhance community-based wellness promotion, and they may also be used with good effect in high-risk groups. They can be used to maintain a state of well-being and/or reduce the risk of disease. Functional foods and their associated health claims are among the more controversial and complex issues being debated by food regulators.[98] Proponents claim that functional foods may reduce health-care expenditure, and health claims are a legitimate nutrition education tool that will help inform consumers of the benefits of certain food products. Opponents respond that it is the total diet that is important for health, not so-called magic bullets. Development of innovative food products while avoiding inappropriate medicalization of the general food supply is a continuing challenge.

> Functional foods offer a particular health advantage and deserve consideration.

NUTRITIONAL WELLNESS: IN SEARCH OF BALANCE

Food, in addition to being one of life's pleasures, is and should remain the dominant source of nutrition. After reviewing the major studies investigating links between antioxidant intake and heart disease, Tran[99] recommended a diet rich in whole grains, fruits, and vegetables rather than prescription of supplements. This recommendation was made in view of the absence of conclusive scientific evidence regarding the efficacy, safety, or appropriate dosage of antioxidants to prevent heart disease. In another study Clarkson and Thompson[100] have reported that although supplementation with vitamins C and E and other antioxidants can reduce the symptoms or indicators of oxidative stress that result from exercise, these supplements do not appear to have a beneficial effect on performance. In fact, because exercise training seems to reduce the oxidative stress of exercise, these researchers have advised physically active individuals to ingest a diet rich in antioxidants and delay supplementation until research fully substantiates that the long-term use of antioxidants is safe and effective. However, good food choices do not necessarily preclude the use of supplements in specific circumstances.

Using Supplements Cautiously

Diet alone may not always suffice. Dietary intake may fail to result in therapeutic nutrient levels. Careful dietary selection may increase the daily intake of vitamin E to 60 IU, a level that exceeds the recommended daily intake (RDI) of 30 IU but fails to constitute an intake that may be optimal for the immune status of the elderly (200 IU/day) or required to reduce the risk of cardiovascular disease (400-800 IU/day).[101] Furthermore, the proposed optimum daily intake of antioxidants for reducing the risk of degenerative diseases exceeds the recommended daily allowance.[102] With respect to coronary heart disease, risk may be reduced with plasma concentrations of at least 27.5 to 30.0 μmol/L vitamin D, 0.4 to 0.5 μmol/L carotene, 40 to 50 μmol/L vitamin C, and 2.2 to 2.8 μmol/L vitamin A.[103]

Nutrient dose may be critical to the clinical outcome. The dose determines whether vitamin E bolsters or suppresses immunity, whether L-glycine protects against cancer or promotes metastasis, or whether retinoic acid is teratogenic or essential for embryogenesis. Supplements can provide known doses; food cannot. Although the dose-response relationship is complex, the efficacy and safety of supplementation with vitamins C and E at recommended levels would seem to be safe.[104] Supplementary intake of vitamin C is safe at levels of up to 600 mg daily; and higher levels, up to 2000 mg daily, are without risk. Similarly, vitamin E has a very low human toxicity, and an intake of 1000 mg daily is without risk, and 3200 mg daily has been shown to be without any consistent risk. However, intake of large amounts of beta-carotene must be viewed with caution, particularly in populations at high risk for lung cancer after many years of smoking. Until further research clarifies the situation, heavy smokers should perhaps avoid supplementary doses of carotenes. Although carotenoids can promote health when taken at dietary levels, there are reservations about supplementation with this nutrient.

A Challenge That Needs Resolution

Discrepancies between epidemiologic findings and results of clinical trials of supplements remain problematic and, despite various explanations,[105] need resolution before supplementation can be recommended confidently. Drugs dominate their cellular environment, but the cellular environment largely determines the action of nutrients. Nutrients, unlike drugs, do not act in isolation. This has clinical consequences. With respect to cancer, although one of four intervention trials of high-dose beta-carotene supplements did not show protective effects, epidemiologic studies have shown an inverse relationship between various cancers and dietary carotenoids or blood carotenoid levels.[106] Beta-carotene, an antioxidant in nonsmokers, assumes the role of a pro-oxidant in the lungs of smokers. Clinical trials in which supplements are used as drugs often provide high doses of single nutrients without the dietary support required to achieve and maintain metabolic balance. The redox environment determines whether serum iron is a pro-oxidant or antioxidant. The high doses achieved by single nutrient supplementation may precipitate metabolic imbalances with untoward clinical consequences. The nutrient mixture of supplements needs to be resolved. A diet rich in fruits and vegetables not only provides an adequate amount of carotene but also supplies desirable biologic ratios and stereoisomers of the various carotenes. Compared with natural beta-carotene, synthetic beta-carotene lacks *cis*-beta-carotene, the carotene that reduces dysplasia.[107]

When synthesized supplements are used, more attention needs to be paid to the biologically active form of the nutrient. Of the eight isomers of synthesized vitamin E, only one has the RRR configuration of natural vitamin E. In animals, the potency of natural versus synthetic vitamin E is 1.36.[108] The different tocol and tocotrienol derivatives α, β, δ, and γ also have varied and specific roles with diverse tissue affinities. γ-Tocopherol has the unique ability to reduce nitrogen dioxide, a radical that can initiate carcinogenesis through inducing mutations, whereas it was the α-tocopheryl acetate that was used in conjunction with beta-carotene in the ATBC trial.[109] Disparity between the clinical outcome achieved by isolated and constitutive isoflavones has also been documented.[110] In various studies soy protein supplements have been reported to decrease LDL cholesterol in proportion to the level of hypercholesterolemia, and furthermore, results of these studies suggest that 20 g of soy protein per 38 mg of isoflavones is the critical dose above which little therapeutic gain can be achieved. In contrast, administration of isoflavones isolated from soy did not appear to have a beneficial effect on cholesterol levels. Postulates for this observed inconsistency range from an imbalance in the relative proportions of individual isoflavones, through absorption differences and a synergistic effect of soy protein, to the presence of unidentified factors.[110]

> Nutrition for optimal health may one day mean a good diet complemented by prudent dietary supplementation.

At the very least, the potency of the isometric form of compounds in neutriceuticals needs to be determined and standardized before predictable clinical outcomes are likely.

An Eclectic Solution

Despite the difficulties of appropriate supplementation, given that contemporary lifestyles may require intakes of certain nutrients that exceed levels provided in an energy-balanced diet, supplementation along with functional foods provide reasonable wellness options. In fact, it has been suggested that "in most diets, inadequate consumption of beneficial dietary components...appears to be more detrimental than is an excessive intake of harmful foods."[111] Certainly, given that older adults are at risk for malnutrition, which may contribute to their increased risk of infection, use of a daily multivitamin or trace-mineral supplement that includes zinc (>20 mg/day) and selenium (100 μg/day), with additional vitamin E, to achieve a total daily dosage of 200 mg deserves consideration.[112] Perhaps it is for reasons such as these that selective supplementation must remain a wellness option. Certainly, as seen in Table 3-1 and in the supplement section of this text, a number of supplements are household names.

SUMMARY

Current recommendations seem to suggest that nutritional health is best achieved by using a diet-focused strategy. Furthermore, in instances when nutritional supplements are indicated, supplementation should be undertaken within the metabolic environment of a nutrient-rich diet. Such recommendations are sound, given the discrepant findings arising from epidemiologic studies and clinical trials. The disappointing results from clinical trials, coupled with the propensity for epidemiologic studies to support an increased intake of particular nutrients such as antioxidants, merely serve to emphasize the need for further investigation.

REFERENCES

1. Prasad C: Food, mood and health: a neurobiologic outlook, *Braz J Med Biol Res* 31:1517-27, 1998.
2. Aarts T: Nutrition industry overview, *Nutr Bus J* 3:1-5, 1998.
3. Frank E, Bendich A, Denniston M: Use of vitamin-mineral supplements by female physicians in the United States, *Am J Clin Nutr* 72:969-75, 2000.
4. Zeisel SH: Is there a metabolic basis for dietary supplementation? *Am J Clin Nutr* 72(suppl 2):507S-11S, 2000.
5. Miller LG, Hume A, Harris IM, et al: White paper on herbal products. American College of Clinical Pharmacy, *Pharmacotherapy* 20:877-91, 2000.
6. Cupp MJ: Herbal remedies: adverse effects and drug interactions, *Am Fam Physician* 59:1239-45, 1999.
7. Yuan CS, Wu JA, Lowell T, Gu M: Gut and brain effects of American ginseng root on brainstem neuronal activities in rats, *Am J Chin Med* 26:47-55, 1998.
8. Linde K, ter Riet G, Hondras M, et al: Systematic reviews of complementary therapies—an annotated bibliography. Part 2: herbal medicine, *BMC Complement Altern Med* 1:5, 2001.
9. Pinn G: Herbal medicine and overview, *Aust Fam Phys* 29:1059-1062, 2000.
10. Mukhtar H, Ahmad N: Tea polyphenols: prevention of cancer and optimizing health, *Am J Clin Nutr* 71(suppl 6):1698S-1702S, 2000.
11. Hill RH, Caudill SP, Philen RM, et al: Contaminants in L-tryptophan associated with eosinophilia myalgia syndrome, *Arch Environ Contam Toxicol* 25:134-42, 1993.
12. Goodman GE: The clinical evaluation of cancer prevention agents, *Proc Soc Exp Biol Med* 216:253-9, 1997.
13. Kurtzweil P: An FDA guide to dietary supplements, *FDA Consumer* 32:28-35, 1998.
14. Morelli V, Zoorob RJ: Alternative therapies: part II. Congestive heart failure and hypercholesterolemia, *Am Fam Physician* 62:1325-30, 2000.
15. Czap A: Supplements facts versus all the facts. What the new label does and doesn't disclose, *Altern Med Rev* 4:5-9, 1999.
16. Kristal AR, Hedderson MM, Patterson RE, et al: Predictors of self-initiated, healthful dietary change, *J Am Diet Assoc* 101:762-6, 2001.
17. Uauy R, Mena P, Valenzuela A: Essential fatty acids as determinants of lipid requirements in infants, children and adults, *Eur J Clin Nutr* 53(suppl 1):S66-77, 1999.
18. Borum PR: Supplements: questions to ask to reduce confusion, *Am J Clin Nutr* 72(suppl 2):538S-540S, 2000.
19. Diamond BJ, Shiflett SC, Feiwel N, et al: Ginkgo biloba extract: mechanisms and clinical indications, *Arch Phys Med Rehabil* 81:668-78, 2000.
20. Ballard-Barbash R, Callaway CW: Marine fish oils: role in prevention of coronary artery disease, *Mayo Clin Proc* 62:113-8, 1987.
21. Guengerich FP: Influence of nutrients and other dietary materials on cytochrome P-450 enzymes, *Am J Clin Nutr* 61(suppl 3):651S-658S, 1995.

22. Kane GC, Lipsky JJ: Drug-grapefruit juice interactions, *Mayo Clin Proc* 75:933-42, 2000.

23. Mills S, Bone K: *Principles and practice of phytotherapy*, Edinburgh, 2000, Churchill Livingstone.

24. Allard JP, Royall D, Kurian R, et al: Effects of beta-carotene supplementation on lipid peroxidation in humans, *Am J Clin Nutr* 59:884-90, 1994.

25. Milner JA: Functional foods: the US perspective, *Am J Clin Nutr* 71(suppl 6): 1654S-9S, 2000.

26. Denke MA: Revisiting the effectiveness of the National Cholesterol Education Program Step 1 and Step 2 diets: cholesterol lowering diets in a pharmaceutically driven world, *Am J Clin Nutr* 69:581-2, 1999.

27. Eastwood MA: Interaction of dietary antioxidants in vivo: how fruit and vegetables prevent disease? *QJM* 92:527-30, 1999.

28. Halliwell B: Why and how should we measure oxidative DNA damage in nutritional studies? How far have we come? *Am J Clin Nutr* 72:1082-7, 2000.

29. Yochum LA, Folsom AR, Kushi LH: Intake of antioxidant vitamins and risk of death from stroke in postmenopausal women, *Am J Clin Nutr* 72:476-83, 2000.

30. Schwenke DC: Does lack of tocopherols and tocotrienols put women at increased risk of breast cancer? *J Nutr Biochem* 13:2-20, 2002.

31. Jiang Q, Christen S, Shigenaga MK, Ames BN: Gamma-tocopherol, the major form of vitamin E in the US diet, deserves more attention, *Am J Clin Nutr* 74:714-22, 2001.

32. Lu QY, Hung JC, Heber D, et al: Inverse associations between plasma lycopene and other carotenoids and prostate cancer, *Cancer Epidemiol Biomarkers Prev* 10:749-56, 2001.

33. Gey KF, Stahelin HB, Eichholzer M: Poor plasma status of carotene and vitamin C is associated with higher mortality from ischemic heart disease and stroke: Basel Prospective Study, *Clin Invest* 71:3-6, 1993.

34. Bub A, Watzl B, Abrahamse L, et al: Moderate intervention with carotenoid-rich vegetable products reduces lipid peroxidation in men, *J Nutr* 130:2200-6, 2000.

35. Arab L, Steck S: Lycopene and cardiovascular disease, *Am J Clin Nutr* 71(suppl 6):1691S-5S, 2000.

36. Kohlmeier L, Hastings SB: Epidemiological evidence of a role of carotenoids in cardiovascular disease prevention, *Am J Clin Nutr* 62(suppl 6):1370S-6S, 1995.

37. Ascherio A: Antioxidants and stroke, *Am J Clin Nutr* 72:337-8, 2000.

38. Pryor WA: Vitamin E and heart disease: basic science to clinical intervention trials, *Free Radic Biol Med* 28:141-64, 2000.

39. Gey KF: Vitamins E plus C and interacting conutrients required for optimal health. A critical and constructive review of epidemiology and supplementation data regarding cardiovascular disease and cancer, *Biofactors* 7:113-74, 1998.

40. Williamson EM: Synergy and other interactions in phytomedicines, *Phytomedicine* 8:401-9, 2001.

41. Chang J: Medicinal herbs: drugs or dietary supplements? *Biochem Pharmacol* 59:211-9, 2000.

42. Beaubrun G, Gray GE: A review of herbal medicines for psychiatric disorders, *Psychiatr Serv* 51:1130-4, 2000.

43. Harris IM: Regulatory and ethical issues with dietary supplements, *Pharmacotherapy* 20:1295-302, 2000.

44. Huijbregts P, Feskens E, Rasanen L, et al: Dietary pattern and 20 year mortality in elderly men in Finland, Italy, and The Netherlands: longitudinal cohort study, *BMJ* 315:13-7, 1997.

45. Wynder EL, Gori GB: Contributions of the environment to cancer incidence: an epidemiological exercise, *J Natl Cancer Inst* 58:825-32, 1977.

46. Hu FB, Rimm EB, Stampfer MJ, et al: Prospective study of major dietary patterns and risk of coronary heart disease in men, *Am J Clin Nutr* 72:912-21, 2000.

47. Kant AK, Schatzkin A, Graubard BI, Schairer C: A prospective study of diet quality and mortality in women, *JAMA* 283:2109-15, 2000.

48. Kant AK, Schatzkin A, Harris TB, et al: Dietary diversity and subsequent mortality in the First National Health and Nutrition Examination Survey Epidemiologic Follow-up Study, *Am J Clin Nutr* 57:434-40, 1993.

49. Weisburger JH: Approaches for chronic disease prevention based on current understanding of underlying mechanisms, *Am J Clin Nutr* 71(suppl 6):1710S-4S, 2000.

50. Pfeuffer M, Schrezenmeir J: Bioactive substances in milk with properties decreasing risk of cardiovascular diseases, *Br J Nutr* 84(suppl 1):S155-9, 2000.

51. Lindmark-Mansson H, Akesson B: Antioxidative factors in milk, *Br J Nutr* 84(suppl 1):S103-10, 2000.

52. Liu S, Manson JE, Lee IM, et al: Fruit and vegetable intake and risk of cardiovascular disease: the Women's Health Study, *Am J Clin Nutr* 72:922-8, 2000.

53. Joffe M, Robertson A: The potential contribution of increased vegetable and fruit consumption to health gain in the European Union, *Public Health Nutr* 4:893-901, 2001.

54. Huang HY, Helzlsouer KJ, Appel LJ: The effects of vitamin C and vitamin E on oxidative DNA damage: results from a randomized controlled trial, *Cancer Epidemiol Biomarkers Prev* 9:647-52, 2000.

55. Miller MR, Pollard CM, Coli T: Western Australian Health Department recommendations for fruit and vegetable consumption—how much is enough? *Aust N Z J Public Health* 21:638-42, 1997.

56. Heber D, Bowerman S: Applying science to changing dietary patterns, *J Nutr* 131(suppl 11):3078S-81S, 2001.

57. Smit E, Nieto FJ, Crespo CJ: Blood cholesterol and apolipoprotein B levels in relation to intakes of animal and plant proteins in US adults, *Br J Nutr* 82:193-201, 1999.

58. Smit E, Nieto FJ, Crespo CJ, Mitchell P: Estimates of animal and plant protein intake in US adults: results from the Third National Health and Nutrition Examination Survey, 1988-1991, *J Am Diet Assoc* 99:813-20, 1999.

59. Kushi LH, Lenart EB, Willett WC: Health implications of Mediterranean diets in light of contemporary knowledge, *Am J Clin Nutr* 61(suppl 6):1416S-27S, 1995.

60. Kouris-Blazos A, Gnardellis C, Wahlqvist ML, et al: Are the advantages of the Mediterranean diet transferable to other populations? A cohort study in Melbourne, Australia, *Br J Nutr* 82:57-61, 1999.

61. Dwyer J: Convergence of plant-rich and plant-only diets, *Am J Clin Nutr* 70(suppl 3):620S-2S, 1999.

62. Ball M: Vegetarian, vegan or meat eater, *Aust Fam Physician* 26:69-74, 1997.

63. Key TJ, Davey GK, Appleby PN: Health benefits of a vegetarian diet, *Proc Nutr Soc* 58:271-5, 1999.
64. Hu FB, Stampfer MJ, Manson JE, et al: Frequent nut consumption and risk of coronary heart disease in women: prospective cohort study, *BMJ* 317:1341-5, 1998.
65. Brown AA, Hu FB: Dietary modulation of endothelial function: implications for cardiovascular disease, *Am J Clin Nutr* 73:673-86, 2001.
66. Awad AB, Chan KC, Downie AC, Fink CS: Peanuts as a source of beta-sitosterol, a sterol with anticancer properties, *Nutr Cancer* 36:238-41, 2000.
67. Wiseman H, O'Reilly JD, Adlercreutz H, et al: Isoflavone phytoestrogens consumed in soy decrease F(2)-isoprostane concentrations and increase resistance of low-density lipoprotein to oxidation in humans, *Am J Clin Nutr* 72:395-400, 2000.
68. Anderson JW, Smith BM, Washnock CS: Cardiovascular and renal benefits of dry beans and soybean intake, *Am J Clin Nutr* 70(suppl 3):464S-74S, 1999.
69. Wang HJ, Murphy PA: Isoflavone content in commercial soybean foods, *J Agric Food Chem* 42:1674-73, 1994.
70. Weaver CM, Plawecki KL: Dietary calcium: adequacy of a vegetarian diet, *Am J Clin Nutr* 59(suppl 5):1238S-41S, 1994.
71. Skibola CF, Smith MT: Potential health impacts of excessive flavonoid intake, *Free Radic Biol Med* 29:375-83, 2000.
72. Coward L, Barnes NC, Setchell KDR, Barnes S: Genistein, daidzein, and their B-glycoside conjugates: antitumour isoflavones in soybean foods from American and Asian diets, *J Agric Food Chem* 41:1961-7, 1993.
73. Potter SM, Baum JA, Teng H, et al: Soy protein and isoflavones: their effects on blood lipids and bone density in postmenopausal women, *Am J Clin Nutr* 68(suppl 6):1375S-1379S, 1998.
74. Wiseman H: Role of dietary phyto-estrogens in the protection against cancer and heart disease, *Biochem Soc Trans* 24:795-800, 1996.
75. Jenkins DJ, Kendall CW, Mehling CC, et al: Combined effect of vegetable protein (soy) and soluble fiber added to a standard cholesterol-lowering diet, *Metabolism* 48:809-16, 1999.
76. Jacobs DR, Murtaugh MA: It's more than an apple a day: an appropriately processed plant-centered dietary pattern may be good for your health, *Am J Clin Nutr* 72:899-900, 2000.
77. Fraser GE, Sabate J, Beeson WL, Strahan TM: A possible protective effect of nut consumption on risk of coronary heart disease. The Adventist Health Study, *Arch Intern Med* 152:1416-24, 1992.
78. Kushi LH, Meyer KA, Jacobs DR: Cereals, legumes, and chronic disease risk reduction: evidence from epidemiological studies, *Am J Clin Nutr* 70(suppl 3):451S-8S, 1999.
79. Slavin JL, Martini MC, Jacobs DR, Marquart L: Plausible mechanisms for the protectiveness of whole grains, *Am J Clin Nutr* 70(suppl 3):459S-63S, 1999.
80. McIntyre A, Gibson PR, Young GP: Butyrate production from dietary fibre and protection against large bowel cancer in a rat model, *Gut* 34:386-91, 1993.
81. Worthington V: Nutritional quality of organic versus conventional fruits, vegetables, and grains, *J Altern Complement Med* 7:161-73, 2001.
82. Marriott BM: Functional foods: an ecological perspective, *Am J Clin Nutr* 71(suppl 6):1728S-34S, 2000.

83. Stacewicz-Sapuntzakis M, Bowen PE, Hussain EA, et al: Chemical composition and potential health effects of prunes: a functional food? *Crit Rev Food Sci Nutr* 41:251-86, 2001.

84. Roberfroid MB: Concepts and strategy of functional food science: the European perspective, *Am J Clin Nutr* 71(suppl 6):1660S-1664S, 2000.

85. Schetchikova N: Functional foods—panacea or plague? *J Am Chiropr Assoc* Oct:20-9, 2001.

86. Ross S: Functional foods: the Food and Drug Administration perspective, *Am J Clin Nutr* 71(suppl 6):1735S-1738S, 2000.

87. Drewnowski A, Gomez-Carneros C: Bitter taste, phytonutrients, and the consumer: a review, *Am J Clin Nutr* 72:1424-35, 2000.

88. Meluzzi A, Sirri F, Manfreda G, et al: Effects of dietary vitamin E on the quality of table eggs enriched with N-3 long-chain fatty acids, *Poult Sci* 79:539-45, 2000.

89. de Lorgeril M, Salen P: Diet as preventive medicine in cardiology, *Curr Opin Cardiol* 15:364-70, 2000.

90. Jariwalla RJ: Rice-bran products: phytonutrients with potential applications in preventive and clinical medicine, *Drugs Exp Clin Res* 27:17-26, 2001.

91. de Jong N, Paw MJ, de Groot LC, et al: Nutrient-dense foods and exercise in frail elderly: effects on B vitamins, homocysteine, methylmalonic acid, and neuropsychological functioning, *Am J Clin Nutr* 73:338-46, 2001.

92. Malinow MR, Duell PB, Irvin-Jones A, et al: Increased plasma homocyst(e)ine after withdrawal of ready-to-eat breakfast cereal from the diet: prevention by breakfast cereal providing 200 microg folic acid, *J Am Coll Nutr* 19:452-7, 2000.

93. Hasler CM, Kundrat S, Wool D: Functional foods and cardiovascular disease, *Curr Atheroscler Rep* 2:467-75, 2000.

94. Fuller R, Gibson GR: Modification of the intestinal microflora using probiotics and prebiotics, *Scand J Gastroenterol* 222(suppl):28-31, 1997.

95. Tuomola E, Crittenden R, Playne M, et al: Quality assurance criteria for probiotic bacteria, *Am J Clin Nutr* 73:393S-398S, 2001.

96. Rolfe RD: The role of probiotic cultures in the control of gastrointestinal health, *J Nutr* 130(suppl 2S):396S-402S, 2000.

97. Scholz-Ahrens KE, Schaafsma G, van Den Heuvel EGE, Schrezenmeir J: Effects of prebiotics on mineral metabolism, *Am J Clin Nutr* 73:459S-464S, 2000.

98. Lawrence M, Rayner M: Functional foods and health claims: a public health policy perspective, *Public Health Nutr* 1:75, 1998.

99. Tran TL: Antioxidant supplements to prevent heart disease, *Postgrad Med* 109:109-14, 2001.

100. Clarkson PM, Thompson HS: Antioxidants: what role do they play in physical activity and health? *Am J Clin Nutr* 72(suppl 2):637S-646S, 2000.

101. Meydani M: Effect of functional food ingredients: vitamin E modulation of cardiovascular diseases and immune status in the elderly, *Am J Clin Nutr* 71:1665S-1668S, 2000.

102. Charleux J: Beta-carotene, vitamin C, and vitamin E: the protective micronutrients, *Nutr Rev* 54:S109-S114, 1996.

103. Gey KF, Moser UK, Joran P, et al: Increased risk of cardiovascular disease at suboptimal plasma concentrations of essential antioxidants: an epidemiological update with special attention to carotene and vitamin C, *Am J Clin Nutr* 57(suppl):787S-797S, 1993.

104. Diplock AT, Charleux JL, Crozier-Willi G, et al: Functional food science and defence against reactive oxidative species, *Br J Nutr* 80(suppl 1):S77-112, 1998.
105. Wheatley C: Vitamin trials and cancer: what went wrong? *J Nutr Environ Med* 8:277-288, 1998.
106. Paiva SA, Russell RM: Beta-carotene and other carotenoids as antioxidants, *J Am Coll Nutr* 18:426-33, 1999.
107. Werbach M: Nutritional influences on illness, *Int J Altern Complement Med* 17:20-1, 1999.
108. Kayden HJ, Wisniewski T: On the biological activity of vitamin E, *Am J Clin Nutr* 72:201-3, 2000.
109. The ATBC Prevention Study Group: The alpha-tocopherol, beta-carotene lung cancer prevention study: design, methods, participant characteristics and compliance, *Ann Epidemiol* 4:1-10, 1994.
110. Lichtenstein AH: Got soy? *Am J Clin Nutr* 73:667-8, 2001.
111. Willett WC: Convergence of philosophy and science: the Third International Congress on Vegetarian Nutrition, *Am J Clin Nutr* 70(suppl 3):434S-438S, 1999.
112. High KP: Nutritional strategies to boost immunity and prevent infection in elderly individuals, *Clin Infect Dis* 33:1892-900, 2000.

■ CHAPTER 5 ■

Supplements: Principles and Practice

Toni Jordan

> It is much more problematic to deliver nutritional magic bullets than to generally increase consumption of plant foods.[1]

Understanding how nutritional medicine works and achieving results as a primary caregiver can be two different things. As with any discipline, success depends on the quality of the tools, as well as the skill of the operator. Although many of the principles of the clinical use of nutraceuticals are the same as those used with more familiar drugs, some rules are different. There are also many common misconceptions about the principles of formulating nutraceuticals, and it is important to understand these principles to achieve the best clinical outcomes.

PRINCIPLES: DIETARY VERSUS THERAPEUTIC

A nutraceutical can exert a physiologic effect in four ways. There are two dietary effects and two therapeutic effects.

The first dietary effect is correction of a gross nutritional deficiency. A nutrient that is currently or usually undersupplied must be supplied to cells to prevent a gross deficiency. The amount of a nutrient required to prevent a gross deficiency is considered the recommended daily allowance (RDA). For example, the RDA for vitamin C was recently raised to 75 mg (for women), 90 mg (for men), plus an additional 35 mg for smokers.[2] This is sufficient to prevent scurvy.

The second dietary effect is correction of a subclinical deficiency. Although gross deficiencies are well understood and not debated, more research is needed in the area of subclinical deficiencies. Is cancer, in fact, a subclinical manifestation of ascorbate deficiency, as Linus Pauling believed?[3] The amounts necessary to correct subclinical deficiencies have not been defined but will be closer to the amount required for a therapeutic effect. This effect also applies when, as a result of an individual variation, a person's requirement for a particular nutrient is greater than average.

Another way a nutrient can exert a physiological effect is by providing the nutrient in a pharmacological rather than physiological dose, thereby exerting a biochemical effect not associated with lower intakes of that nutrient. The therapeutic effect is only achieved once a specific concentration of the substance has been reached. For example, vitamin C at amounts in excess of 1000 mg per day helps to reduce the duration and symptoms of colds and flu. This is in addition to its antiscurvy action, as we understand it today, but perhaps is better understood in an evolutionary context. It is estimated that early human beings' daily intake of vitamin C was closer to 2000 to 3000 mg per day.

The other therapeutic effect is to provide a substance not normally required by the cell but which is capable of altering cellular function. This is the function of herbal medicines. We do not normally have echinacosides and hyperforin as part of our cellular biochemistry, but they exert a chemical effect when they are present. This is often due to an agonist- or antagonist-mimicking effect.

It is also important to remember that herbs can be sources of nutrients, just as fruits and vegetables can. When evaluating a formula, the clinician needs to decide whether the amount of an herb included is sufficient for a therapeutic effect, nutritive effect, or neither. Some formulas contain substances that have neither a nutritive nor a therapeutic benefit; these are included simply to contribute to an impressive-looking list of active ingredients. The clinician should disregard these ingredients.

LACK OF "SCIENTIFIC" DATA

When a clinician first begins practicing nutritional and herbal medicine, one of the most frustrating and discouraging obstacles is a lack of good scientific data, validations, and evidence-based examples. Several factors contribute to this lack.

Data Are No Longer Being Delivered

A busy primary caregiver is not able to do as much research and reading as he or she would like. Often, new and interesting information is drawn to his or her attention by the marketing and sales staff of pharmaceutical companies. With rare examples, the counterpart of the pharmaceutical company, the vitamin company, generates a much larger proportion of its revenue from sales to the general public. The vitamin company's marketing budget may not include detailing health care professionals. What good data are available may not be delivered to the primary care clinician.

Vitamins and Minerals Are Not Patentable

The hundreds of millions of dollars invested by a pharmaceutical company in research and development of a new drug can be recouped, because novel substances can be patent-protected. A vitamin company has no incentive to invest in research for a widely available substance, because there is no safeguard for the investment. This also affects the pricing structure. The margin on a natural substance is much smaller than that on a pharmaceutical agent, because the competitive activity in the complementary health industry brings prices down.

Although therapeutic claims for natural substances can be researched, patented, and registered (e.g., contains substance X, which has been shown in clinical trials to do Y), this probably does not confer any marketing advantage to the vitamin company. The next product on the shelf could also contain substance X, and the consumer's buying decision would likely not rest on the claim.

Individual Nature of Treatments

In complementary medicine, the skill of the clinician and the suitability of his or her tools are paramount. In contrast to orthodox medicine, it is often simply not appropriate to give a large group of people exactly the same regimen to prevent or treat an illness. The decisions of the primary caregiver in complementary medicine are often more complex; for example, exactly how much of this substance is appropriate? Should it be given by itself or with something else? Is there something about this patient's physiology that requires a different substance all together? Does the patient have another condition that must be addressed first? Will success be influenced by diet, stress level, sleep pattern, or other lifestyle factors? The one-size-fits-all standard double-blind, placebo-controlled trial is not always the most appropriate means of providing good information about complementary medicines.

WATER-SOLUBLE VITAMINS

Vitamin C

The forms of vitamin C include ascorbic acid, the mineral ascorbates (calcium ascorbate, sodium ascorbate, and magnesium ascorbate), and ascorbyl palmitate. The mineral ascorbates are not acids and are more suitable than ascorbic acid for subjects with sensitive stomachs and as chewable preparations for children. They also have the advantage of delivering an amount of the mineral carrier. Vitamin C solutions and topical preparations are generally unstable.[4] Ascorbic acid should be used as the reference for dosage calculations.

Bioflavonoids

Bioflavonoids are often considered with vitamin C, but they have a wider range of variations and indications than is often realized. Some examples of bioflavonoids are:

- Rutin, hesperidin, and quercetin. These can be found singly or combined in a bioflavonoid complex.
- Flavanols. These include catechins, and oligomeric proanthocyanidins, which are pairs and triples (dimers and trimers) of catechin, and tannins, which are quadruples (tetramers) of catechins. Flavanols are found in grape seeds, tea, and pine bark, among other sources; and indications for use include antioxidant effects, hypoxia, inflammation, and ischemia.
- Flavonoid glycosides. These include anthocyanosides, or anthocyanidins, found in the herb bilberry. Anthocyanosides are used in ophthalmology and in the treatment of altered microcirculation and peripheral venous insufficiency, among other indications.

Vitamin B Complex

The vitamin B complex—comprising thiamin, riboflavin, niacin, pyridoxine, pantothenic acid, folic acid, biotin, and cyanocobalamin and the factors choline, inositol, and para-aminobenzoic acid—is also found in various forms. *Niacin*, a general term for vitamin B_3, is available in different forms. The most common forms are niacinamide (or nicotinamide) and nicotinic acid. The nicotinic acid form of vitamin B_3 causes the side effect of flushing. In the United States, the term *niacin* means the nicotinic acid form.

Laetrile, a glucoside found in apricot kernels, is sometimes called vitamin B_{17}. Controversially used in nonorthodox cancer therapies, laetrile is not considered part of the B complex.

FAT-SOLUBLE VITAMINS

Concerns about vitamin toxicity generally involve the fat-soluble vitamins because of their ability to be stored by the body. This is why the treatment rationale and dosage are especially important.

Usually, rather than being expressed in milligrams or grams as other nutrients are, fat-soluble vitamins are expressed in international units (IU). Although the use of the term *international units* was technically abandoned in 1981 in the ninth edition of the *Recommended Dietary Allowances*, it is still used in practice. Rather than weight, international units express the amount of work that a vitamin will perform. It is helpful to think of international units as expressing the distance a car will travel, whereas milligrams express the amount of gas in the tank.

Vitamin E

Vitamin E is available in many forms. One way to distinguish the various forms of the vitamin is by the prefix *d*-(RRR, or natural) versus *dl*-(all-*rac*, or synthetic). Natural vitamin E consists of one stereoisomer, which is highly bioavailable. Synthetic vitamin E consists of eight stereoisomers, only one of which is RRR (natural) vitamin E. Because the *d*-form has a higher biopotency, the amounts required when given by weight vary for the same strength. This has been already included in the calculation to convert milligrams to international units: the ratio is currently accepted as being 1.36 for the biopotency of the *d*-form versus the *dl*-form of Vitamin E (tocopherol), although other studies suggest that natural vitamin E delivers at least twice the activity of synthetic vitamin E.[5]

Vitamin A

Although it is beginning to be acknowledged that much of the recent hysteria about vitamin A toxicity is not scientifically based and that vitamin A toxicity has been overstressed,[6] many primary caregivers prefer to prescribe beta-carotene rather than retinol. The difficulty lies in the uncertain conversion ratio, which can differ according to biochemical individuality, type and amount of fiber in the diet, and current vitamin A status, among other variables.[7] The conversion ratio of beta-carotene to vitamin A has been quoted as anywhere between 2:1 and 26:1, and many points in between, including the 6:1 suggested by the World Health Organization.[8] Although beta-carotene is a valuable therapeutic substance in its own right, it is not vitamin A, and rates of conversion to vitamin A can vary greatly.[9]

Vitamin D

Vitamin D is generated through exposure to UV radiation, and in some climates during winter, blood levels of vitamin D can drop.[10] Low levels are also associated with some countries and ethnic groups.[11] Other lifestyle factors such as use of sunscreen, reduced sun exposure, and UV-resistant glass can also reduce endogenous levels of vitamin D.

MINERALS

Minerals can be very difficult to utilize, especially in elderly people or those with low stomach acid. As a rule, minerals are better absorbed as chelates. This binding to another substance, often an amino acid, makes the mineral more like a normal foodstuff. There are some specific rules about mineral absorption; for example, calcium citrate is about 25% better absorbed than calcium carbonate.[12] Selenomethionine appears to be the most desirable form of selenium.[13]

When products are compared for mineral content, the elemental amount should always be used. Even in seemingly identical complexes such as magnesium oxide, there are light and heavy variations that alter the amount of available magnesium.

NUTRIENTS

The bioequivalence of coenzyme Q10 has been compared in two common forms, a powder-filled capsule and an oil-based formulation. Both formulations showed similar poor and slow absorption characteristics.[14] When any oil-based product is taken, absorption will be improved if it is consumed with an oily meal.

ESSENTIAL FATTY ACIDS

The importance of essential fatty acids (EFAs) and their clinical actions are just beginning to be understood. There are many types, and it is important to be clear about their specific functions.

The two main types of EFAs are omega-3 (ω-3) and omega-6 (ω-6). The number refers to the position of the first carbon-double bond. Omega-6 fatty acid is generally supplied as evening primrose oil, a source of γ-linolenic acid. Evening primrose oil is commonly used to alleviate skin disorders and premenstrual syndrome, but other sources of ω-6 fatty acids include black currant seed oil and borage oil.

The two ω-3 EFAs commonly prescribed are eicosapentaenoic acid (EPA) and docosahexaenoic acid (DHA). Omega-3 oils are usually found in three types: α-linolenic acid (from flaxseed oil), EPA, or DHA. EPA is found is salmon oil and is often marketed as *MaxEPA*. DHA is found in tuna oil. EPA or DHA is required clinically, and the drawback to using the precursor, α-linolenic acid, is that all the subsequent reactions and cofactors must be working well. However, for vegetarians, α-linolenic acid from flaxseed oil may be the only option.

EPA is indicated more for cardiovascular conditions and arthritis because of its action in reducing the proportion of series 2 prostaglandins. DHA is used more for its action on nerve cell membranes and brain function. Fish liver oils do not contain useful amounts of EFAs and are a source of vitamins A and D only.

Human research on ω-9 fatty acids, such as nervonic acid, is limited.

HERBS

When one is determining the form of herbs to be prescribed, it is important to consider the following:

- Plant part. Is the plant part used the same as the one found to have therapeutic benefit?
- Species. A cheaper species may have been substituted for the correct one.
- Dosage. Is the amount relevant, either therapeutically or nutritively?
- Type. For example, *Ginkgo biloba* extract EGb761 has been shown to have therapeutic value in dementia.[15]

• Standardized/non-standardized. Standardized herbs have a guaranteed amount of a marker chemical.

If this information is not on the label, the supplement is not necessarily reliable. (A nonstandardized herbal extract will be described as "extract equivalent to..." or in similar wording without stating an amount of marker compound.) Not all herbs are available as standardized extracts.

Standardized Versus Non-standardized Herbs

Supporters of standardized herbs argue that guaranteeing the amount of a marker chemical provides assurance that the herb is of defined strength and quality. If the marker substance used is the active ingredient, the actual therapeutic potency of the herb is being controlled. It enables more accurate dosing, results that are more consistent, and a greater potential for scientific justification of herbal medicine. In fact, some herbal medicines, such as *Ginkgo biloba* leaf, have no history of traditional use. The herb's clinical indications for treatment of dementia and memory loss are primarily related to the standardized *Ginkgo* extract EGb761.

Those who disapprove of the use of standardized herbs argue that herbal medicine is not like conventional drug therapy and that there are many individual phytochemicals in the herb that exert a therapeutic effect. Standardizing the amount of a market chemical may have no relevance to therapeutic outcomes, because standardization does not guarantee standardization of all phytochemicals—or even preservation of all of the herb's relevant phytochemicals. Practitioners of traditional herbal medicine use a non-standardized extract, and they argue that standardized herbs are closer to drug therapy than herbal medicine.

ADMINISTRATION OF THE SUPPLEMENT

Dosage Form

The *United States Pharmacopeia* requirement for disintegration of oral dosage forms is a maximum of 30 minutes in water at 37°C with disks, which are small plastic weights placed on top of the tablet or capsule in the disintegration tester. The rationale is that if disintegration takes place in less than 30 minutes in water, the time required would be considerably shorter in stomach acid. The temperature of the water is the same as body temperature. Often it is assumed that the use of the disks limits the amount of movement of the tablets to make disintegration more difficult; but when the disks are removed, disintegration times increase markedly.[16]

However, disintegration time is a poor indicator of bioavailability. In a comparison of vitamin C tablets with mean disintegration times ranging from 9 to 120 minutes, it was demonstrated that tablets with a mean disintegration time of 60 minutes had the highest bioavailability. These tablets would fail to meet the current *United States Pharmacopeia* requirement. It has been suggested that for a relatively unstable substance such as vitamin C, a formulation that is released more slowly would make a larger amount physiologically available.[17]

Hard-Shell Capsules or Tablets?

It is commonly believed that hard-shell capsules are preferable to tablets. Three issues are relevant to this argument.

Ease of Digestion. Although it is commonly believed that tablets are harder to digest, one indicator of digestion is disintegration time. Assuming an equivalent disintegration time, there is no reason to believe that tablets would be any more difficult to digest than either hard or soft-shell capsules. In fact, in manufacturing hard-shell capsules, sometimes a "slug," or heavily compressed pellet, of the powder is formed. This slug is then inserted into the capsule casing. In this case there is little difference between the compression of a tablet and a hard-shell.

Therapeutic Amounts. On average, a tablet can contain more active substance than a hard-shell capsule. Tablets are usually larger and can be made in a variety of shapes. Hard-shell capsules are available in only a few sizes.

Animal Products. Although tablets are not guaranteed to be free of animal products, hard-shell capsules are often made from gelatin, although vegetable sources such as potato starch are available. All manufacturers should be able to provide certificates as to the BSE (bovine spongiform encephalopathy)-free status of their capsules. Awareness of the presence of gelatin in capsules is also important for patients following Halal, Kosher, or vegetarian diets.

Route. The bioavailability of some nutrients varies enormously according to delivery route, and this can affect dosage. For example, oral administration of vitamin B_{12} is at least as effective as intramuscular administration even in the absence of intrinsic factor, but the oral dosage must be higher and more frequent. Oral doses of 2000 µg daily are as effective in raising cobalamin levels as weekly intramuscular injections of vitamin B_{12} for 6 weeks, followed by monthly intramuscular injections of B_{12}.[18,19] Sublingual administration of 1000 µg of vitamin B_{12} twice daily raises serum vitamin B_{12} levels fourfold to therapeutic values within 7 to 12 days.[20]

In humans, about 85% of an intravenous dose of vitamin C can be recovered in urine as ascorbic acid and its major metabolites, as compared with 30% of the same dose delivered orally.[21] There is considerable intersubject variation in ascorbic acid absorption, and it has been suggested that the amount of individual variability shown might explain inconsistent trial results for vitamin C. It seems that there are good and poor absorbers of the vitamin.

When rates of elimination of vitamin C were compared in sheep, injections given intramuscularly produced greater areas under the curve than those given intravenously. The same researchers concluded, in a comparison of dosages given intravenously, that the higher the dose, the greater is the rate of elimination.[22]

In general, vitamin C is very effective when given intravenously. Up to 12 g is the usual dose. When injected, B complex vitamins are usually given intramuscularly (in the gluteal muscles).

POSITIVE INTERACTIONS

Nutraceuticals

A combination of vitamin C (2000 mg daily) and vitamin E (1000 IU daily), taken orally, reduces the tendency to sunburn, which may indicate a lowered risk for the long-term effects of UV damage.[23] This has not been noted for either of these substances taken separately.

Vitamin C is usually recommended to be taken with bioflavonoids, which are found together with ascorbic acid in nature. It has recently been shown that flavonoids inhibit intracellular accumulation of vitamin C,[24] so the effect of taking the two together may be to maintain higher extracellular levels of vitamin C.

Despite the current practice of giving women large amounts of folic acid before conception and during pregnancy and giving women with premenstrual syndrome large amounts of pyridoxine, it is recommended that B-group vitamins be taken together, as they are found in food. The balance of the B vitamins is important, and an excessive amount of one can lead to a relative deficiency of another.[25]

When calcium supplements are taken, vitamin D, preferably in the form of cholecalciferol, is generally accepted to be required.

Experts vary on the best way to take calcium and magnesium supplements. There are two strongly held points of view.

- *It is essential to take calcium and magnesium supplements apart from each other.* Some experts believe that although both minerals are important, their role as competitive channel blockers means that they should be taken separately, at different times of the day.
- *It is essential to take calcium and magnesium supplements together, in some defined ratio.* Other experts believe that the minerals need to be taken in balance to avoid constipation and cramping. Opinions vary on the required ratio, from 2.5:1 (the current RDA ratio) to 2:1, to 1:1.[26]

Experts strongly disagree about whether calcium and magnesium supplements should be taken together or separately.

Diet

Vitamin C enhances the absorption of iron.[27]

NEGATIVE INTERACTIONS

Nutraceuticals

The absorption of iron is negatively affected by other minerals, including calcium.[27]

Diet

As a rule, all vitamins and fat-soluble nutrients should be taken with food. The longer the nutrient is in contact with intestinal mucosa, the more complete is the absorption. Food slows down transit time, increasing the amount of nutrient absorption. Minerals, on the other hand, are often absorbed better away from food. For example, plant components, such as polyphenols and phytates, can block the absorption of iron, so iron supplements should not be taken with meals. Instead, iron supplements should be taken with a vitamin C supplement or a glass of orange or black currant juice, because vitamin C helps iron absorption. However, tea should be consumed between meals[27] because its high phytate content can block absorption of minerals from food. Some people find that mineral supplements, especially zinc, can cause nausea when taken on an empty stomach, so it is often recommended to take them at night before bed. If this does not help, they should be taken with food, because at least some will be absorbed.

Probiotics should also be taken away from food, because increased stomach acid will reduce the viable count of most strains. If a probiotic in tablet or capsule form is chosen, the viability of the product must be ensured. Often the heat generated in the formation of tablets and capsules can damage the bacteria. Most probiotics require refrigeration.

COMBINATIONS (COFACTORS)

Nutritional Status and Diet

The amount of a substance required to exert a therapeutic effect is often dependent on the baseline amount of that substance. When a primary caregiver prescribes an antibiotic, for example, he or she assumes that the patient's baseline level of the antibiotic is zero. This enables a reasonably precise calculation of the dosage required.

However, when a nutritional doctor is prescribing, for example, a vitamin, he or she does not know the patient's baseline level of this vitamin. To gauge this, the doctor may order analytical testing (which may be expensive, depending on the number of substances to be measured) or question the patient extensively about his or her diet (which often provides unreliable information). Depletion of stores can increase absorption (e.g., iron), and the body adapts the rate of elimination to ensure homeostasis.

> The lower the baseline level of a substance, the lower is the amount required to exert a therapeutic effect.

A person who is poorly nourished generally requires a lower dosage before an effect is achieved. A primary caregiver with more clinical experience will often be able to correctly judge dosage requirements using volunteered and observed symptoms.

Other aspects of the diet can also affect the pharmacodynamics of nutritional supplements, just as the proportion of carbohydrates to protein in the diet can change the rate of urinary clearance of drugs.[28] The clinical significance of this has not been determined.

Herb-Drug Interactions

Currently, there is much debate about the effects of herbs and nutrients taken with prescribed medications. Some common forms of interaction between drugs and herbs and nutrients are physical interaction, cumulative function, and induction of liver enzymes by herbs.

Physical Interaction.   Some herbs interact in a physical way with prescription drugs. They may reduce absorption either by binding drugs in the intestine (e.g., some gums and fibers) or by increasing gut transit time (e.g., some natural laxatives).

Cumulative Function.   Cumulative function involves an herb or nutrient and a drug having a similar physiologic function. This can mean that the effect of both taken together can greatly increase the intended effect, thereby causing adverse effects. An example of this is serotonin syndrome, which has been reported in patients taking selective serotonin reuptake inhibitors with the antidepressant herb *Hypericum perforatum. Hypericum perforatum* is believed to act by increasing brain serotonin levels, as do selective serotonin reuptake inhibitors. Serotonin syndrome involves tremors, restlessness, twitching, nausea, and flushing caused by excessive serotonin levels.

The difficulty for the primary caregiver is that these side effects are not uncommon when the drug is used in isolation. Thirteen percent of patients in worldwide clinical trials of paroxetine withdrew because of adverse reactions.[29]

Herbs as Inducers of Liver Enzymes.   Much of the popular literature on herb-drug interactions focuses on the role of herbs as potent inducers of liver enzymes. Although some reports discuss drugs such as those necessary to control transplant rejection, a great many reports involve warfarin. The herbs and nutrients that are theoretically able to interfere with the action of warfarin because of a variety of mechanisms include angelica root, arnica flower, anise, asafetida, bogbean, borage seed oil, bromelain, capsicum, celery, chamomile, clove, fenugreek, feverfew, garlic, ginger, ginkgo, horse chestnut, licorice root, lovage root, meadowsweet, onion, parsley, passionflower herb, poplar, quassia, red clover, rue, sweet clover, turmeric, willow bark, coenzyme Q10, danshen, devil's claw, dong quai, ginseng, green tea, papain, and vitamin E.[30]

Two acknowledgments should be made. First, a great many diet and lifestyle factors also induce liver enzymes, including consumption of broccoli,[31] alcohol,[32] char-grilled beef, and red wine and exposure to cigarette smoke. Second, warfarin is an extremely problematic drug because of its extreme sensitivity to interactions with foods[33] and other drugs.

Although the question of drug-herb interactions is a valid one for the primary caregiver, the focus should be returned to the drug and its interactions with all dietary, lifestyle, and natural medicine factors, rather than the interactions of the specific herb. This would produce safer and better care for patients.

Age

Often, nutrient requirements are reduced in older people. A lower dosage may be required to produce a result. However, other aspects of aging can affect pharmacodynamics e.g., in rats, aging decreases the ability of the blood-brain barrier to transport the amino acid tryptophan. If this is also true for humans, a higher dosage of tryptophan may be required to exert an effect in older people.

Some older people may have less exposure to direct sunlight. Combined with an increased requirement for vitamin D that is associated with aging, this lack of sun exposure may lead to a vitamin D deficiency, and many older people may benefit from vitamin D supplementation. Also, poor dentition and reduced stomach acid may contribute to lower nutrient absorption, from food as well as supplements.

Children also have some specific needs for different levels of nutrients. Children with learning disabilities have been shown to respond well to supplementation.[34] Poor diets in children, caused by fussy eating, can lead to micronutrient deficiencies.[35] Sufficient calcium during childhood is important to provide an adequate "calcium bank" for later life.

Children also have unique dosage requirements. Assuming that a child is a miniature adult with no specific changes to hepatic or renal clearance, children's dosages can be calculated either by weight or age. Many rules exist for both methods of calculation, such as Clark's Rule and Young's Rule.

> Clark's Rule: Child's approximate dose =
> Child's Weight in Kilograms/60 × Adult Dose
>
> Young's Rule: Child's approximate dose =
> Child's Age/ (Age + 12) × normal adult dose

MEDICAL CONDITIONS AND SURGERY

Existing medical conditions alter the amount of nutrients required and lead to questions that are more difficult to answer. Thinking more broadly about the optimum health of humans can lead to a reevaluation of many medical conditions. Is homocysteine a risk factor for heart disease or a marker for insufficient vitamin B_{12} and folic acid?

Individuals preparing for surgery would benefit from B complex supplementation to reduce ischemia.[36] Additional zinc and vitamin C are also often recommended during recovery. Use of supplements designed to reduce blood clotting, such as vitamins E and C and *Ginkgo biloba*, should be discontinued before surgery.

Pregnancy

The use of herbal medicines and supplements in pregnancy continues to be a source of much controversy. However, in many cases and with the correct advice, these medicines are safer and more effective than prescription drugs, for both the unborn baby and the mother. Data continue to accumulate on the importance and effectiveness of supplements during pregnancy, and this research will continue as rates of infertility, birth defects, and miscarriage rise. Supplements that are safe and helpful during pregnancy include probiotic bacteria, multivitamins, antioxidants, multiminerals, DHA, and vitamin A.

Probiotic Bacteria.   In a landmark double-blind, randomized, placebo-controlled trial, published in the *Lancet* in 2001, Kalliomaki et al[37] reported that mothers with a family history of atopic disease halved their risk of having a child with chronic recurring atopic eczema by taking *Lactobacillus* GG during pregnancy and giving it to their infants for the first 6 months of life. The authors propose that gut microflora are a source of natural immunomodulators.

Multivitamins.   It is common knowledge that women intending to conceive, as well as pregnant women, should take folic acid to reduce the risk of neural tube defects. How much longer will it take before public health policy reflects the importance of all vitamins before conception for the health of both mothers and babies? Preliminary results already suggest that one in four major cardiac defects could be prevented by periconceptual vitamin use.[38] A number of multivitamins are especially designed for pregnant women, and choosing one of these can increase the confidence of the clinician and the patient.

Antioxidants.   Vitamins C (1000 mg) and E (400 IU) have been shown to reduce the incidence of preeclampsia in at-risk women.[39] In this trial women did not begin receiving supplements until between 16 and 22 weeks of gestation. An interesting sequel would be a placebo-controlled study of the risk of preeclampsia when the vitamin administration was begun before conception.

Multiminerals.   Although iron supplements are often routinely recommended for pregnant women, they should not be prescribed without a medical diagnosis of iron deficiency. Many investigators believe that unusual food cravings are a sign of mineral deficiency. Early research is showing that women who miscarry may be deficient in selenium[40]; however, the results are not conclusive. Deficiencies in zinc, magnesium, copper, and calcium have also been reported to have negative effects on pregnancy and the health of the baby.[41] Male infertility is also a growing problem, and there is evidence that zinc has a vital role in protecting healthy sperm from superoxide anions. Infertile men have significantly lower seminal plasma zinc concentrations.[42]

Docosahexaenoic Acid.   EFAs are important for sperm health and cell membrane formation and for visual and cortical function. Supplementation with DHA during pregnancy has become popular, especially during the last trimester. If any oils are recommended, it is important that fat-soluble antioxidants also be included. Additional oils can have a pro-oxidant effect.

Vitamin A.   Vitamin A is usually avoided during pregnancy and substituted with beta-carotene. However, vitamin A and beta-carotene do not perform the same biochemical functions. Some countries enforce compulsory warnings on the labels of vitamin A supplements to limit their use in pregnancy. Despite these common beliefs, evidence that vitamin A supplementation causes malformations is lacking. In one study it was shown that infants exposed to "high" amounts of vitamin A (greater than 50,000 IU/day) did not have an increased risk of malformations.[6] Recommending amounts between 2500 IU and 10,000 IU per day would appear to be conservative.

Individual Variability

Some other reasons that supplementation might be necessary include poor digestion; consumption of hot coffee, tea, spices, and alcohol; smoking; and the use of laxatives. Men sometimes have greater requirements than women; often this is simply due to an assumption of a greater body weight, but sometimes there is a biochemical foundation. In addition, some geographic areas are endemically low in some minerals, and this is reflected in the health of the inhabitants in that region. One example of this is the selenium deficiency found in some parts of China.

Quality

How can the primary caregiver be confident about the quality of the products he or she is prescribing? Some countries, notably Australia and Canada, have strict, government-monitored criteria for quality and safety (although not for efficacy). This system involves adherence to a code of good manufacturing practice (GMP).

The GMP is an international code involving the highest standards in cleanliness, accuracy, and high-level controls of the manufacturing process. In these countries, a product cannot be registered with the relevant health department without evidence of adherence to this code. In Australia, the appropriate registration is represented by a number on the front panel of the product. This number is either AUST LXXXXX (for substances considered low risk with a lesser information requirement) or AUST RXXXXX. This shows the product has been manufactured under GMP, with independent inspections by a government body.

The United States has no requirement for GMP manufacturing of complementary medicines, and this has repercussions for the quality of the product. An example of this occurred in 2000, when the US Food and Drug Administration tested 45 commercial products containing the hormone supplement dehydroepiandrosterone (DHEA). The amounts of active ingredients found in the products ranged from 0% to 109% of the declared amounts.[43] Before a primary caregiver prescribes or recommends a product not approved for sale in his or her home country, he or she should consider carefully the medicolegal ramifications of poor product quality.

NUTRACEUTICALS

Dehydroepiandrosterone

DHEA is a hormone manufactured by the adrenal cortex. Its primary endogenous function is as an androgenic precursor in men and women, although precise mechanisms of action of both DHEA and its active metabolite, DHEA sulfate, are not fully understood. As a nutraceutical, it is used primarily for life extension and slowing of the aging process, based on the premise that DHEA levels decrease naturally with age.[44]

DHEA has a wide variety of actions. It does seem to protect against cancer,[45] at least in mice and rats, especially against cancer of the breast, colon, lung, liver, and skin and lymphomas.[46] It improves many immune markers, in both quantity and quality, and sometimes by very large amounts.[47] DHEA is an antioxidant and increases energy in some people.

DHEA is used to treat fibromyalgia, to increase muscle growth and lean body mass, especially in the elderly, and to prevent osteoporosis[47]; and it is administered both orally and topically. Patients with Alzheimer's disease have significantly lower DHEA levels than healthy people of the same age,[48] but causality is not proven. Other indications for use include amnesia, stress, anxiety, and poor sleep quality. It is also used to treat sexual dysfunction, most notably to improve libido in older women.[44]

Side effects of DHEA are mostly anecdotal. Illegal in most countries, DHEA is most commonly used in the United States, where it is categorized as a dietary supplement and is available over-the-counter. It is by no means certain that all side effects are captured. Those that have been reported include acne, hirsutism, hair and nail growth, and seborrhea. These side effects may be dose-dependent.

For some time, it was considered that an enlarged prostate or the risk of prostate cancer or any other hormonally-controlled cancer was an absolute contraindication for DHEA use. This is due to DHEA being a precursor for testosterone and dehydrotestosterone, which may promote prostate cell proliferation. Recently, some researchers have challenged this theory by suggesting that DHEA actually protects against prostate cancer, at least in rats.[49]

When treatment with any hormone is contemplated, the existence of a negative feedback mechanism must always be considered. It is possible that endogenous production could be largely shut down by exogenous supplementation.

Phosphatidyl Serine

Phosphatidyl serine (PS) is a phosphoglyceride phospholipid found in brain tissue. Phosphatidyl choline is a similar substance, but it contains choline instead of serine. PS concentrates in cell membranes where it is intricately involved in their repair, strength, permeability, elasticity, and maintenance of structural integrity. This is important, especially in the brain. It is the dominant phospholipid in the myelin sheath.

The key indications for use of PS are nervous system problems—age-associated memory impairment,[50] Alzheimer's disease,[51] and dementia.[52] In one study baby mice were supplemented with PS from birth for two months. After one month of supplementation, the mice had higher intelligence than control mice, and after two months, the supplemented mice learned faster and more accurately than adult control mice. The improved learning ability has also been demonstrated in older mice.

PS is also reported to improve mood in the elderly, help repair neuron damage, restore plasticity to synapses, increase the number of neurotransmitter receptors, and improve reflexes. It is reported to have some anticoagulant activity, so it should not be taken with warfarin or other prescribed anticoagulants. PS is generally well-tolerated, but there have been some reports of nausea and increased sleep latency. PS should be taken with food, but not at bedtime.

Melatonin

Melatonin is a neurohormone, produced mainly by the pineal gland during daylight hours. Key indications for melatonin are jet lag and sleep disorders, and it is believed to have anti-aging and life-extension effects. Endogenous secretion of melatonin declines rapidly with age. Mice treated with melatonin live longer than untreated mice and have thicker, more lustrous fur and firmer and more streamlined bodies. Untreated mice have flabby bodies, wrinkled necks, and scruffy coats that are graying in patches.

Melatonin's most studied effects are on the nervous system. It is widely used in the treatment of jet lag and seasonal affective disorder and for improvement of sleep quality. It has been reported to reduce the number of nighttime movements, sleep latency,[53] sleep duration,[54] and core temperature during sleep and to improve the subjective quality of sleep without increasing next-morning drowsiness. Melatonin increases the percentage of rapid eye movement (REM) sleep and increases the amount of slow-wave sleep. It is used therapeutically for insomnia.

Because of melatonin's role in tryptophan metabolism, it is not recommended for use with antidepressants, cortisone, or cannabis. Adverse effects of melatonin have been reported. Young mice that received long-term supplementation had shortened life spans. Depression occurs in 2% of users; 5% of users report nightmares, especially in dosages of more than 1 mg, and 5% complain that their sleep is worse. Headaches have also been reported, as has decreased libido with long-term use. It is contraindicated in kidney disease, autoimmune diseases, and pregnancy and lactation; but as with DHEA, there is a lack of research and reports of side effects.

Although melatonin is widely available as a hormonal substance in the United States, concerns about melatonin are similar to those associated with DHEA.

Methylsulfonylmethane

Methylsulfonylmethane (MSM) is a natural compound and popular supplement mainly used for arthritis, interstitial cystitis, pain relief, reduction of scar tissue, and skin conditions. MSM is a highly available source of sulfur, so conditions in which sulfur is indicated would respond to MSM. Horses are given MSM to strengthen the tissues of the hoof.

No drug interactions have been noted with MSM. No median lethal dose has been established. In humans, diarrhea and headaches have been reported. No allergic reactions have been reported, and there are no known contraindications.

Alpha-Lipoic Acid

Alpha-lipoic acid is an endogenously produced, sulfurous antioxidant[55] which is a component of several enzyme systems. Also known as *thioctic acid*, it is found in many foods. Alpha-lipoic acid is an unusual antioxidant in that it functions in both watery and fatty sections of cells.

It has been reported to prevent high blood pressure,[56] probably as a result of its action in increasing glutathione levels. This action leads to the supposition that lipoic acid will help prevent cataracts.[57] Lipoic acid's action in protecting cells from oxidative stress is quite well-researched,[58] and it has become a logical adjunct to therapy for diabetes. It has also been reported to protect the heart[58] and cardiovascular system from oxidative stress.

S-adenosylmethionine

S-adenosylmethionine (SAMe) is a thiol-containing compound with antioxidant properties that is an important source of methyl groups in the brain. The exact mechanism is not known, but it is believed to revolve around its action as a methyl donor, and possibly its action on the fluidity of cell membranes. It is a methioinine derivative, and it shows some evidence of nervous system effects. The best indication for SAMe is depression; results of good trials and clinical experience promise impressive possibilities.

Of particular importance in depression is the speed at which SAMe acts, often in 7 days at a dosage of 400 mg,[60] and sometimes in as little as 4 days. Also important is the apparent lack of side effects, which have been described as being mild and transient. Because side effects of prescription antidepressants are one of the main reasons for noncompliance, SAMe has the potential to be an effective and safe antidepressant. Early research is also showing promising results in liver disease, especially cirrhosis, and in arthritis and migraines. SAMe is contraindicated in bipolar disorder, because endogenous SAMe increases in manic states, and it can induce manic states.

Glutathione

Glutathione is a tripeptide composed of cysteine, glutamine, and glycine; in its reduced form it is a major antioxidant. It is perhaps best known for its role as a substrate in phase II liver detoxification. Although it is known that glutathione decreases in a number of conditions such as Alzheimer's disease, human immunodeficiency virus infection, and asthma, no causality has been proven.

Phase II detoxification is highlighted as a major key to cancer prevention. Most chemicals, both endogenous and exogenous, undergo phase I detoxification first, producing highly reactive and carcinogenic by-products, which then proceed to pass through phase II detoxification. The timing of these reactions is crucial to cancer prevention. An overly fast phase I produces a large amount of these by-products faster than phase II can water-solubilize them. Thus substances that increase the speed of phase I, such as cigarette smoke, are cancer-inducing. Substances that speed up phase II, such as broccoli, are defensive against cancer. Glutathione falls into this category; however, because selenium is part of the enzyme glutathione peroxidase, adequate levels of selenium are also necessary.

Unfortunately, at present, there are not enough data to prove that glutathione is absorbed whole from the gut. Like most peptides, it is broken down in the gut into its individual constituents. There is little evidence that oral administration of glutathione is any better than administration of cysteine, one of its constituents.

EXAMPLES OF FORMULAS

There are supplement formulas for a wide range of conditions, from stress to depression, from coughing to arthritis. A listing of these formulas and points to consider when they are used follows.

Stress

A formula commonly used to alleviate stress is listed in Table 5-1. Several points must be considered in evaluation of the stress formula, as follows:

- Taking large amounts of one B vitamin can cause deficiencies in the others. For this reason, as a rule, taking a balanced combination of B vitamins is preferred to taking large amounts of one alone.
- This formula contains very high potency B vitamins, including a total of 210 mg of vitamin B_3, sometimes proposed as the endogenous ligand for benzodiazepine receptors. Only 10 mg of this total vitamin B_3 is nicotinic acid, so flushing, a sometimes distressing side effect, is unlikely.
- This formula also contains lithium, an essential trace mineral. Better known for its role in psychiatric disorders at much higher doses (about 900 mg), lithium in this amount is nutritive only.
- The amounts of vitamin C and calcium are too low to be considered adequate therapeutic supplements. This is because the amounts required of both would simply not fit in a tablet with these other ingredients. Both these amounts are purely nutritive.
- Both beta-carotene and vitamin A are included, for their different functions.
- Folic acid in this formula is only 150 µg below the amount required for prevention of neural tube defects before conception and during the first trimester of pregnancy.
- Vitamin E is included as d-α-tocopheryl acid succinate. The "d" prefix denotes natural vitamin E, the preferred form.
- Zinc is included in two forms, as sulfate and gluconate. Some people have difficulties absorbing zinc, so the rationale for this was probably to aid zinc utilization.
- Betaine hydrochloride is an enzyme from pineapple. It is included in this formula to help increase digestion and assist in the absorption of minerals.

TABLE 5-1 ■ Formula to Alleviate Stress

SUPPLEMENT	DOSAGE
Thiamine hydrochloride (vitamin B$_1$)	50 mg
Riboflavin sodium phosphate (vitamin B$_2$)	20 mg
Nicotinamide	200 mg
Nicotinic acid	10 mg
Calcium pantothenate	100 mg
Pyridoxine hydrochloride (vitamin B$_6$)	50 mg
Cyanocobalamin (vitamin B$_{12}$)	100 μg
Folic acid	150 μg
Retinyl palmitate (vitamin A)	750 IU
Beta-carotene	3 mg
Ascorbic acid (vitamin C)	50 mg
Cholecalciferol (vitamin D$_3$ 100 IU)	2.5 μg
d-α-Tocopherol acid succinate (natural vitamin E 25 IU)	20.66 mg
Biotin	20 μg
Inositol	25 mg
Choline bitartrate	50 mg
Lysine hydrochloride	10 mg
Glutamine	50 mg
Calcium (as amino acid chelate 50 mg)	10 mg
Magnesium (magnesium phosphate 34 mg & potassium-magnesium aspartate 20 mg)	7.6 mg
Potassium (potassium phosphate 30 mg & potassium-magnesium aspartate 20 mg)	15.6 mg
Zinc sulfate (zinc 7.6 mg)	21 mg
Zinc gluconate (zinc 1.3 mg)	10 mg
Copper (as amino acid chelate 100 μg)	1.96 mg
Lithium (as carbonate 750 μg)	140 μg
Cobalt (as chloride 100 μg)	25 μg
Aminobenzoic acid	20 mg
Betaine hydrochloride	10 mg
Extracts equiv dry	
Valerian (*Valeriana officinalis*) root	100 mg
Scullcap (*Scutellaria lateriflora*) herb	100 mg

- These high-dose B vitamins, combined with minerals, can cause nausea. These tablets should be taken with food. Should nausea occur, administration of 1/2 tablet may be recommended, with an increase to one tablet after 1 week. Many drug-nutrient interactions are not known, so this tablet should not be taken at the same time as other prescribed medicines.
- These amounts of the nervine herbs valerian and scullcap are below the therapeutic range. When used in this way, herbal medicines are nutritive only, like vegetables in the diet. They provide useful phytochemicals but not in medicinally relevant amounts.

Pain and Inflammation

A commonly used remedy for pain and inflammation is listed in Table 5-2. Several points must be considered in evaluation of the effectiveness of this formula, as follows:

- The enzyme bromelain and the bioflavonoid quercetin have been included because of their inhibitory action on proinflammatory prostaglandins, leukotrienes, and other inflammatory mediators. Together with the minerals zinc and copper, this formula would be likely to cause nausea on an empty stomach; therefore, it should be taken with food.
- Zinc and copper compete for absorption. In this formula copper is included because of its antiinflammatory action. Zinc has a lesser action in this area and is probably included to prevent a zinc deficiency caused by excess copper.
- Feverfew inhibits the release of inflammatory mediators from platelets and leukocytes.
- Although the dosage of this product is one tablet, three times a day, this is more suitable for chronic conditions. If taken soon after an injury, up to three tablets three times a day could be taken.
- For best results, this formula should be combined with more vitamin C (if the inflammation is musculoskeletal), glucosamine (if the inflammation is arthritic), *Lactobacillus* bacteria (taken separately, if the inflammation is intestinal), and more zinc (again taken separately, if the inflammation is of the skin).

Premenstrual or Postmenstrual Tension and Menopause

A formula commonly used to relieve premenstrual or postmenstrual tension and pain associated with menopause is listed in Table 5-3. Several points must be kept in mind when use of this formula is considered.

TABLE 5-2 ■ Remedy for Pain and Inflammation

SUPPLEMENT	DOSAGE
Quercetin	50 mg
Bromelain	50 mg
Ascorbic acid (vitamin C)	60 mg
Zinc	3 mg
Copper	1 mg
Feverfew (*Tanacetum parthenium*)	50 mg

TABLE 5-3 ■ Premenstrual or Postmenstrual Tension Relief

SUPPLEMENT	DOSAGE
Angelica polymorpha (dong quai) root	200 mg
Zingiber officinale (ginger) root	50 mg
Cimicifuga racemosa (black cohosh) root & rhizome	250 mg
Cnicus benedictus (blessed thistle) herb	150 mg
Chamaelirium luteum (false unicorn) root	150 mg
Viburnum opulus (cramp bark) bark	100 mg
Mitchella repens (squaw vine) whole plant	50 mg
Dioscorea villosa (wild yam) root	50 mg

- This is a purely herbal formula. For premenstrual syndrome, additional B vitamins (especially B_6) and magnesium may be required.
- The use of wild yam is controversial. Its use is supported by anecdotal evidence only.
- Ginger is included here as a mild circulatory stimulant and antiinflammatory agent.
- As described here, all herbal formulas should include the full species name and plant part. Formulas that do not disclose these details should be considered highly suspect.
- Naturopathic principles suggest that lower amounts of herbs can be used when herbs are combined.
- Many herbs, including the hormonal herbs in this formula, as well as the immune stimulant golden seal, are contraindicated during pregnancy.
- These herbs are traditional extracts, not standardized extracts.

Osteoporosis

A formula used to treat osteoporosis is listed in Table 5-4. Several points should be considered when this formula is used.

- The formula contains 1 mg of elemental boron. Boron is included for its beneficial effects in osteoporosis and arthritis. Boron toxicity occurs at daily intakes of about 100 mg.
- Of the many forms of calcium available, hydroxyapatite is one of the best absorbed. This is calcium derived from whole bone, so the entire mineral matrix of bone, not just calcium, is included. Normally it is derived from cattle. A reputable supplier should be chosen to ensure that it is not contaminated with heavy metals. Before any cattle products are imported, most countries' quarantine and inspection services will demand evidence that the product is BSE (bovine spongiform encephalopathy)-free.
- The hydroxyapatite form of calcium is not suitable for vegetarians. Calcium citrate is also very well absorbed and could be recommended as an alternative. Calcium carbonate is poorly absorbed in most people.
- Vitamin D_3 is very important in calcium absorption and utilization. All calcium formulae should contain vitamin D_3.

TABLE 5-4 ■ Osteoporosis Formula

SUPPLEMENT	DOSAGE
Hydroxyapatite	500 mg
Calcium hydrogen phosphate	150 mg
Calcium (from microcrystalline hydroxyapatite)	115 mg
Vitamin D_3 (as cholecalciferol, 1.25 mg)	50 IU
Manganese chelate (equiv to 5 mg of manganese)	50 mg
Zinc chelate (equiv to 3 mg of zinc)	30 mg
Copper chelate (equiv to 300 µg)	5 mg
Boron (as sodium borate; equiv to 1 mg of boron)	8.8 mg

TABLE 5-5 ■ Nausea Treatment

SUPPLEMENT	DOSAGE
Zingiber officinale Roscoe (ginger) dried rhizome	400 mg

- Copper and manganese are both essential for bone development.
- This formula does not include magnesium, because a therapeutic dose of magnesium and calcium would be too large for one tablet. Magnesium is essential to bone health and should also be recommended for osteoporosis.

Nausea

A formula used to relieve nausea is listed in Table 5-5. When this formula is used, the following points should be considered:

- Ginger is traditionally used to ease the symptoms of nausea. In pregnancy, it appears to be a highly effective and safe therapy, at a dose of 1 g per day.[61] In fact, in the United States, it has been reported that more than 50% of obstetricians and gynecologists recommend ginger to their patients with morning sickness.[62]
- Ginger is also commonly used for motion sickness.

Immunity

Table 5-6 lists a formula to use for boosting immunity to disease. When this formula is used, the following points should be kept in mind:

- Echinacea is still the first choice of many clinicians for stimulating immunity.
- Each of the three species (*Echinacea pallida*, *E. angustifolia*, and *E. purpurea*) has different phytochemicals,[63] as does each different plant part.[64] Although opinion varies as to the correct species for specific situations, most experts agree that the root contains a higher concentration of immune stimulants. As to species, the clinician should at least confirm that the product contains the species he or she intended.
- Recent studies have shown that echinacea is safe to use during pregnancy.[65]

TABLE 5-6 ■ Immunity Boosters

SUPPLEMENT	DOSAGE
Echinacea (*Echinacea angustifolia*) root, dry	750 mg
Arizona garlic	100 mg
Biotin	200 μg
Beta-carotene	6 mg
Pyridoxine hydrochloride (vitamin B_6)	10 mg
Ascorbic acid	500 mg
Vitamin E (equivalent to 84 mg)	100 IU
Zinc chelate (equivalent to zinc 2.15 mg)	21.5 mg

- Garlic is another very important immune modulator, perhaps because it stimulates lymphocyte proliferation[66]; however, it is unlikely that 100 mg would be sufficient to have this effect. A high-potency garlic supplement, standardized to allicin, could be added to the regimen.
- This amount of zinc, although a useful addition if taken four times a day, is not sufficient. In many trials, zinc in lozenge form has been successfully used acutely, often at a dosage of up to 13 mg every two hours.[67]
- Other substances commonly used for boosting immunity include *Cordyceps sinensis*, the Chinese caterpillar fungus, *Astragalus membranaceus*, and the probiotics *Lactobacillus rhamnosus* and *Bifidobacterium longum*. *Astragalus* and *Cordyceps* species are especially indicated for chronic conditions.

Attention Deficit Hyperactivity Disorder

A formula used in controlling attention-deficit/hyperactivity disorder is listed in Table 5-7. Two important points should be considered when this formula is used:

- Specific formulas, usually in liquid form, have had anecdotal success in controlling attention-deficit/hyperactivity disorder, as well as poor behavior and poor concentration. Although recent trials of DHA have not been positive,[68] it may be other ingredients in these mixtures that help alleviate the condition. In fact, it may be simply zinc that is helpful in this formula.[69]
- This formula includes the essential oils thyme and rosemary, which are highly concentrated plant derivatives. Caution is advised when essential oils are administered internally. They are included here in very small amounts, but research on oral use is only beginning.

Coughing

Table 5-8 lists a formula used to alleviate coughing. When this formula is used, the following points should be considered:

TABLE 5-7 ■ Attention Deficit Hyperactivity Disorder Formula

SUPPLEMENT	DOSAGE
Tuna oil, natural	937.5 mg
−Equivalent to ω-3 marine triglycerides	290 mg
−As Docosahexaenoic acid (DHA)	235 mg
−Eicosapentaenoic acid (EPA)	55 mg
Evening primrose oil	312.5 mg
−Equivalent to γ-Linolenic acid (GLA)	29.5 mg
d-α-Tocopherol acetate (natural vitamin E, 100 IU)	73.5 mg
Zinc gluconate (zinc 1.8 mg)	13 mg
Pyridoxine hydrochloride (vitamin B₆)	3.1 mg
Thyme oil	630 μg
Rosemary oil	130 μg

TABLE 5-8 ■ Cough Mixture

SUPPLEMENT	DOSAGE
Each 5-mL dose contains	
Glycyrrhiza glabra (licorice) root	125 mg
Inula helenium (elecampane) root	100 mg
Euphorbia hirta (euphorbia) herb	50 mg
Achillea millefolium (yarrow) herb	50 mg
Echinacea angustifolia (echinacea) root	50 mg
Thymus vulgaris (thyme) leaf	30 mg
Sambucus nigra (elderberry)	30 mg
Eupatorium perfoliatum (boneset) herb	25 mg
Plantago major (plantain) leaf	18 mg
Prunus serotina (wild cherry) bark	12 mg
Ethanol 780 µL\5 mL (16% vol/vol)	

- Cough mixtures are an extremely appropriate way to use herbal medicines. Standard over-the-counter antitussive agents have side effects and a potential for abuse, and there is no evidence for their efficacy, according to the Cochrane Review.[70]
- This mixture of herbs is a logical mix of respiratory relaxants and antitussive herbs and should be effective. However, it also contains alcohol and licorice (contraindicated in patients with hypertension).

Heart/Cardiovascular Health

Table 5-9 lists a formula that can be used to improve heart health and treat cardiovascular complaints. It is important to remember the following points when this formula is used:

TABLE 5-9 ■ Cardiovascular Health Formula

SUPPLEMENT		DOSAGE
Each capsule contains		
Coenzyme Q10		50 mg
Taurine		150 mg
Hawthorn berries (*Crataegus monogyna*) extract equiv		500 mg
-Ginkgo biloba (10 mg) extract equiv.	500 mg	
Standardized to contain ginkgo flavoneglycosides		2.4 mg
-Ginkgolides	300 µg	
-Bilobalide	250 µg	
Natural mixed carotenoids		3 mg
Mixed tocopherols including trienols		50 IU
Thiamine (vitamin B_1)		50 mg
Nicotinic acid (vitamin B_3)		10 mg
Pyridoxine hydrochloride (vitamin B_6)		15 mg
Cyanocobalamin (vitamin B_{12})		25 µg
Folic acid		150 µg
d-α-Tocopherol (natural vitamin E)		50 IU
Chromium picolinate (equiv 15 µg chromium)		120 µg
Zinc gluconate (equiv 5 mg zinc)		38.4 mg
Selenomethionine (equiv selenium 8 µg)		20 µg

- Coenzyme Q10 is becoming increasingly popular for the prevention and treatment of all types of cardiac complaints. Although there is evidence for its role in treatment of essential hypertension[71] and cardiac failure,[72] especially interesting are the data concerning the role of coenzyme Q10 and lipid-lowering agents (statins).
- Statin drugs block the production of coenzyme Q10, which is important in many biochemical reactions. It is becoming more widely acknowledged that statin drugs cause coenzyme Q10 deficiency, which may be remedied by supplementation.[73]
- Although this formula contains enough coenzyme Q10 to prevent deficiency during therapy with statins and to be used as a general formula for heart health, it does not contain enough to treat cardiac failure, breast cancer, or chronic fatigue syndrome.
- This formulation is presented as a soft gelatin capsule. It should be taken with an oily meal to maximize the absorption of coenzyme Q10.
- The conversion of ubiquinone (the supplemental form of coenzyme Q10) to ubiquinol (the antioxidant form) is zinc-dependent.[73] Zinc is included in this formula and should be included whenever coenzyme Q10 is prescribed to ensure adequate zinc status.
- Taurine, hawthorn, and *Ginkgo* are included for their general benefits to heart health. The *Ginkgo* extract here is a standardized one, providing a guarantee as to the amounts of flavonglycosides and ginkgolides in the formula. Low selenium levels may be associated with cardiovascular risk factors.[75]
- Until recently, the therapeutic use of vitamin E was limited to α-tocopherol, and the therapeutic use of the carotenes was limited to beta-carotene. The use of mixed tocopherols and mixed carotenoids in this formula is an acknowledgment that there are important forms of these two nutrients other than just vitamin E and beta-carotene.

Depression and Anxiety

Listed in Table 5-10 is a remedy used to treat depression. There are several important points to consider when this remedy is used:

- From a nutritional perspective, depression has special features of which a primary care provider must be aware. In addition to the biochemical features of the actual condition, many persons with depression neglect their diets and have poor eating habits. This may have been occurring over a long period, well before the patient first sought treatment. The resulting deficiencies, especially in B vitamins, amino acids, and the essential minerals such as zinc, can contribute to the seriousness of the condition and affect treatment success rates.
- The vitamin and mineral amounts in this formula are the minimum required in deficiency states, and the holistic health care professional should not treat depression without giving some thought to broad based

TABLE 5-10 ■ Depression Formula

SUPPLEMENT	DOSAGE
Each tablet contains	
Hypericum perforatum (St. John's wort) herb, standardized to contain hypericin 600 µg	1.2 g
Eleutherococcus senticosus (Siberian ginseng) root	100 mg
Fucus vesiculosus (kelp) whole plant equiv iodine 50 µg	50 mg
Ascorbic acid (vitamin C)	100 mg
Folic acid	200 µg
Thiamine hydrochloride (vitamin B_1)	10 mg
Riboflavin (vitamin B_2)	10 mg
Nicotinamide	20 mg
Calcium pantothenate	10 mg
Pyridoxine hydrochloride (vitamin B_6)	10 mg
Cyanocobalamin (vitamin B_{12})	250 µg
Biotin (vitamin H)	10 µg
d-α-Tocopheryl acid succinate (natural vitamin E 10 IU)	8.27 mg
Magnesium oxide-heavy (magnesium 150 mg)	250 mg
Potassium sulfate (potassium 10 mg)	22.35 mg
Zinc sulfate monohydrate (zinc 5 mg)	13.8 mg
Manganese sulfate monohydrate (manganese 2 mg)	6.16 mg
Ferrous fumarate (iron 1.6 mg)	4.9 mg
Copper gluconate (copper 10 fg)	71.5 µg

vitamin and mineral supplementation. Depression can be a result of deficiencies of some of the B vitamins and in vitamin C.

• *Hypericum* is one of the most widely used herbs in the world, especially in Europe. Although the data for the use of the herb in treatment of mild and moderate depression are impressive, the data for severe depression are poor. This formula would be ideal as a first treatment for mild or moderate depression.

Arthritis

A formula used to alleviate arthritis pain is listed in Table 5-11. When this remedy is used, the following points should be considered:

TABLE 5-11 ■ Arthritis Treatment

SUPPLEMENT	DOSAGE
Each tablet contains	
Glucosamine hydrochloride (glucosamine 480 mg)	600 mg
Ext equiv *Boswellia serrata* gum oleoresin dry	1.37 g
Equiv boswellic acid	148 mg
Hydroxyapatite (calcium 23 mg)	100 mg
Manganese amino acid chelate (manganese 5 mg)	50 mg
Copper gluconate (copper 300 µg)	2.14 mg
Zinc amino acid chelate (zinc 3 mg)	15 mg
Cholecalciferol (vitamin D_3 50 IU)	1.25 µg

- Glucosamine is an extremely popular supplement for the treatment of arthritis. There are two different forms commercially available, glucosamine hydrochloride, as used in this formula, and glucosamine sulfate. In most of the early research, the sulfate form, which is manufactured from the hydrochloride form and is sometimes stabilized with sodium chloride, was used. The hydrochloride form has a higher percentage of glucosamine and is considered by most practitioners to be the preferred form.
- Glucosamine is manufactured from seafood, so it is not recommended for people with seafood allergies. Also, some patients with diabetes report that glucosamine interferes with their blood glucose levels, so this formula should be used with caution.
- *Boswellia serrata* is an Ayurvedic herb used for inflammation. Minerals, especially copper, are very valuable in the treatment of arthritis.

Diabetes

A formula used to improve blood glucose control is listed in Table 5-12. It is important to consider the following points:

- This formula is intended to improve blood glucose control and prevent diabetic neuropathies, especially in type two diabetes. It is not intended to replace prescription medication for the treatment of these diseases.
- *Gymnema sylvestre* and *Momordica charantia* (bitter melon) are Ayurvedic herbs traditionally used in the treatment of diabetes. *G. sylvestre* inhibits glucose uptake,[76] and *M. charantia* is believed to increase the liver's utilization of glucose.
- B group vitamins, vitamin E, and zinc are designed to protect blood vessels from diabetic neuropathy.
- Chromium is the most important mineral in diabetes management. Although this is a balanced and helpful formula, more chromium is

TABLE 5-12 ■ Diabetes Formula

SUPPLEMENT	DOSAGE
Each tablet contains	
Gymnema sylvestre leaf	2500 mg
Standardized to contain gymnemic acids	62.5 mg
Momordica charantia fruit	1125 mg
Thiamine hydrochloride (vitamin B₁)	20 mg
Nicotinamide	100 mg
Pyridoxine hydrochloride (vitamin B₆)	10 mg
d-α-Tocopheryl acid succinate (natural vitamin E 50 IU)	41.3 mg
Magnesium amino acid chelate (magnesium 30 mg)	150 mg
Manganese amino acid chelate (manganese 50 µg)	500 µg
Zinc amino acid chelate (zinc 2 mg)	10 mg
Copper gluconate (copper 25 µg)	357 µg
Chromium picolinate (chromium 25 µg)	202 µg
Hesperidin	50 mg

required. While debate about the benefits of the picolinate form over a chelate continues, patients with diabetes would need 800 µg per day, rather than the 25 µg here. If 800 mcg is used, a chelate should be recommended, since results of toxicity studies on high doses of picolinic acid are not conclusive.

Prostate Health

Table 5-13 lists a formula used to promote prostate health. The following points are important to remember when this formula is used:

- This formula contains saw palmetto and *Epilobium parvifolum*, both well-respected herbs in the treatment of prostate conditions.
- Although sufficient and helpful as an herbal formula, this would not be sufficient to treat benign prostatic hyperplasia by itself. Certainly, more zinc would need to be added, and also selenium and lycopene.

Essential Fatty Acids

Table 5-14 lists a formula that provides EFAs to maintain a balanced diet. Before using this product, the patient should consider the following:

- This is a balanced formula containing ω-3, ω-6, and ω-9 fatty acids.
- Flaxseed oil is mainly ω-3; pumpkin seed oil is 45% linoleic acid, (ω-6), 15% ω-linolenic acid (ω-3), and 32% monounsaturated oleic fatty acids (ω-9); and borage oil is mainly ω-6.

TABLE 5-13 ■ Prostate Formula

SUPPLEMENT	DOSAGE
Each tablet contains	
Serenoa serrulata (saw palmetto) fruit	300 mg
Epilobium parvifolum herb	150 mg
Cucurbita pepo (pumpkin) seed	1000 mg
Urtica dioica (nettle) root	100 mg
Eleutherococcus senticosus (Siberian ginseng) root	50 mg
Centella asiatica (gotu kola) seed	100 mg
Smilax officinalis (sarsaparilla) root	150 mg

TABLE 5-14 ■ Essential Fatty Acid Blend

SUPPLEMENT	DOSAGE
Each capsule contains	
Linseed oil	500 mg
Borage seed oil	50 mg
Blackcurrant seed oil	50 mg
Vitamin E (*d*-α-tocopherol), (equiv vitamin E 50 IU)	33.6 mg
Rosemary oil	10 mg
In a base of pumpkin seed oil	400 mg

TABLE 5-15 ■ Headache Remedy

SUPPLEMENT	DOSAGE
Each tablet contains	
Tanacetum parthenium (feverfew) herb top flowers.	156 mg
Standardized to contain parthenolide	607 µg
Vinca minor (lesser periwinkle) root	1 g
Salix alba (white willow) bark inner.	250 mg
Thiamine hydrochloride (vitamin B$_1$)	50 mg
Riboflavin (vitamin B$_2$)	50 mg
Nicotinamide (vitamin B$_3$)	100 mg
Pyridoxine hydrochloride (vitamin B$_6$)	25 mg
Magnesium (as amino acid chelate)	100 mg
Homeopathic ingredient: *Nux vomica* 6C	5 mg

- Although all sources of the oils are all vegetarian, if the capsule is made from gelatin, the product is not suitable for vegetarians.

Headache/Migraine

A formula commonly used to alleviate headaches is shown in Table 5-15. Some points to consider in evaluating the effectiveness of the formula are:

- The herbal ingredients in this formula are well supported. Feverfew has a long history of use in the prevention of migraines because of its involvement in blocking the release of histamine, which causes vasodilation of blood vessels.[77] The active principle of *Vinca minor* is vincamine, which normalizes the cerebral vascular system. White willow is a source of salicin, from which aspirin was first derived.
- B group vitamins are included here to raise the pain threshold.[78]
- Magnesium is used successfully by many health care professionals in the treatment of migraines and other headaches, and there is evidence to support its use.[79]
- *Nux vomica* is a homeopathic ingredient traditionally used to relieve headache, especially headache associated with nausea.
- Although this formula is primarily designed for prophylaxis, the white willow, magnesium, and *Nux vomica* would also be suitable for acute headaches. For acute attacks, two tablets taken every two hours could be prescribed.

REFERENCES

1. Potter JD: Food and phytochemicals, magic bullets and measurement errors: a commentary, *Am J Epidemiol* 144:1026-7, 1997.
2. Institute of Medicine: *Dietary reference intakes for vitamin C, vitamin E, selenium and beta carotene and other carotenoids*, Washington, DC, 2000, National Academy Press.

3. Cameron E, Pauling L, Leibovitz B: Ascorbic acid and cancer: a review, *Cancer Res* 39:663-81, 1979.

4. Austria R, Semenzato A, Bettero A: Stability of vitamin C derivatives in solution and topical formulations, *J Pharm Biomed Anal* 15:795-801, 1997.

5. Burton GW, Traber MG, Acuff RV, et al: Human plasma and tissue alpha-tocopherol concentrations in response to supplementation with deuterated natural and synthetic vitamin E, *Am J Clin Nutr* 67:669-84, 1998.

6. Mastroiacovo P, Mazzone T, Addis A, et al: High vitamin A intake and early pregnancy in major malformations: a multicenter prospective controlled study, *Teratology* 59:7-11, 1999.

7. Deming DM, Boileau AC, Lee CM, Erdman JW Jr: Amount of dietary fat and type of soluble fiber independently modulate postabsorptive conversion of beta-carotene to vitamin A in Mongolian gerbils, *J Nutr* 130:2789-96, 2000.

8. Olson JA: Bioavailability of carotenoids, *Arch Latinoam Nutr* 49(3 suppl 1): 21S-5S, 1999.

9. Borel P, Grolier P, Mekki N, et al: Low and high responders to pharmacological doses of beta-carotene: proportion in the population, mechanisms involved and consequences on beta-carotene metabolism, *J Lipid Res* 39:2250-60, 1998.

10. Guillemant J, Le HT, Maria A, et al: Wintertime vitamin D deficiency in male adolescents: effect on parathyroid function and response to vitamin D3 supplements, *Osteoporos Int* 12:875-9, 2001.

11. Bahijri SM: Serum 25-hydroxy cholecalciferol in infants and preschool children in the Western region of Saudi Arabia. Etiological factors, *Saudi Med J* 22:973-9, 2001.

12. Sakhaee K, Bhuket T, Adams-Huet B, Rao DS: Meta-analysis of calcium bioavailability: a comparison of calcium citrate with calcium carbonate, *Am J Ther* 6:313-21, 1999.

13. Schrauzer GN: Nutritional selenium supplements: product types, quality, and safety, *J Am Coll Nutr* 20:1-4, 2001.

14. Kommuru TR, Ashraf M, Khan MA, Reddy IK: Stability and bioequivalence studies of two marketed formulations of coenzyme Q10 in beagle dogs, *Chem Pharm Bull (Tokyo)* 47:1024-8, 1999.

15. Le Bars PL, Kieser M, Itil KZ: A 26-week analysis of a double-blind, placebo-controlled trial of the ginkgo biloba extract EGb 761 in dementia, *Dement Geriatr Cogn Disord* 11:230-7, 2000.

16. Bhagavan HN, Wolkoff BI: Correlation between the disintegration time and the bioavailability of vitamin C tablets, *Pharm Res* 10:239-42, 1993.

17. Zia H, Amini H, Hekmatyar F, et al: In vivo and in vitro availability of commercial vitamin C tablets, *Pahlavi Med J* 8:414-8, 1977.

18. Elia M: Oral or parenteral therapy for B_{12} deficiency, *Lancet* 352:1721-2, 1998.

19. Kuzminski AM, et al: Effective treatment of cobalamin deficiency with oral cobalamin, *Blood* 92:1191-8, 1998.

20. Delpre G, et al: Sublingual therapy for cobalamin deficiency as an alternative to oral and parenteral cobalamin supplementation, *Lancet* 354:740-1, 1999.

21. Yung S, Mayersohn M, Robinson JB: Ascorbic acid absorption in humans: a comparison among several dosage forms, *J Pharm Sci* 71:282-5, 1982.

22. Black WD, Hidiroglou M: Pharmacokinetic study of ascorbic acid in sheep, *Can J Bet Res* 60:216-21, 1996.

23. Eberlein-Konig B, Placzek M, Przybilla B: Protective effect against sunburn of combined systemic ascorbic acid (vitamin C) and d-alpha-tocopherol (vitamin E), *J Am Acad Dermatol* 38:45-8, 1998.

24. Park JB, Levine M: Intracellular accumulation of ascorbic acid is inhibited by flavonoids via blocking of dehydroascorbic acid and ascorbic acid uptakes in HL-60, U937 and Jurkat cells, *J Nutr* 130:1297-302, 2000.

25. Bosy-Westphal A, Holzapfel A, Czech N, Muller MJ: Plasma folate but not vitamin B(12) or homocysteine concentrations are reduced after short-term vitamin B(6) supplementation, *Ann Nutr Metab* 45:255-8, 2001.

26. Reavley N: *Vitamins etc*, Melbourne, 1998, Bookman Press.

27. Zijp IM, Korver O, Tijburg LB: Effect of tea and other dietary factors on iron absorption, *Crit Rev Food Sci Nutr* 40:371-98, 2000.

28. Pantuck EJ, et al: Effects of protein and carbohydrate content of the diet on drug conjugation, *Clin Pharmacol Ther* 50:254-8, 1991.

29. 1999 MIMS Annual, Medi Media, Sydney.

30. Heck AM, DeWitt BA, Lukes AL: Potential interactions between alternative therapies and warfarin, *Am J Health Syst Pharm* 57:1221-30, 2000.

31. Kall MA, et al: Effects of dietary broccoli or human in vivo drug metabolizing enzymes: evaluation of caffeine, estrone and chlorzoxazone metabolism, *Carcinogenesis* 17:793-9, 1996.

32. Murray RK, et al: *Harper's biochemistry*, ed 24, Stamford, 1996, Appleton & Lange.

33. Booth SL, Centurelli MA: Vitamin K: a practical guide to the dietary management of patients on warfarin, *Nutr Rev* 57:288-96, 1999.

34. Carlton RM, Ente G, Blum L, et al: Rational dosages of nutrients have a prolonged effect on learning disabilities, *Altern Ther Health Med* 6:85-91, 2000.

35. Skinner JD, Carruth BR, Houck KS, et al: Longitudinal study of nutrient and food intakes of white preschool children aged 24 to 60 months, *J Am Diet Assoc* 99:1514-21, 1999.

36. Badner NH, Freeman D, Spence JD: Preoperative oral B vitamins prevent nitrous oxide-induced postoperative plasma homocysteine increases, *Anesth Analg* 93:1507-10, 2001.

37. Kalliomaki M, et al: Probiotics in primary prevention of atopic disease: a randomized placebo-controlled trial, *Lancet* 357:1076-9, 2001.

38. Botto LD, Mulinare J, Erickson JD: Occurrence of congenital heart defects in relation to maternal mulitivitamin use, *Am J Epidemiol* 151:878-84, 2000.

39. Chappell LC, Seed PT, Briley AL, et al: Effect of antioxidants on the occurrence of pre-eclampsia in women at increased risk: a randomized trial, *Lancet* 354:810-6, 1999.

40. Al-Kunani AS, Knight R, Haswell SJ, et al: The selenium status of women with a history of recurrent miscarriage, *BJOG* 108:1094-7, 2001.**

41. Black RE: Micronutrients in pregnancy, *Br J Nutr* 85(suppl 2):S193-7, 2001.

42. Chia SE, et al: Comparison of zinc concentrations in blood and seminal plasma and the various sperm parameters between fertile and infertile men, *J Androl* 21:53-7, 2000.

43. Thompson RD, Carlson M: Liquid chromatographic determination of dehydroepiandrosterone (DHEA) in dietary supplement products, *J AOAC Int* 83:847-57, 2000.

44. Baulieu E, et al: Dehydroepiandrosterone (DHEA), DHEA sulfate, and aging: contribution of the DHEAge study to a sociobiomedical issue, *Proc Natl Acad Sci U S A* 97:4279-84, 2000.

45. Nyce JW, Magee PN, Hard GC, Schwartz AG: Inhibition of 1,2-dimethylhydrazine-induced colon tumorigenesis in Balb/c mice by dehydroepiandrosterone, *Carcinogenesis* 5:57-62, 1984.

46. Schwartz AG, Pashko LL: Cancer prevention with dehydroepiandrosterone and non-androgenic structural analogs, *J Cell Biochem Suppl* 22:210-7, 1995.

47. Khorram O, Vu L, Yen SS: Activation of immune function by dehydroepiandrosterone (DHEA) in age-advanced men, *J Gerontol A Biol Sci Med Sci* 52:M1-7, 1997.

48. Nasman B, et al: Serum dehydroepiandrosterone sulfate in Alzheimer's disease and multi-infarct dementia, *Biol Psychiatry* 30:684-90, 1991.

49. Rao KV, Johnson WD, Bosland MC, Lubet RA, Steele VE, Kelloff GJ, McCormick DL: Chemoprevention of rat prostate carcinogenesis by early and delayed administration of dehydroepiandrosterone. *Cancer Res* Jul 1;59(13):3084-9, 1999.

50. Crook TH, et al: Effects of phosphatidylserine in age-associated memory impairment, *Neurology* 41:644-9, 1991.

51. Crook T, et al: Effects of phosphatidylserine in Alzheimer's disease, *Psychopharmacol Bull* 28:61-6, 1992.

52. Cenacchi T, et al: Cognitive decline in the elderly: a double-blind, placebo-controlled multicentre study on efficacy of phosphatidylserine administration, *Aging* Apr; 5(2):123-33, 1993.

53. Zhdanova IV, et al: Sleep-inducing effects of low doses of melatonin ingested in the evening, *Clin Pharmacol Ther* 57:552-8, 1995.

54. Attenburrow ME, et al: Low dose melatonin improves sleep in healthy middle-aged subjects, *Psychopharmacology* 126:179-81, 1996.

55. Arivazhagan P, Ramanathan K, Panneerselvam C: Effect of DL-alpha-lipoic acid on the status of lipid peroxidation and antioxidants in mitochondria of aged rats, *J Nutr Biochem* 12:2-6, 2001.

56. Vasdev S, Ford CA, Parai S, et al: Dietary lipoic acid supplementation prevents fructose-induced hypertension in rats, *Nutr Metab Cardiovasc Dis* 10:339-46, 2000.

57. Head KA: Natural therapies for ocular disorders, part two: cataracts and glaucoma, *Altern Med Rev* 6:141-66, 2001.

58. Maddux BA, See W, Lawrence JC Jr, et al: Protection against oxidative stress-induced insulin resistance in rat L6 muscle cells by mircomolar concentrations of alpha-lipoic acid, *Diabetes* Feb; 0(2):404-10, 2001.**

59. Suh JH, Shigeno ET, Morrow JD, et al: Oxidative stress in the aging rat heart is reversed by dietary supplementation with (R)-(alpha)-lipoic acid, *FASEB J* 15:700-6, 2001.

60. Fava M, Giannelli A, Rapisarda V, et al: Rapidity of onset of the antidepressant effect of parenteral S-adenosyl-L-methionine, *Psychiatry Res* 56:295-7, 1995.

61. Vutyavanich T, Kraisarin T, Ruangsri R: Ginger for nausea and vomiting in pregnancy: randomized, double-masked, placebo-controlled trial, *Obstet Gynecol* 97:577-82, 2001.

62. Power ML, Holzman GB, Schulkin J: A survey on the management of nausea and vomiting in pregnancy by obstetrician/gynecologists, *Prim Care Update Ob Gyns* 8:69-72, 2001.**

63. Sloley BD, Urichuk LJ, Tywin C, et al: Comparison of chemical components and antioxidants capacity of different Echinacea species, *J Pharm Pharmacol* 53: 849-57, 2001.

64. Mazza G, Cottrell T: Volatile components of roots, stems, leaves, and flowers of Echinacea species, *J Agric Food Chem* 47:3081-5, 1999.

65. Gallo M, Sarkar M, Au W, et al: Pregnancy outcome following gestational exposure to echinacea: a prospective controlled study, *Arch Intern Med* 160: 3141-3, 2000.

66. Colic M, Savic M: Garlic extracts stimulate proliferation of rat lymphocytes in vitro by increasing IL-2 and IL-4 production, *Immunopharmacol Immunotoxicol* 22:163-81, 2000.

67. Marshall S: Zinc gluconate and the common cold. Review of randomized controlled trials, *Can Fam Physician* 44:1037-42, 1998.

68. Voigt RG, Llorente AM, Jensen CL, et al: A randomized, double-blind, placebo-controlled trial of docosahexaenoic acid supplementation in children with attention-deficit/hyperactivity disorder, *J Pediatr* 139:189-96, 2001.

69. Arnold LE, Pinkham SM, Votolato N: Does zinc moderate essential fatty acid and amphetamine treatment of attention-deficit/hyperactivity disorder? *J Child Adolesc Psychopharmacol* 12:111-7, 2000.

70. Schroeder K, Fahey T: Over-the-counter medications for acute cough in children and adults in ambulatory settings (Cochrane Review), *Cochrane Database Syst Rev* 3:CD001831, 2001.

71. Langsjoen P, Willis R, Folkers K: Treatment of essential hypertension with coenzyme Q10, *Mol Aspects Med* 15(suppl):S265-72, 1994.

72. Mortensen SA: Perspectives on therapy of cardiovascular diseases with coenzyme Q10 (ubiquinone), *Clin Invest* 71(suppl 8):S116-23, 1993.

73. Crane FL: Biochemical functions of coenzyme Q10, *J Am Coll Nutr* 20:591-8, 2001.

74. Xia L, Bjornstedt M, Nordman T, et al: Reduction of ubiquinone by lipoamide dehydrogenase. An antioxidant regenerating pathway, *Eur J Biochem* 268:1486-90, 2001.

75. Miettinen TA, Alfthan G, Huttunen JK, et al: Serum selenium concentration related to myocardial infarction and fatty acid content of serum lipids, *Br Med J (Clin Res Ed)* 287:517-9, 1983.

76. Shimizu K, Iino A, Nakajima J, et al: Suppression of glucose absorption by some fractions extracted from Gymnema sylvestre leaves, *J Vet Med Sci* 59:245-51, 1997.

77. Ernst E, Pittler MH: The efficacy and safety of feverfew (Tanacetum parthenium): an update of a systematic review, *Public Health Nutr* 3:509-14, 2000.

78. Schoenen J, et al: High-dose riboflavin as a prophylactic treatment of migraine: results of an open pilot study, *Cephalalgia* 14:328-32, 1994.

79. Peikert A, et al: Prophylaxis of migraine with oral magnesium: results from a prospective, multi-centre, placebo-controlled and double-blind randomized study, *Cephalalgia* 16:257-63, 1996.

■ CHAPTER 6 ■

ASSESSMENT OF NUTRITIONAL STATUS

PAUL HOLMAN

> There is no gold standard for determining nutritional status.

This chapter considers issues of nutritional assessment through history-taking, examination, and biochemical investigation. It is important to note at this stage that there are no absolute standards by which we may define malnutrition. The onset of nutritional deficiency is usually insidious and often obscured by coexistent illness, medication, and drug use. No one assessment technique, either clinical or biochemical, is a reliable indicator of deficiency except in the most severe cases. There is also a lack of comparative data among different assessment approaches.

DIETARY ASSESSMENT

Figure 6-1 is a shorthand overview of nutritional biochemistry that is useful to bear in mind when thinking about nutrients and their roles, but it is not an exhaustive treatment. The middle equation describing structure and regulation is particularly useful in summing up the rationale behind many of our nutritional interventions.[1] It explains that essential fatty acids and amino acids are converted into structural and regulatory substances by means of enzymes that are usually dependent on B group vitamins and trace minerals. Temperature, pH, and antioxidant status are all variables that affect the process. A host of other endogenous and exogenous substances including toxins, hormones, and phytochemicals may influence any one enzymatic process.

In the assessment of nutritional intake, there are two areas for consideration: the quantity of nutrients ingested and the adequacy of this intake for the individual. Genetic makeup is an important factor here (see Organic Acid Analysis).

The estimation of actual dietary intake is fraught with difficulties. Retrospective methods of data collection, such as 24-hour recall, are dependent on memory and one can assume that there is underreporting of energy and nutrient intake by as much as 20%—even when a computer-assisted method is used. Accuracy may be improved somewhat by food frequency

ENERGY

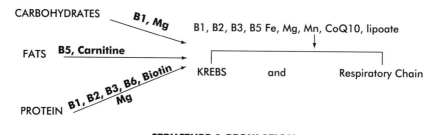

STRUCTURE & REGULATION

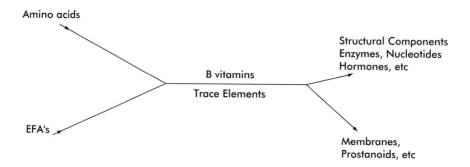

PROTECTION & DETOXIFICATION

FREE RADICAL CONTROL   LIVER DETOX

A   B gp
C   C
E   Mo
Se   S aminos
Zn   phytonutrients
Phytonutrients

FIG. 6-1 Overview of nutritional biochemistry. *EFAs,* Essential fatty acids; *Se,* selenium; *Zn,* zinc.

questionnaires, but this is time-consuming and still dependent on the vagaries of recall. Prospective methods such as food diaries may cause the subject to change eating habits or to consciously or unconsciously edit the record.

Having obtained an estimate of the dietary intake, one must decide how to process it. The data can be analyzed with a computer or "eyeballed" for a general impression of the number of portions from major food groups and the quality of food eaten. The former method is obviously more accurate but is still compromised by a number of factors including the following:

• The adequacy of the database for local conditions
• The variation in the nutrient content of foods and changing bioavailability

- Changing fortification patterns
- The production of "new" foods
- The use of supplements
- Many other confounding variables

In practice, I use 24-hour recall and then ask for a five-day diary before the next visit. I then "eyeball" the records for adequacy of portions and supplement this evaluation with a more detailed estimate of protein intake, using an abbreviated table of protein values. I emphasize protein because it is frequently inadequate in the patients that I encounter most often (i.e., women with chronic fatigue syndrome [CFS] or depression).

An estimate of nutrient intake level says nothing, of course, about the bioavailability of a nutrient for a particular individual. Usually, we cannot know about the issues of absorption, transport, cellular utilization, and loss. Ultimately, an answer can only be found through a therapeutic trial of the nutrient concerned. The recommended daily allowance (RDA) is a very approximate guide to adequacy in any one individual. RDAs set by different expert committees across the world vary by a factor of two or greater. This reflects the ambiguity inherent in a blanket recommendation that is then applied to individuals. Thus the RDA is a sort of necessary fiction against which we can test the therapeutic and potentially toxic effects of our prescriptions.

It is almost routine for clients to be taking either herbal or nutritional supplements. It is essential for one to actually look at the bottles for content figures, because there is a vast array of preparations that go by generic titles such as *B complex*. The actual content of similar-sounding preparations can vary 20-fold or more.

While discussing a client's dietary pattern, it is also useful to ask about hypoglycemic symptoms. I do not attribute a great deal of etiologic significance to functional hypoglycemia but do regard it as an indicator of the adequacy of protein/carbohydrate ratios, as well as a manifestation of excess refined carbohydrate intake, stimulant use, and stress. Functional hypoglycemia most commonly manifests as tiredness, irritability, and carbohydrate or caffeine craving in the late morning or afternoon.

At this point, it is usually convenient to ask about medication and drug use, especially in view of the frequency and significance of medication-nutrient interactions. Possible problems should be flagged at this point in the history.

Nutrient Deficiency Symptoms

Figure 6-2 is a schema representing the progressive development of malnutrition. Clinical symptoms of deficiency arise at a fairly advanced stage of the process. In prosperous, urbanized populations, gross deficiency symptoms and signs will be uncommon. The subtle manifestations of deficiency will appear as changes in subjective feelings of well-being, especially in regard to psychologic state and energy levels. The often progressive and insidious nature of nutritional deficiency means there is no clear-cut point at which malnutrition can be defined. There is no gold standard for determining nutritional status because[2]:

- There is no universally accepted definition of malnutrition.
- Assessment parameters are affected by illness and injury.
- It is difficult to isolate the effects of malnutrition (on outcome) from coexistent diseases.
- It is not clear which of the commonly used nutritional assessment techniques is the most valuable because of the paucity of comparative data.

As physicians, we must bear in mind these caveats while remaining cognizant of the fact that the symptoms and signs that we gather in our history-taking may be a reflection of disordered nutrition and may require further

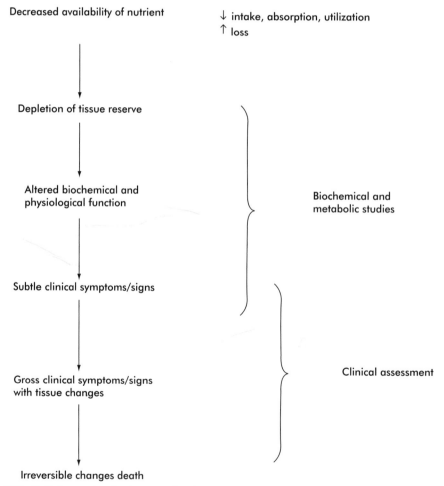

FIG. 6-2 Progressive development of malnutrition.

investigative effort. Ultimately, however, it is the process of enlightened experimentation that will guide our therapeutic direction.

Table 6-1 is a list of symptoms and signs of deficiency compiled from a variety of sources, but especially textbook descriptions of classic severe deficiency syndromes such as beriberi and scurvy. Readers are strongly advised to familiarize themselves with the basic deficiency syndromes. The best and most detailed descriptions are to be found in older textbooks. Lonsdale[3] found that the older descriptions provided a wealth of detail for his research into the effects of vitamin B_1 deficiency. The greater one's familiarity with a deficiency syndrome, the more likely it is that one will recognize the highly attenuated versions of the syndromes that we see in everyday practice. Occasionally, one will see an unambiguous deficiency sign such as angular stomatitis, especially among at-risk populations such as alcoholics or the elderly.

This table is not meant to be comprehensive and should be supplemented with other available information.[4] It has also been necessary to draw some arbitrary boundaries in a simple format like this. Thus the symptom of "dull hair" is mentioned with only protein and essential fatty acid deficiencies. Since other nutrients, such as vitamin B_6 and zinc, contribute to healthy protein synthesis, deficiencies of vitamin B_6 and zinc might also be associated with lusterless hair. It is axiomatic that nutrients work in teams and that there will frequently be overlap in their activities and therefore in the manifestations of their deficiency. However, for clarity's sake, I have largely confined myself to symptoms and signs that are described in the classic deficiency states. It is also for this reason that I have omitted a specific sign, white spots on the nails, because this manifestation is probably less specifically attributable to zinc deficiency than originally thought.[5]

A number of anthropometric measures can be useful. Weight and height can be related in the body mass index (BMI), which acts as a guide to risks associated with obesity. Changes in body weight can result from a number of factors, including differences in hydration, edema, and fullness of the gastrointestinal (GI) tract and bladder. Loss of muscle mass may be obscured by an increase in fat, as in age-related sarcopenia.

$$BMI = Weight\ (kg)\ /\ Height\ (m^2)$$

Subcutaneous fat measurements do not necessarily reflect body stores. There are numerous technical sources of error conspiring to produce inter- and intra-observer error. There is, of course, considerable research on skinfold thickness variation, with triceps skinfold thickness tending to correlate with estimates of total body fat in women and children and subscapular skinfold thickness correlating with total body fat in men. Individuals with values above the tenth percentile for waist/hip ratio are at very high risk for adverse health consequences, especially cardiovascular disease and diabetes.

In a detailed constitutional assessment, triceps, subscapular and supraspinale (above the anterior superior iliac spine) are the key skinfold

TABLE 6-1 ■ Nutritional Deficiency: Symptoms and Signs

SYMPTOM	PR	EFA	B₁	B₂	B₃	B₅	B₆	B₁₂	FOL	BIOT	C
Fatigue	✓		✓		✓	✓		✓		✓	✓
Mental Slowness	✓		✓	✓				✓	✓		✓
Poor Memory			✓					✓	✓		
Depression		✓	✓	✓	✓	✓	✓	✓	✓	✓	
Anxiety			✓	✓							
Irritability			✓								
Insomnia			✓	✓	✓	✓	✓		✓		
Sensitive to light				✓							
Sensitive to sound			✓								
Headache			✓		✓						
Burning sensation					✓	✓					
↓ Taste/smell											
Night blindness											
Burning eyes				✓							
↓ Appetite	✓		✓		✓			✓			
Indigestion			✓		✓	✓		✓			✓
Nausea			✓		✓						
Constipation			✓		✓			✓			
Diarrhea			✓		✓			✓	✓		
Bleeding gums											✓
Muscle pain										✓	
Leg cramps						✓					
Calf pain			✓								
Muscle weakness											
Muscle twitching						✓					
Joint pain											✓
↓ Wound healing	✓	✓			✓						✓
Dry skin		✓									
Oily skin/acne					✓						
Dermatitis	✓				✓		✓				
Sebomhoeic dermatitis		✓			✓		✓			✓	
Excess perspiration											
Hair loss	✓									✓	
Dull hair	✓	✓									
SIGN											
Anemia	✓							✓	✓		
↓ Blood pressure			✓		✓						
Cardiac arrhythmia			✓								
Glossitis				✓	✓	✓	✓	✓	✓	✓	
Angular stomatitis	✓			✓	✓				✓		
Magenta tongue				✓	✓					✓	
Papillary atrophy				✓	✓			✓			
Koilonychia											
Brittle nails		N	O	N		S	P	E	C	I	F
Follicular keratosis		✓									
Petechiae											✓
Perifollicular hemorrhage											✓
Hyperpigmentation	✓				✓			✓	✓		
Parotid gland enlargement	✓										
Peripheral neuropathy			✓		✓	✓	✓	✓	✓		

E	A	D	CA	MG	NA	K	ZN	MN	CU	FE	SE	CR
✓	✓	✓			✓	✓	✓			✓		
							✓					
		✓	✓	✓								
		✓	✓	✓							✓	
		✓	✓	✓								
		✓	✓	✓								
✓	✓	✓	✓	✓								
	✓						✓					
							✓					
	✓						✓					
	✓											
			✓			✓	✓					
										✓		
				✓						✓		
				✓			✓			✓		
		✓								✓		
			✓	✓								✓
			✓	✓	✓	✓	✓					
			✓	✓	✓	✓	✓					
			✓	✓								
								✓	✓			
								✓				
	✓											
	✓											
							✓					
							✓		✓			
							✓					
				✓								
							✓			✓		
									✓	✓		
		✓	✓	✓		✓				✓		
										✓		
										✓		
										✓		
										✓		
I	C											
	✓											
	✓											

measurements; maximum calf and biceps circumferences are taken for indices of muscle development and biepicondylar breadth of the femur and humerus as indices of bone size.[6] Height divided by the cube root of weight is taken as an index of linearity. However, for most clinical purposes, this measure of detail is not required to form an idea of constitutional type.

Since there is a relationship between enzyme kinetics and temperature, it would seem logical to get an idea of a patient's average daily reading. Surprisingly, there is little information on the relationship between body temperature and health; thus, we must rely on the clinical experience of the few investigators who have examined this topic. Barnes and Galton,[7] on the basis of results of metabolic studies, considered that early morning temperature reflected the basal metabolic rate and therefore thyroid function. This seems to be true in some cases, but it is apparent that low early morning temperatures may also reflect a poor adrenal response or a phase shift in the daily temperature cycle resulting from severe mood or sleep disturbance. Low energy intake, a low early morning blood sugar level, or iron deficiency may produce a slight temperature change. Barnes and Galton recommend that the underarm temperature be taken with a mercury thermometer for 10 minutes before the individual leaves bed or stirs around much. Menstruating women should do this on days 2, 3, and 4 of their cycle; all other individuals may record their temperature at any time. Temperatures below 36.5°C are considered less than optimal.

Wilson[8] prefers temperatures to be taken during the day 3 hours after rising and at two subsequent 3-hour periods. Menstruating women should not record their temperature 3 days before menstruation when it is highest. Wilson's benchmark is 37.0°C, taken orally with a mercury thermometer for 5 minutes. The problem with this approach is that there are clearly many variables that affect daytime temperature, including activity level, environmental temperature, food intake, body build, circadian and reproductive rhythms, and stress levels. However, Wilson believes that with a chart of sufficient duration, one can discern a pattern of substantially low temperatures, which can be used to guide therapy.

One can use both approaches, asking patients to record early morning temperature and having them obtain two subsequent readings at 3-hour intervals. A persistently low temperature tends to indicate hypometabolism, the cause of which needs to be investigated within the context of the other aspects of the clinical picture. Thus a modestly overweight, unstressed, adequately nourished, 40-year-old woman who has low temperatures in summer is likely to have hypothyroidism. On the other hand, low temperatures in a chronically stressed, young, ectomorphic woman on a low-protein diet are likely to be of a nutritional or adrenal origin. Daily temperature recording can also be very useful for monitoring treatment. Successful treatment strategies are often reflected in an increase in average body temperature, a testimony to overall improvement in metabolic efficiency. The accurate laboratory determination of basal metabolic rate would be ideal for assessment and follow-up, but this is not usually practical.

Acid-base balance is the other crucial factor that can affect enzyme function and many other facets of biochemical activity. Naturopathic literature, as well as some of the metabolic typing methods, places great emphasis on acid-base balance, often suggesting that unhealthy diets produce unfavorable acidic conditions in the body. There is no evidence for these assertions. The main determinant of blood and tissue pH is the blood carbon dioxide level, which is controlled largely by respiration. Carbon dioxide contributes 15 to 20 moles of volatile acid per day to the body. Contributions from other sources are minimal—about 1 mmol/kg from lactic acid with only 20 to 30 mmol from dietary protein. This underscores the importance of assessing respiration. Individuals with transient or chronic hyperventilation may experience a significant respiratory alkalosis with widespread effects on metabolism.[9,10]

Desktop capnometers that give a good estimate of lung arterial carbon dioxide levels are available. Individuals who are stressed frequently have alkalosis, and breath re-education is an absolute priority in their rehabilitation. In fact, other treatment methods will be of little value until a very faulty breathing pattern is corrected.

Typical Day

It is important to get a sense of the shape and content of daily life. A simple chronological account from waking to retiring can be filled out with appropriate detail as necessary. It is particularly relevant to know whether a person eats regularly in a relaxed way or erratically in a rushed manner. Are there mini-breaks during the day or does the person plough through till the evening in a mad rush? Does the person have time for herself and her enjoyment, or is she over-focused and constantly moving on to the next task?

The sleep history is conveniently taken at this point. Dement,[11] who is probably the world's leading authority on sleep disorders, has concluded that 50% of the North American population mismanage their sleep to the point at where it negatively affects health and safety. Dement also notes that Westerners tend to sleep 1 to 1½ hours less than their great-grandparents. He believes that the majority of individuals need 1 hour of sleep for every 2 hours spent awake. Individuals apparently needing less are often building a massive sleep debt whose consequences may be anything from a serious accident to health problems such as myocardial infarction or CFS.

An individual's biorhythmic style, whether that of a "lark" or an "owl," may give some idea as to his or her resilience to seasonal changes and travel over different time zones. Larks seem to be able to adjust their clocks rapidly, whereas owls need extra help to adapt to a new rhythm; consequently they may experience more sleep, mood, and health problems with a change in season, especially during autumn and spring. Seasonal mood changes are, of course, very common, and it is essential to ask whether an individual experiences a lowering of mood during the winter months.

The account of an individual's typical day will also give some idea of the sort of stress levels that he or she is experiencing. One can draw conclusions about coping style and resilience as one gets to know the person concerned.

Food Sensitivity

Food sensitivity is an important and vast subject, and the summary here is only of an introductory nature. This section does not cover the areas of inhalant and chemical problems, but it is important to remember that difficulties in these areas can precipitate or exacerbate food sensitivity.

The terms *food allergy, intolerance,* and *sensitivity* are often confused. Normally, a distinction is made between food *allergy* and food *intolerance.* The term *food allergy* describes an immediate reaction to small amounts of a food or food substance, and such reactions are usually immunoglobulin E mediated and persist for life. Individuals are usually well aware that they have the problem, and a limited number of foods such as fish, shellfish, eggs, nuts, milk, strawberries, and soy are involved. Physical manifestations involve atopic dermatitis, oral allergy syndrome, urticaria, asthma, upper respiratory problems, GI disturbance, migraines, and anaphylaxis. Food intolerance, on the other hand, tends to involve a larger number of foods and a delayed onset of symptoms. It involves foods consumed regularly in the diet, and symptoms will disappear if the food is avoided. There is a much broader range of clinical manifestations, and symptoms seem to fluctuate and affect different organ systems over time. Most of our discussion here concerns the phenomenon of food intolerance, although it should be said that the distinction between food allergy and food intolerance is not clear-cut.

The incidence of food intolerance in the general population is unknown but may be up to 25%. There is increasing evidence from well-controlled investigations that food sensitivity plays a role in a wide spectrum of conditions. Particularly strong evidence is to be found in studies on irritable bowel syndrome, eczema, migraine, rheumatoid arthritis, and serous otitis media. However, it is important to remember that almost any medical condition may involve food intolerance as a contributing factor.

Any food may be involved and some are more commonly implicated than others (e.g., gluten, cow's milk, egg, orange, yeast, soy, and peanuts), although there is no completely safe food. Most individuals react to less than six or so foods, although there is a tendency for the phenomenon to generalize. Symptoms may appear up to several hours after ingestion, and a delay of 48 hours is not unusual in the case of GI symptoms. In the overall course of food intolerance, onset may be gradual, beginning with, for example, headaches and progressing to slow deterioration of general health with symptoms referable to different body systems. On the other hand, onset may be acute after a viral illness, administration of antibiotics, psychological stress, or inhalant or chemical exposure. Fluctuation is the rule, with psychological stress playing a major part. Sometimes the problem disappears even with continued exposure, and symptoms may disappear during child-hood only to reappear later in a different form. Food craving affects up to 50% of patients, and patients who experience craving are more likely to have a history of atopy.

Clues to a food intolerance problem may be found in the family, child-hood, or medical history. Problem foods are those that are likely to be eaten regularly and that the individual would sorely miss during a fast.

The definitive diagnosis of a food intolerance can only be achieved by elimination and challenge. There are a wide variety of approaches, varying from complete elimination in the form of a fast to a modest elimination in the form a whole-food diet in which excess dietary junk is eliminated. The fol-lowing diet is acceptable to most people:

- Fresh white fish
- Lamb
- Venison and rabbit
- Biodynamic rice (brown or white)
- Pears/pear juice
- Vegetables, but not the following, which have high amine/salicylate con-tent: cauliflower, broccoli, broad beans, eggplant, tomato, olive, capsicum, alfalfa, cucumber, onion, spinach, mushroom, and zucchini
- Mineral or filtered water.

Some practitioners would exclude potatoes on the basis of their botanical relationship to the tomato-capsicum family.

If a person is able to follow such a diet for 2 to 3 weeks, it forms one of the most useful tools we have in nutritional medicine. Individuals almost invari-ably experience improvement on the diet. This strongly reinforces their per-sistence with such a regimen and the rather tedious process of food challenge that follows. Withdrawal symptoms from foods may be experienced, partic-ularly in the first few days, and often take the form of headaches, GI distur-bances, and irritability.

In the process of food challenge,[12] it is usual to test one food per day, except in the case of grain and milk products, which may require a 2- to 3-day interval after challenge. Incriminated foods need not be eliminated for-ever, and individuals should always be encouraged to test small quantities of these foods later to see whether there is a lower threshold of consumption that their system can tolerate. If dietary liberalization is not emphasized, there is always a danger that sensitivity will begin to generalize and a per-son may become more restricted in lifestyle as he or she begins to react to more foods and environmental chemicals as a result of deteriorating adap-tive mechanisms.

Serologic tests such as immunoglobulin G panels may be useful as a screen in circumstances in which elimination diets are difficult to implement (e.g., with children) but should not be used as a sole guide to treatment. Specific immunoglobulin A tests such as antiendomysial antibodies may be relevant when specific conditions such as gluten intolerance are investigated, and antigliadin antibodies may be useful in monitoring dietary compliance in gluten-sensitive individuals. Little credence can be given to the widespread practice of food intolerance diagnosis through electrodermal methods.

Assessment of Gastrointestinal Function

Assessment of GI function is clearly a very important part of the nutritional history. Some relevant areas of inquiry include:

- Pain and discomfort—timing, quality, and location
- Bloating and flatus—quantity and quality
- Timing of bowel movements—frequency and regularity
- Quality of stool—quantity, color, odor, consistency, presence of undigested food, whether it floats or sinks
- Relationship of the above to particular foods or food groups

Such information may enable one to form an idea of possible deficits in:

- Gastric acid production
- Fat emulsification, digestion, and absorption
- Enzyme function
- Gut ecology

In practice, these areas are so interrelated that one may be left with only the broad conclusion that GI function is inadequate and that more definitive information will require investigations such as gastric acid monitoring and stool analysis and culture.

Assessment of Hormonal Function

In our current state of knowledge, the assessment of endocrine parameters is one of the few ways in which we can obtain direct measures of control and regulatory functions. There is an intimate relationship between endocrine function and nutrition, with the thyroid, adrenal, and reproductive glands assuming special importance. Biochemical testing may be a poor guide to hormonal balance, and clinicians should acquaint themselves with both the subtle and gross manifestations of endocrine imbalances and the reciprocal relationships between nutritional status and glandular function.

Good accounts of hypothyroidism,[13] subclinical hypoadrenocorticalism,[14,15] and the relationships among some hormones, vitamins, and minerals[16] are available.

MANAGING THE INFORMATION

Hopefully, we are now in a position to begin to order the many facts that have been gleaned from the history into a coherent formulation. The initial history-taking may require up to 3 hours and is often still incomplete. However, after the first two or three sessions with a patient, we are in a position to develop a problem list, a probable diagnosis, and a provisional formulation.

The problem list will remain the connecting link throughout the diagnostic and therapeutic processes. The problem-oriented method of record-keeping is a good way of tracking the vicissitudes of a patient's medical progress. The provisional diagnosis, the conventional nosologic category, is an essential part of the formulation, even though it may be of limited explanatory value.

The initial formulation is a working hypothesis that seeks to explain the patient's situation in terms of organism-environment interactions. Its emphases will often reflect the particular interests and biases of the clinician concerned. The formulation also attempts to order the temporal profile of events in terms of predisposing, precipitating, and perpetuating (PPP) factors.

An example of an initial formulation follows the case of Susanna below.

Susanna is a 35-year-old teacher who had experienced moderately severe chronic fatigue in the months after a neck injury at work. She met diagnostic criteria for CFS and also had moderately severe depression, which has responded partially to moclobemide prescribed by her general practitioner. Her neck pain had never completely resolved despite extensive treatments for the original injury whose exact nature was never fully established, except that there was no obvious bony or soft tissue disease.

Before her injury, she described herself as "the life and soul of the party," as well as a compulsive organizer and someone who "never stopped." She also described herself as highly emotionally sensitive with a tendency to take on other people's problems.

Her general health had always been good, although she had a life-long tendency to GI problems that had partially responded to wheat avoidance. She had been a vegetarian for several years and had chronic sleep difficulties which preceded her accident. These difficulties were partly related to her husband's snoring. Examination revealed a mesomorphic ectomorph with no obvious nutritional deficiency signs. Blood pressure was low with a marked postural drop. There was no evidence of hypothyroidism in the history or on examination. Respiratory rate was increased at 20 breaths/min.

The problem list for Susan is as follows:

- Chronic fatigue
- Moderately severe depression
- Pain/residual physical disability
- Chronic GI problems
- Low blood pressure

The diagnosis would seem to be CFS with secondary depression. The picture in terms of PPP factors might be formulated as in Figure 6-3 in relation to problem number 1.

In listing potential PPP factors, we are generating hypotheses to be tested. In this case, there seem to be a number of areas in which the organism has

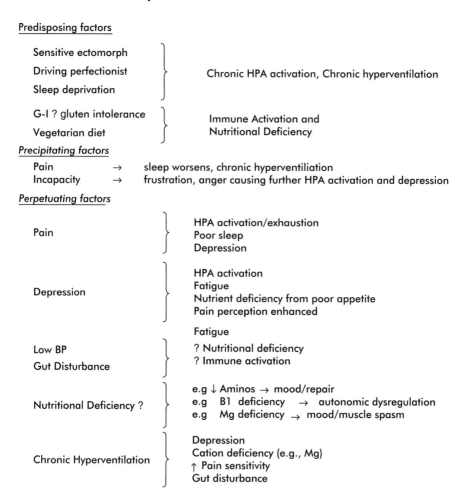

Predisposing factors

Sensitive ectomorph
Driving perfectionist ⎱ Chronic HPA activation, Chronic hyperventilation
Sleep deprivation

G-I ? gluten intolerance ⎱ Immune Activation and
Vegetarian diet ⎰ Nutritional Deficiency

Precipitating factors

Pain   →   sleep worsens, chronic hyperventiliation
Incapacity   →   frustration, anger causing further HPA activation and depression

Perpetuating factors

Pain
    HPA activation/exhaustion
    Poor sleep
    Depression

Depression
    HPA activation
    Fatigue
    Nutrient deficiency from poor appetite
    Pain perception enhanced

Low BP
Gut Disturbance
    Fatigue
    ? Nutritional deficiency
    ? Immune activation

Nutritional Deficiency ?
    e.g ↓ Aminos → mood/repair
    e.g B1 deficiency → autonomic dysregulation
    e.g Mg deficiency → mood/muscle spasm

Chronic Hyperventilation
    Depression
    Cation deficiency (e.g., Mg)
    ↑ Pain sensitivity
    Gut disturbance

FIG. 6-3 A picture of predisposing, precipitating, and perpetuating factors. *BP,* Blood pressure; *G-I,* gastrointestinal; *HPA,* hypothalamo-pituitary-adrenocortical system.

been stressed beyond its adaptational capacities so that our formulation might be represented as a matrix of interacting factors (see Figure 6-4).

Oversimplified though this formulation is, it provides clear avenues for investigation. Initially, it would be reasonable to check adrenal and thyroid gland function; to look for major nutritional problems such as deficiencies in vitamin B_{12}, folate, iron, magnesium, and amino acids; and to investigate the whole issue of food sensitivity and possible gluten intolerance, as well as GI function. While these avenues are being pursued, some inroads on the sleep problem could be made. Later on, it would be appropriate to look at lifestyle issues in terms of the person's temperament and character traits.

In this matrix, sleep occupies a central position because it has probably been important in predisposing, precipitating, and perpetuating the other

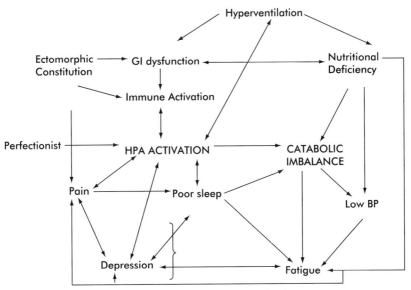

FIG. 6-4 Formulation as matrix of interacting factors. *BP,* Blood pressure; *G-I,* gastrointestinal; *HPA,* hypothalamo-pituitary-adrenocortical system.

problems. However, we could equally place disturbed nutrition at the center and explore some of the widespread ramifications of different nutritional deficiencies (see Figure 6-5).

It is possible that magnesium is of central importance here, because it is linked with GI dysfunction, hyperventilation, insomnia, depression, and musculoskeletal pain. We also remember the teamwork concept and magnesium's important relationship with other vitamins and minerals (e.g.,

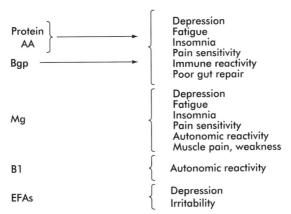

FIG. 6-5 Widespread ramifications of different nutritional deficiencies. *Bgp,* B group vitamins; *EFAs,* essential fatty acids.

calcium and B vitamins). The process thus follows the scheme detailed in Figure 6-6.

In following this process, considerable amounts of information may be collected. As one proceeds, summary sheets can be used to keep track of all the information. The principal summary involves tracking each problem and the accompanying investigations and interventions. This is especially useful in reminding one that interventions in one problem area will often have ramifications in another. Thus in the case of Susanna, one could lose sight of the low blood pressure and forget to regularly monitor it and thus miss the interventions that might be having a positive effect on it.

It is also useful to keep an investigation summary sheet (see Figure 6-7). Laboratories will often provide summary data over time, but these data are seldom in the short-hand form that is useful for examining the big picture. It is useful to look at the detail of a test when it is done and then summarize for the purposes of later review. A mass of data that must be scrutinized in detail every time one looks over the testing history is not efficient and can lead to oversights.

Testing for food and other sensitivities requires a detailed diary. The patient and clinician should keep a copy of the testing process and its results for future reference; it is an essential baseline when the reintroduction of foods is considered or the emergence of inexplicable symptoms occurs.

ENLIGHTENED EXPERIMENTATION

Keeping recommendations simple when prescribing changes can help pinpoint the effective therapies in each situation.

In recommending dietary changes or prescribing specific nutrients, it is important to keep things simple. It is only by doing one thing at a time that we can get any idea as to what is essentially therapeutic. It is worthwhile to

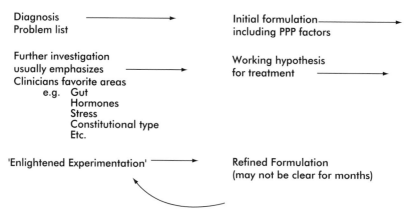

FIG. 6-6 Reforming the formulation. *PPP,* Predisposing, precipitating, and perpetuating factors.

Date			
FBE			
U & E			
LFTs			
Glucose			
GTT			
Cholesterol			
TGs			
TFTs			
Thyroid Antibodies			
Other Serology			
B12			
Folate			
Other B			
Other Vitamins			
Ca			
Mg			
Fe			
Other Mineral			
Oestradiol			
Progesterone			
Testosterone			
DHEA			
Cortisol			
Miscellameous			
HMA			
EFA			
CDSA			
Amino/Organic acid			
CO_2			
Temperature			

FIG. 6-7 Example of an investigation summary sheet.

consider that each nutrient or dietary substance has a number of effects, including the following:

- Physiological effects
- Pharmacological effects
- Toxic effects
- Interaction effects (drugs and other nutrients)

These effects are particularly evident with B vitamins, which, when given in higher doses, can exert marked metabolic effects, as well as produce potentially dangerous side effects. Vitamins B_3 and B_6 are well known in this respect. Similarly, an individual who is a particular metabolic type may react favorably to some B vitamins but not to others (see the section on metabolic typing). These considerations oblige us to be careful with dosage and, when possible, to test B vitamins individually before we consider broad-spectrum supplementation at doses well over the RDA. Marked effects on brain function or metabolism are not seen on a short-term basis with all nutrients, of course; but B vitamins, individual amino acids, essential fatty acids, calcium, and magnesium are examples of nutrients that can be tested individually as appropriate.

Against this approach, we must weigh the injunction that nutrients work in teams and that it is overall dietary change that is crucial. Testing teams of nutrients is fine as long as one clearly defines the testing boundaries (e.g., giving a broad-spectrum amino acid mixture for a while is a test of protein/amino acid deficiency), but it is unwise to continue use of such supplements without careful periodic review and further investigation.

Applying too many therapeutic strategies at once may provide a good short-term effect, but when difficulties or relapses occur, one will have little idea about how to intervene with elegant minimalism. Nowhere is this better seen than in the strategies for GI rehabilitation. It is not uncommon to see patients who have been prescribed enzymes, acidifiers, probiotics, and a long list of adjuvant nutrients when only scant information from history or testing is available. It is possible to gradually wean an individual off one item at a time after a suitable therapeutic effect has been observed, but this is both clumsy and costly. Better to start, for example, in the case of the GI tract, with only those factors that appear necessary from the history and results of laboratory tests.

The subject of nutrient interaction is complex and often paid insufficient attention by practitioners. Obvious interactions such as those between calcium and iron or zinc and copper are well known, but we should be aware that all supplements send a ripple of interaction through the system; and it is virtually impossible to imagine, let alone delineate, all the consequences. Watts and Rosenthal[16] have attempted to expand our appreciation of this area; even cursory inspection of their interaction diagrams gives us greater respect for the far-reaching beneficial and harmful effects of providing large doses of supplemental nutrients. We are now beginning to see the down side of nutrients once considered totally nontoxic (e.g., vitamin C). These effects may appear only in the long term and manifest subtly, but they do remind us of the dynamic relationship of yin and yang (e.g., an antioxidant can become pro-oxidant in the appropriate circumstance, or a nutrient originally given to make up a deficiency may become excessive).

These findings also point to the ultimate goal of dietary therapy, which is to establish a mix of foods that is supportive of optimal balance in an individual's constitution. In the final analysis, we want to wean off supplements as much as possible and instinctively balance our diets as circumstances in our lives change and our bodies adapt to the different phases of the life cycle. In short, appropriate eating for health is preferred to supplementation for a high-tech fix or life extension miracle.

BIOCHEMICAL TESTS

Biochemical testing covers a spectrum of investigation varying in complexity from simple static tests, such as measurement of serum vitamin levels, to the sophisticated monitoring methods of the metabolic unit. Static tests have their place, but in general, there is a trend toward functional tests that involve measuring the activity of an enzyme or metabolic pathway in which a particular nutrient is a critical component. Even so, it must be remembered that in biochemical testing, we are taking an isolated snapshot of a very limited facet of a particular nutrient's total spectrum of activity. Also relevant is the fact that body chemistry is constantly shifting in accord with biorhythmic cycles, environmental challenge, and dietary change. In test-retest situations, we should at least try to control for simple factors, such as time of day or even the day of the week and season.

Many confounding variables affect results of biochemical tests. These include age, sex, ethnicity, pregnancy, hormone status, organ disease (especially liver and kidney disease), medications, other nutrients, and generalized disease (especially infection). It is essential to have a friendly pathologist with whom one can consult to put test results within the context of the whole clinical picture. It is important not to get into the habit of treating patients primarily on the basis of their test results.

Protein Status

Total serum protein and serum albumin levels are not considered sufficiently sensitive indicators of protein status. Plasma transport proteins such as transferrin, retinol-binding protein, and thyroid-binding prealbumin have a shorter half-life and smaller pool size than albumin and are consequently better indicators of current protein status. Because they are negative acute-phase reactants, their levels tend to be lowered by infection.

Retinol-binding protein tends not to respond to depletion if there is vitamin A or zinc deficiency, and transferrin is affected by iron status. Pregnancy, exercise, and insulin level may also affect plasma transport protein levels. Kidney failure may increase levels and liver failure may decrease them.

Urinary 3-methylhistidine and urinary creatinine values are not very useful markers but insulin-like growth factor I may prove to be a sensitive indicator of protein status.

The meaningful interpretation of amino acid profiles, either plasma or urinary, is exceedingly complex, and practitioners need to form liaisons with laboratories that specialize in such analyses. Information relevant to a number of areas can be obtained by such investigation. These include dietary intake, GI function, renal function, liver detoxification, inborn errors of metabolism, and adequacy of vitamin and mineral status.[17]

As a rule, morning or 24-hour urine levels will reflect metabolic relationships and body pools better than the "snapshot" of a serum level. Blood levels, on the other hand, obviate the compounding effects of kidney function (normal and abnormal) and may be a better measure of the nutritional status of individual amino acids, especially those like methionine and tryptophan, which may be barely present in urine.

Exciting and clinically relevant research in the area of CFS and amino acid profiling is being done by the Collaborative Pain Research Unit at University of Newcastle, Australia.[18] Richards et al[19] studied a large group of patients with CFS and healthy control subjects; after subjects fasted overnight, amino acid and organic acid profiles were determined from first morning urine specimens. They found six distinctly different profiles of urinary amino acids in both patients with CFS and control subjects and concluded that six discrete types of amino acid homeostasis could be described with minimal within-group variance. This implies that in the population as a whole, there is a set of amino acid phenotypes that have different requirements for amino acid intake, including "semi-essential" amino acids. The emphasis of this research on assessing metabolic profiles as opposed to seeing amino acids as individual entities is important and highlights the necessity for systemic thinking in the area of organismic homeostasis. In short, it is a significant step toward a metabolic typology.

Alanine, glycine, glutamine/glutamic acid, and serine are the principal metabolites used by the clustering technique to divide the groups. Tyrosine, 3-methylhistidine, and 1-methylhistidine were excluded from the profiles because they are catabolic markers often increased in exercise, psychologic stress, trauma, or infection. Healthy control subjects and patients with CFS were distinguished by the extent of the characteristic amino acid deficiencies or excesses and by their profiles of organic acid and unidentified urine components.

Organic Acid Analysis

Like amino acid analysis, organics profiling is a nascent science in which rigorous research has not yet caught up with clinical use and commercial hype. The subject has been reviewed by Bralley and Lord.[20] The term *organic acid profile* was originally confined to analyses of water-soluble organic acids with ninhydrin negativity (thus excluding amino acids). However, with the inclusion of neutral compounds of fungal origin, we are better advised to use the term *organics profiling*.

In the recent history of clinical biochemistry, a significant impetus to the study of organic acids came through attempts to elucidate inborn errors of metabolisms. Lonsdale[21] has given us a fascinating and highly readable account of the evolution of his clinical philosophy from his early days as a researcher and pediatrician working with inborn errors to his later experience as a fully fledged practitioner of nutritional medicine. In common with other nutritional pioneers, he realized that nutritionally responsive, inherited disorders were but one end of a spectrum of biochemical competence and that many individuals had conditions that could be viewed as attenuated versions of the fully blown classical picture. His earlier account of thiamine dependency and the role of energy metabolism in the protean manifestations of dysautonomia is a modern medical classic.[3]

Organics profiling usually covers the areas outlined in the following sections, although space permits only a few examples of individual tests under each heading.

Energy Metabolism.   Assay of citric acid cycle intermediates may provide insight into metabolic deficits that are potentially correctable by supplying nutrient cofactors. Thus high citrate and *cis*-aconitate levels with low or lownormal isocitrate levels could imply an inefficiency in the enzyme aconitase, which affects the two-step conversion from citrate to isocitrate. This defect might be ameliorated by cysteine (as a glutathione enhancer), iron, or both.

The Newcastle Group (see Collaborative Pain Research Unit above) has found that a high citrate level is the most common organic acid abnormality in CFS and has the potential to deplete positive ions such as calcium and magnesium.[18]

A number of amino acids feed into the citric acid cycle. This means that a low level of α-ketoglutarate, for example, can potentially be corrected by added glutamine.

Fatty acid transport into mitochondria for oxidation may be impaired as a result of carnitine deficiency. This results in an alternative oxidation pathway, which leads to the production of adipic and suberic acids.

Vitamin Deficiency.   Methylmalonic acid is probably the best known example of an organic acid marker of vitamin deficiency. In this case, a lack of vitamin B_{12} compromises the activity of methylmalonyl-CoA mutase, which converts methylmalonyl coenzyme A to succinyl coenzyme A. The inherited form of methylmalonic acidemia is amenable to high-dose vitamin B_{12} therapy. An acquired increase in level as a result of poor vitamin B_{12} intake or absorption is a relatively late marker of deficiency.[22]

3-Hydroxyisovaleric acid is one of the characteristic organic acids excreted in excess when carboxylase activity is compromised as a result of an isolated genetic defect, multiple carboxylase deficiency, or dietary insufficiency of biotin. Urinary biotin and organic acid excretion have greater utility in diagnosing biotin deficiency than plasma and serum concentrations.[23]

A number of branched-chain keto acids (e.g., 2-ketoisovalerate from valine) can provide evidence of functional B group deficiency, especially thiamine.

Gut Dysbiosis. A number of organic acids may arise from the metabolic activities of gut microflora. 4-Hydroxyphenylacetic acid, for example, results from tyrosine breakdown in conditions of abnormal bacterial overgrowth.

Shaw[24] has drawn attention to abnormal products from yeast or fungal overgrowth, which may interfere with glucose metabolism, citric acid cycle activity, protein synthesis, and cofactor binding. These substances include arabinose, tartaric acid, citric acid, and citramalic acid.

Detoxification. Glucaric acid is a principal compound in phase II liver detoxification, and levels may be increased as a result of toxic exposure. Hippuric acid levels may be elevated with toluene exposure (but can be abnormal as a result of gut dysbiosis), and orotic acid is a sensitive measure of poor ammonia disposal.

Miscellaneous. Organic profiles usually contain far more compounds than have been listed here, but the clinical utility of many of these measurements has yet to be established. We should be cautioned by the years of research expended on neurotransmitter metabolites such as 5-hydroxyindoleacetic acid (from serotonin). Originally mooted as a possible marker of brain 5-hydroxytryptamine activity, the test came under increasing scrutiny with the discovery that cerebral spinal fluid 5-hydroxyindoleacetic acid seemed largely to be a product of the spinal cord and to reflect general activity level rather than brain serotonin release. How much less valid then is the idea that urinary 5-hydroxyindoleacetic acid may reflect something about the central nervous system and mood?

Vitamins and Minerals

The body, with its hierarchy of systems, is like a community of citizens. Events such as famine or epidemic disease that have adverse consequences for the community as a whole will have different effects on individual members; some will be affected greatly and some, minimally. The part can never reliably reflect the whole, and so it is with biochemical testing.

A number of tests are potentially available for each nutrient, and we are concentrating on those that are endorsed by scientific consensus as representing best current practice. However, these do not necessarily reflect the current pattern of use among a majority of clinicians or the profile of tests offered by laboratories.

It is also important to remember that the sum value of two poor or mediocre tests does not provide a result of superior inferential validity (e.g., a low hair magnesium level does not add weight to a low serum level).

Vitamin A.   Direct assessment of vitamin A stores by means of liver biopsy is the most accurate, although usually undesirable, method. Plasma measurements are not helpful because levels tend to be maintained until liver reserves are exhausted. Conjunctival impression cytology is a rapid, cheap, and non-invasive way of screening populations at risk (e.g., children in underprivileged communities). It evaluates the development of squamous metaplasia and loss of goblet cells from the conjunctiva but may be confounded by eye infections or other sources of irritation. The relative dose-response test has also been successfully used in human population studies. It depends on the release of holo–retinol-binding protein by the liver after the administration of a large dose of retinyl acetate; the difference between baseline and 5-hour levels of serum retinol gives an index that is elevated in deficiency states. Confounding factors include protein and zinc deficiency and liver disease.

Thiamine.   Thiamine level is best estimated by the erythrocyte transketolase stimulation test with stimulation in vitro by addition of thiamine pyrophosphate. Confounding variables include long-term alcohol consumption, diabetes, pernicious anemia, negative nitrogen balance, and infection.

Riboflavin.   Riboflavin level is usually measured by erythrocyte glutathione reductase activity with stimulation by flavin adenine dinucleotide. Confounding variables include alcohol consumption; diabetes; thyroid, liver, or kidney disease; glucose-6-phosphate dehydrogenase deficiency; vitamin B_1, B_3, or B_6 deficiency; and stress. Measurement of the whole-blood flavin adenine dinucleotide level can be a useful confirmatory test of long-term status.

Niacin.   The urinary ratio of 2-pyridone to N-methylnicotinamide is usually taken as a measure of niacin status. However, it has been found that this ratio is strongly affected by protein intake.[25] Studies suggest that the erythrocyte nicotinamide adenine dinucleotide concentration may serve as a sensitive indicator, especially when measured in relation to the concentration of nicotinamide adenine dinucleotide phosphate, which does not seem to decline in subjects on low-niacin diets.[26]

Pantothenic Acid.   Pantothenic acid is seldom assayed because of the resistance of humans to vitamin B_5 deficiency of dietary origin. Urinary excretion of the vitamin probably correlates best with intake.

Pyridoxine.   The urinary pyridoxic acid concentration is probably the best indicator of current intake because the plasma pyridoxal-5-phosphate (PLP) level tends to be maintained in the face of deficient intake.[27] Whole-blood or erythrocyte pyridoxal-5-phosphate (PLP) are probably better measures of B_6 reserve.[28] All of the tests mentioned so far can be confounded by medications, pregnancy, exercise, alcohol, smoking, or liver disease. Erythrocyte amino-transferase activity with PLP stimulation is attended by a number of problems. It is affected by B_1, B_2, and B_3 deficiency; liver and kidney disease; alcohol; high protein intake; stress and genetic polymorphism of the alanine aminotrans-ferase enzyme. Its activity may reflect longer-term B_6 status.[29] This is probably a reflection of the fact that pyridoxine-dependent enzymes avidly retain their coenzyme and a fall in aminotransferase activity may have to wait for new ery-throcytes containing less B_6 to be gradually released into the circulation.

Folic Acid. The serum folate concentration indicates recent intake of folic acid, whereas erythrocyte levels correlate better with long-term status and body stores. Confounding factors include alcohol, smoking, pregnancy, medications, and organ disease. Iron deficiency may affect red blood cell folate content.** Although homocysteine levels can reflect folate status, this measurement is also influenced by B_6 and B_{12} levels.[30]

Vitamin B_{12}. Vitamin B_{12} is routinely assayed as serum total cobalamins. The test can be affected by liver disease, myeloproliferative disorders, and medications. There is growing evidence that, especially in the elderly, there is a danger of neurologic damage if the usually accepted normal range (low limit = 150-200 pg/mL) is accepted as evidence of adequate B_{12} status. Thus Goodman et al[31] noted neuropsychological deficits that were reversible with B_{12}, despite levels being in the 250 to 400 pg/mL range. Similarly, in an examination of an elderly population in the Framingham study investigators concluded, from the use of the methylmalonic acid assay, that a better cut-off point would be 350 pg/mL.[32] The earliest marker of B_{12} deficiency is a low level of the transport protein holotranscobalamin II; this can be detected before a low serum B_{12} level. It is affected by liver disease and is not a rou-tine test as yet.

Vitamin C. The plasma vitamin C level falls rapidly in response to low vitamin C intake with a slower decline in leukocyte concentrations. However, measurement of leukocyte ascorbate tends to be the favored method of determining vitamin C levels, because levels correlate with con-centrations in other tissues. A problem in interpretation may arise because different leukocyte classes accumulate different levels of ascorbate; for example, granulocytes contain less ascorbate than mononuclear leukocytes. Thus trauma or inflammation, which increase granulocyte levels, may decrease total leukocyte ascorbate levels. Measurement of leukocyte vitamin C should therefore be accompanied by a differential count.

Vitamin D. 25-Hydroxycholecalciferol is generally accepted as a good measure of vitamin D status. In early vitamin D deficiency, there is a normal fasting calcium level, low to low/normal phosphorous level, low 25-hydroxy-cholecalciferol level, increased parathyroid hormone level and increased alkaline phosphatase level, and raised 1,25 dihydroxycholecalciferol level. With chronic deficiency, this pattern remains the same, except that there is a fall in 1,25 dihydroxycholecalciferol.

Vitamin E. Because there is a close relationship between serum vitamin E and lipid levels, measurements are best expressed in terms of vitamin E/lipid ratios. Platelet vitamin E is probably a more sensitive indicator of dietary tocopherol intake, but this assay requires more blood and a more elaborate laboratory procedure. A number of functional tests that rely on vitamin E's protective action against oxidation exist. However, measures of oxidative susceptibility are not necessarily indices of vitamin E status alone.

Calcium. Total serum calcium is maintained within close limits despite a negative calcium balance, and abnormalities are usually found only when there is marked disease such as hypoparathyroidism. Ionized calcium may be a more sensitive indicator of calcium balance but is difficult to measure and is affected by venous stasis and pH. It may give the first indication of a change in parathyroid function.

Twenty-four hour measurement of urinary calcium levels can be used to monitor calcium supplementation, but isolated readings are affected by too many variables including renal function. Alkaline dietary loads and metabolisable organic anions such as citrate, for example, reduce calcium excretion, whereas the opposite is true for acid loads and sodium.

The state of bone storage may be monitored through bone density estimation and indirectly through urinary telopeptides.

Magnesium. Muscle or bone levels are the best guide to magnesium status, because serum levels can be maintained at the expense of the limited stores. The magnesium load test correlates well with results obtained from tissue biopsy.[33] This test relies on the fact that a deficient subject will retain a greater than expected proportion of an intravenous magnesium load. A 1-hour version of the test is now available, and this may make its regular application more practicable.[34]

Urinary magnesium may be useful for monitoring repletion, but erythrocyte levels are probably not superior to results from serum.[35]

Iron. The three stages in the development of iron deficiency are well known. Initially, body iron stores fall and this is reflected in decreasing serum ferritin levels. There can be confounding effects from lymphoma, liver disease, infection, thalassemia, age, and sex. In the second stage, the lack of sufficient iron supply is reflected in a low serum iron level, decreased transferrin saturation, and increased erythrocyte protoporphyrin levels. Confounding effects for serum iron include alcoholism; infection; malignancy; deficiencies of B_6, B_{12}, folate, and vitamin C; and viral hepatitis. For total iron-binding capacity, the confounding effects include infection, protein-calorie malnutrition, alcoholic cirrhosis, malignancy, pregnancy, and viral hepatitis.

In the third stage, there is frank anemia, usually of a microcytic type. Confounding effects include infection, B_{12} and folate deficiency, chronic diseases, hemoglobinopathies, sex, and altitude.[36]

It is now standard practice to provide a panel of results for iron, including serum iron, transferrin, transferrin saturation, derived total iron-binding capacity, and ferritin. Taken together, these results provide a very good picture of iron status. However, as with B_{12}, it is important to remember that values of ferritin, for example, in the low-normal range may be associated with some measure of impaired energy or cognitive performance.[37]

Zinc.   There is no completely satisfactory test for zinc status, and the proliferation of static and functional tests over the years is adequate testimony to this fact. A low serum zinc level is a late marker of zinc deficiency, and in fact, all tests of tissue or tissue fluid level (including red and white blood cells, hair, nails, saliva, sweat, and urine) have marked limitations.

Zinc-loading tests are not routinely performed, and functional tests of zinc-related enzymes or proteins (e.g., thymulin) are still largely research tools. We may still conclude that the best way to test for zinc deficiency is through a therapeutic trial.[38]

Copper.   Serum or plasma copper levels are quite resistant to copper depletion. The assessment of copper levels in the blood is complicated by the fact that more than 90% of circulating copper is bound to ceruloplasmin, which is an acute-phase reactant whose level will be influenced by inflammation and a number of pathologic conditions. Pregnancy, hormone replacement therapy, and the contraceptive pill all tend to raise copper levels, which, even under normal circumstances, tend to be higher in women. Red blood cell superoxide dismutase is a potentially useful but not widely available test.

Manganese.   There are no reliable indicators of manganese deficiency in humans.[39] Whole blood levels reflect the soft tissue concentration in rats, but the situation in humans is less clear. Urinary manganese is not useful. Lymphocyte manganese superoxide dismutase can be affected by a number of disease states and inflammation.

Chromium.   There is no reliable method of chromium estimation, and as with other micronutrients, the best test is often a therapeutic trial. Thus glucose, insulin, and lipid values should be monitored before and after supplementation.[40] Response in blood glucose levels may be seen in 2 weeks, with significant effects on lipid levels taking several months.

Selenium.   Plasma selenium gives a fairly good guide to short-term selenium status and whole-blood or erythrocyte selenium to longer-term status.

Glutathione peroxidase (GSH-Px) activity can be monitored in plasma, erythrocytes, or platelets. Plasma activity is only useful in populations with low intakes, and erythrocyte GSH-Px responds only slowly to changes in selenium intake. Platelet GSH-Px is rapidly responsive and provides a good measure of short-term changes.

There are good correlations between selenium levels in whole blood and hair, and thus hair mineral analysis (HMA) may be a useful tool in monitoring selenium treatment[41] or occupational exposure.[42]

Iodine.   The urinary iodine test is enjoying a revival of interest because of the growing realization that there is a return of widespread iodine deficiency in the community.[43]

Hair Mineral Analysis

Hair mineral analysis (HMA) must be approached with caution, because there are many problems associated with the reliability of testing procedures and with interpretation of the resulting profiles. With respect to the first problem, split hair samples were sent to six laboratories in the United States, and the results were compared.[44] There were wide disparities in reported mineral concentrations, laboratory calibration standards, reference ranges, and dietary and supplement advice. The researchers recommended practitioners refrain from using HMA to assess nutritional status or environmental exposures. Although this conclusion is probably far too sweeping, it must be acknowledged that the interpretation of HMA results is governed by a number of difficulties.

Literature on HMA is often conflicting, and the author is not familiar with any recent review that attempts to summarize the current state of research. For many of the trace nutrients, however, one can find evidence to support good correlations with other parameters of nutrient status. There is a good correlation between hair and plasma selenium levels in healthy children.[45] Hair zinc content can be a good indicator of nutriture in children.[46] Hair is a good index of liver copper stores in experimental animals.[26] However, for each of these findings, evidence from other sources can be presented introducing caveats, contradictions, and complexities. This leaves the practitioner who wishes to use HMA no choice but to study the literature in detail for each element before braving the world of clinical application.

Accumulation of minerals in hair involves very different processes from those that are reflected, for example, in erythrocyte mineral levels. Hair minerals accumulate over time, and their concentrations are influenced by endocrine and dietary factors. Hair zinc levels increased in experimental animals when the protein/carbohydrate ratio increased.[47] Some endocrine relationships have been outlined.[16] It is not unreasonable to expect, then, that some aspects of HMA reflect metabolic activities and patterns not shown by other chemical tests. Watts[16] claims a relationship between certain mineral ratios and metabolic type. Practitioners who use metabolic typing systems must conduct their own research projects to investigate these possibilities further.

External contamination of hair with elements, such as copper, is a problem that cannot be completely eliminated by laboratory processing.

Overall, there seems to be some consensus among practitioners who use HMA that

- Hair mineral profiles are useful when performed by a reputable experienced laboratory that publishes material on its techniques and interpretive methodologies.
- HMA is a good screening tool for the initial assessment of patients. It is particularly useful in alerting one to the possibilities of toxic metal accumulation and in identifying trace nutrient deficiencies (e.g., calcium) that cannot be detected by other screening methods. However, HMA should never be used in isolation; it works best as a lead into other types of testing.
- Some HMA patterns correlate well with clinical realities (e.g., the low, flat profile of individuals with poor digestion/hypochlorhydria).
- The interpretation of mineral ratios (e.g., zinc/copper, calcium/magnesium) is probably more important than the absolute level of individual nutrients.

On a personal note, I have performed serial HMAs on myself over the past 20 years and have had the opportunity to observe the relationship of these profiles with other biochemical tests, with nutrient supplementation, and with my overall diet and health. I have been impressed with the consistency of the profiles, the correlation of low nutrient levels with other, corroborative tests, and the response of hair levels to mineral supplementation.

The often uncanny match between profiles from couples who share similar diets is further anecdotal evidence to support the idea that HMA reflects a genuine dietary reality.

Thyroid Function

Of all the endocrine systems, the thyroid merits special attention because of the significant incidence of thyroid problems and also the far-reaching effects of even minimal thyroid dysfunction. This discussion is confined to hypothyroid rather than hyperthyroid states. Hypothyroidism is not an all-or-nothing phenomenon, and it is becoming increasingly clear that thyroid failure encompasses a spectrum of dysfunction from overt myxoedema to subtle problems of cellular responsiveness manifesting in ill-defined clinical ways.

To do justice to this variety of clinical presentation, testing methods must be appropriately sensitive. Hypothyroidism is graded as shown in Table 6-2.[48] The presence of antibodies alone is sometimes referred to as *grade 4 hypothyroidism*, and the term *subclinical hypothyroidism* has been defined in ways that encompass grades 2 and 3 or only grade 3. One could add another

TABLE 6-2 ■ Grades of Hypothyroidism

	T_4	TSH	dTSH TO TRH	ANTIBODIES
Grade 1 *(overt)*	↓	↑	↑	+/–
Grade 2 *(SCH)*	N	↑	↑	+/–
Grade 3 *(SCH)*	N	N	↑	+/–

↓ Decreased; ↑ increased

grade (5) to describe a situation in which there is a reduced cellular sensitivity to thyroid hormones, which manifests with hypothyroid symptoms and a persistent reduction in body temperature.[8]

The thyrotropin-releasing hormone (TRH) test, which measures the change in thyroid-stimulating hormone (TSH) levels as a result of an injection of TRH, is becoming less available as more reliance is placed on thyrotropin levels alone. However, the normal range for TSH is almost certainly misleading, since TSH levels greater than 2 mU/I are associated with an increased risk of developing hypothyroidism.[49] In light of this, it would seem reasonable to conclude that high normal TSH levels, in conjunction with low normal thyroxine/triiodothyronine levels, might be an indication for a trial of thyroid hormone replacement. Further supporting evidence can be obtained from the temperature recording method described previously.

The urinary level of triiodothyronine may prove a good indicator of subtle thyroid dysfunction,[50] and the urinary iodine level should not be forgotten as part of the overall thyroid testing.

Results of other tests, such as measurements of total cholesterol and creatine phosophokinase, may be abnormal, but they lack specificity.

REFERENCES

1. Rudin D: The three pellagras, *J Orthomolecular Psychiatry* 12:91-110, 1983.
2. Meguid M, Laviano A: Clinical examination. In Sadler MJ, editor: *Encyclopaedia of human nutrition*, San Diego, 1998, Academic Press.
3. Lonsdale D: *A nutritionist's guide to the clinical use of vitamin B_1*, Tacoma, WA, 1987, Life Sciences Press.
4. McLaren DS: *Color atlas of nutritional disorders*, Chicago, 1981, Year Book.
5. Pfeiffer CC: *Mental and elemental nutrients: a physician's guide to nutrition and health care*, Chicago, 1976, Keats Publishing.
6. Carter JEL, Heath BH: *Somatotyping development and applications*, Cambridge, 1990, Cambridge University Press.
7. Barnes BO, Galton L: *Hypothyroidism: the unsuspected illness*, New York, 1978, Thomas Y Crowell.
8. Wilson ED: *Doctor's manual for Wilson's syndrome*, ed 3, 1997, Muskeegee Medical Publishing.
9. Fried R: *The psychology and physiology of breathing*, New York, 1993, Plenum Press.
10. Gardner WN: The pathophysiology of hyperventilation disorders, *Chest* 109:416-534, 1996.

11. Dement W: *The promise of sleep*, London, 2001, Pan Books.
12. Brostoff J, Gamlin L: *The complete guide to food allergy and intolerance*, London, 1989, Bloomsbury Publishing.
13. Arem R: *The thyroid solution*, New York, 1999, Ballantine Books.
14. Tintera J: The hypoadrenocortical state and its management, *N Y State J Med* 35(13), 1955. (Reproduced in Light MH, editor: *Hypoadrenocorticism*, 1974, Adrenal Metabolic Research Society.)
15. McK W, Jefferies MD: *Safe uses of cortisol*, Springfield, IL, 1981, Charles C Thomas.
16. Watts DL, Rosenthal BE: *Trace elements and other essential nutrients: clinical application of tissue mineral analysis*, Houston, TX, 1995, Longevity Press.
17. Pangborn J: *When should amino acids be measured?* Chicago, 1994, Bionostics West.
18. McGregor NR, Dunstan RH, Zerbes M, et al: Preliminary determination of a molecular basis to chronic fatigue syndrome, *Biochem Mol Med* 57:73-80, 1996.
19. Richards RS, Roberts TK, McGregor NR, et al: Blood parameters indicative of oxidative stress are associated with symptom expression in chronic fatigue syndrome, *Redox Rep* 5:35-41, 2000.
20. Bralley JA and Lord RS: Organic Acid Profiling. In Pizzorno JE, Murray MT, editors: *Textbook of Natural Medicine*, 1999, Churchill Livingstone.
21. Lonsdale D: *Why I left orthodox medicine: healing for the 21st century*, Charlottesville, VA, 1994, Hampton Roads Publishing.
22. Herbert V: Vitamin B_{12}. In Brown M, editor: *Present knowledge in nutrition*, Washington, DC, 1990, International Life Sciences Foundation.
23. Mock DM: Biotin. In Brown M, editor: *Present knowledge in nutrition*, Washington, DC, 1990, International Life Sciences Foundation.
24. Shaw W: *Biological treatments for autism and PDD*, Lenexa, KS, 2001, Great Plains Laboratory.
25. Shibata K, Matsuo H: The relationship between protein intake and the ratio of N methyl -2-pyridone and N methylnicotinamide, *Agric Biol Chem* 52:2747-52, 1988.
26. Jacob RA, Swendseid ME, McKee RW, et al: Biochemical markers for assessment of niacin status in young men: urinary and blood levels of niacin metabolites, *J Nutr* 119:591-8, 1989.
27. Powers JS, Zimmer J, Meurer K, et al: Direct assay of vitamins B_1, B_2, and B_6 in hospitalized patients: relationship to level of intake, *J Parenter Enteral Nutr* 17:315-6, 1993.
28. Vermaak WJ, Ubbink JB, Barnard HC, et al: Vitamin B_6 nutritional status and cigarette smoking, *Am J Clin Nutr* 51:1058-61, 1990.
29. Leklem JE: Vitamin B_6: a status report, *J Nutr* 120(suppl 11):1503-7, 1990.
30. Bates CJ, Pentieva KD, Prentice A, et al: Plasma pyridoxal phosphate and pyridoxic acid and their relationship to plasma homocysteine in a representative sample of British men and women aged 65 years and over, *Br J Nutr* 81:191-201, 1999.
31. Goodman M, Chen XH, Darwish D: Are US lower normal B_{12} limits too low? *J Am Geriatr Soc* 44:1274-5, 1996.
32. Lindenbaum J, Rosenberg IH, Wilson PW, et al: Prevalence of cobalamin deficiency in the Framingham elderly population, *Am J Clin Nutr* 60:2-11, 1994.
33. Hessov IB: Magnesium deficiency in Crohn's disease, *Clin Nutr* 9:297-8, 1990.

34. Rob PM, Dick K, Bley N, et al: Can one really measure magnesium deficiency using the short-term magnesium loading test? *J Intern Med* 246:373-8, 1999.
35. Basso LE, Ubbink JB, Delport R: Erythrocyte magnesium concentration as an index of magnesium states: a perspective from a magnesium supplementation study, *Clin Chim Acta* 291:1-8, 2000.
36. Fidanza F: Biochemical assessment. In Sadler MJ, editor: *Encyclopedia of human nutrition, vol 2,* San Diego, 1999, Academic Press.
37. Tucker DM, Sandstead HH, Penland JG, et al: Iron status and brain function: serum ferritin levels associated with asymmetries of cortical electrophysiology and cognitive performance, *Am J Clin Nutr* 39:105-13, 1984.
38. Evans GW: Zinc and its deficiency diseases, *Clin Physiol Biochem* 4:94-8, 1986.
39. Keen CL, Jodi L, Zidenberg-Cherr E, Ziedenberg-Cherr S: Manganese. In Sadler MJ, editor: *Encyclopedia of human nutrition, vol 3,* San Diego, 1999, Academic Press.
40. Anderson RA: Chromium, glucose tolerance, diabetes and lipid metabolism, *J Adv Med* 8:37-49, 1995.
41. Terada A, Nakada M, Nakada K, et al: Selenium administration to a ten year old boy receiving long term parenteral nutrition—change in selenium concentration in blood and hair, *J Trace Elem Med Biol* 10:1-5, 1996.
42. Srivastava AK, Gupta BN, Bihari V: Hair selenium as a monitoring tool for occupational exposure, *J Toxicol Environ Health* 51:437-45, 1997.
43. Eastman CJ: Where has all our iodine gone? *Med J Aust* 171:455-6, 1999.
44. Seidel S, Kreutzer R, Smith D, et al: Assessment of commercial laboratories performing hair mineral analysis, *JAMA* 285:67-72, 2001.
45. Mengubas K, Diab NA, Gokmen G, et al: Selenium status of healthy Turkish children, *Biol Trace Elem Res* 54:163-72, 1996.
46. Weber CW, Nelson GW, Vasquez de Vaquera M, et al: Trace elements in the hair of healthy and malnourished children, *J Trop Pediatr* 36:230-4, 1990.
47. Gershoff S, McGandy R, Nondastuda A, et al: Trace minerals in human and rat hair, *Am J Nutr* 30:868-72, 1977.
48. Haggerty JJ, Prange AJ: Borderline hypothyroidism and depression, *Annu Rev Med* 46:37-46, 1995.
49. Weetman AP: Hypothyroidism: screening and subclinical disease, *BMJ* 314:1175-8, 1997.
50. Baisier WV, Hertoghe J, Eeckhaut W: Thyroid insufficiency: is TSH measurement the only tool? *J Nutr Environ Med* 10:105-15, 2000.

■ CHAPTER 7 ■

LABORATORY DIAGNOSIS AND NUTRITIONAL MEDICINE

COLM BENSON

> Laboratory investigations do not always provide definitive answers; "In food tolerance . . . all responsible authorities accept that we have no reliable test and that the diagnosis rests on a purely clinical elimination and challenge."[1]

INTRODUCTION

Subtle biochemical and tissue changes can be detected long before signs and symptoms suggest the presence of disease. Laboratory investigations are used to predict disease and to confirm a working diagnosis in persons with suspected disease. Biochemical testing covers a wide spectrum of investigation and includes both simple and sophisticated testing methods.

Body chemistry is constantly shifting in accord with biorhythmic cycles, environmental challenge, and dietary change. Because these variables can affect the results of biochemical tests, it is wise to schedule tests so that these conditions, including time of day and season, are parallel. It is essential to put test results within the context of the whole clinical picture.

This chapter focuses on how measurement of various chemicals can serve as diagnostic markers. Particular attention is paid to how these various laboratory assessments can be used as a guide to disease prevention and patient care. The assessments detailed describe those test most frequently requested by practitioners. These assessments are available to both medical and non-medical practitioners.

ESSENTIAL FATTY ACIDS (EFAS)

Edible fats and oils, which have been used for thousands of years by mankind for cooking or adding taste to food, are mainly triglycerides. These consist of one part glycerol and three parts fatty acids, with the latter accounting for about 95% of the weight of triglycerides. The fatty acids are either saturated (solid at room temperature) or unsaturated (liquid at room temperature). The unsaturated group can be further divided into the *cis*-monounsaturated type (one double bond), as in olive oil, or polyunsaturated fatty acid (PUFA) with two or more *cis*-double bonds, as in common vegetable and fish oils.[2]

There are also *trans*-monounsaturated fatty acids found at a relatively low level (<5%) in fats from ruminant animals (cattle, sheep, and goats) and in partially hydrogenated oils found in some margarines. The PUFAs can also be subdivided into two types, the omega-6 type (as in most common vegetable oils) and the omega-3 type (as in fish oils and certain vegetable oils). The PUFAs are essential for humans.[3]

Of all the fatty acids found in foods, only linoleic acid (LA) and alpha-linolenic acid (ALA) cannot be made in the body; thus these two are essential, like most vitamins. Discovered in the 1930s, LA is the parent or precursor for the omega-6 (or n-6) series of PUFA. The omega, or n-6, notation means that the first double bond in this family of PUFA is 6 carbons from the methyl end of the molecule. ALA is the parent fatty acid for the omega-3 (or n-3) PUFA. ALA is called alpha-linolenic acid to distinguish it from gamma-linolenic acid (GLA), found in the omega-6 series.

The EFAs are converted in the liver to long-chain PUFA with more carbon atoms and more double bonds. These long-chain PUFA retain the omega type of the parent EFA; thus the body forms a series of omega-6 and omega-3 PUFA. The speed or efficiency of processing the EFA to long-chain PUFA, particularly in the case of the omega-3 PUFA series, is slow in humans. Furthermore, there is competition between LA and ALA for metabolism to the long-chain PUFA at the first delta-6-desaturase step, so that diets rich in LA and relatively poor in ALA lead to substantially enhanced tissue levels of the long-chain omega-6 PUFA relative to long-chain omega-3 PUFA. The ratio of omega-6 to omega-3 PUFA in red blood cells, platelets, plasma, and plasma phospholipids can be used to diagnose low dietary intakes of omega-3 PUFA. A raised level of 22:5 n-6 relative to docosahexaenoic acid (DHA) (22:6 n-3) is also an index of omega-3 deficiency.[4,5]

> The ratio of omega-6 to omega-3 PUFA can be used to diagnose low dietary intakes of omega-3 PUFA.

The Effect of Fatty Acids

Diets rich in fats and oils containing saturated and *trans*-fatty acids raise plasma cholesterol levels, leading to an increased risk for coronary heart disease.[6] The *cis*-unsaturated fatty acids generally counteract this effect, so there has been much emphasis on reducing the intake of saturated and *trans*-monounsaturated fats (found in animal fats, pastry, biscuits, margarine, etc.) and increasing the intake of *cis*-monounsaturated oils (olive and canola oils) and PUFA (flaxseed, sardine, tuna). The ratio of saturated plus *trans* fatty acids to unsaturated fatty acids in plasma can indicate the type of diet being consumed.[7]

Essential Fatty Acids and Health

The functions of LA and other omega-6 PUFA include a role in growth, reproduction, skin and hair condition, and wound healing. These effects occur largely through the actions of LA or other omega-6 PUFA in cell membranes (structure and function). LA also reduces plasma cholesterol levels, reduces platelet aggregation, and serves as a precursor of cell membrane arachidonic acid (AA), which in turn is a substrate for the hormone-like substances known as eicosanoids (formerly known as prostaglandins) and leukotrienes. These substances play vital roles in the regulation of tissue function, cell signaling, and, in particular, gene transcription events.[8]

The omega-3 PUFA were neglected as essential dietary nutrients for 50 years; however, it is now recognized that they play an essential role in human health in regulating or balancing the effects of the omega-6 PUFA. There are three main omega-3 PUFA: ALA (the parent of this series), eicosapentaenoic acid (EPA), and DHA. The latter are particularly effective in lowering plasma triglyceride levels, and they play a structural role in cell membranes in the brain and retina; in ion transport in tissues, including the heart; and in the regulation of inflammatory conditions. EPA competes with AA for metabolism by the cyclooxygenase to thromboxane, prostacyclin, and leukotrienes, leading to a downregulation of proinflammatory eicosanoid-related cellular events.[8]

Diets relatively poor in omega-3 PUFA are considered to have an exaggerated metabolism of AA to proinflammatory eicosanoids, whereas those rich in EPA are considered to reduce this conversion. With diets rich in EPA and DHA, for example, there is a reduction in thromboxane A_2 (TXA$_2$) formation and a decreased TXA2/prostacyclin ratio, which is associated with reduced platelet aggregation. Vitamin E is also considered to reduce the production of proinflammatory eicosanoids by inhibition of the release of AA from membrane phospholipids and to reduce platelet aggregation.[9] There is widespread interest in the role of omega-3 PUFA in maternal health and neurologic function in infants, heart disease, psoriasis, asthma, depression, attention deficit hyperactivity disorder (ADHD) in children, bowel cancer, non-insulin dependent diabetes mellitus, schizophrenia, the learning performance of school children, transplantation, bone formation, and the reduction of the severity of symptoms of arthritis.[10,11]

Balance in the Diet

The diets of Australians and people in most Western societies contain relatively high levels of omega-6 fatty acids and low levels of omega-3 fatty acids. Typically, the omega-6 intake is about 20 g/day and the omega-3 intake not more than 2 g/day. Within this 2 g/day, the DHA and EPA content is about

100 mg/day because of low fish intake, which is a major source of the long-chain omega-3 fatty acids.[12] Many organizations, including the NHMRC,[13] recommend an increased intake of DHA and EPA. A figure of 210 mg/day has been recommended in the United Kingdom.[13] However, a recent ISS-FAL[14] meeting recommended the intake of long-chain omega-3 PUFA be increased to 650 mg/day on the results of the GISSI Prevenzione Trial of 1999. In addition, there are suggestions that our diet should have a balance of omega-6 to omega-3 type of less than 5:1,[14] whereas presently it is between 10:1 to 20:1 in many countries. It has been estimated that humans evolved eating diets in which the omega-6 to omega-3 ratio was close to 1:1.[14]

Biochemistry

When diets lack the EFAs, oleic acid is converted to a novel PUFA (Mead acid, MA, or 20:3 n-9) via the same enzymatic pathways used to metabolize LA and ALA. The measurement of the MA/AA ratio in plasma and red blood cells can be used to indicate EFA deficiency.[4,5]

Use the MA/AA ratio to detect EFA deficiency.

The major site of EFA metabolism is in the liver, although it is believed that other tissues may have the capacity to synthesize DHA from 22:5 n-3 produced by the liver (e.g., brain, and retina). The long-chain PUFA can be transported to the peripheral tissues from the liver via the plasma lipoproteins. The rate-limiting enzyme for production of long-chain PUFA is the first step, the delta-6-desaturase. Factors considered to reduce the activity of the delta-6-desaturase include fasting, glucagon, glucocorticoids, diabetes, aging, and alcohol.[10,11]

Gamma-Linolenic Acid (GLA)

The reason for the interest in GLA is that it is an omega-6 PUFA, which enters the metabolic pathway after the first delta-6-desaturase step, thus bypassing this rate limiting. Oils rich in GLA, such as evening primrose oil, can increase the blood levels of dihomogammalinolenic acid (20:3 n-6), which is the precursor of prostaglandin E_1 (PGE_1). This eicosanoid has antagonistic actions to eicosanoids derived from AA (e.g., PGE_2). Evening primrose oil is currently used to treat atopic eczema and there is evidence that it improves nerve function in a safe and effective manner in patients with established diabetic neuropathy.[3]

Deficiency of Essential Fatty Acids (EFAs)

Adult humans were not thought to develop EFA deficiency; however, this condition does occur in situations of malabsorption (short-bowel syndrome, leaky gut, etc.). The classical symptoms of EFA deficiency are those related to skin (dry, scaly, poor wound healing) and hair (dull, dandruff); however, confirmation is required biochemically by assay of red blood cell, platelet, plasma, and plasma phospholipid fatty acids.[15]

Deficiency of the EFA results in the synthesis of significant quantities of MA (20:3 n-9/5,8,11-eicosatrienoic acid), which is a metabolite of oleic acid, a nonessential 18-carbon fatty acid. Oleic acid is only converted to MA when there are low levels of the usual EFA substrates, because it is a poor competitor for the delta-6-desaturase enzyme. Typically, an EFA-deficient pattern shows raised levels of MA (a ratio of MA/AA > 0.4), low levels of LA and ALA, and raised levels of palmitoleic (16:1 n-7) and oleic acids (18:1n-9). A scheme has been proposed for examining fatty acid data to allow for interpretation of cases of EFA deficiency based on ratios of essential/nonessential fatty acids.[16]

The omega-6 to omega-3 balance in tissues can be assessed by analysis of red blood cells, platelet, plasma, and plasma phospholipid fatty acids. In particular, the omega-3 status can be assessed by examining the ratio of omega-6/omega-3 PUFA, the AA/EPA ratio, the 22:5 n-6 to 22:6 n-3 ratio and the total proportion or concentration of omega-3 PUFA.[16]

High intakes of saturated or *trans* fatty acids are reflected by increases in the levels of these fatty acids in plasma and platelet lipids.[16]

cis-Monounsaturated Fatty Acids and Cellular Aging

The mitochondrial theory of aging suggests that this phenomenon is the consequence of random somatic mutations in mitochondrial deoxyribonucleic acid (DNA), induced by long-term exposure to free radical attack. There are two potential dietary means of delaying the effects of free radicals on cellular aging, enrichment of mitochondrial membranes with monounsaturated fatty acids, and supplementation with antioxidants.[9,17]

Blood Fatty Acid Level Assessment

Plasma fatty acids have been considered to reflect short-term dietary changes, whereas red blood cells and platelets are considered to give a longer term view of fatty acid status. Recent data have shown that plasma phospholipids can provide a long-term view of intake.[18]

Analysis of total plasma fatty acids can allow determination of ratios of essential to nonessential fatty acids to determine EFA status and conditions of high intakes of saturated and *trans*-monounsaturated fatty acids. Red blood cell fatty acids can be used to detect EFA deficiency and omega-3 PUFA deficiency. Platelet fatty acids can be used to detect EFA deficiency, omega-3 PUFA deficiency, and conditions of high intakes of saturated fatty acids. Plasma phospholipid fatty acids can be used to detect EFA deficiency and omega-3 PUFA deficiency.[18]

The expression of the results from fatty acid analyses has usually been as a percentage composition of all fatty acids detected in the sample rather than as a specific concentration of individual fatty acids. The former method is still in widespread use, with most reference ranges throughout the world reported this way. However, concentration data is becoming prevalent for total plasma fatty acids and phospholipid fatty acids. In the case of red blood cells and platelets, the data is usually expressed as a percentage composition, because the total number of cells extracted is not normally determined.

Therapies

Linoleic Acid (LA).   Deficiency of the EFA or of the omega-3 PUFA alone can be corrected by consumption of oils and foods rich in these PUFA. Most vegetable oils contain LA, and rich sources include sunflower, safflower, grape seed, corn, peanut, canola, and cottonseed oil. The requirement for LA is of the order of 2% of total dietary energy. This equates to approximately 5 g/day and 7 g/day for women and men, respectively. Deficiency can be corrected within 14 days. If oral administration is not the preferred route, then the oil can be rubbed onto the skin. This approach has corrected EFA deficiency in children.[3]

Gamma-Linolenic Acid (GLA).   The main oils containing GLA are evening primrose oil, borage oil, and black currant seed oil. A dose rate of 12 g/day has been used for treatment of atopic eczema.[3]

Omega-3 Oils: Fish Oils and Selected Vegetable Oils.   The main oils containing omega-3 PUFA include the EPA-rich fish oils (cod liver oil, sardine oil), the DHA-rich fish oils (tuna oil), and the ALA-rich vegetable oils (flaxseed, canola, walnut, soy oils). The potency of EPA and DHA is many times that of ALA because of the inefficient conversion of ALA to EPA and DHA in humans. Consumption of rich sources of omega-3 from fish or fish oils leads to increases in the blood EPA and DHA levels within 7 days.[19]

There are a number of different brands of fish oil capsules available in Australia, which usually indicates the EPA and DHA content, with a common value being 180 mg of EPA and 120 mg DHA. There appears to be a similar response in accumulation of EPA and DHA in blood whether the source is fish or fish oils. Because the long-chain omega-3 PUFAs contain highly unsaturated fatty acids, which are susceptible to oxidation, it is desirable to consider the vitamin E status of the patient if high doses of fish oils are recommended. Most fish oil capsules contain 1 to 2 mg of vitamin E, which is about 10% of the recommended daily intake (RDI) (10 mg/day).[9]

The specimen requirements for EFAs are outlined in Table 7-1.

URINARY TELOPEPTIDES: OSTEOPOROSIS RISK MARKER

Osteoporosis is preventable and/or reversible when detected early. A specific urine test is available to detect the onset of osteoporosis. Osteoporosis

TABLE 7-1 ■ Specimen Requirements for Essential Fatty Acids

SPECIMEN	AMOUNT REQUIRED	TUBE SPECIFICATION	SPECIAL REQUIREMENTS
Total plasma	2 mL plasma FROZEN	Lithium heparin/EDTA	Fasting from 10 PM
Plasma			
phospholipids	2 mL plasma FROZEN	Lithium heparin/EDTA	Fasting from 10 PM
Red cell	10 mL whole blood	EDTA	Fasting from 10 PM
Platelet	10 mL whole blood	EDTA	Fasting from 10 PM

EDTA, ethylenediaminetetraacetic acid.

can progress without symptoms for many years to advanced stages in which debilitating fractures are the first symptoms of the disease. If detected early, osteoporosis can be treated by intervention therapy (i.e., antiresorptive agents) and prevent further development of the disease.[20] According to recently collected statistics, osteoporosis affects over 75 million people, men and women, worldwide and puts 1 out of every 2 women at risk of developing fractures. The risk to women of developing osteoporosis approximates to the combined risk of breast, ovarian, and endometrial cancers.

Clinical Features

The most common risk factors for osteoporosis are as follows:

- Estrogen deficiency
- Hairline and stress bone fractures resulting from estrogen deficiency
- Chronic low intake of dietary calcium
- Cigarette smoking
- High caffeine consumption
- Dietary faddism, resulting in below average body weight
- Early menopause
- Family history (genetic)
- Sedentary lifestyle
- Certain medications (e.g., corticosteroids)

The rate of bone loss is the most effective measurement for early detection of those people at risk of developing osteoporosis. Bone mineral density (BMD) changes slowly over medium to long periods, especially in younger women. The inherent imprecision of bone density measurements therefore can result in patients not being identified as being at risk of developing osteoporosis at a stage in which early intervention therapy may be most effective.[21]

The processes of bone turnover (deposition and resorption) are critical in bone density and stability.

Bone Remodeling

Bone is continuously remodeled through a coupled process of bone resorption and bone formation. Osteoclasts degrade bone during the resorption phase by excavating small pits; osteoblasts (formation cells) then replace the bone collagen removed by osteoclasts. Net bone loss may result when resorption outpaces formation, often occurring in women after menopause as estrogen production falls.[21,22]

A biochemical test on first morning urine samples is now available; it allows practitioners to measure the bone remodeling process. As bone is continuously broken down and rebuilt, products of bone matrix (mainly type I collagen and minerals) are released into the circulation. Cross-linked N-telopeptides (NTx), specific to bone type I collagen, are released by osteoclasts as they break down bone. NTx is then released into circulation and excreted in urine, where it can be measured by the NTx test as an indicator of bone resorption.[20]

Elevated levels of NTx indicate elevated bone resorption. NTx results can be used to do the following:

- Predict skeletal response to antiresorptive therapy in postmenopausal women
- Determine probability for decrease in BMD in postmenopausal women not on therapy
- Counsel patients about compliance and continuation of therapy
- Monitor response to therapy as early as 3 months after initiation

Although some postmenopausal women are taking standard doses of hormone replacement therapy (HRT) for menopausal symptoms, the measurement of NTx levels in urine helps to determine whether doses of HRT are adequate to prevent bone resorption in the individual woman. It is important to note that the effective doses for bone loss prevention may be significantly higher than the dosage prescribed for mild menopausal symptoms.[22] Elevated bone resorption is exhibited by patients taking certain drugs such as oral steroids or GnRh analogues and by most patients with thyroid disease (hyperthyroidism and hyperparathyroidism).[23] Published data indicates that bone loss rate measurements are helpful in deciding which postmenopausal patients are likely to have a good response to antiresorptive therapy and in monitoring the effectiveness of that therapy.[23,24] The patient groups who would benefit most from NTx measurements are perimenopausal and postmenopausal women, amenorrheic premenopausal women, thyroid patients, oral steroid-treated patients, GnRh treated patients, immunosuppressed patients, those with a family history of osteoporosis, osteoporotic patients, Paget's disease patients, and cancer patients (bone metastases). Detection of patients with cancer and micrometastatic disease, before clinical symptoms of bone metastases develop, would reduce the lead time of the disease and allow more aggressive therapy earlier.

Monitoring antiresorptive therapy to adjust dosage and encourage patient compliance is important in those patients who are early postmenopausal women, individuals diagnosed with osteoporosis, those with Paget's disease, and those who are on estrogen-suppressing therapies.

Predicting skeletal response (BMD) to hormonal antiresorptive therapy in early postmenopausal women is necessary.

The specimen requirements for urinary telopeptides are outlined in Table 7-2.

SALIVARY HORMONE PROFILE: ESTRADIOL, PROGESTERONE, TESTOSTERONE, DEHYDROEPIANDROSTERONE-SULFATE (DHEA-S), CORTISOL, AND MELATONIN

Reliable, accurate, and reproducible measurements of hormone levels are a powerful tool to support clinical decision making and the therapeutic management of patients. Salivary hormone profiles are used by complementary healthcare practitioners to assist with patient treatment and management.

Hormones are messenger molecules, which are secreted by many glands and tissues in the body and act on distant cells at target sites called receptors. These receptors transduce the message into intracellular commands. This process is used to regulate the activity of the target cells and coordinate their interaction. Hormones may be small molecular weight molecules (steroids, thyroxin, histamine, epinephrine) or small or large molecular weight peptides (enkephalins, endorphins, releasing factors, stimulating hormones).

Hormones are primarily produced in glandular tissue and may act on the cell from which they are released (autocrine) or on other local cells (paracrine). Secretion may be into the exterior environment, which includes the gut lumen (exocrine), or into the internal environment, where they are distributed widely following secretion and equilibrate throughout virtually all extracellular space, including formed saliva stored in the salivary glands. These hormones include the steroid hormones estradiol, progesterone, testosterone, cortisol, DHEA-S, and melatonin. These hormones are conveniently measured in saliva.

Once a hormone is bound to its receptor, the transduction of the message may initiate a wide range of intracellular events, including protein synthesis and secretion, lipid metabolism, and carbohydrate turnover. Because hormones act over a range of distances, many of their functions are integrative and are aimed at coordinating the wide variety of functions required to maintain optimal overall wellness.

Estrogen is the term used for a group of several different but related hormones that perform the functions normally attributed to estrogen. In adult women, three different natural estrogens predominate. They are estrone

TABLE 7-2 ■ Specimen Requirements for Urinary Telopeptides

SPECIMEN	AMOUNT REQUIRED	TUBE/KIT	SPECIAL REQUIREMENTS
Urine	10 mL	Special laboratory collection kit	Second morning void

(approximately 10% to 20% of circulating estrogens), estradiol (10% to 20%), and estriol (60% to 80%). Under normal circumstances, hormone levels vary according to the stage of the menstrual cycle, but the amount of each hormone usually fluctuates within the proportions listed previously.

Within a population of individuals, there may be a wide range of hormone levels that can be termed normal. This is because of genetic and somatic differences across the population. The term normal can be divisive in a clinical situation. Reference ranges, which are statistically derived and are aimed at providing the practitioner with a starting point for clinical decision making, are a better determinant.

When hormone levels have been measured, the practitioner is in a position to assess whether some intervention is required to bring the hormone level back into the normal range. This may include drug therapies, the use of complementary therapies, or simply lifestyle changes. Repeat measurements assist in determining if the intervention is succeeding in treatment and whether it must be altered or continued.

Measurement or determination of hormone levels and comparison with reference range data assist in establishing the complete picture for the individual. In a holistic approach to patient care, this is critical for long-term success. In specific situations, where a known pathologic condition exists (e.g., a hormone-secreting tumor), hormone measurement can allow the practitioner to measure the extent of the pathologic disorder. Table 7-3 lists many

TABLE 7-3 ■ Hormones Measured in Saliva: Site of Production and Major Effects

HORMONE	SITE OF PRODUCTION	MAJOR EFFECTS
Testosterone (males)	Testis	Maturation of male sex organs, development of male sexual characteristics
Testosterone (females)	Adrenal cortex	Androgen balancing role, feedback control factor
Progesterone (males)	Adrenal cortex	Feedback control factor
Progesterone (females)	Ovary (CL), placenta	Cellular differentiation, placental development, mammary (alveolar) development
Oestradiol (males)	Adrenal cortex	Estrogen balancing role, feedback control factor
Oestradiol (females)	Ovary (CL), placenta	Cellular differentiation, development of female sexual characteristics, control of cyclicity, mammary (duct) development
Cortisol (both sexes)	Adrenal cortex	Effects on metabolism of carbohydrates, lipids and proteins, immune function and immune status, and stress responsiveness
Melatonin (both sexes)	Pineal gland	Light-dark cycle adaptation, circadian rhythms, antioxidant effect
Dehydroepiandro-sterone-sulfate (DHEA-S) (both sexes)	Multiple	General endocrine status regulator

of the hormones that can be measured in saliva and what roles they play in the body.

Many factors may contribute to altered hormone levels. These include both environmental and lifestyle-induced factors and specific conditions. These range from pathology at the site of production (e.g., tissue damage leading to reduced secretion), altered feedback control (e.g., decreased receptor responsiveness leading to elevated levels of hormones), deficiencies in precursor availability (e.g., low estrogen levels in women with very low adiposity because of decreased cholesterol availability), or transient nonspecific effects (e.g., unrelated illness, fever, or infection). The altered hormone levels may result from adaptive responses to a triggering factor (e.g., feedback control by the same or a related hormone) or from direct disturbance of correct hormonal control by an external agent (drug, pathogen, environmental factor).

Factors that Alter Hormone Levels

Salivary hormone levels may be altered in many common conditions. The following are also the conditions in which measurement of the salivary hormone levels can provide the practitioner with valuable data for making clinical decisions.

In females, the conditions that can be measured through hormone profiling include amenorrhea (absence of menstrual bleeding); dysmenorrhea (pain in association with menstrual bleeding); vaginal atrophy (loss of vaginal tissue mass because of decreased cell volume); luteal phase defects (altered luteal phase length and/or duration); menopause, hot flushes, and/or night sweats (rapid rise in basal body temperature coupled with sensation of heat, sweating, and sometimes disorientation); infertility and miscarriage; endometriosis (diffuse endometrial cells in extraendometrial abdominal locations that bleed in parallel with normal menstrual cycling); hirsutism (excessive hair growth or hair growth in atypical locations); and breast and other cancers.[25,26]

It is important to further mention hot flushes and hirsutism. Hot flushes have become an increasingly common feature of the development of menopause in many women. The genesis of flushing is thought to lie in rapid alteration of thermoregulatory set points in response to transient changes in hormone levels. Measurement of hormone levels may be useful in establishing basal levels to determine whether hormone supplementation may be useful in reducing flush severity or frequency. In hirsutism, hair growth in response to elevated adrenal secretion of androgen (usually testosterone) in women may indicate an adrenal tumor or may be a defect in control of secretion. Saliva hormone measurement allows the differentiation of these diagnoses and indicate appropriate intervention.

The conditions that can be monitored in males include hirsutism, premature hair loss, impotence, infertility, prostate and other cancers, and sleep disturbances.[27]

Saliva hormone levels are also useful indicators for a wide range of primary conditions for which altered hormone levels are the secondary response, such as gut dysbiosis, increased gut permeability, altered hepatic liver detoxification pathways (e.g., degradation of hormone conjugation), and allergic or inflammatory states.

In addition to specific conditions, many other factors contribute to altered hormone levels. Measurement and correct practitioner interpretation of the hormone levels can assist in making a decision to consider lifestyle changes as part of a management protocol.

Baseline and peak stress levels and the individual's physiologic ability to manage stressful situations can alter hormone levels. Measurement of cortisol levels assists, for example, in determining the individual's stress responsiveness.[26]

Diet, including correct hydration (fluid intake and cellular uptake), correct macronutrient balance, correct micronutrient availability, estrogens leading to menstrual symptoms, and the use of known hormone receptor-active foods such as soy protein and herbal foods preparations, will influence hormone levels.

Also influencing hormone levels are the frequency, intensity, and duration of appropriate exercise, according to patient variables such as age, sex, current state of fitness, body mass index, and contraindications. Intense exercise and low body mass index are factors as well.

Past history or current exposure to environmental xenoestrogenic toxins (xenobiotics with estrogen-like activity) such as plastics, pesticides, and petroleum products should be considered.

Lastly, individual lifestyle decisions, including the use and/or abuse of cigarettes, alcohol, caffeinated coffee, refined sugar, nonprescription, and recreational drugs, and current use of prescription drugs for related and nonrelated conditions can alter the level of hormones.

Menopause

Menopause is defined as the cessation of menstruation. This suggests an abrupt halt to cyclic bleeding, but in many women it is a progressive process that occurs over months and, in some cases, years. The period of time when menstrual irregularities (changes in cycle length, alteration in menstrual bleeding, etc.) occur is termed perimenopause. In Western women, this typically occurs in the age range 40 to 60 years.

Apart from changes to menstrual periods, symptoms such as hot flushes, night sweats, insomnia, and mood disturbances often occur. This is the consequence of large reductions in progesterone and estrogen levels. For instance, at menopause, estradiol levels reduce drop to subfunctional levels in most women. Historically, postmenopausal women maintained lower but adequate levels of progesterone and estrogens. However, in recent years, many women are experiencing much more severe symptoms, which parallel the much-reduced levels of these hormones. There has been suggested evidence that increased lifetime (and perhaps more importantly prenatal) exposure to xenoestrogens has altered the set point for postmenopausal secretion and also changed receptor sensitivity to the actions of these hormones.[28]

The most common symptoms of menopausal difficulties are hot flushes and night sweats. In clinical practice it is important to differentiate a hormonal hot flush with a fever flush. The latter, common in individuals with low-grade, subclinical infections (often arising in the bowel), usually begin in the head and neck and move downward through the body to the feet. They occur most often at night and can be stress-induced. A true hormonal hot flush generally begins in the lower abdomen and moves up to the head and neck. Rarely are the lower extremities involved. Please note that these are guidelines only, and, as self-reporting is often a poor way to collect patient data, additional investigation is suggested.

The decision between the range of treatment and management options for the symptomatic menopausal woman depends very much on patient preference and practitioner knowledge. This is a controversial area and one that is currently the focus of much research. The choice between conventional treatment, natural therapies, and an integrated approach is not clear-cut, but salivary hormone measurement offers an excellent tool for assisting with these decisions.

Collecting Samples

The decision to measure saliva or serum samples is based on several factors. Saliva hormone levels have been shown to accurately reflect the biochemically available fraction of circulating hormone for both progesterone and estradiol. The correlation between serum and salivary hormones is very high. For example, serum and saliva progesterone levels demonstrate a correlation coefficient of $r = 0.94$.[29]

Estradiol and progesterone found in serum is largely protein-bound and is not readily bioavailable to receptors in target tissues throughout the body. These bound hormones are on their way to the liver to be metabolized and excreted in bile. Thus estradiol and progesterone measured in serum is mostly a measure of hormone that is not going to be used by the body. A serum test is useful to measure how much total hormone is being produced by the body.[28]

Progesterone is a highly lipophilic (fat-loving) molecule and is well absorbed through the skin into the underlying fat layer. It is, in fact, one of the most lipophilic of the steroid hormones. From the fat layer, the progesterone is taken up gradually by red blood cell membranes in capillaries passing through the fat. The progesterone transported by red blood cell membranes is readily available to all target tissues and to saliva. This progesterone is completely bioavailable and readily measured by saliva testing. Obviously, serum testing is not a good way to measure transdermal progesterone absorption.

Saliva samples, especially serial samples, improve the overall clinical picture. They are easy to collect and the collection method circumvents the problems associated with dissociation from binding proteins and handling losses that can occur with blood collection. Saliva collection is noninvasive and does not require specialized equipment; thus it ideally suits complementary practice. Samples may be collected by the patient at home and stored before dispatch for assay testing. Serum measurement may be preferable in situations in which total circulating hormone levels need to be measured. A concurrent saliva sample can be useful to allow rapid estimation of bioavailable versus protein-bound fractions to assess for aberrant binding protein levels or affinities to determine binding protein defects.

The timing of collection depends to a great extent on the nature of the investigation, but, generally, a baseline level may be determined from a single sample. To conduct a full investigation, serial samples are recommended. Serial samples allow a full profile of cyclic changes in hormone levels to be assessed. The cyclic nature of hormonal secretion, which is a reflection of many factors including the pulsatile secretion of releasing factors, diurnal variation, and menstrual cyclicity, make serial sampling the collection method of choice. Table 7-4 indicates some typical protocols for specific investigations.

General Testing Information

The standard protocol for testing cortisol is to collect two samples. The first sample should be collected on rising (0600 to 0800 hours) and the second sample at 1800 hours. The protocol for testing melatonin is to collect one sample at midnight (0000 hours) in a darkened room. The person must be in a room with a low light level for at least 30 minutes before the specimen is collected. If the person is in a brightly lit room, the production of melatonin will be affected and an accurate result cannot be obtained. The second sample for melatonin should be collected on rising (0600 to 0800 hours).[30]

It is important to wash one's hands thoroughly before beginning, especially if topical hormone creams have been used. Hormone residues left on hands from creams may contaminate the saliva during collection, resulting in elevated test results.

Saliva samples should be collected on rising, between 0600 to 0800 hours, before the person eats, drinks, or applies makeup, and so forth (except for the midnight collection for melatonin). Hormone production is optimal in the early morning and is susceptible to variation caused by stress, eating, drinking, and exercise. The patient should be instructed to (1) rinse the mouth out with water and (2) not eat, drink, brush or floss teeth, or apply makeup before collecting the saliva sample. As mentioned previously, eating or drinking can cause variations in test results. Brushing or flossing teeth can cause the gums to bleed, which may also affect test results.

If the person uses a hormone cream, the sample should be collected 12 hours after the last application. If a hormone cream is applied at night, it

TABLE 7-4 ■ Protocols for Sample Collection

CONDITION	PROTOCOL
Premenopausal Women (Regular/Irregular Menstrual Cycle)	
Follicular phase investigation	5 samples equally spaced between days 1-14
First day	Estradiol, progesterone, testosterone, DHEA-S
Other 4 days	Estradiol, progesterone
Total	12 hormones
Luteal phase investigation	5 samples equally spaced between days 14-28/30
First day	Estradiol, progesterone, testosterone, DHEA-S
Other 4 days	Estradiol, progesterone
Total	12 hormones
Full cycle investigation	5 samples equally spaced between days 1-28/30
First day	Estradiol, progesterone, testosterone, DHEA-S
Other 4 days	Estradiol, progesterone
Total	12 hormones
Perimenopausal Women (Irregular Menstrual Cycle)	
Luteal phase investigation	3 samples equally spaced between days 14-28/30
First day	Estradiol, progesterone, testosterone, DHEA-S
Other 2 days	Estradiol, progesterone
Total	8 hormones
Menopausal and postmenopausal Women (No Menstrual Cycle)	
Baseline investigation	1 sample collected on any day
Any day	Estradiol, progesterone, testosterone, DHEA-S
Total	4 hormones
Men	**1 sample collected on any day**
Any day	Estradiol, progesterone, testosterone, DHEA-S
Total	4 hormones

DHEA-S, dehydroepiandrosterone-sulfate.

should be applied at least 12 hours before the saliva specimen is collected in the morning. If a hormone cream is applied in the morning, the saliva sample should be collected before the cream is applied.

If the person uses a troche, he or she must wait 4 days. If a hormone troche (a small lozenge placed in the mouth) is used, there must be a 4-day break from using the troche before the saliva samples are collected.

COMPLETE DIGESTIVE STOOL ANALYSIS

"You are what you eat" is a common saying that is referred to in the context of general health. However, it is an oversimplification of an individual's potential to achieve optimal health. It assumes that he or she consumes a balanced nutritional diet, lives and works in a clean environment, is stress and infection free, and has inherited defective-free genes. A balanced diet alone should act as the foundation for excellent health and well-being—if only it were that simple. For example, it is well-established that some foods are grown in nutrient deficient soils!

The manifestation of chronic ill health is determined, in most instances, by the low-level impact of prevailing factors causing a cascade of interrelated stresses on physiologic processes and organ functions, which results in critical disturbances to homeostasis and health. The major organs governing the initiation and progression of these processes are the gastrointestinal (GI) tract and the liver, respectively.

The GI tract must digest and process food, selectively absorb essential nutrients and biochemicals and eliminate toxic, allergenic, and inflammatory compounds. The microflora in the small and large intestine must be in balance to ensure the health and function of the intestinal mucosa. Imbalances in microflora can alter the immunologic and mechanical integrity of the mucosa ("leaky gut"), thus permitting absorption of inflammatory, allergenic, and toxic molecules.

The liver must detoxify the body by removing endogenous waste products (i.e., end products of metabolism), xenobiotics (i.e., ingested, inhaled, and dermally absorbed toxic chemicals), and absorbed endotoxins (i.e., GI products absorbed through a leaky gut).[31]

Gastrointestinal Health

Optimal health is every individual's desired state, in which well-being is achieved by a balance between nutrition and lifestyle. Lifestyle essentially includes physical condition, psychologic disposition, and the physical environment. The many nutrients, which are absorbed by the GI tract, act to maintain the body's homeostasis in optimal balance.[32]

The synergy of balanced nutrition and lifestyle are fundamental to the control of predisposing factors involved in the onset and progress of disease. Normal human bacterial microflora in the small and large intestine maintain a delicate balance. Their metabolic and enzymatic activity is critical in the metabolism, biotransformation, and absorption of nutrients. These nutrients include all compounds taken orally and all substances entering the intestine via the biliary tract or by direct secretion into the lumen. When the microflora balance is disturbed (dysbiosis), these metabolic and enzymatic activities can be severely compromised. Dysbiosis is a state in which imbalances in intestinal flora cause changes to normal GI processes, manifesting in clinical and preclinical conditions, which can lead to varying degrees of unwellness. The symptoms of dysbiosis can vary significantly between individuals; however, the causes can be placed into four major categories, namely, putrefaction, fermentation, deficiency, and sensitization.

Infection by viruses, bacteria, fungi, and parasites and chemical attack (intoxication) by xenobiotics and therapeutic agents (drugs, etc.) can also be implicated. Dysbiosis can lead to the breakdown of mucosal integrity (leaky gut), contributing to increased absorption and compromised liver function. The complete digestive stool analysis (CDSA) offers a practical and economical noninvasive assessment of the functional health of the entire GI tract. The CDSA may provide an important opportunity in the assessment of chronic disorders and imbalances in the GI tract by investigating biochemical and microbiologic parameters resulting from altered digestion, absorption, motility, microflora imbalance, metabolic activity, immune function, and disease processes such as infection and inflammation.

The GI tract is arguably the body's most strategic organ for metabolism, biotransformation, and absorption of nutrients. Microbiologic and biochemical enterohepatic functions are important factors in human health and may be etiologic agents in the onset of disease. Therefore assessment of chronic health issues should include a thorough evaluation of GI tract and enterohepatic status.[33]

> The CDSA provides baseline diagnostic information on which current and future GI well-being can be gauged. The CDSA is not indicated as a procedure for the diagnosis of underlying disease.

The GI tract, for the purposes of understanding the process of digestion and absorption, can be divided into four main areas: the mouth, stomach, small intestine, and large intestine. The mouth is responsible for mastication and the physical break up of food. Saliva and enzymes mix with food to facilitate transit, digestion, and protection of the pharyngeal and esophageal mucosa. The stomach mixes and digests food by gastric juices (emulsifiers, enzymes, acids) and orders delivery to the small intestine. In turn, the small intestine is the major site for digestion and absorption, mediated by pancreatic enzymes and bile acids. Residency time of nutrients is crucial to efficiency of absorption. The large intestine is responsible for the absorption of water and microbial fermentation of soluble fiber, resistant starch, and undigested carbohydrates, as well as the production of short-chain fatty acids (SCFA) and pH control of feces.

The GI tract provides an ideal environment for a vast and diverse array of normal flora. These bacteria exert positive effects and are vital for well-being and health. As a consequence of their metabolic activities and when dysbiosis occurs, they may also exert negative effects.

Few of the bacteria ingested with food or drink or which originate in the nose, mouth, or oropharynx survive the very acidic conditions in the stomach. Hence, colonization of the stomach is an infrequent event (<10 viable organisms/mL of stomach contents is the norm), although it may occur when *Helicobacter pylori* invade the stomach mucosa.

Putrefactive dysbiosis is more likely when diets high in animal protein and fat and low in fiber are consumed. Significant imbalances in stool bacteria populations occur (i.e., increased *Bacteroides* sp. and decreased *Bifidobacterium* sp.) with consequent major disturbances to enzyme activity and metabolism, causing the following: decarboxylation of amino acids (production of vasoactive and neurotoxic amines like histamine, octopamine, tyramine), catalysis of tryptophan by bacterial enzyme tryptophanase (production of indoles, skatoles, phenols, etc.), hydrolysis of urea to ammonia by increased bacterial urease (*Bacteroides* sp., *Proteus* sp., *Klebsiella* sp. activity) that results in raised stool pH and yeast/fungal overgrowth, hydrolysis of conjugated bile acids and hormones by bacterial enzymes (increased stool levels of bile acids and increased plasma levels of estrogens), bacterial reduction of primary bile acids (production of secondary bile acids such as deoxycholate), reduced production of SCFAs (impaired energy synthesis in colonic epithelial cells), and compromised liver detoxification enzyme systems.

> Putrefactive dysbiosis is strongly implicated in the pathogenesis of colon and breast cancer.

Fermentation (Bacterial Overgrowth). Fermentation is a condition of overgrowth of endogenous bacteria and yeasts in the stomach and small intestine. It is exacerbated by gastric hypochlorhydria (stomach hydrochloric acid deficiency), abnormal motility, immune deficiency, and poor nutrition. Bacterial overgrowth can also occur without any specific symptoms. Fermentation increases the risk of systemic infection and gastric cancer in individuals with hypochlorhydria and can increase intestinal permeability in susceptible individuals. Bacterial overgrowth (fermentation dysbiosis) may cause mucosal damage (degradation of intestinal brush border enzymes by bacterial proteases), pancreatic insufficiency, altered fat absorption, reduced vitamin B_{12} availability (bacterial consumption of cobalamin), bacterial conversion of nitrates to nitrites and nitrosamines, and elevated levels of SCFAs.

Deficiency. Reduced concentration of normal fecal flora such as *Bifidobacterium* sp., *Lactobacillus* sp., and *Escherichia coli* create an imbalance that leads to deficiency dysbiosis. An unfavorable alteration in the balance of normal flora can be caused by antibiotic therapy or a diet depleted in soluble fiber. In rare situations, chronic exposure to ingested xenobiotics can have the same effect. Individuals suffering from symptoms of irritable bowel syndrome (IBS) and food intolerance may have imbalance of fecal flora (decreased ratio of anaerobes to aerobes) and decreased fecal SCFAs. Deficiency dysbiosis and putrefactive dysbiosis are conditions generally treated using similar protocols.[34]

Sensitization. Inappropriate immunologic responses to organisms inhabiting the gut lumen and adhering to the intestinal mucosal surface can be triggered by products of dysbiosis and components of normal intestinal flora. Such responses lead to inflammatory conditions, which are associated with IBS and inflammatory bowel disease (IBD), and increased intestinal permeability, which permits the absorption of enterotoxins, bacterial and food antigens, and bacterial debris. Increased intestinal permeability is involved in the cause of inflammatory joint diseases (arthropathies) and allergy (asthma, eczema).[35]

Infection.   Susceptibility to infection by viruses, bacteria, fungi, and parasites is higher in dysbiosis. The prevalence of these infectious agents has increased dramatically in recent years, because of factors such as international travel, contaminated processed foods, and increased antibiotic use. Changes in global climatic conditions may also have an effect on the normal balance and the abundance of infectious agents.[36]

Intoxication.   Chemical poisoning of vital biochemical and microbiologic processes by xenobiotics and therapeutic agents (e.g., antibiotics) can cause physiologic imbalances and contribute to dysbiosis. A detailed assessment of a patient's history should identify whether intoxication is implicated.[37]

CDSA Profile

The CDSA profile is recommended for an initial, thorough evaluation of GI tract function. The information provided includes the following:

- Macroscopic (color, form, consistency, mucus, blood, pus, fibers, food remnants)
- Microscopic (starch, meat fibers, vegetable cells and fibers, red blood cells, white blood cells, fat globules)
- Biochemical (pH, occult blood, chymotrypsin, cholesterol, triglycerides, total fecal fat, long-chain fatty acids, SCFAs)
- Parasitology (all pathogenic and nonpathogenic parasites)
- Bacteriology (normal flora, imbalanced flora, potential pathogens)
- Mycology (yeasts and molds, specifically *Candida albicans*)

A CDSA comprises the stool parasitology and culture and the microscopy and biochemistry panels. The stool parasitology and culture provides an analysis of parasitology, bacteriology, and mycology. A 3-day follow-up analysis is performed when a parasitic infection is detected in the CDSA. The stool microbiology follow-up provides an analysis of bacteriology and mycology.

Patients should be instructed on the importance of proper specimen collection (refer to collection instructions). Only those specimens collected in appropriate kits (provided by the laboratory) should be analyzed. To obtain the most accurate laboratory results, specimens must arrive at the laboratory within 72 hours of collection. Delay in samples reaching the laboratory can cause bacterial overgrowth or death and biochemical changes that may produce inaccurate results and diagnoses.

The CDSA interpretive guidelines are shown in Table 7-5.

Short Chain Fatty Acids (SCFAs) and Bowel Health

SCFAs (acetate, propionate, and butyrate) are produced by bacterial fermentation of dietary carbohydrate. Their specific effects and benefits are outlined in Table 7-6. They are the main fuel source for the cells lining the small intestine

TABLE 7-5 ■ **Interpretive Guidelines**

RESULT	POSSIBLE CAUSE	CONSIDERATIONS
Macroscopic		
Color		
Brown/light brown		Normal
Yellow	↑Triglycerides steatorrhea	↑Pancreatic enzymes
	Food—curcuminoids	
	Antibiotic abuse	
Green	↑Bile	Gall bladder support
	Diarrhea	↑Probiotics
Black	Oxidized blood	Investigate upper GI bleeding
	Charcoal/iron tablets	
Form		
Unformed/liquid	↓Digestion	↑Pancreatic enzymes
	Inflammation/infection	↑Probiotics
Consistency		
Soft	Overgrowth of anaerobic	↑probiotics
	bacteria in upper GI tract	Tx mucosal support
	resulting in poor fat	
	absorption	
	↑Candida	
	Allergy/food intolerance	↑Probiotics/antimicrobials
	↑Laxative use	Elimination diet
	↑Vitamin C	Stop laxative use
	↑Stress	↓vitamin C intake
		Exercise, yoga, meditation,
		St. John's wort
Watery	Bacterial (*Shigella, Salmonella,*	Tx antimicrobial support
	enterotoxigenic *Escherichia*	↑Probiotics
	coli, Vibrio cholera,	
	Clostridium difficile) infection	
	Viral infection	
	Amoebae, Giardia infection	Elimination diet, mucosal
	Laxative abuse	support, exercise, yoga,
	Alcohol and/or coffee	meditation, St. John's wort
	Irritable bowel syndrome (IBS)	
	(mucus may also be present)	
	↑Stress	
Mucus		
3+ to 4+	Inflammation/infection	↑EFAs, antiinflammatory,
		herbal support
Occult Blood		
Positive	Consider immediate investigation	
	to identify source	
Pus		
3+ to 4+	Inflammation	↑EFAs, antiinflammatory,
	Infection	herbal support
	Malignancy	Further investigation
Fibers		
3+ to 4+	↓Digestion	↑Pancreatic enzymes
Food remnants		
3+ to 4+	↓Digestion	↑Pancreatic enzymes

TABLE 7-5 ■ Interpretive Guidelines—cont'd

RESULT	POSSIBLE CAUSE	CONSIDERATIONS
Microscopic (×400 Magnification)		
Starch		
3+ to 4+	↓CHO fermentation	
	↑Artificial sweetener use	
WBC		
Positive	Infection, ulceration, hemorrhage	
RBC		
Positive	Infection, ulceration, hemorrhage	
Fat globules		
	↓Digestion	↑Pancreatic enzymes
Digestive Markers		
↑**Triglycerides**	↓Chewing time	↑Mastication time
	↓Gastric acid	↑Bitter herbs, HCl
	↓Pancreatic enzymes	↑Lipase
	↓Bile salts	↑Cholagogues
↓**Chymotrypsin**	↓GI tract motility	↑Water, fiber, HCl
	↓Pancreatic enzymes	↑Pancreatic enzymes,
	↓HCl	↓Refined CHO
		↓Saturated fats
		↓Soft drinks, coffee, alcohol
↑**Chymotrypsin**	↑GI tract motility	↑Water, fiber
		↑Minerals, vitamins
		↑Mucosal support
		Tx diarrhea
↑**Meat fibers**	↓Chewing time	↑Mastication time
3+ to 4+	↓Gastric acid	↑Digestive herbs, HCl
	↓Pancreatic enzymes	↑Pancreatic enzymes
↑**Vegetable fibers**	↓Chewing time	↑Mastication time
3+ to 4+	↓Gastric acid	↑Digestive herbs, HCl
	↓Pancreatic enzymes	↑Pancreatic enzymes
	↓Bile salts	↑Cholagogues
↑**pH**	↓SCFA production	↑Fiber, water
	↓Acid producing flora	↑Probiotics
	↓HCl	↑Digestive herbs, HCl
	↓Transit time	Assess colon cancer risk
	↑Laxative use	
↓**pH**	↑Bacterial overgrowth	↑Probiotics
	↓Lipid absorption	↑Pancreatic enzymes support
	↓CHO absorption	↑Fiber, water
	↑Transit time	
↑**Valerate/**	↓Protein digestion (check if ↑	↑Pancreatic enzymes, HCl,
isobutyrate	meat and vegetable fibers or	digestive herbs
	↓chymotrypsin)	Tx mucosal support
	↓Absorption	Tx food intolerance,
		infection, flora imbalance
Absorption		
↑**Cholesterol/**	↓Absorption	Tx mucosal support, digestive
LCFAs		herbs
	↑Bacteria/parasites	Tx food intolerance, elimination
		diet
		Tx infection, flora imbalance,
		↑minerals, vitamins, EFAs

TABLE 7-5 ■ Interpretive Guidelines—cont'd

RESULT	POSSIBLE CAUSE	CONSIDERATIONS
↑Total fecal fat ↑Total SCFAs	↓Digestion	↑Pancreatic enzymes
	↑SI bacterial overgrowth	↑Probiotics ↓Abx
	↓Absorption	Tx mucosal support
	↑Transit time	Tx food intolerance, ↑fiber, water
	↓Pancreatic enzymes	↑Pancreatic enzymes
↓Total SCFAs	↑Antibiotic use	↑Probiotics
	↓Fiber, water	↑Fiber, water
	↓Transit time	↑Fiber, water
	↓Mucosal integrity	Assess colon cancer risk
	↓Anaerobic organisms ulcerative colitis colonic neoplasia	

CHO, carbohydrate; EFAs, essential fatty acids; GI, gastrointestinal; HCl, hydrochloric acid; LCFAs, long-chain fatty acids; RBC, red blood cell; SCFAs, short-chain fatty acids; SI, Tx, treatment; WBC, white blood cell.

(enterocytes) and help prevent breach of the paracellular spaces by supporting cellular integrity and decreasing inflammation. Other acidic products of fermentation are found in the colon, such as branched-chain fatty acids, isobutyrate, and isovalerate, which are products of amino acid fermentation.

Starches give the highest SCFA yield and the most butyrate, whereas nonstarch polysaccharides (e.g., pectins) produce mostly acetate and propionate. Butyrate is protective against colorectal cancers and ulcerative colitis. Increased levels of SCFAs may reflect malabsorption or bacterial overgrowth. It may also indicate disordered fluid, electrolyte, and acid-base balances of the body. Decreased levels reflect disruption of the normal intestinal ecology.[34]

Treatment considerations for conditions affecting GI health include digestive herbs and nutrients, antiinflammatory herbs and nutrients, antiparasitic and antimicrobial herbs, therapeutic oils, prebiotics and probiotics, fiber, water, and mucosal support. A more complete listing is detailed in Box 7-1. Digestive enzymes are contraindicated for individuals with inflammation of the stomach lining.

H. PYLORI

The importance of *H. pylori* in GI diseases has increased greatly since Marshall and Warren described the presence of Campylobacter-like organisms in the antral mucosa of patients with histologic evidence of antrum gastritis and peptic ulcers, especially duodenal ulcers.[38] Although a causative relationship has not yet been fully established, the strong correlation

TABLE 7-6 ■ Short Chain Fatty Acids: Effects and Benefits

SHORT CHAIN FATTY ACIDS (SCFA)	SPECIFIC EFFECT	BENEFITS
Total SCFA	Lowering of pH	Diminished bioavailability of alkaline cytoxic compounds
		Inhibition of growth of pH-sensitive organisms
Acetate	Possible ↑ in Ca & Mg absorption	Diminished fecal loss of Ca & Mg
	Relaxation of resistance vessels	Greater colonic and hepatic portal venous blood flow
	Enhanced colonic muscular contraction	Easier laxation, relief of constipation
Propionate	Relaxation of resistance vessels	Greater colonic and hepatic portal venous blood flow
	Stimulation of colonic electrolyte transport	Greater ion and fluid absorption, prevention of diarrhea
	Colonic epithelial proliferation	Possible greater absorptive capacity
Butyrate	Relaxation of resistance vessels	Greater colonic and hepatic portal venous blood flow
	Metabolism by colonocytes	Maintenance of mucosal integrity, repair of diversion and ulcerative colitis, colonocyte proliferation
	Maintenance of normal colonocyte phenotype	Diminished risk of malignancy
	Stimulation of colonic electrolyte transport	Greater ion and fluid absorption, prevention of diarrhea

Topping DL: Short-chain fatty acids produced by intestinal bacteria, *Asia Pacific J Clin Nutr* 5:15-9, 1996.

■ Box 7-1 ■

TREATMENT CONSIDERATIONS

Digestive herbs/Nutrients
Hydrastis canadensis (goldenseal root)
Gentiana lutea (gentian root)
Betaine hydrochloride
Bromelain
Papain

Antiinflammatory herbs/Nutrients
Curcuma longa (tumeric)
Zingiber officinale (ginger)
Uncaria tomentosa (cat's claw)
Tanacetum parthenium (feverfew)
Boswellia serrata (boswellia)
Quercetin
Zinc and copper

Antiparasitic and Antimicrobial Herbs
Juglans nigra (black walnut)
Artemisia annua (wormwood)
Berberis vulgaris (bearberry)
Allium sativum (garlic)
Pau d'arco

Therapeutic Oils
Eicosapentaenoic acid (EPA) (n-3)—salmon, mackerel, sardine
Docosahexaenoic acid (DHA) (n-3)
Gamma-linoleic acid (GLA) (n-6)—evening primrose oil, borage oil
Alpha-linolenic acid (ALA) (n-3)—linseed oil, pumpkin see oil,

Prebiotics and Probiotics
Fructo-oligosaccharieds
Lactobacillus acidophilus
Bifidobacterium bifidum

Fiber (35-40 g/day)
Psllium husks
Slippery elm
Wheat, oat, and rice bran

Water
Drink 1.5 L of filtered water daily

Mucosal Support
L-glutamine
Zinc

■ Box 7-1 ■
TREATMENT CONSIDERATIONS—CONT'D
Vitamin A
Vitamin E
Vitamin C
Pantothenic acid
Folic acid
Glycyrrhiza
Gamma oryzanol
Slippery elm
Aloe vera
Cat's claw
Selenium
Carotenoids
N-acetyl cysteine
Bioflavonoids
Essential Fatty Acids (EFAs)

between the presence of *H. pylori* and histologically confirmed gastritis, peptic ulcer disease, and gastric carcinoma can no longer be debated.[39]

The ecologic niche for *H. pylori* in humans appears to be restricted to the stomach and duodenum. Patients who harbor the organism are divided into two basic groups. The first are those who are said to be colonized. These patients carry the organism but have no signs of GI disease. Those with symptoms and detectable levels of *H. pylori* are considered to be infected. The process by which patients become colonized is still under investigation and the process by which a colonized individual becomes infected remains unclear.[40]

The diagnostic strategies for the determination of *H. pylori* have been developed along two lines. The first involves direct detection of the organism and, to date, is invasive. The second, noninvasive approach involves the detection of antibodies made against *H. pylori* or by the detection of the organism's urease activity.[41]

The invasive route requires that a biopsy be taken from the upper GI tract. The presence of *H. pylori* is then confirmed by direct microscopic examination or by culturing of the organism from the biopsy material. This strategy has the advantage of being able to detect active infections and is highly specific with a very high positive predictive value. The difficulty associated with this approach is that there is risk and discomfort to the patient. In addition, *H. pylori* tends to colonize in patches and may be missed totally by the biopsy. Culturing of *H. pylori* from biopsy material tends to be difficult and time-consuming. These technical difficulties may lead to false-negative results.[42]

The urea breath test (using ^{14}C or ^{13}C urea) is a noninvasive method that detects *H. pylori* by exploiting its highly active urease.[43] Although highly sensitive and specific, the test has limitations. It is time-consuming and requires specialized instrumentation for the detection of ^{14}C or ^{13}C.

The most common noninvasive approach to the detection of *H. pylori* is the serologic identification of specific antibodies in the sera of infected patients. The correlation between histologic gastritis, the presence of *H. pylori*, and seropositivity is extremely strong. The disadvantage of these tests is that they require expertise for interpretation and have a lower specificity because of cross reactions from other organisms. Their major advantage is that they are rapid and offer a high sensitivity.

Specimen samples require 100 mg of fresh stool transported in a sterile feces container at room temperature; the specimen must reach the laboratory within 48 hours of collection. Only fresh stool samples should be submitted. No preservative should be used. This test can be performed as an optional parameter on specimens collected for a CDSA.

A positive result indicates active infection by *H. pylori*. An equivocal result may indicate colonization rather than infection in asymptomatic patients. Patients receiving this result should wait 1 month and submit a further sample for analysis. A negative test result indicates the absence of *H. pylori* antigen or an antigen level that is below the test's level of detection. Test results should be used in conjunction with the patient's clinical history.

Studies on the epidemiology of *H. pylori* have shown that this organism is present worldwide.[44] Gastritis caused by *H. pylori* has been shown to correlate with age, ethnic background, family size, and socioeconomic class.[45] Although the epidemiologic studies on *H. pylori* infection and colonization are ever expanding, the route by which individuals acquire this organism is, at present, unknown.[40]

Studies indicate that the incidence of infection in the United States may increase 1% to 2% annually.[43] It is not uncommon to see positivity rates of 50% in those who are 60 years or older. The frequency of *H. pylori* infection in patients diagnosed with duodenal ulcers, however, is approximately 80% for patients in every age group.[44] The positivity rates seen with *H. pylori* clearly depend on the sample population and how that population is defined.

The rate of positivity may vary depending on geographic location, method of specimen collection, handling and transportation, test employed, and general health environment of the patient population under study.

INTESTINAL PERMEABILITY

In the past few years, the interest in changes to gut permeability has risen as the association among intestinal inflammation, increased permeability, and autoimmune disease has become well established. The penetration of the intestinal mucosal barrier appears to correlate with clinical disease manifested as infection, food allergy, Crohn's disease, coeliac disease, dermatologic conditions, colitis, or autoimmune diseases (such as rheumatoid arthritis, ankylosing spondylitis, Reiter's syndrome, eczema, and other allergy disorders). Decreased permeability appears as a fundamental cause of malnutrition, malabsorption, and failure to thrive.[46]

The small intestine has the paradoxical, dual function of being a digestive and absorptive organ as well as a barrier to the penetration of toxic compounds and macromolecules. The mucosal membranes accomplish this barrier function through a combination of intestinal immune function and mechanical exclusion. Elaborate immunologic and mechanical processes for excluding harmful dietary antigens, bacterial products, and viable microbial organisms are present at the mucosal level.

The distal intestine contains numerous dietary and bacterial products with toxic properties, including actual bacterial cell wall polymers, chemotactic peptides, bacterial antigens capable of inducing antibodies that cross react with host antigens, and bacterial and dietary antigens that can form systemic immune complexes.[47]

Abnormalities of the immune system or mechanical barriers lead to enhanced uptake of inflammatory mediators and pathogenic bacteria. With clinical intestinal injury, mucosal absorption of substances that are normally excluded increases dramatically. Intestinal inflammation enhances the uptake and systemic distribution of potentially injurious macromolecules. Peters and Bjarnason,[48] in an excellent review of uses of permeability testing noted, "Measurement of intestinal permeability will play an increasing role in clinical investigation and monitoring of intestinal disease."

The measurement of passive permeability using the dual sugar technique (lactulose and mannitol) may be the most useful and precise noninvasive method for assessing mucosal integrity in the small bowel. Mannitol (a monosaccharide) and lactulose (a disaccharide) are water-soluble molecules that are not metabolized by the body. Mannitol (molecular weight 182) is readily absorbed, and lactulose (molecular weight 360) is only slightly absorbed. An oral dose containing 5 g lactulose and 3 g mannitol in 10 g of glycerol is given and a timed urine sample is analyzed for the ratio of the percentage recovery of lactulose and mannitol.

Clinical Significance

Studies on a wide range of illnesses have demonstrated alterations in the uptake of monosaccharides, disaccharides, or both and have correlated these changes with clinical and pathologic conditions. These illnesses, which disrupt the structural barrier of the GI tract, often result in pathologic changes in distant organs and tissues.[49,50]

The clinical conditions associated with altered intestinal permeability include IBD, irritable bowel disease, malnutrition and malabsorption, accelerated aging, Crohn's disease, intestinal infections, ulcerative colitis, endotoxemia, autism, nonsteroidal antiinflammatory drug (NSAID) enteropathy, celiac disease, chemotherapy, inflammatory joint disease, giardiasis, food allergy, trauma, alcoholism, and human immunodeficiency virus (HIV) positive status. Some of the symptoms associated with increased intestinal permeability include abdominal pain, arthralgias, cognitive and memory deficits, diarrhea, fatigue and malaise, fevers of unknown origin, food intolerances, myalgias, poor exercise tolerance, shortness of breath, skin rashes, and toxic feelings.

Interpretive Guidelines

The permeation of water-soluble molecules through the intestinal mucosa can occur either through cells (transcellular uptake) or between cells (paracellular uptake). Small molecules (mannitol) readily penetrate cells and passively diffuse through them. Larger molecules such as disaccharides (lactulose) normally are excluded by cells. The rate-limiting barrier in this case is the tight junction between cells, which help maintain epithelial integrity.

The intestinal permeability test directly measures the ability of two non-metabolized sugar molecules, mannitol and lactulose, to permeate the intestinal mucosa. Lactulose is only slightly absorbed and serves as a marker for mucosal integrity. Mannitol is readily absorbed and serves as a marker for transcellular uptake. Low levels of mannitol and lactulose indicate malabsorption. Elevated levels of mannitol and lactulose are indicative of general increased permeability and leaky gut. Permeability to mannitol may decrease, which is indicative of malabsorption of small molecules.

The lactulose/mannitol ratio is a useful parameter. An elevated ratio indicates that the effective pore size of the gut mucosa has increased, allowing access (to the body) of larger, possibly antigenic, molecules. One should consider the possibility of mild IBD or gluten enteropathy in these cases.[48]

Clinical Therapeutics

Treatment of altered intestinal permeability is very important for several reasons. Increased permeability can contribute to, or cause, a wide range of systemic reactions. Decreased permeability can cause malabsorption and malnutrition, leading to a wide range of systemic effects. Correcting the altered permeability can have an immediate effect on relief of symptoms and a gradual improvement on the underlying condition. Eliminating the cause can often stop the pathologic process, allowing the body to heal and return to homeostasis.

One of the first considerations is to identify and eliminate the cause of altered permeability. Some of the most common causes of increased permeability are NSAID use, intestinal infection, dysbiosis, parasites, maldigestion, deficient immunoglobulins, allergenic foods, alcoholism, toxic chemicals, trauma, and endotoxemia. Decreased permeability may be caused by chemotherapy, gastroenteritis, IBS, food allergy, and ulcerative colitis. Identifying the cause is an important first step in reversing altered permeability.

There are a number of therapeutic substances, such as L-glutamine; zinc; vitamins A, E, and C; pantothenic acid; folic acid; glycyrrhiza; gamma oryzanol; slippery elm; aloe vera; cat's claw; selenium; carotenoids; N-acetyl cysteine; bioflavonoids; and EFAs, which can be used for mucosal support to lower intestinal permeability. In determining which substance to use, it is helpful to understand the proposed mechanism of action. Administration of therapeutic substances must be carried out under the supervision of a medical practitioner. Application of this test to children between the ages of 2 to 12 must be conducted under the supervision of a medical practitioner, as well.

FUNCTIONAL LIVER DETOXIFICATION PROFILE (FLDP)

The liver is metabolically the most complex organ in the body and serves numerous vital functions. These functions include energy balance regulation, blood protein synthesis, and immune modulation.[51] Efficient liver function is necessary for the processing and excretion of endotoxic and exotoxic chemicals (hormones, drugs, chemicals, etc.), which are commonly referred to as xenobiotic chemicals.

Inefficient liver function can lead to metabolic poisoning, which is a nondescript term referring to the buildup within cells, tissues, and organs of metabolic end products and xenobiotics that have not been processed by the liver and excreted. These end products alter the pH gradient and electrolyte profile within cells and can serve as competitive enzyme inhibitors that ultimately interrupt effective bioenergetics within the cell. The symptoms of metabolic poisoning at the elevated level are reflective of poor energy dynamics and include fatigue, hypotonia, and brain biochemical disturbances. Recent studies have reported a relationship between impaired detoxification capability, mitochondrial dysfunction, and chronic fatigue syndrome.[52]

These reports suggest that oxidative damage to mitochondria and the detoxification process is itself a fundamental mechanism in the development of chronic fatigue syndrome. Well-recognized examples of metabolic poisoning include the symptoms of uremia or hepatic encephalopathy. Both of these conditions are associated with fatigue and central nervous system disturbances and are a consequence of this metabolic poisoning of specific tissues.

The liver possesses two mechanisms for the removal of unwanted chemicals from the body. In general, these unwanted substances are lipophilic in nature and are therefore difficult to transport across the cell membranes for excretion. The liver can chemically alter the compound by either an oxidation reaction (Phase I), or a conjugation reaction that adds a small molecule (Phase II). The interpretive guidelines for Phase I and II reactions are outlined in Box 7-2. These reactions have the effect of making the compound more polar or water-soluble, thereby allowing it to be more easily excreted

■ **Box 7-2** ■

FUNCTIONAL LIVER DETOXIFICATION PROFILE (FLDP) INTERPRETIVE GUIDELINES

Phase I: P-450 Detoxification
Low caffeine clearance (Phase I)
Indicates slow P-450 enzyme activity due to enzyme inhibitors (e.g., drugs, toxic metals, enterotoxins, liver damage, and/or insufficient nutrient cofactors)
High caffeine clearance (Phase I)
Reflects excessive P-450 enzyme induction, possibly resulting from exposure to cigarette smoking, alcohol, drugs (prescribed and illicit), and absorption of enterotoxins (i.e., leaky gut)
Note: High Phase I can indicate an increased risk of free radical damage.
Low Sulphate/Creatinine Ratio
Reflects low amount of glutathione and sulphate available for detoxification. Excess exposure to xenobiotics. Increased free radical activity
Molybdenum deficiency (required for conversion of sulfites to sulfates)
High Sulphate/Creatinine Ratio
A high sulphate/creatinine ratio suggests adequate levels of glutathione and efficient sulfation conjugation

Phase II: Conjugation Pathways
Low Glutathionation
Indicates low levels of glutathione available for removal of toxic intermediate metabolites and increased risk of free radical activity
Low Sulfation
Inadequate sulphate reserves for conjugation of biotransformed molecules, especially steroid hormones, drugs, xenobiotics and phenolic compounds
Low Glucuronidation
May also indicate low sulfation or glycination. Glucuronidation is an important pathway when sulfation and/or glycination are compromised
Low Glycination
Limited glycine available for salicylate conjugation. Increased risk of free radical activity
High Phase II Result
Indicates increased burden for specific conjugation pathways. Prolonged stress on a particular pathway will cause an increase in free radical damage that, in turn, will reduce liver function in the long term

in the urine or bile. This biotransformation process occurs for a great number of xenobiotics, such as enterotoxins (potentially toxic chemicals endogenously generated by gut bacteria), endobiotics (intermediate and end products of normal metabolism and enzymolysis), and exotoxins (ingested, inhaled, and absorbed toxic chemicals).[53,54]

Phase I reactions use the mixed microsomal enzymes designated as the cytochrome P-450 mixed function oxidase (MFO) enzymes. This intensively studied class of enzymes resides on the endoplasmic reticulum membrane system of hepatocytes. The primary function of these enzymes is to oxidize unwanted chemicals for excretion. Human liver cells possess the genetic code for many isoenzymes of P-450, whose synthesis can be induced on exposure to specific chemicals. This provides a mechanism of protection from a wide variety of toxic chemicals. As a result of this oxidative process, oxygen free radicals can be generated in substantial quantities, which, in some instances, can change harmless compounds into potential carcinogens. Consequently, an overactive or induced P-450 system can be a potent source of damaging free radical pathology, necessitating antioxidant therapy such as vitamin E, C, and beta-carotene.

Phase II reactions involve the addition of a small, polar molecule to the chemical. This conjugation step may or may not be preceded by a Phase I reaction. The conjugation molecules are acted on by specific enzymes to catalyze the reaction step. Molecules used by the liver for this purpose include glutathione, sulphate, glycine, acetate, cysteine, and glucuronic acid. Adequate amounts of these molecules are necessary for proper detoxification ability. Table 7-7 lists nutritional therapies during the different phases.

> Standard liver function tests (LFTs) only assess existing pathologic damage to hepatocytes.

Test Procedure

Low doses of caffeine, aspirin, and paracetamol are taken orally. Saliva and urine samples are collected at timed intervals and sent to the laboratory for analysis. An average dose of 200 mg of caffeine (equivalent to two cups of strong coffee) is taken in the morning and its clearance rate (Phase I) is determined by analyzing two saliva samples taken at prescribed time intervals

TABLE 7-7 ■ Nutritional Support Summary

PHASE I	INTERMEDIATE PHASE	PHASE II
Vitamins B_2, B_3, B_6, B_{12}, folic acid	Vitamin A, C, E, Se, Cu, Zn, Mn	Amino Acids (glutathione, glycine, cysteine, glutamine, methionine, taurine, arginine, N-acetyl cysteine)
Glutathione	Co Q10	
Branched-chain amino acids (leucine, isoleucine, glycine)	Garlic and onions	Vitamins B_2, B_5, B_{12}, C, E, folic acid
	Bioflavonoids	
Flavonoids	Silymarin	Selenium, zinc, molybdenum, magnesium
Phospholipids	Pycnogenol	Fish oils
		Cruciferous vegetables (cabbage, broccoli, Brussels sprouts)
		Green tea
		An adequate protein diet

after ingestion. Aspirin (650 mg) and paracetamol (750 mg) are taken before going to bed, and urine is collected over the following 10 hours. The total volume of urine is noted and a subsample taken off for analysis. Again, administration of therapeutic substances and application of this test to children must be carried out under the supervision of a medical practitioner.

The FLDP provides valuable information for patients with altered intestinal permeability, autoimmune disease, chronic fatigue syndrome, encephalopathy, food allergies, headaches, hepatitis, infectious bowel disease, intestinal toxemia, chemical sensitivities, premenstrual tension, and exposure to xenobiotics.

REFERENCES

1. Eaton K: Position statement and fungal-type dysbiosis, *J Nutr Env Med* 12:5-9, 2002.
2. Brenner RR: Factors influencing fatty acid chain elongation and desaturation. In Vergroessen AJ, Crawford MA, editors: *The role of fats in human nutrition,* London, 1989, Academic Press.
3. Burton JL: Essential fatty acids in atopic eczema. Clinical. In Horrobin DF, editor: *Omega-6 essential fatty acids: pathophysiology and roles in clinical medicine,* 1990, Wiley-Liss.
4. Horrobin DE: *Omega-6 essential fatty acids: pathophysiology and roles in clinical medicine,* 1990, Wiley-Liss.
5. Hauman BF: Inform 1997. Nutritional aspects of n-3 fatty acids, *Am Oil Chem Soc* May:428-447.
6. Connor SL, Connor WE: Are fish oils beneficial in the prevention and treatment of coronary artery disease? *Am J Clin Nutr* 66 (4 suppl)1020S-31S, 1997.
7. Mansour MP, Sinclair AJ: Changes in the levels of plasma trans fatty acids reflect changes in dietary intake, *Proc Nutr Soc* 19:48, 1995.
8. 4th International congress on essential fatty acids and eicosanoids, *Prostaglandins Leukot Essent Fatty Acids* 57:181-268, 1997.
9. Allard JP, Kurian R, Aghdassi E, et al: Lipid peroxidation during n-3 fatty acid and vitamin E supplementation in humans, *Lipids* 32:535-41, 1997.
10. Kalmijn S, Feskens EJ, Launer LJ, et al: Polyunsaturated fatty acids, antioxidants, and cognitive function in very old men, *Am J Epidemiol* 145:33-41, 1997.
11. Ma J, Folsom AR, Shahar E, et al: Plasma fatty acid composition as an indicator of habitual dietary fat intake in middle-aged adults. The Atherosclerosis Risk in Communities (ARIC) Study Investigators, *Am J Clin Nutr* 62:564-71, 1995.
12. Makrides M: Essential fatty acids in infancy: nutritional requirements, problems and practicalities, *Proc Nutr Soc Austr* 21:21-7, 1997.
13. NHMRC: Report of working party. The role of polyunsaturated fatty acids in the Australian diet, 1992, Australian Government Publishing Service.
14. Fatty acids and lipids from cell biology to human disease. Proceedings of the 2nd international congress of the ISSFAL. Bethesda, MD, June 7-10, 1995, *Lipids* 31(suppl):S1-S325, 1996.

15. Salem N, Ward GR: Are omega-3 fatty acids essential nutrients? In Simopoulos AP, editor: *Nutrition and fitness in health and disease, World Review of Nutrition and Dietetics,* Vol 72, Washington, DC, 1993, Karger Publishing.

16. Simopoulos AS: Summary of the NATO advanced research workshop on dietary omega-3 and omega-6 fatty acids: biological effects and nutritional essentiality, *J Nutr* 119:521-8, 1989.

17. Siscovick DS, Raghunathan TE, King I, et al: Dietary intake and cell membrane levels of long chain. n-3 polyunsaturated fatty acids and the risk of primary cardiac arrest, *JAMA* 274:1363-7, 1995.

18. Sinclair AJ, O'Dea K, Johnson L: Estimation of the n-3 status in a group of urban Australians by the analysis of plasma studies: phospholipid fatty acids, *Aust J Nutr Dietet* 51:53-6,1994.

19. Daviglus ML, Stamler J, Orencia AJ, et al: Fish consumption and the 30-year risk of fatal myocardial infarction, *N Engl J Med* 336:1046-53, 1997.

20. Parviainen MT, Jaaskelainen K, Kroger H, et al: Urinary bone resorption markers in monitoring treatment of symptomatic osteoporosis, *Clin Chim Acta* 279:145-54, 1999.

21. Taguchi Y, Gorai I, Zhang MG, et al: Differences in bone resorption after menopause in Japanese women with normal or low bone mineral density: quantitation of urinary cross-linked N-telopeptides, *Calcif Tissue Int* 62:395-9, 1998.

22. Chaki O, Yoshikata I, Kikuchi R, et al: The predictive value of biochemical markers of bone turnover for bone mineral density in postmenopausal Japanese women, *J Bone Miner Res* 15:1537-44, 2000.

23. Bonn D: Parathyroid hormone for osteoporosis, *Lancet*, 1996.

24. Creighton DL, Morgan AL, Boardley D, et al: Weight-bearing exercise and markers of bone turnover in female athletes, *J Appl Physiol* 90:565-70, 2001.

25. Aardal E, Holm AC: Cortisol in saliva—reference ranges and relation to cortisol in serum, *Eur J Clin Chem Clin Biochem* 33:927-32, 1995.

26. Heim C, Ehlert U, Hanker JP, et al: Abuse-related posttraumatic stress disorder and alterations of the hypothalamic-pituitary-adrenal axis in women with chronic pelvic pain, *Psychosom Med* 60:309-18, 1998.

27. Christiansen K, Knussmann R: Sex hormones and cognitive functioning in men, *Neuropsychobiology* 18:27-36, 1987.

28. Wren B, McFarland K, Edwards L, et al: Effect of sequential transdermal progesterone cream on endometrium, bleeding pattern, and plasma progesterone and salivary progesterone levels in postmenopausal women, *Climacteric* 3(3):155-60, 2000.

29. Vining RF, McGinley RA: The measurement of hormones in saliva: possibilities and pitfalls, *J Steroid Biochem* 27:81-94, 1987.

30. Brzezinski A: Melatonin in humans, *N Engl J Med* 336:186-95, 1997.

31. Drossman DA, Li Z, Andruzzi E, et al: U.S. householder survey of functional GI disorders: prevalence, sociodemography and health impact, *Dig Dis Sci* 38: 1569-80, 1993.

32. Johnson LR: Gastric secretion. In Johnson LR, editor: *Gastrointestinal physiology,* ed 5, St. Louis, 1997, Mosby.

33. Lipski E: *Digestive wellness,* New Canaan, CT, 1996, Keats.

34. Topping DL: Short-chain fatty acids produced by intestinal bacteria, *Asia Pacific J Clin Nutr* 5:15-9, 1996.

35. Cooper R, Fraser SM, Sturrock RD, et al: Raised titres of anti-Klebsiella IgA in ankylosing spondylitis, rheumatoid arthritis and inflammatory bowel disease, *Br Med J* (Clin Res Ed) 296:1432-4, 1988.
36. Russo AR, Stone SL, Taplin ME, et al: Presumptive evidence for Blastocystis hominis as a cause of colitis, *Arch Intern Med* 148:1064, 1988.
37. Montecucco C, Schiavo G: Mechanisms of action of tetanus of botulinum neurotoxins, *Mol Microbiol* 13:1-8, 1994.
38. Murray DM: Clinical relevance of infection by *Helicobacter pylori, Clin Microbiol Lett* 15:33-7, 1993.
39. Parsonnet J, Friedman GE, Vandersteen DP, et al: *Helicobacter pylori* infection and the risk of gastric carcinoma, *N Engl J Med* 325:1127-31, 1991.
40. Malaty HM, Graham DY, Klein PD, et al: Transmission of *Helicobacter pylori* infection. Studies in families of healthy individuals, *Scand J Gastroenterol* 26: 927-32, 1991.
41. Westblom TU, Madan E, Kemp J, et al: Evaluation of a rapid urease test to detect *Campylobacter pylori* infection, *J Clin Microbiol* 26:1393-4, 1988.
42. Barthel JS, Everett ED: Diagnosis of *Campylobacter pylori* infections: the "gold standard" and the alternatives, *Rev Infect Dis* 12(suppl 1):S107-14, 1990.
43. Graham DY, Malaty HM, Evans DG, et al: Epidemiology of *Helicobacter pylori* in an asymptomatic population in the United States. Effect of age, race, and socioeconomic status, *Gastroenterology* 100:1495-501, 1991.
44. Loffeld RJ, et al: The prevalence of anti-*Helicobacter (Campylobacter) pylori* antibodies in patients and healthy blood donors, *J Med Microbol* 32:105-9, 1991.
45. Fiedorek SC, Malaty HM, Evans DL, et al: Factors influencing the epidemiology of *Helicobacter pylori* infection in children, *Pediatrics* 88:578-82, 1991.
46. Crissinger KD, Kvietys PR, Granger DN: Pathophysiology of gastrointestinal mucosal permeability, *J Intern Med Suppl* 732:145-54, 1990.
47. Deitch EA: The role of intestinal barrier failure and bacterial translocation in the development of systemic infection and multiple organ failure, *Arch Surg* 125:403-4, 1990.
48. Peters TJ, Bjarnason I: Uses and abuses of intestinal permeability measurements, *Can J Gastroenterol* 2:127-32, 1988.
49. Rooney PJ, Jenkins RT, Buchanan WW: A short review of the relationship between intestinal permeability and inflammatory joint disease [see comments], *Clin Exp Rheumatol* 8:75-83, 1990.
50. Munkholm P, Langholz E, Hollander D, et al: Intestinal permeability in patients with Crohn's disease and ulcerative colitis and their first degree relatives, *Gut* 35:68-72, 1994.
51. Berne RM, Levy MN: *Physiology,* ed 4, St. Louis, 1998, Mosby.
52. Rea WJ: *Chemical sensitivity: tools of diagnosis and methods of treatment,* Vol 4, Boca Raton, FL, 1997, Lewis Publishers.
53. Anderson KE: Dietary regulation of cytochrome P450, *Annu Rev Nutr* 11:141-67, 1991.
54. Bland JS: Nutritional upregulation of hepatic detoxification enzymes, *J Appl Nutr* 44(3-4):2-15, 1992.

PART TWO

DISEASE MANAGEMENT

■ CHAPTER 8 ■

ACNE

Acne vulgaris is a common skin condition characterized by inflammation of sebaceous glands. There is no cure for acne. Gradual improvement occurs over time. Factors believed to trigger acne include emotional stress, oral contraceptives, and corticosteroids. The prevalence of acne peaks during adolescence, and males are more severely affected than females.

CLINICAL DIAGNOSIS

Androgens stimulate keratin turnover, and keratin plugs block drainage of sebum from the sebaceous glands. Open comedones (blackheads) and closed comedones (whiteheads) form as sebum is trapped in the duct of the gland. Lipid in the trapped sebum is broken down into inflammatory fatty acids by lipases produced by *Propionibacterium acnes*. Papules and pustules are formed. Breakdown of the sebum results in cyst formation; in severe cases, scarring may cause permanent disfigurement. The face, neck, upper chest, back, and shoulders are commonly involved. Emotional problems and social withdrawal may result.

THERAPEUTIC STRATEGY

Acne is the result of four distinct processes: increased proliferation, cornification, and shedding of follicular epithelium; increased sebum production; colonization of the follicle with *P. acnes*; and induction of inflammatory responses by bacterial antigens and cell signals.[1] The focus of disease management has shifted toward earlier treatment targeting these fundamental processes. The aims of treatment are to unblock sebaceous ducts, inactivate bacteria responsible for releasing inflammatory fatty acids from sebum, decrease sebaceous gland activity, and/or change the consistency of sebum.

LIFESTYLE CHANGES

Good skin care involves gentle washing with normal soap, but no more than twice a day. The area may be exposed to moderate sunlight, but oil-based cosmetics should be avoided; and the lesions should not be scrubbed, picked, or squeezed. Squeezing can burst the gland, dispersing fatty acids into the surrounding tissue, thereby increasing inflammation and scarring.

Beneficial dietary modification seems to be largely limited to increasing dietary fiber. Fat and refined carbohydrates are postulated to increase sebum production. However, investigations of modified sugar intake have had contradictory outcomes. Chocolate, shellfish, nuts, fatty foods, and soft drinks are not scientifically recognized causes of acne. Food sensitivity, although long suspected, has yet to be scientifically validated. Nonetheless, it may be wise to avoid foods suspected to aggravate acne.

NUTRIENT THERAPY/DIETARY SUPPLEMENTS

Nutritional intervention may dampen the inflammatory response.[2] Attempts to change the composition of sebum may be made by increasing dietary essential fatty acids, such as flaxseed oil (20 mL in the morning) or evening primrose oil (1 g taken twice a day with food). This change favors production of less inflammatory eicosanoids. Supplementation with vitamin E (200 IU twice a day), selenium (200 ug/day), zinc (135 mg/day combined with copper, 2 mg/day) may also reduce inflammation. In Swedish studies[3] depressed glutathione peroxidase levels have been found in patients with acne, and clinical trials with selenium supplementation have had some positive results.

Vitamin A is involved in the maintenance of epithelial tissue; deficiency of vitamin A is associated with hyperkeratinization. Patients with acne may have relatively low serum and skin levels of vitamin A. Synthetic vitamin A derivatives (e.g., isotretinoin) are used in pharmacologic doses in severe cases. Doses of 25,000 to 100,000 IU of vitamin A are effective; the dose is then reduced. Because of the potential for hepatotoxicity, vitamin A in doses greater than 10,000 IU should be avoided. Doses of no more than 2500 IU a day should be taken by women who may become pregnant. Acute toxic effects should be suspected in patients who experience headache, nausea, ataxia, or depression. Prolonged use of vitamin A at levels of 25,000 IU and greater is associated with evidence of long-term toxic effects. Patients may complain of blurred vision, skin desquamation, and hair loss. On physical examination, hepatosplenomegaly may be detected. Treatment needs to be continued for at least 4 weeks before results can be expected. Retinoic acid may also be applied as a cream or gel to comedones. Although retinoids are the mainstay of modern acne treatment,[4] medical intervention includes a combination of retinoids and antimicrobials. Topical retinoids have comedolytic and, in some cases, anti-inflammatory effects, but because they lack any direct effect on *P. acnes,* use of antibiotics is warranted.[1]

The nutrient alternative to antibiotics is zinc. Zinc acetate appears to be an effective antibacterial in the short-term treatment of acne.[5] Clinical trials support the use of 135 mg of zinc per day.[2] Persons with pustular acne and zinc deficiency benefit most. However, zinc is less effective than antibiotics in eliminating the bacteria that trigger fatty acid breakdown.

For acne that worsens just before menstruation, vitamin B_6 offers a clinically supported natural intervention.[2] Premenstrual acne may respond to daily vitamin B_6 in doses of 50 mg, starting 7 days before and continued during the menstrual period. Topical plus systemic pantothenic acid (10 g/day in divided doses) has also been shown to be effective.[6]

HERBAL THERAPY

Attempts to unblock glands can be made by drying the lesion; and topical application of 5% to 15% tea tree oil is reputed to achieve this effect. Four clinical trials have provided promising, but by no means compelling, evidence that tea tree oil may be an effective treatment for acne.[7] Within a few days to several months, tea tree oil undergoes photo-oxidation, leading to the creation of degradation products that are moderate to strong sensitizers. Photo-oxidation occurs regardless of whether tea tree oil is kept in open or closed bottles or other containers. Patients using tea tree oil topically may become sensitized to this natural remedy.[8]

PRACTICE TIPS

- Acne does not result from oily hair touching the forehead or face; therefore, bangs or fringes need not be cut.
- Open comedones are not dirt to be removed by scrubbing; they result from oxidation of inspissated sebum blocking the duct of the sebaceous gland.
- Local applications tend to cause redness and drying of the skin.
- High doses of vitamins A, E, and B_5 may be effective.
- Lavender oil—with its antibacterial, anti-inflammatory, and astringent effects—may help if it is applied to blemishes.

CASE STUDY BY IAN BRIGHTHOPE

J.J. is a 17-year-old boy who had had acne vulgaris for the past 3 years. The acne was getting worse over the previous 6 months and topical applications were not helping. Administration of broad-spectrum antibiotics improved the condition but caused an irritable bowel–type syndrome and was stopped. Oral contraceptives and isotretinoin were considered, but the family had a philosophical objection to both medications and decided to seek alternative medical advice. J.J. consumed approximately 2/3 L of milk per day and had a fondness for cheese and chocolate. A full hair analysis revealed low levels of zinc, chromium, and selenium; and radioallergosorbent test results were highly positive for cow's milk and positive for chocolate and yeast. He was started on a low-stress diet, including increased intake of vegetables, brown rice, fish, and a green juice complex. He eliminated all dairy food, chocolate, and yeast from the diet. He was encouraged to drink 2 liters of water per day. Within 2 weeks, there was a marked improvement in his skin with a 20% decrease in the formation of new comedones and a 10% decrease in nodules. Pustules remained the same because of the time it takes for them to resolve. The level of inflammation in the skin had diminished. These changes may have occurred without any dietary intervention, but this level of change had not been apparent for more than 12 months. J.J. wished to go to the next phase of treatment and took some nutritional supplements. The following program has been found to be most useful.

1. Vitamin A: 500,000 units immediately, then 50,000 units daily for 3 months, then 50,000 units on alternate days (watch for dry skin, headaches, and diplopia)
2. Vitamin C: 1000 mg 4 times a day; intravenous vitamin C, 15 to 30 g per day if acne is severe
3. Natural vitamin E: 250 to 500 IU, per day orally, which can also be applied locally to healing lesions to reduce scarring
4. Zinc chelate: 30 mg of elemental zinc 3 times a day, reducing after 1 week to two times a day, reducing after 1 month to once a day (watch for nausea and joint pains)
5. Selenium: 200 mcg per day of elemental selenium as either sodium selenite or selenomethionine (higher doses must be monitored with a monthly blood test)
6. High-potency B complex vitamin: one daily, more B_6 may be needed (>50 mg)
7. Yeast-free chromium chelate: 600 mcg of elemental chromium per day, especially if there are cravings for sugar
8. *Lactobacillus rhamnosus* and *Bifidobacterium species*; with bacteriocins, 5 billion organisms three times a day, preferably before meals; give if patient has been taking antibiotics
9. Greens Powder (green juice complex): 2 to 4 g of green juice complex daily in juice or water
10. Evening primrose oil with γ-linolenic acid: 1000 mg, three times a day, which may be doubled, if necessary; do not give during acute flare-ups; best used when lesions are disappearing and resolving

J.J. received the first six supplements in the list for 6 weeks, during which time his acne almost completely disappeared. He was still getting a few whiteheads and his skin was blotchy. The dosages of these supplements were halved, and he stopped taking the vitamin A. He was then given a rotation of items 7 to 10 for an additional 3 months; he took each formula for 2 weeks or until no further improvement could be observed. His skin continued to improve, and the scarring that had occurred was notably less severe. His general well-being also dramatically improved: he had increased energy levels and more enthusiasm for his university studies. Incidentally, some long-standing warts on his hands, which had been intractable to any therapy, resolved by resorption.

REFERENCES

1. Shalita A: The integral role of topical and oral retinoids in the early treatment of acne, *J Eur Acad Dermatol Venereol* 15(suppl 3):43-9, 2001.
2. Wernbach MR: *Textbook of nutritional medicine*, Tarzana, CA, 1999, Third Line Press
3. Bruce A: Swedish views on selenium, *Ann Clin Res* 18:8-12, 1986.
4. Zouboulis CC: Exploration of retinoid activity and the role of inflammation in acne: issues affecting future directions for acne therapy, *J Eur Acad Dermatol Venereol* 15(suppl 3):63-7, 2001.
5. Fluhr JW, Bosch B, Gloor M, Hoffler U: In-vitro and in-vivo efficacy of zinc acetate against propionibacteria alone and in combination with erythromycin, *Zentralbl Bakteriol* 289:445-56, 1999.
6. Leung LH: Pantothenic acid deficiency as the pathogenesis of acne vulgaris, *Med Hypotheses* 44:490-2, 1995.
7. Ernst E, Huntley A: Tea tree oil: a systematic review of randomized clinical trials, *Forsch Komplementarmed Klass Naturheilkd* 7:17-20, 2000.
8. Hausen BM, Reichling J, Harkenthal M: Degradation products of monoterpenes are the sensitizing agents in tea tree oil, *Am J Contact Dermat* 10:68-77, 1999.

CHAPTER 9

ALLERGIC RHINITIS

Perennial allergic rhinitis is an immunoglobulin (IgE)–mediated inflammatory disorder of the nasal mucosa. Predisposing factors include a family disposition, environmental agents (e.g., dust mites, animal dander, pollen, and grasses), and food allergy. The immediate-response phase of allergic rhinitis is triggered by an allergen-IgE reaction in the nasal mucosa. Food sensitivities, some environmental agents, structural abnormalities, metabolic conditions, or drugs may trigger the condition. Approximately 2 to 8 hours after initial exposure, a delayed-response phase, characterized by increased sensitivity to the allergen, occurs. Mast cell degranulation in the immediate-response phase and basophil release of histamine in the delayed-response phase account for many of the symptoms. Histamine binding to H_1-receptors increases vasodilatation, capillary permeability, and smooth muscle contraction, resulting in a watery nasal discharge from a swollen, nasal mucosa.

Patients with allergic rhinitis experience a decline in physical and mental health status. The coexistence of asthma and allergic rhinitis is frequent, with allergic rhinitis usually preceding asthma. The prevalence of allergic rhinitis in asthmatic patients is 80% to 90%.[1] The shared immunologic pathogeneses in allergic rhinitis and asthma are the nasal bronchial reflex and allergen sensitization.[2]

CLINICAL DIAGNOSIS

Allergic rhinitis is characterized by paroxysms of sneezing, nasal congestion, pruritus, and rhinorrhea. Conjunctival, nasal, and pharyngeal congestion may be present. Nasal polyps may develop.

THERAPEUTIC STRATEGY

Intervention consists of preventing exposure to dietary and environmental triggers and changing the internal environment to one that is less pro-inflammatory.

LIFESTYLE CHANGES

Dietary triggers should be avoided. Food allergy triggers include eggs, nuts, fish, shellfish, dairy products, and wheat.[3] Chickpeas have also been found to trigger respiratory allergic reactions in populations in which they are a staple food.[4]

In view of the links with atopy, it is not surprising that a consistent negative relationship has been detected between prevalence rates of wheezing, allergic rhinoconjunctivitis, and atopic eczema and the intake of starch, cereals, and vegetables.[5] However, another study showed that, unlike asthma, which was found to be directly related to saturated fat intake and inversely related to intake of monounsaturated fat and vitamins C and E, none of these nutritional factors were associated with allergic rhinitis.[6]

NUTRIENT THERAPY/DIETARY SUPPLEMENTS

Current thinking suggests that bromelain, quercetin, N-acetylcysteine, and vitamin C are safe, natural remedies that may be used as primary therapy or in conjunction with conventional methods.[7] Quercetin, by stabilizing membranes, exerting a potent antioxidant effect, and inhibiting hyaluronidase, inhibits inflammatory processes attributed to neutrophils activated. Membrane stabilization results in prevention of mast cell and basophil degranulation and decreases inflammation by inhibition of neutrophil lysosomal enzyme secretion and leukotriene production. The recommended dosage of quercetin for patients with allergic rhinitis ranges from 250 to 600 mg, three times daily, 5 to 10 minutes before meals.[7] At an equivalent dose, quercetin is a more potent membrane stabilizer than sodium cromoglycate.

More dubious is the use of vitamin C and N-acetylcysteine.[7] Vitamin C has been found to exert a number of effects on histamine. Histamine levels were found to increase exponentially as ascorbic acid levels in the plasma decreased. Vitamin C appears to prevent the secretion of histamine by leukocytes and increase its detoxification. Patients with nasal pH values closer to 8.0 (normal range, 5.5 to 7) seem to respond more favorably to vitamin C therapy. For treatment of allergic rhinitis, a dosage of at least 2 g per day should be administered. N-acetylcysteine, a natural, sulfur-containing amino acid derivative, detoxifies and protects cells against oxidative stress and is an effective mucolytic agent in doses of 200 mg, twice daily. Its usefulness in allergic rhinitis has yet to be investigated. Recommended therapeutic dosages range from 500 to 2000 mg daily.

Other nutrients that may be helpful are selenium and vitamins A, B, and E.

HERBAL THERAPY

A review of herbal interventions revealed that some herb-based medicines specifically reduced histamine-induced reactions (e.g., rhinorrhea, sneezing, and itching).[8] Various herbs are helpful.[9] Anticatarrhal herbs such as goldenseal and immune-enhancing herbs such as echinacea deserve consideration. *Urtica dioica* (stinging nettle), an antiallergic herb, contains histamine, serotonin, and acetylcholine in the fresh stinging hairs on its leaves. In a randomized, double-blind study, more than half of the patients who were given 300 mg of freeze-dried *U. dioica* per day regarded it as helpful.[10] The benefits may be attributable to histamine acting as an autocoid (a local hormone) to modulate the immune response.

Bromelain may be helpful as a mucolytic and anti-inflammatory agent. The therapeutic dose of bromelain for allergic rhinitis ranges from 400 to 500 mg (1800-2000 mcu potency) three times daily.[11] Bromelain is taken concomitantly with quercetin.

Other natural interventions that may be useful for the treatment of allergic rhinitis include chamomile, elderflower, eyebright, garlic, goldenrod, feverfew, yarrow, royal jelly, ephedra, hydrangea root, *Ligusticum porteri*, and olive leaf. Chinese herb formulas are also beneficial and appear to control perennial allergic rhinitis by modulating the function of lymphocytes and neutrophils.[12]

Because stress is perceived to aggravate rhinitis, an herbalist may consider using ginseng.

PRACTICE TIPS

• In patients with seasonal rhinitis, herbal and nutrient intervention should be initiated some 6 weeks before the start of the hay fever season.

REFERENCES

1. Leynaert B, Neukirch F, Demoly P, Bousquet J: Epidemiologic evidence for asthma and rhinitis comorbidity, *J Allergy Clin Immunol* 106(suppl 5):S201-S205, 2000.
2. DuBuske LM: The link between allergy and asthma, *Allergy Asthma Proc* 20:341-5, 1999.
3. Sampson HA, Ho DG: Relationship between food-specific IgE concentrations and the risk of positive food challenges in children and adolescents, *J Allergy Clin Immunol* 100:444-51, 1997.
4. Patil SP, Niphadkar PV, Bapat MM: Chickpea: a major food allergen in the Indian subcontinent and its clinical and immunochemical correlation, *Ann Allergy Asthma Immunol* 87:140-5, 2001.
5. Ellwood P, Asher MI, Bjorksten B, et al: Diet and asthma, allergic rhinoconjunctivitis and atopic eczema symptom prevalence: an ecological analysis of the International Study of Asthma and Allergies in Childhood (ISAAC) data. ISAAC Phase One Study Group, *Eur Respir J* 17:436-43, 2001.
6. Huang SL, Pan WH: Dietary fats and asthma in teenagers: analyses of the first Nutrition and Health Survey in Taiwan (NAHSIT), *Clin Exp Allergy* 31:1875-80, 2001.

7. Thornhill SM, Kelly AM: Natural treatment of perennial allergic rhinitis, *Altern Med Rev* 5:448-54, 2000.

8. Bielory L, Lupoli K: Herbal interventions in asthma and allergy, *J Asthma* 36: 1-65, 1999.

9. Mills S, Bone K: *Principles and practice of phytotherapy*, Edinburgh, 2000, Churchill Livingstone.

10. Mittman P: Randomized, double-blind study of freeze dried *Urtica dioica* in the treatment of allergic rhinitis, *Planta Med* 56:44-7, 1990.

11. Kelly GS: Bromelain: a literature review and discussion of its therapeutic applications, *Altern Med Rev* 1:243-57, 1996.

12. Yang SH, Hong CY, Yu CL: Decreased serum IgE level, decreased IFN-gamma and IL-5 but increased IL-10 production, and suppressed cyclooxygenase 2 mRNA expression in patients with perennial allergic rhinitis after treatment with a new mixed formula of Chinese herbs, *Int Immunopharmacol* 1:1173-82, 2001.

■ CHAPTER 10 ■

ALZHEIMER'S DISEASE

About 7% of the population aged 65 years and older has Alzheimer's disease. Alzheimer's disease is the most common form of dementia in the elderly; the incidence of this disease doubles roughly every 5 years after the age of 65.[1] Mortality rates rise with increasing levels of cognitive deficit.

What begins with cognitive deficiencies progresses to impaired orientation and disordered behavior with loss of independence. Alzheimer's disease should be suspected in persons of 55 years or older who present with deterioration of short-term memory, personality changes, and atypical mood changes. Such changes should be taken seriously in anyone older than 40 years.

CLINICAL DIAGNOSIS

In patients with Alzheimer's disease, memory problems, characterized by poor concentration and faulty short-term memory, gradually develop over months and years. Long-term memories are better retained. Patients cannot recall recent events but can reminisce about the past. Familiar tasks are well performed, but learning new tasks is daunting. Progressive intellectual impairment is manifested by an inability to solve problems, poor judgment, and impaired insight. Patients have a rigid outlook. Language deterioration presents as disordered speech and difficulty in reading and writing. Mood changes are encountered, and despite a normal level of consciousness, patients are inattentive. Patients demonstrate gradual disintegration of their personality with blunting of affect, increasing tactlessness, apathy, and loss of initiative. Social withdrawal is inevitable. Results of laboratory investigations are normal.

Although numerous other associations have been found, only four risk factors, namely, increasing age, the presence of the apolipoprotein E–epsilon 4 allele, familial aggregation of cases, and Down syndrome, are firmly established.[1] The epsilon 4 allele of the apolipoprotein E gene (*APOE4*) on chromosome 19 is regarded as a true susceptibility factor for the onset of the late and prevalent form of Alzheimer's disease.[2]

THERAPEUTIC STRATEGY

Although there is currently no cure for Alzheimer's disease, there may be ways of preventing it, slowing its progression, and reducing symptom severity, especially in its early stages. Overall potential therapeutic targets include enhancing cholinergic transmission, restricting oxidative stress and inflammation, preventing B-amyloid formation and toxicity, and elevating circulating levels of estrogens and other neurotrophic agents, such as nerve growth factor.[3] From a natural medicine perspective, once a treatable cause of dementia has been excluded, enhancing cholinergic transmission, reducing inflammation, and avoiding neurotoxins become important intervention strategies.

Genetic and environmental factors have been shown to interact in the development of both early- and late-onset forms of the disease. One potential intervention strategy is to reduce oxidative stress. Neurons are extremely sensitive to attacks by destructive free radicals. Apolipoprotein E is subject to attacks by free radicals, and apolipoprotein E peroxidation has been correlated with Alzheimer's disease. However, apolipoprotein E can also act as a free radical scavenger, and this behavior is isoform-dependent. Although inheritance of *APOE4* increases the risk of disease and decreases the age of onset,[4] the *APOE2* allele appears to be protective, lowering the risk of disease and increasing the age at onset. Free radicals have been linked with β-amyloid in a positive feedback cycle closely associated with the locally induced, nonimmune-mediated, chronic inflammatory responses seen relatively early in the brains of patients with Alzheimer's disease. The neurodegenerative plaques of Alzheimer's disease are characterized by a self-sustaining acute-phase reaction in which both interleukin-1 (IL-1) and IL-6 are upregulated. Sex hormones, nitric oxide, and eicosanoid precursors (e.g., fish oil) may all potentially alter this inflammatory process.[5] Vascular nitric oxide has an autocrine anti-inflammatory impact on endothelium and inhibits macrophage IL-6 production. Estrogen promotes vascular nitric oxide synthesis and potentially blocks IL-6 production in brain glia and astrocytes and limits brain IL-1 activity. Likewise, testosterone can inhibit IL-6 induction in androgen-responsive cells, which may include brain glia and astrocytes. Results of epidemiologic studies suggest that anti-inflammatory drugs prevent or retard Alzheimer's disease.[6,7]

Cell membranes of patients with Alzheimer's disease appear to have low polyunsaturated fatty acids levels,[8] and ω-3 fatty acids are potent neuroprotectors that can inhibit the synthesis and release of proinflammatory cytokines, such as tumor necrosis factor-α.[9] Whether inflammation alone is sufficient to cause neurodegeneration remains uncertain.

With respect to sporadic or nonfamilial Alzheimer's disease, in addition to controlling inflammation, elimination of neurotoxins should also be considered. Aluminum is a neurotoxin linked with Alzheimer's disease.[10] Although results of animal studies support this postulate,[11] aluminum remains a controversial risk factor for sporadic Alzheimer's disease.[12]

LIFESTYLE CHANGES

Establishing simple daily routines is the key to prolonging the patient's independence. Patients with Alzheimer's disease often demonstrate unexplained weight loss and cachexia. Abnormally elevated levels of physical activity and energy expenditure, rather than a hypermetabolic state, need to be considered as possible causes.[13] Because weight loss increases the risk of infection, skin ulcers and falls increase, a management system that ensures that these patients eat regular nutritious meals and undertake controlled, rather than exhaustive, physical activity is recommended. Physical activity appears beneficial, although a diet with high levels of vitamins—particularly B_6, B_{12}, and folate—and a moderate intake of red wine also appear to be protective.[1]

NUTRIENT THERAPY/DIETARY SUPPLEMENTS

Although causal links have not been proven, regular use of aluminum cookware is probably not a good idea. Furthermore, although no particular diet has been shown to prevent Alzheimer's disease, it may be prudent to regularly eat fish, fresh fruits, and vegetables. Fish is a good source of docosahexaenoic acids, the fatty acids, which are depleted in the brains of patients with Alzheimer's disease. Supplementation with fish oil and evening primrose oil may favorably redress the eicosanoid balance.

Fruits and vegetables are good sources of antioxidants. Longitudinal and cross-sectional comparisons of 442 subjects showed that higher ascorbic acid and beta-carotene plasma levels are associated with better memory performance in people aged 65 and older.[14] Good dietary antioxidants include citrus fruits, peppers, pineapple, squash, and cantaloupe. In addition to a diet rich in antioxidants, supplementation with vitamin C (2000 mg), carotenoids (25,000 IU retinol equivalents), and vitamin E may further boost free radical scavenging.

A placebo-controlled, clinical trial of 2000 IU (1342 α-tocopherol equivalents) of vitamin E per day in patients with moderately advanced Alzheimer's disease indicated that vitamin E may slow functional deterioration.[15] A double-blind, placebo-controlled, randomized, multicenter trial in patients with Alzheimer's disease of moderate severity demonstrated that α-tocopherol slowed the progression of disease by 670 days.[16] Vitamin E also prevents the oxidative damage induced by β-amyloid in cell culture and delays the onset of memory deficits in animal models. However, in a review of all unconfounded, double-blind, randomized trials in which treatment with vitamin E at any dose was compared with placebo, Tabet et al[17] concluded there was insufficient evidence for efficacy of vitamin E in the treatment of people with Alzheimer's disease. Because an excess of falls occurred in the vitamin E group, vitamin E supplementation may require further evaluation.

Another study investigating the relationship of plasma antioxidants to reduced functional capacity in the elderly showed that women with low lycopene and low low-density lipoprotein (LDL) cholesterol levels had more dependencies (3.6:1) than women with high lycopene and low LDL cholesterol levels.[18] Good sources of lycopene are tomatoes, guavas, and watermelon. Results of animal and in vitro studies suggest that reducing cholesterol may reduce β-amyloid deposits and production.[19] A selective fat diet may be prudent.

It has been suggested that apolipoprotein E–related differences in insulin metabolism in Alzheimer's disease may be related to disease pathogenesis.[20] There is a growing body of evidence to suggest that carbohydrate neurochemistry, particularly thiamin neurochemistry, is disrupted in Alzheimer's disease.[21,22] Recently, daily supplementation of thiamin at levels of 8 g, but not 3 g, had a mild beneficial effect.[23] However, despite a significant correlation between vascular dementia and the intake of vitamins B_1 and B_{12}, zinc, and selenium and total blood antioxidant capacity, no links have been demonstrated in Alzheimer's disease.[24]

The plasma homocysteine level is another significant predictor of the severity of dementia: elevated levels are detected in 45% of patients with dementia.[25] In view of their relationship to the production of hyperhomocysteinemia, vitamin B_{12} and folate have a potential role in the pathophysiology of Alzheimer's disease.[26] Foods enriched with physiologic doses of vitamins and folate-supplemented breakfast cereal (200 µg per serving) have been shown to correct abnormalities of folate in the elderly[27] and reverse elevation of homocysteine levels.[28] Food-based supplementation deserves consideration.

HERBAL THERAPY

In humans, many free radical scavengers, including vitamin E, selegiline, and *Ginkgo biloba* extract EGb 761, have produced promising results.[29] Of the herbal remedies, gingko holds the greatest promise. Specific ginkgolides interact with the cholinergic system and have neuroprotective or regenerative capabilities, and flavonoids, present in ginkgo, act as antioxidants.[2] The published evidence suggests that, although ginkgo is of questionable use for memory loss, it has some effect on dementia.[30] All but one of 40 controlled trials of ginkgo extracts in the treatment of dementia demonstrated clinically significant improvement in memory and concentration and reduction in fatigue, anxiety, and depressed mood; but in most studies of gingko, patient populations were poorly defined, sample sizes were small, and nonstandard measures were used.[31] A recent, well-designed, multicenter study showed significantly less decline in cognitive function among patients with dementia receiving gingko. A 26-week trial of 120 mg (40 mg, three times a day) of ginkgo extract was conducted with mildly to severely impaired patients who been given a diagnosis of uncomplicated Alzheimer's disease or multi-infarct dementia.[32] This double-blind, placebo-controlled, parallel-group study demonstrated that although the placebo group showed a statistically significant worsening in all domains of assessment, the group receiving ginkgo extract showed slight improvement in assessments of cognition, daily living, and social behavior. No differences between ginkgo extract and placebo were observed with respect to safety. In contrast, in another trial, ginkgo at a dose of 240 mg or 160 mg per day was not found to be an effective treatment for older people with mild to moderate dementia or age-associated memory impairment.[33] Nonetheless, a review of trials indicated that ginkgo extracts are effective in managing minor cognitive impairment, but more evidence is needed to ascertain its efficacy in more severe forms of dementia.[34] The efficacy of gingko may well be related to the cause of the dementia.

Ginseng deserves a brief mention. A ginkgo/ginseng combination was found to have a somewhat positive effect on cognitive function in a 90-day, double-blind, placebo-controlled, parallel-group study involving 64 persons aged 40 to 65 years.[35] The extent to which this outcome was attributable to ginseng rather than gingko is unknown. Indian ginseng (*Withania somniferum*) modulates cholinergic activity and has a neuroprotective effect in vitro.[2]

It should be noted that a number of potential interactions between herbal and conventional drugs place older people at risk for an adverse drug event.[36]

PRACTICE TIPS

- The earlier natural intervention measures are implemented, the more beneficial is the clinical impact.
- Dietary, nutritional, and herbal interventions in the prodromal stages are more likely to favorably influence the progression of Alzheimer's disease.
- Select fish oil supplement in which 1 g fish oil contains 120 mgDHA and 180 mgEPA.

CASE STUDY BY IAN BRIGHTHOPE

Brian was a 68-year old former cleric who had experienced deteriorating short-term memory and extreme restlessness with depression for 12 to 18 months. He had been given a diagnosis of Alzheimer's disease with moderate cortical atrophy and ventricular enlargement 5 months before presentation. His general physical health was excellent, and he intermittently maintained quite a positive attitude toward life. His family was advised that he was seriously affected and that they should consider his admission to a nursing home, if not immediately, within the next 3 months. His wife was 72 years of age and had managed to cope with him, with assistance, at home.

The family sought nutritional assistance and was advised that it might be helpful but that change would be slow and the result might not be much better than his current condition. Additional pathology tests with abnormal results included the following:

1. Low normal serum vitamin B_{12} levels
2. Low normal serum folic acid levels
3. Low normal thyroid function
4. Subnormal basal body temperature
5. Low intracellular magnesium levels
6. Low normal serum zinc levels
7. Total heavy metal overload in hair analysis (including lead, mercury, aluminum, and cadmium)
8. Increased antigluten and antigliadin antibodies

Brian began receiving a gluten-free diet consisting of:

1. Pure water, 1.5 L daily
2. Fish, three times a week
3. Lecithin, 20 to 50 g daily
4. Vegetables, six to eight portions daily
5. High-protein soy-based "shake," one daily
6. Other unprocessed foods

His nutritional supplementation plan consisted of:

1. Natural vitamin E, 250 IU four times a day
2. Vitamin C with quercetin, 1000 mg three times a day
3. High docosahexaenoic acid (DHA) tuna fish and evening primrose oil capsules, 2000 mg three times a day
4. Niacinamide, 500 mg two times a day
5. High-potency B complex vitamin, one daily (50-100 mg of each main B vitamin)
6. Halibut liver oil capsules, two daily
7. Magnesium aspartate/chelate, 200-300 mg of elemental magnesium at night
8. Zinc chelate, 30 mg of elemental zinc in the morning

He was also prescribed 10 mcg of tertroxin (thyroid hormone, triiodothyronine) for his clinical hypothyroidism.

In addition, the following substances were administered:

1. Intravenous ethylenediamine tetraacetic acid (EDTA) chelation therapy (2 g of EDTA in 5% dextrose, 3-hour infusions twice weekly, 10 weeks of treatment, weekly to monthly infusions thereafter)
2. Intravenous sodium ascorbate (5 g after EDTA infusions)
3. Intravenous magnesium (200-500 mg per infusion)
4. Intramuscular injections (B complex, 50-200 mg of the main vitamins biweekly; 15 mg of folic acid twice weekly)

A review of his condition after 6 weeks suggested that he was less depressed and less agitated and was sleeping better. He was also more active and showed a greater interest in current affairs and in his old church. There was no change in memory.

At this time, he was given an extract of *Gingko biloba*. A review in another 8 weeks by an independent assessor showed that his short-term memory had improved significantly, and this correlated with his clinical presentation and family reports.

Brian, despite strong vociferous objections to all the "pills" he had to swallow, continued with this program until he died in his sleep at the age of 77. He remained at home and was never admitted to a nursing home. He gardened and helped his wife, who survived him, until the end. Exercise, such as walking, is extremely important in patients with early Alzheimer's disease, if they can do it.

A note on the use of *Gingko biloba*: It is very effective and its effects are evident sooner, within a couple of weeks, if patients who are as ill as Brian are given an appropriate nutritional program.

This program, or a modified version, should be prescribed for anyone older than 40 years who shows the early mental symptoms of dementia. The nutrients will also help those patients who may have other forms of dementia such as vascular (fish oils and vitamin E), multi-infarct (vitamin E, selenium, and essential fatty acids), Parkinson's-associated dementia (vitamin E), and alcoholic brain disease (antioxidants and B group vitamins).

REFERENCES

1. McDowell I: Alzheimer's disease: insights from epidemiology, *Aging (Milano)* 13:143-62, 2001.
2. Oliveira JR, Zatz M: The study of genetic polymorphisms related to serotonin in Alzheimer's disease: a new perspective in a heterogenic disorder, *Braz J Med Biol Res* 32:463-7, 1999.
3. Ernst E: *Herbal medicine: a concise overview for professionals*, Oxford, 2000, Butterworth Heineman.
4. Saunders AM: Apolipoprotein E and Alzheimer disease: an update on genetic and functional analyses, *J Neuropathol Exp Neurol* 59:751-8, 2000.
5. McCarty MF: Vascular nitric oxide, sex hormone replacement, and fish oil may help to prevent Alzheimer's disease by suppressing synthesis of acute-phase cytokines, *Med Hypotheses* 53:369-74, 1999.
6. Eikelenboom P, Rozemuller AJ, Hoozemans JJ, et al: Neuroinflammation and Alzheimer disease: clinical and therapeutic implications, *Alzheimer Dis Assoc Disord* 14(suppl 1):S54-S61, 2000.
7. Rogers J, Webster S, Lue LF, et al: Inflammation and Alzheimer's disease pathogenesis, *Neurobiol Aging* 17:681-6, 1996.
8. Youdim KA, Martin A, Joseph JA: Essential fatty acids and the brain: possible health implications, *Int J Dev Neurosci* 18:383-99, 2000.
9. Das UN: Beneficial effect(s) of ω-3 fatty acids in cardiovascular diseases: but, why and how? *Prostaglandins Leukot Essent Fatty Acids* 63:351-62, 2000.

10. Strong MJ, Garruto RM, Joshi JG, et al: Can the mechanisms of aluminum neurotoxicity be integrated into a unified scheme? *J Toxicol Environ Health* 48:599-613, 1996.

11. Exley C: A molecular mechanism of aluminum-induced Alzheimer's disease? *J Inorg Biochem* 76:133-40, 1999.

12. Yokel RA: The toxicology of aluminum in the brain: a review, *Neurotoxicology* 21:813-28, 2000.

13. Poehlman ET, Dvorak RV. Energy expenditure, energy intake, and weight loss in Alzheimer disease. *Am J Clin Nutr* 2000; 71:650S-655S.

14. Perrig WJ, Perrig P, Stahelin HB: The relation between antioxidants and memory performance in the old and very old, *J Am Geriatr Soc* 45:718-24, 1997.

15. Grundman M: Vitamin E and Alzheimer disease: the basis for additional clinical trials, *Am J Clin Nutr* 71:630S-636S, 2000.

16. Sano M, Ernesto C, Thomas RG, et al: A controlled trial of selegiline, alpha-tocopherol, or both as treatment for Alzheimer's disease. The Alzheimer's Disease Cooperative Study, *N Engl J Med* 336:1216-22, 1997.

17. Tabet N, Birks J, Grimley Evans J: Vitamin E for Alzheimer's disease (Cochrane Review), *Cochrane Database Syst Rev* 4:CD002854, 2000.

18. Snowdon DA, Gross MD, Butler SM: Antioxidants and reduced functional capacity in the elderly: findings from the Nun Study, *J Gerontol A Biol Sci Med Sci* 51:M10-M16, 1996.

19. Sparks DL, Martin TA, Gross DR, Hunsaker JC: Link between heart disease, cholesterol, and Alzheimer's disease: a review, *Microsc Res Tech* 50:287-90, 2000.

20. Craft S, Asthana S, Schellenberg G, et al: Insulin effects on glucose metabolism, memory, and plasma amyloid precursor protein in Alzheimer's disease differ according to apolipoprotein-E genotype, *Ann N Y Acad Sci* 903:222-8, 2000.

21. Blass JP, Sheu RK, Gibson GE: Inherent abnormalities in energy metabolism in Alzheimer disease. Interaction with cerebrovascular compromise, *Ann N Y Acad Sci* 903:204-21, 2000.

22. Heroux M, Raghavendra Rao VL, Lavoie J, et al: Alterations of thiamine phosphorylation and of thiamine-dependent enzymes in Alzheimer's disease, *Metab Brain Dis* 11:81-8, 1996.

23. Meador K, Loring D, Nichols M, et al: Preliminary findings of high-dose thiamine in dementia of Alzheimer's type, *J Geriatr Psychiatry Neurol* 6:222-9, 1993.

24. Tabet N, Mantle D, Walker Z, Orrell M: Vitamins, trace elements, and antioxidant status in dementia disorders, *Int Psychogeriatr* 13:265-75, 2001.

25. Nilsson K, Gustafson L, Hultberg B: The plasma homocysteine concentration is better than that of serum methylmalonic acid as a marker for sociopsychological performance in a psychogeriatric population, *Clin Chem* 46:691-6, 2000.

26. Reynish W, Andrieu S, Nourhashemi F, Vellas B: Nutritional factors and Alzheimer's disease, *J Gerontol A Biol Sci Med Sci* 56:M675-M680, 2001.

27. de Jong N, Paw MJ, de Groot LC, et al: Nutrient-dense foods and exercise in frail elderly: effects on B vitamins, homocysteine, methylmalonic acid, and neuropsychological functioning, *Am J Clin Nutr* 73:338-46, 2001.

28. Malinow MR, Duell PB, Irvin-Jones A, et al: Increased plasma homocyst(e)ine after withdrawal of ready-to-eat breakfast cereal from the diet: prevention by breakfast cereal providing 200 microg folic acid, *J Am Coll Nutr* 19:452-7, 2000.

29. Christen Y: Oxidative stress and Alzheimer disease, *Am J Clin Nutr* 71: 621S-629S, 2000.

30. Ernst E: The risk-benefit profile of commonly used herbal therapies: Ginkgo, St. John's Wort, Ginseng, Echinacea, Saw Palmetto, and Kava, *Ann Intern Med* 136:42-53, 2002.

31. Beaubrun G, Gray GE: A review of herbal medicines for psychiatric disorders, *Psychiatr Serv* 51:1130-4, 2000.

32. Le Bars PL, Kieser M, Itil KZ: A 26-week analysis of a double-blind, placebo-controlled trial of the *Ginkgo biloba* extract EGb 761 in dementia, *Dement Geriatr Cogn Disord* 11:230-7, 2000.

33. van Dongen MC, van Rossum E, Kessels AG, et al: The efficacy of ginkgo for elderly people with dementia and age-associated memory impairment: new results of a randomized clinical trial, *J Am Geriatr Soc* 48:1183-94, 2000.

34. Linde K, ter Riet G, Hondras M, et al: Systematic reviews of complementary therapies—an annotated bibliography. Part 2: herbal medicine, *BMC Comp Alter Med* 1(1):5, 2001.

35. Wesnes KA, Faleni RA, Hefting NR, et al: The cognitive, subjective, and physical effects of a *Ginkgo biloba/Panax ginseng* combination in healthy volunteers with neurasthenic complaints, *Psychopharmacol Bull* 33:677-83, 1997.

36. Gold JL, Laxer DA, Dergal JM, et al: Herbal-drug therapy interactions: a focus on dementia, *Curr Opin Clin Nutr Metab Care* 4:29-34, 2001.

■ CHAPTER 11 ■

ANXIETY

One in four people is affected by anxiety at some point in life. Anxiety may result from trying to meet family or work demands perceived as excessive, or it may be self-imposed through attempts to meet unrealistic personal expectations.

In a survey on the use of complementary and alternative therapies for anxiety and depression, one in five subjects said they visited a complementary medicine therapist, but more than half reported using alternative therapies to treat anxiety or severe depression during the past 12 months.[1] In this survey, two of three patients who saw a conventional provider because of anxiety attacks or severe depression also reported that they used alternative therapies to treat their condition.

CLINICAL DIAGNOSIS

Generalized anxiety manifests as a pervading, persistent sense of apprehension in the absence of an identifiable threat. Characterized by intense concern about trivial or unrealistic problems, anxiety is aggravated by somatic awareness. It is perpetuated and escalated by awareness of physical symptoms such as a dry mouth, pounding heart, or tense muscles, induced by autonomic and motor changes. A sleep disturbance is common. In addition to chronic anxiety, acute anxiety may manifest as a panic attack. Panic attacks are experienced as recurrent, unexpected episodes of intense anxiety. Figure 11-1 provides a self-screen for the detection of clinical anxiety.

THERAPEUTIC STRATEGY

Anxiety has cognitive, emotional, and physical elements. In addition to attempts to change cognitive and somatic perceptions by behavioral means, chemical interventions can used to modify neurotransmitters. Monoamine changes in the brain are believed to be associated with anxiety disorders.[2] The major monoamine neurotransmitters are the catecholamines— dopamine, norepinephrine, and epinephrine—and the indolamine, serotonin. Both serotonin and γ-aminobutyric acid (GABA), another inhibitory

❑ Am I clinically anxious?

SELF-SCREEN FOR GENERALISED ANXIETY

Indicate if you regularly experience:

❑ *Feelings of apprehension.* This may present as:
  ❑ an exaggerated startle response (e.g. in response to a loud noise)
  ❑ hypervigilance
  ❑ an exaggerated sensitivity to bright lights, sound or pain
  ❑ generalised unease and restlessness

❑ *Feelings of frustration.* This may present as:
  ❑ irritability
  ❑ impatience

❑ *Cognitive difficulties.* This may be manifest as:
  ❑ difficulty in concentrating
  ❑ mental 'blanks'
  ❑ confusion

❑ *Sleep disturbance.* This may present as:
  ❑ difficulty falling asleep
  ❑ early waking
  ❑ interrupted sleep
  ❑ excess sleep (hypersomnia)

❑ *Autonomic dysfunction.* This may present with:
  ❑ palpitations or a pounding heart
  ❑ shallow, rapid breathing
  ❑ dizziness, lightheadedness and tingling
  ❑ a tight throat/lump in the throat
  ❑ diarrhea
  ❑ hyperventilation and dizziness
  ❑ urinary frequency
  ❑ a clammy skin
  ❑ a dry mouth

❑ *Motor tension.* This may present as:
  ❑ restlessness
  ❑ a tremble
  ❑ aching muscles
  ❑ headache
  ❑ fatigue
  ❑ residual muscle tension (see Handout 12.9)

Professional help is recommended if you have ticked at least three boxes and are regularly troubled by six or more of the above symptoms.

PANIC ATTACKS

I have episodes of intense anxiety during which I experience:

❑ acute breathlessness
❑ dizziness and lightheadedness
❑ palpitations or a pounding heart
❑ trembling

❑ flushes, chills or sweating
❑ paraesthesia and tingling
❑ feelings of unreality (depersonalisation)

Professional help is indicated if you experience episodes of intense unease associated with four of the above.

FIG. 11-1 Self-screen for anxiety. From www.jamisonhealth.com, Elsevier Science.

neurotransmitter, affect mood, anxiety, and sleep. These two neurotransmitters are believed to control anxiety, depression, and pain perception. Interventions that enhance the action of GABA appear to encourage skeletal muscle relaxation and modulate emotional activity, reducing anxiety without significantly depressing respiratory or vasomotor centers.

LIFESTYLE CHANGES

Stress management techniques, ranging from improved problem solving to relaxation strategies, deserve consideration. Pets have been found to enhance well-being and decrease anxiety. Regular aerobic exercise is beneficial, and food sensitivity should routinely be ruled out.

Food choices may influence anxiety. Avoidance of excess caffeine, alcohol, and sugar has long been surmised to be helpful. More recently, ingestion of fats has been recognized as influencing behavioral responses. Consumption of lard and a vegetable margarine with a high content of saturated fatty acids was found to decrease hypothalamic serotonin levels, whereas ingestion of a sunflower oil and an olive oil–enriched margarine, both high in polyunsaturated fatty acids, did not significantly affect serotonin levels.[3]

In animal studies, researchers have found that a phytoestrogen-rich diet fed to adult rats produces anxiolytic effects.[4] These experiments showed that consumption of dietary phytoestrogens results in very high plasma isoflavone levels, which could significantly alter sexually dimorphic brain regions and affect anxiety, learning, and memory. These changes were noted even when consumption occurred over a relatively short period in adulthood. Further investigation is required before any firm recommendations can be made.

NUTRIENT THERAPY/DIETARY SUPPLEMENTS

Controlled clinical trials have demonstrated that any one of the following is helpful in treating anxiety: L-5-hydroxytryptophan (200-900 mg/day), inositol (500-1200 mg/day), or correction of selenium deficiency (200 μg daily).[5] Tryptophan is the precursor of serotonin. Despite abundant evidence that serotonin is involved in anxiety in both animals and humans, acute tryptophan depletion, although it enhanced the effect of a panic attack, was found to have little effect on general levels of anxiety.[6] Another study confirmed that tryptophan depletion did not induce a significant general change in subjective anxiety but tended to induce anxiety in females.[7]

Diverse nutrients, including calcium, magnesium, ω-3 fatty acids, vitamins C, E, and B complex, are believed to be helpful. A double-blind, randomized, controlled trial of healthy male volunteers showed that Berocca (Roche), a multivitamin mineral supplement, was associated with consistent and statistically significant reductions in anxiety and perceived stress.[8] Various explanations for this outcome can be surmised. Vitamin B_6 facilitates production of serotonin from tryptophan, and the nutritional status of vitamin B_6 has a significant and selective modulatory impact on central production of both serotonin and GABA.[9] Furthermore, although selective serotonin reuptake inhibitors are considered the first-line treatment option for premenstrual syndrome, a recent double-blind, placebo-controlled study of women indicated that calcium was effective in reducing emotional, behavioral, and physical premenstrual symptoms.[10]

Alterations in calcium homeostasis, hypocalcemia, and hypercalcemia have long been associated with many affective disturbances. Clinical trials in women with premenstrual syndrome have shown that calcium supplementation effectively alleviates the majority of mood and somatic symptoms.[11] Calcium supplementation of 1200 to 1600 mg daily is recommended for women who experience premenstrual syndrome. Inclusion of 100 mg of pantothenic acid as part of a B complex has also been suggested for particularly stressful periods.[12]

HERBAL THERAPY

Herbs appear to be the superior natural option for the management of anxiety. Valerian and kava hold particular promise.

Valerian is a popular over-the-counter anxiolytic. In humans, it seems to be quite safe.[13,14] Valerian extracts cause both central nervous system depression and muscle relaxation. Aqueous extracts of the root contain appreciable amounts of GABA, which may directly cause sedation; or sedation may result from an interaction of valerian constituents with central GABA receptors (e.g., valerenic acid has been shown to inhibit enzyme-induced breakdown of GABA in the brain).[15] In one study a commercially mixed herbal formulation containing *Valeriana officinalis*, a valerian-only aqueous extract (400 mg), was compared with placebo in the treatment of subjects with various sleep difficulties.[16] Both valerian preparations produced a significant decrease in subjectively evaluated sleep latency scores and improved sleep quality. A sleep laboratory study demonstrated that although the effects of 900 mg of valerian on sleep were not significantly different from those of placebo, it did decrease subjective feelings of somatic arousal without affecting physiologic activation.[17] A laboratory study of healthy volunteers showed that valerian, as well as kava, may be beneficial to health by reducing physiologic reactivity during stressful situations.[18]

Although several double-blind, placebo-controlled trials have demonstrated the anxiolytic efficacy of kava, these studies had ill-defined patient populations, small sample sizes, and short treatment duration.[19] Nonetheless, in a systematic review and meta-analysis, Pittler and Ernst[20] concluded that kava extract deserved consideration as a symptomatic treatment for anxiety. Kava may achieve its sedative effect by a number of mechanisms. It appears that kava may improve vagal control in generalized anxiety disorder.[21] Anxiety disorders are associated with decreased vagal control of heart rate and increased risk of death from heart disease and sudden cardiac death. A preliminary study suggested that kava may exert a favorable effect on reflex vagal control of heart rate in generalized anxiety disorders. The improved baroreflex control of heart rate induced by kava paralleled the patient's clinical improvement.[21] In addition to the anxiolytic effect of kava being achieved by modulation of a peripheral nervous system trigger, central nervous system modification may also play a role.

Kava extract has been reported to affect neurotransmission at the level of GABA receptors, without modifying GABA or benzodiazepine binding. The kavapyrones affect the glutamate systems and inhibit sodium and calcium channels, resulting in centrally acting skeletal muscle relaxation and an anticonvulsant effect. The uptake of norepinephrine, a "feel good" neurotransmitter, is also inhibited. Clinical trials have shown that kava is superior to placebo, and roughly equivalent to oxazepam, 15 mg/day, or bromazepam, 9 mg/day.[22] A 5-week randomized, placebo-controlled, double-blind study showed that kava was well tolerated and reduced symptoms of anxiety, tension, and restlessness after benzodiazepine treatment was withdrawn.[23] Kava does not show the tolerance problems associated with benzodiazepines. At a daily therapeutic dose of around 200 mg, kava may cause mild gastrointestinal complaints and/or allergic skin reactions in up to 1.5% of people.[17] Other side effects caused by using kava are discussed more thoroughly in chapter 77. Kava extract is increasingly regarded as an effective alternative to antidepressants and tranquilizers in the treatment of anxiety of nonpsychotic origin. It has emerged as an efficacious short-term treatment for anxiety.[24]

A number of other herbs warrant investigation. The adaptogenic qualities of Siberian ginseng (100-300 mg three times a day) may benefit anxious patients who are stressed and fatigued. In animal studies *Hypericum perforatum* and *Panax ginseng* were found to be associated with significant and qualitatively comparable antistress activity as judged by a variety of behavioral and physiologic changes in rats exposed to long-term stress.[25] There is also some scientific support for combination herbal therapy. Findings from animal studies have indicated that a combination of *Ginkgo biloba* and *Zingiber officinale* (ginger) has anxiolytic effects comparable to those of diazepam; however, in high doses, anxiogenic properties were also noted.[26] Herbal combinations of *Crataegus, Ballota, Passiflora*, and *Valeriana* species, with their mild sedative effects, and *Cola* and *Paullinia* species, which mainly act as mild stimulants, fared better than placebo in a multicenter, double-blind, general practice study of outpatients with anxiety disorders.[27]

PRACTICE TIPS

- Patients taking sedatives or tranquilizers (e.g., diazepam, tricyclic antidepressants) may be become excessively drowsy if they are also taking black cohosh, kava, melatonin, valerian, or serotonin.
- Addition of a dozen drops of lavender to a warm bath is relaxing.

CASE HISTORY BY PAUL HOLMAN

Merran is a 55-year-old office manager who, 3 months before our initial consultation, had suddenly felt unwell at work. She had experienced an abrupt onset of dizziness, lightheadedness, and uncomfortable "electric sensations" in her trunk and limbs. These symptoms were followed by moderately severe anxiety, verging on panic, and a feeling of breathlessness. Over the next few weeks, these sensations followed a fluctuating course with an overall increase in severity, but neurologic and cardiologic investigation failed to demonstrate any identifiable problem. Left with no clear-cut diagnosis and continuing to have inexplicable symptoms, Merran began having frank panic attacks, and she was referred to me.

The history revealed that Merran was an artistic and highly sensitive person (HSP) with a tendency toward perfectionism, a desire to help others before attending to her own needs and a disposition to worry. She had not been treated for psychological problems before, but neither had her life been as stressful as it had been in the previous 18 months with worry over her depressed, unemployed husband and a mildly anorexic daughter preparing for final year school examinations.

Merran's general health was good, and she had passed smoothly through menopause 2 years previously without significant physical or psychologic symptoms. She took no medication or supplements except calcium carbonate as an osteoporosis preventive, although results of a recent bone density test had been normal. Her digestion was good, but her dietary history revealed a low protein intake in the context of a very light breakfast and lunch and animal protein at tea time on only three to four occasions per week. There were no nutritional or thyroid deficiency symptoms or signs, although a tendency to dry skin might have indicated essential fatty acid (EFA) deficiency. At our first interview, her original symptoms were still prominent, together with marked initial and middle insomnia and some mild depressive symptoms, such as loss of confidence and drive and occasional tearfulness.

On examination, Merran showed herself to be a quiet, likeable, intelligent woman who expressed herself well, was psychologically minded, and appeared tense but not clinically depressed. Her blood pressure was on the low side, 110/70 mm Hg sitting, and she appeared to be a chest breather with occasional sighs.

We discussed her symptoms in terms of stress overload and chronic habitual hyperventilation (HV) as a possible factor in producing dizziness and breathlessness.

A provisional formulation is shown in Table 11-1.

TABLE 11-1 ■ Provisional Formulation

PREDISPOSING	PRECIPITATING	PERPETUATING
HSP	Stress overload	Insomnia
Low on-self care	(Rescuing/helping)	HV
Low protein intake	HV	Tense, needy home atmosphere
? Other nutrient deficiency	Insomnia	? Nutrient deficiency (incl. Mg deficiency)

Merran was not keen on taking any medication, even for temporary night sedation, so we decided initially on tryptophan, 500 mg, at night with a low dose (<25 mg) multi-B vitamin, pending further nutritional investigation. Merran did not want an elaborate and expensive investigative effort, so we decided on the following:

- Determination of vitamin B_{12} and erythrocyte folate levels (obligatory in evaluation of anxiety and depression)
- Determination of erythrocyte magnesium level (may be lowered during hyperventilation)
- Determination of plasma EFA level (dry skin and often deficient in anxiety/depression)
- Hair mineral analysis (HMA) (an overall look at trace element status and mineral ratios within the constraints mentioned in the section on assessment)
- Thyroid function tests (previously done and normal [thyroid-stimulating hormone level <2.0])

At subsequent follow-up, capnometry revealed a low resting pCO_2 of 28 mm Hg, which rapidly dropped to 20 mm Hg with ventilatory provocation. At the same time, symptoms of dizziness and chest tightness appeared but rapidly resolved with rebreathing from cupped hands. The vitamin B_{12}/folate level was normal, magnesium level was low normal, and EFA showed a low $\omega 3/\omega 6$ ratio. HMA revealed an increased calcium/magnesium ratio and low levels of selenium, manganese, and boron. Tryptophan (500 mg) had not improved sleeping greatly, but more protein at lunchtime had reduced her tendency to experience more prominent symptoms later in the afternoon.

At this point, there seemed to be no reason to revise any points in the original formulation, and so the daily supplement regimen became the following:

- Tryptophan, 1000 mg at night
- Magnesium, 100 mg elemental at night
- Calcium - stop pro tem
- Multi B 1 mane
- Selenium 100 mcg
- EPA/DHA 1000 mg
- Vitamin E 250 IU

Omega-3 EFAs can be specifically helpful in relief of panic or anxiety, if these are deficient, as can selerum in depression.

When prescribing tryptophan, I always explain the history and symptoms of eosinophilia-myalgia syndrome so that patients can recognize the symptoms in the (extremely) unlikely event that they experience this problem.

Breath re-education was obviously a priority for Merran; she agreed to undertake this with instruction from me (with the help of a biofeedback device) and also in the ongoing context of a yoga class.

At the 3-month mark, she had improved greatly and was not experiencing any further panic attacks and had only minimal anxiety or somatic manifestations of anxiety when overtired or unable to preserve her daily personal space and quiet time. Ongoing issues related to the following:

- Counseling with respect to self-assertion and limit setting
- Ongoing management of her diet and the establishment of an ideal protein/carbohydrate ratio
- Further review of her osteoporosis risk and the need for further supplementation with calcium and trace elements such as manganese and boron

REFERENCES

1. Kessler RC, Soukup J, Davis RB, et al: The use of complementary and alternative therapies to treat anxiety and depression in the United States, *Am J Psychiatry* 158:289-94, 2001.
2. Cameron OG: Psychopharmacology, *Psychosom Med* 61:585-90, 1999.
3. Orosco M, Rouch C, Dauge V: Behavioral responses to ingestion of different sources of fat. Involvement of serotonin? *Behav Brain Res* 132:103-9, 2002.
4. Lephart ED, West TW, Weber KS, et al: Neurobehavioral effects of dietary soy phytoestrogens, *Neurotoxicol Teratol* 24:5-16, 2002.
5. Werbach MR: *Textbook of nutritional medicine*, California, 1999, Third Line Press.
6. Anderson IM, Mortimore C: 5-HT and human anxiety. Evidence from studies using acute tryptophan depletion, *Adv Exp Med Biol* 467:43-55, 1999.
7. Monteiro-dos-Santos PC, Graeff FG, dos-Santos JE, et al: Effects of tryptophan depletion on anxiety induced by simulated public speaking, *Braz J Med Biol Res* 33:581-7, 2000.
8. Carroll D, Ring C, Suter M, Willemsen G: The effects of an oral multivitamin combination with calcium, magnesium, and zinc on psychological well-being in healthy young male volunteers: a double-blind placebo-controlled trial, *Psychopharmacology (Berl)* 150:220-5, 2000.
9. McCarty MF: High-dose pyridoxine as an 'anti-stress' strategy, *Med Hypotheses* 54:803-7, 2000.
10. Pearlstein T, Steiner M: Non-antidepressant treatment of premenstrual syndrome, *J Clin Psychiatry* 61(suppl 12):22-7, 2000.
11. Thys-Jacobs S: Micronutrients and the premenstrual syndrome: the case for calcium, *J Am Coll Nutr* 19:220-7, 2000.
12. Diefendorf D, Healey J, Kalyn W, editors: *The healing power of vitamins, minerals and herbs*, Surry Hills, Australia, 2000, Readers Digest.
13. Fugh-Berman A, Cott JM: Dietary supplements and natural products as psychotherapeutic agents, *Psychosom Med* 61:712-28, 1999.
14. Kuhlmann J, Berger W, Podzuweit H, Schmidt U: The influence of valerian treatment on "reaction time, alertness and concentration" in volunteers, *Pharmacopsychiatry* 32:235-41, 1999.
15. Houghton PJ: The scientific basis for the reputed activity of valerian, *J Pharm Pharmacol* 51:505-12, 1999.

16. Leathwood PD, Chauffard F, Heck E, Munoz-Box R: Aqueous extract of valerian root (*Valeriana officinalis* L.) improves sleep quality in man, *Pharmacol Biochem Behav* 17:65-71, 1982.

17. Kohnen R, Oswald WD: The effects of valerian, propranolol, and their combination on activation, performance, and mood of healthy volunteers under social stress conditions, *Pharmacopsychiatry* 21:447-8, 1988.

18. Cropley M, Cave Z, Ellis J, Middleton RW: Effect of kava and valerian on human physiological and psychological responses to mental stress assessed under laboratory conditions, *Phytother Res* 16:23-7, 2002.

19. Beaubrun G, Gray GE: A review of herbal medicines for psychiatric disorders, *Psychiatr Serv* 51:1130-4, 2000.

20. Pittler MH, Ernst E: Efficacy of kava extract for treating anxiety: systematic review and meta-analysis, *J Clin Psychopharmacol* 20:84-9, 2000.

21. Watkins LL, Connor KM, Davidson JR: Effect of kava extract on vagal cardiac control in generalized anxiety disorder: preliminary findings, *J Psychopharmacol* 15:283-6, 2001.

22. Cauffield JS, Forbes HJ: Dietary supplements used in the treatment of depression, anxiety, and sleep disorders, *Lippincotts Prim Care Pract* 3:290-304, 1999.

23. Malsch U, Kieser M: Efficacy of kava-kava in the treatment of non-psychotic anxiety, following pretreatment with benzodiazepines, *Psychopharmacology (Berl)* 157:277-83, 2001.

24. Ernst E: The risk-benefit profile of commonly used herbal therapies: Ginkgo, St. John's Wort, Ginseng, Echinacea, Saw Palmetto, and Kava, *Ann Intern Med* 136:42-53, 2002.

25. Kumar V, Singh PN, Bhattacharya SK: Anti-stress activity of Indian *Hypericum perforatum* L, *Indian J Exp Biol* 39:344-9, 2001.

26. Hasenohrl RU, Nichau CH, Frisch CH, et al: Anxiolytic-like effect of combined extracts of *Zingiber officinale* and *Ginkgo biloba* in the elevated plus-maze, *Pharmacol Biochem Behav* 53:271-5, 1996.

27. Bourin M, Bougerol T, Guitton B, Broutin E: A combination of plant extracts in the treatment of outpatients with adjustment disorder with anxious mood: controlled study versus placebo, *Fundam Clin Pharmacol* 11:127-32, 1997.

■ CHAPTER 12 ■

ASTHMA

Asthma is characterized by episodes of acute breathlessness. This multifactorial disease results from the interaction of genetic, allergic, environmental, infectious, emotional, and nutritional factors. The underlying pathophysiology involves bronchial inflammation associated with airway hyperresponsiveness and increased mucus production.

Although few well-controlled studies support the efficacy of complementary therapies in the treatment of asthma or other atopic disorders, such interventions are popular self-care measures among patients.[1] However, patients are often not inclined to tell their primary care provider about their self-treatment regimen. Such omission is of clinical relevance because herbal preparations have been cited as the third most popular complementary treatment modality by British patients with asthma.[2]

CLINICAL DIAGNOSIS

Patients with asthma experience attacks of wheezing, coughing, and shortness of breath.

THERAPEUTIC STRATEGY

Asthma attacks are frequently triggered by airborne allergens, including dust mites. They may also be triggered by factors as diverse as food and psychosocial stress. Regardless of the trigger, the pathophysiologic changes in asthma are characteristic. Intervention focuses on modulating an immune-based inflammatory response.

An imbalance between an exaggerated humoral and suppressed cell-mediated immune system may influence genetic susceptibility to asthma.[3] An aberrant or inadequately regulated CD4+ T-cell immune response has been postulated. The T-helper 2 subset produces cytokines, including various interleukins that stimulate the growth, differentiation, and recruitment of mast cells, basophils, eosinophils, and B cells. Interleukin 4 (IL-4) promotes the synthesis of immunoglobulin E (IgE). IgE, plentiful in mast cells and basophils, mediates bronchospasm, a characteristic of asthma.

Cromolyn sodium, a drug used prophylactically in asthma, inhibits IL-4–induced bronchoconstriction. Prostaglandin E_2 (PGE_2) acts on T lymphocytes, reducing the formation of interferon-γ, which suppresses the synthesis of IgE. Linoleic acid is a dietary precursor of PGE_2. Over the last 20 years, an increased intake of linoleic acid has coincided with an increased prevalence of asthma, eczema, and allergic rhinitis[4] and has also paralleled a decrease in fish consumption. Fish is rich in eicosapentaenoic acid, which inhibits the formation of PGE_2.

A decreased cellular capacity to cope with oxidative stress is a potential risk factor for an asthma attack.[5] Free radicals may precipitate bronchospasm, induce mucus secretion, and cause microvascular leakage. This can be caused by direct inflammatory damage or induction of an autonomic imbalance between muscarinic receptor-mediated contraction and the β-adrenergic–mediated relaxation of pulmonary smooth muscle. Reduction of platelet glutathione peroxidase activity in the most severe cases suggests a diminished capacity to restore part of the antioxidant defenses; however, a case-control study failed to demonstrate any association between antioxidant intake and asthma.[6]

LIFESTYLE CHANGES

Although less than 10% of nonasthmatic children have subnormal levels of gastric acid, 80% of asthmatic children have hypochlorhydria. However, food sensitivities are only likely to contribute to asthmatic symptoms in a few people and only those with nonseasonal asthma. A practical approach to managing perennial asthma is to initially remove all foods eaten at least twice a week from the diet. Certain patients believe that avoidance of shellfish, chocolate, eggs, nuts, milk, cheese, certain liquors, and food additives such as metabisulfites, tartrazine (FD&C Yellow Dye #5), sodium benzoate, and sulfur dioxide is helpful. However, in a review Ardern and Ram[7] concluded that routine tartrazine exclusion may not benefit most patients, except those few individuals with proven sensitivity. Despite conflicting evidence as to whether tartrazine causes exacerbations of asthma, some studies have demonstrated a positive association, especially in individuals with cross-sensitivity to aspirin. Overall, IgE-mediated reactions to food are a minor cause of respiratory symptoms, particularly in children.

Although the role of food intolerance in asthma is well recognized, it is not the major cause of asthma, and there are no available data to support the use of nutritional supplements in the treatment of chronic asthma.[8] Although suboptimal intake of dietary nutrients may enhance bronchial inflammation, available data are insufficient to implicate any casual relationships. Nonetheless, a diet that favors fish (ω-3 fatty acids) rather than meat (ω-6 fatty acids) may be helpful. Results of a population-based, cross-sectional survey indicated that protein-rich and fat-rich or high-fat foods of animal origin were associated with a higher incidence of asthma in teenagers.[9]

Drinking coffee benefits patients with asthma. In fact, sudden elimination of caffeinated drinks can result in rebound bronchoconstriction. Theophylline, a popular bronchodilating prescription drug, is a metabolite of caffeine. A double-blind study demonstrated that a cup of coffee containing 150 mg of caffeine produced as much as a 15% increase in the volume of air asthmatic patients were able to expire in 1 second (FEV_1).[10] In patients with severe asthma, two cups of strong coffee (10 mg/kg) had efficacy and side effects (headache, dizziness, and tremor) similar to those of theophylline (5 mg/kg).[11] The minimal effective threshold to prevent exercise-induced bronchoconstriction seems to be around 7 mg/kg of caffeine.[12] If professional treatment is unavailable, emergency relief from an acute asthma attack may be obtained by drinking at least three large cups of brewed coffee.

A high-salt diet is associated with increased bronchial reactivity.[13] Although it may be logical to recommend avoidance of excess salt,[14] analysis of available evidence suggests that dietary salt intake is unrelated to allergic asthma.[15]

NUTRIENT THERAPY/DIETARY SUPPLEMENTS

Nutrients that have the potential to provide a measure of relief include the following: antioxidants, especially vitamins C and E, selenium, and zinc; vitamins B_6 and B_{12}; ω-3 fatty acids from fish; the flavonoid quercetin; and botanicals *Tylophora asthmatica*, *Boswellia serrata*, and *Petasites hybridus*.[3]

Although epidemiologic studies support a diet rich in ω-3 polyunsaturated fatty acids (PUFAs),[16] clinical trials have been more problematic. Eight randomized, controlled trials, six of parallel design and two cross-over studies, produced little evidence to recommend that people with asthma supplement or modify their dietary intake of fish oil to improve their asthma control.[17] Nonetheless, a diet that shifts the fatty acid ratio away from ω-6 fatty acids shunts eicosanoid production away from the arachidonic acid pathway and decreases the production of bronchoconstrictive leukotrienes. After taking 3 g of ω-3 PUFA daily for 30 days, seven atopic patients reported significant improvement.[18] It is possible that fish oil is only helpful in certain cases. A urinary ratio of 4-series to 5-series leukotrienes of less than 1, induced by ω-3 PUFA ingestion, may prove a useful predictor of respiratory benefit and discriminate between responders and nonresponders.[19] It should be noted that getting an adequate dietary intake may be problematic; at least two and probably four servings a week of cold water fish may be necessary to be effective.[20]

Suboptimal intake of dietary nutrients is believed to enhance inflammation and contribute to bronchial hyperreactivity in asthma; however, the role of the antioxidant vitamins A, C, and E and selenium, sodium, and magnesium requires clarification.[14] Results of epidemiologic studies suggest that vitamin C is beneficial. As vitamin C intake rises, forced expiratory volume in 1 second (FEV_1) and forced vital capacity increase. However, clinical studies in patients with asthma have yielded contradictory results.[3] Although current evidence from randomized, controlled trials is insufficient to recommend a specific role for vitamin C in the treatment of asthma,[21] it is worth noting that some studies suggest that vitamin C supplementation of 2 g improves FEV1, reduces exercise-induced brochospasm, and prevents airway reactivity induced by a metacholine challenge test.[22] Other antioxidant associations that lack clinical confirmation include the possibility that vitamin E and selenium could regulate the autonomic balance of bronchial smooth muscle receptors. Controlled clinical trials have demonstrated that supplementation with 100 µg of selenium and/or 400 mg of magnesium provides symptomatic relief but may not modify objective parameters.[22] Hypomagnesemia is common in patients with asthma, being lowest in those with more severe cases. A high magnesium intake is negatively associated with and a low zinc intake is positively associated with bronchial hyperreactivity.[20] Theoretically, zinc, plant sterols, and sterolins are all promising treatments that may address an immune imbalance in asthma.[18]

HERBAL THERAPY

Evaluation of 17 randomized clinical trials identified no definitive evidence for any of the herbal preparations investigated.[2] Some herbs have an anti-inflammatory effect, and others, an antispasmodic effect. Ephedra is one option because its sympathomimetic action favors bronchodilatation. However, it may cause insomnia and aggravate hypertension and anxiety. Turmeric, aloe vera, and *Boswellia serata* may reduce inflammatory mediators (e.g., leukotrienes) in asthma, whereas *Ginkgo biloba* may block platelet-activating factor.[23] Historically, ginkgo has been used to treat asthma. The ginkgolides have the capacity to antagonize bronchoconstriction, bronchial hyperresponsiveness, and the allergic response effects of platelet-activating factor.

Allergic wheezing may be caused by echinacea, psyllium, and isphagula.

PRACTICE TIPS

- Pyridoxal 5′-phosphate, found in lower concentrations in patients with asthma, may reduce symptoms of asthma and the side effects of theophylline when administered in the form of pyridoxine hydrochloride (at doses of 50 mg twice daily for adults and at doses of 100 mg twice daily for children).
- Vitamin B_6 may reduce the frequency and severity of acute asthmatic attacks. Tryptophan should be avoided; it is the precursor of serotonin, a bronchoconstrictor in patients with asthma.
- High doses of vitamin C reduce bronchospasm after exercise.

- A trial of betaine or glutamic hydrochloride should be considered for patients who have hypochlorhydria as determined by gastric acid testing.

REFERENCES

1. Graham DM, Blaiss MS: Complementary/alternative medicine in the treatment of asthma, *Ann Allergy Asthma Immunol* 85:438-47, 2000.
2. Huntley A, Ernst E: Herbal medicines for asthma: a systematic review, *Thorax* 55:925-9, 2000.
3. Miller AL: The etiologies, pathophysiology, and alternative/complementary treatment of asthma, *Altern Med Rev* 6:20-47, 2001.
4. Black PN, Sharpe S: Dietary fat and asthma: is there a connection? *Eur Respir J* 10:6-12, 1997.
5. Greene LS: Asthma and oxidant stress: nutritional, environmental, and genetic risk factors, *J Am Coll Nutr* 14:317-24, 1995.
6. Picado C, Deulofeu R, Lleonart R, et al: Dietary micronutrients/antioxidants and their relationship with bronchial asthma severity, *Allergy* 56:43-9, 2001.
7. Ardern KD, Ram FS: Tartrazine exclusion for allergic asthma (Cochrane Review), *Cochrane Database Syst Rev* 4:CD000460, 2001.
8. Monteleone CA, Sherman AR: Nutrition and asthma, *Arch Intern Med* 157:23-34, 1997.
9. Huang SL, Lin KC, Pan WH: Dietary factors associated with physician-diagnosed asthma and allergic rhinitis in teenagers: analyses of the first Nutrition and Health Survey in Taiwan, *Clin Exp Allergy* 31:259-64, 2001.
10. Gong H, Simmons MMS, Tashkin DP, et al: Bronchodilator effects of caffeine in coffee. A dose-response study of asthmatic subjects, *Chest* 89:335-42, 1986.
11. Becker AB, Simons KJ, Gillespie CA, Simons FE: The bronchodilator effects and pharmacokinetics of caffeine in asthma, *N Engl J Med* 310:743-6, 1984.
12. Kivity S, Ben Aahron Y, Man A, Topilsky M: The effect of caffeine on exercise-induced bronchoconstriction, *Chest* 97:1083-5, 1990.
13. Brighthope I: Nutritional medicine—its presence and power, *J Aust College Nutr Env Med* 17:5-18, 1998.
14. Baker JC, Ayres JG: Diet and asthma, *Respir Med* 94:925-34, 2000.
15. Ardern KD, Ram FS: Dietary salt reduction or exclusion for allergic asthma (Cochrane Review), *Cochrane Database Syst Rev* 4:CD000436, 2001.
16. Schwartz J: Role of polyunsaturated fatty acids in lung disease, *Am J Clin Nutr* 71(suppl 1):393S-396S, 2000.
17. Woods RK, Thien FC, Abramson MJ: Dietary marine fatty acids (fish oil) for asthma (Cochrane Review), *Cochrane Database Syst Rev* 4:CD001283, 2000.
18. Villani F, Comazzi R, De Maria P, Galimberti M: Effect of dietary supplementation with polyunsaturated fatty acids on bronchial hyperreactivity in subjects with seasonal asthma, *Respiration* 65:265-9, 1998.
19. Broughton KS, Johnson CS, Pace BK, et al: Reduced asthma symptoms with n-3 fatty acid ingestion are related to 5-series leukotriene production, *Am J Clin Nutr* 65:1011-7, 1997.
20. Hackman RM, Stern JS, Gershwin ME: Complementary/alternative therapies in general medicine: asthma and allergies. In Spencer JW, Jacobs JJ, editors:

Complementary/alternative medicine: an evidence-based approach, St. Louis, 1998, Mosby.

21. Kaur B, Rowe BH, Ram FS: Vitamin C supplementation for asthma (Cochrane Review), *Cochrane Database Syst Rev* 4:CD000993, 2001.

22. Werbach MR: *Textbook of nutritional medicine*, Tarzana, CA, 1999, Third Line Press.

23. Pinn G: Herbal therapy in respiratory disease, *Aust Fam Phys* 30:775-8, 2001.

■ CHAPTER 13 ■

BENIGN PROSTATIC HYPERTROPHY

Benign prostatic hypertrophy begins at around 40 to 45 years of age and continues slowly until death. It is an androgen-dependent metabolic disorder associated with increased levels of dihydrotestosterone within the prostate. Increased conversion of testosterone to dihydrotestosterone may result from an increase in 5-α-reductase caused by drugs or pesticides. However, although the exact etiology remains poorly defined, 5-hydroxytestosterone is thought to have a permissive rather than causative role in benign prostatic hypertrophy.[1]

With increasing age, up to 70% of men are affected. Only 50% of men with an enlarged prostate require therapy.

CLINICAL DIAGNOSIS

Patients with prostatic hypertrophy present with prostatism and an enlarged, firm prostate with a smooth lateral border. Prostatism presents clinically with the following:

- Obstructive symptoms such as hesitancy, a weak intermittent urinary stream, straining, and terminal dribbling
- Irritative symptoms including urgency, frequency, nocturia, urge incontinence, and a small voided volume

THERAPEUTIC STRATEGY

Aging is associated with a progressive decline in plasma testosterone levels; estrone and estradiol levels remain unchanged, and the sex hormone-binding globulin level increases. Dihydrotestosterone emerges as the most important bioavailable testosterone in prostatic tissue, and levels of intraprostatic estrogens and their receptors are elevated in benign prostatic hyperplasia.[2] Prostate hyperplasia is thought to be hormone-mediated, and intervention focuses largely on modulation of hormonal balance. Phytonutrients are capable of altering sex hormone levels. Phytosterols, in addition to having anti-inflammatory and immune-modulating effects, inhibit the action of testosterone. Genistein, an isoflavone, is an estrogen analogue that inhibits growth of benign prostate hypertrophy tissue in culture, possibly by impairing conversion of testosterone by 5-α-reductase to the more active androgen, dihydrotestosterone.[3]

Symptoms may be improved by tempering sympathetic nervous system activity. Sympathetic dominance increases prostatic smooth-muscle tone and prostatic symptoms. Walking at least 3 hours each week may reduce sympathetic nervous system activity.[4]

Intervention focuses on modulating the hormonal and autonomic nervous system balance in the prostate.

LIFESTYLE CHANGES

A low-fat, high-fiber diet seems beneficial. Fruits are negatively, but butter and margarine are positively, related to an increased risk of benign prostatic hyperplasia.[5] Although there is a lack of clinical evidence,[6] a diet rich in phytoestrogens (e.g., isoflavonoids, and lignans) is also recommended.[5,7] Good sources of flavonoids are apples and onion; isoflavonoids are plentiful in soy products; and lignans are found in flaxseed, cereals, whole grains, fruits, and vegetables. Depending on the source, the concentration of isoflavones varies from 1 to 3 mg per gram of soy protein. One serving of traditional soy foods provides 25 to 40 mg of isoflavones.[8]

Avoiding sympathetic triggers such as decongestants, coffee, alcohol, and nicotine may reduce symptoms. Curtailing fluids after 5:00 PM is also helpful.

NUTRIENT THERAPY/DIETARY SUPPLEMENTS

A combination of L-alanine (200 mg), L-glutamic acid (530 mg), and glycine (90 mg) three times a day is generally accepted as an intervention that will reduce obstructive symptoms, possibly by shrinking the prostate.[9]

Evidence from controlled clinical trials supports the use of β-sitosterol (130 mg), a phytosterol, in the management of benign prostatic hyperplasia. Two randomized, placebo-controlled trials that lasted 6 months with dosages of β-sitosterol from 60 to 130 mg daily resulted in improved peak urinary flow rate and an improvement in subjective symptoms.[10,11] A multicenter, double-blind, placebo-controlled, clinical trial with β-sitosterol showed that the beneficial effects of β-sitosterol treatment demonstrable at 6 months were maintained for 18 months.[12] Longer-term safety and effectiveness are still unknown.[10]

Zinc sulfate, 220 mg twice a day, may be beneficial.[9] Zinc alters hormonal binding in the prostate and inhibits the activity of 5-α-reductase.

HERBAL THERAPY

Saw palmetto, *Panax ginseng*, and nettle root are all used for this condition.[13] A review of trials indicated that there is good evidence for the efficacy of saw palmetto (*Serenoa repens*) in the treatment of benign prostatic hyperplasia.[14] In fact, saw palmetto (160 mg twice a day between meals) is considered a safe option with no recognized adverse effects for treating this condition.[15-17] As an alternative to the usual 160 mg of fat-soluble extract (standardized to 85% to 95% fatty acid sterols) twice daily, administration of 1 to 2 g of saw palmetto berry for more than 4 to 6 weeks may provide symptomatic relief.[18]

Saw palmetto has also been used in various combinations. Although a nutritional supplement that included saw palmetto, androstenedione, and dehydroepiandrosterone did not prevent the conversion of ingested androstenedione to estradiol and dihydrotestosterone,[19] a randomized, multicenter, double-blind, clinical trial of patients with early benign prostatic hyperplasia showed that a fixed combination of extracts of saw palmetto fruit and nettle root (*Urtica dioica*) was as effective as the synthetic 5-α-reductase inhibitor finasteride and was better tolerated.[20] Saw palmetto may be taken in combination with nettle (250 mg of standardized root extract twice a day).[21] Nettle contains phytoestrogens and has an anti-inflammatory effect.

Nettle and pumpkin seed have both been approved by the German Commission E for use in the treatment of benign prostatic hypertrophy.[22] Pumpkin seed contains phytosterols, which inhibit the action of testosterone and may also have a diuretic effect.

PRACTICE TIPS

- If zinc is supplemented for longer than 30 days, copper should be prescribed at a dosage of 2 mg/day.
- Although unlikely to be causally linked, prostate cancer often coexists with prostatic hypertrophy.
- Prostate cancer should be ruled out before amino acid supplements are prescribed.
- Herbal supplements with phytoestrogens may have estrogenic side effects.
- Patients should eat of lot of cooked tomatoes and at least three servings of cruciferous vegetables per week.

REFERENCES

1. Oesterling JE: Benign prostatic hyperplasia: a review of its histogenesis and natural history, *Prostate Suppl* 6:67-73, 1996.
2. Sciarra F, Toscano V: Role of estrogens in human benign prostatic hyperplasia, *Arch Androl* 44:213-20, 2000.
3. Messina MJ: Legumes and soybeans: overview of their nutritional profiles and health effects, *Am J Clin Nutr* 70(suppl 3):439S-450S, 1999.
4. Platz EA, Kawachi I, Rimm EB, et al: Physical activity and benign prostatic hyperplasia, *Arch Intern Med* 158:2349-56, 1998.
5. Lagiou P, Wuu J, Trichopoulou A, et al: Diet and benign prostatic hyperplasia: a study in Greece, *Urology* 54:284-90, 1999.

6. Lowe FC, Ku JC: Phytotherapy in treatment of benign prostatic hyperplasia: a critical review, *Urology* 48:12-20, 1996.
7. Denis L, Morton MS, Griffiths K: Diet and its preventive role in prostatic disease, *Eur Urol* 35:377-87, 1999.
8. Coward L, Barnes NC, Setchell KDR, Barnes S: Genistein, daidzein, and their B-glycoside conjugates: antitumor isoflavones in soybean foods from American and Asian diets, *J Agric Food Chem* 41:1961-7, 1993.
9. Werbach MR, Moss J: *Textbook of nutritional medicine*, Tarzana, CA, 1999, Third Line Press.
10. Klippel KF, Hiltl DM, Schipp B: A multicentric, placebo-controlled, double-blind clinical trial of beta-sitosterol (phytosterol) for the treatment of benign prostatic hypertrophy, *Br J Urol* 80:427-32, 1997.
11. Berges RR, Windeler J, Trampisch HJ, Senge T: Randomized, placebo-controlled, double-blind clinical trial of beta-sitosterol in patients with benign prostatic hyperplasia, *Lancet* 345:1529-32, 1995.
12. Wilt T, Ishani A, MacDonald R, et al: Beta-sitosterols for benign prostatic hyperplasia, *Cochrane Database Syst Rev* 2:CD001043, 2000.
13. Mills S, Bone K: *Principles and practice of phytotherapy*, Edinburgh, 2000, Churchill Livingstone.
14. Linde K, ter Riet G, Hondras M, et al: Systematic reviews of complementary therapies—an annotated bibliography. Part 2: Herbal medicine, *BMC Complement Altern Med* 1:5, 2001.
15. Gerber GS: Saw palmetto for the treatment of men with lower urinary tract symptoms, *J Urol* 163:1408-12, 2000.
16. Marks LS, Partin AW, Epstein JI, et al: Effects of a saw palmetto herbal blend in men with symptomatic benign prostatic hyperplasia, *J Urol* 163:1451-6, 2000.
17. Wilt TJ, Ishani A, Stark G, et al: Saw palmetto extracts for treatment of benign prostatic hyperplasia: a systematic review, *JAMA* 280:1604-9, 1998.
18. Glisson J, Crawford R, Street S: The clinical applications of *Ginkgo biloba*, St. John's wort, saw palmetto, and soy, *Nurse Pract* 24:30-49, 1999.
19. Brown GA, Vukovich MD, Martini ER, et al: Effects of androstenedione-herbal supplementation on serum sex hormone concentrations in 30- to 59-year-old men, *Int J Vitam Nutr Res* 71:293-301, 2001.
20. Sokeland J: Combined sabal and urtica extract compared with finasteride in men with benign prostatic hyperplasia: analysis of prostate volume and therapeutic outcome, *BJU Int* 86:439-42, 2000.
21. Diefendorf D, Healey J, Kalyn W, editors: *The healing power of vitamins, minerals and herbs*, Surry Hills, Australia, 2000, Readers Digest.
22. Pinn G: Herbal medicine in renal and genitourinary disease, *Aust Fam Physician* 30:974-7, 2001.

CHAPTER 14

BREAST DISEASE

Benign breast conditions affect about half of all women. Fibrocystic breast disease typically presents as any combination of breast nodularity, swelling, and pain. Breast cancer is the third major cause of death and the second leading cause of death from cancer in adult women. The breast is the leading site of new cancers in adult women. Risk increases with age, and about one in 20 breast cancers are inherited.

CLINICAL DIAGNOSIS

All women should perform regular breast self-examination (see Figure 14-1).

Women with fibrocystic breast disease may have lumpy or nodular breasts that change with the phase of the menstrual cycle; thickened breast tissue; solitary or multiple cysts; and/or rubbery, smooth, mobile, painless fibroadenomas.

Breast cancer presents as a hard, nontender mass that later may become fixed and distort the breast, nipple, or overlying skin. Axillary lymphadenopathy indicates early spread, and evidence of distal metastases (e.g., bone pain) is found later in the disease. Breast cancer is detected in the early stages by mammography and in later stages by breast palpation.

Inherited breast cancer is most likely to occur at an earlier age, be bilateral, and be encountered among close relatives.

THERAPEUTIC STRATEGY

Prevention is the key. Breast disease seems to be linked to the cyclic hormonal responses of breast tissue. To date, no satisfactory mechanism explaining the pathogenesis of benign breast disease has been provided. In the interim, intervention seeks to avoid exposure to variables that may trigger breast tissue proliferation. Mechanisms determining breast carcinogenesis also remain unclear; however, certain nutrients that have a particularly important impact on breast tissue have been identified.

Phytoestrogens are phytochemicals with estrogenic activity. Because some types of breast cancer are stimulated by estrogen, uncertainty has dogged their influence on female health. However, clinical studies have not, to date, attributed an unacceptable risk to consumption of dietary

245

❑ How can I reduce my risk of female cancers?

Examination guidelines:

❑ Strip to the waist
❑ Visually examine the breasts in front of a mirror
❑ Palpate all the breast tissue
  • examine small breasts standing or lying
  • examine medium and large breasts lying

This procedure requires exploring an area that extends from the collar bone at the top to the bra line below, from midway between the breasts to the middle of the armpit. The breast area may be systematically covered by palpating imaginary parallel vertical strips. It takes 3–5 minutes to palpate uniformly up and down through the defined area on each side.

An approved palpation technique advocates:

❑ Use the flat part of the fingers, which includes the sensitive finger pads, and work in 5 cm (2 in) circles to cover each imaginary vertical strip in the area marked.

❑ Using two pressures at each spot:
  • *light pressure*: for feeling anything near the surface, the patient should hold her fingers together and flat, and make a circle firm enough to dent the skin
  • *firm pressure*: a second circle, pressing firmly in order to feel any deep lumps, should be superimposed on the original spot. Pressure should not cause discomfort but should be hard enough to feel the ribs.

❑ Check for a nipple discharge.

Seek professional advice if any abnormality is detected.

FIG. 14-1 Breast self-examination checklist.

phytoestrogens. In a review of cost-to-benefit analysis, data suggesting that consumption of soy affected the risk of developing, or of surviving, breast cancer in adult women were not found to be impressive.[1] Soy beans and red clover are rich sources of estrogenic isoflavones, such as genistein and daidzein. Flaxseed is a rich source of estrogenic lignans. Enterodiol and enterolactone are formed from intestinal bacterial action on diglucoside precursors in flaxseed. Lignans and isoflavones may protect against breast cancer by:

• Competing strongly with estradiol for the β-estrogen receptors found in reproductive organs, as well as in bone, prostate, and brain. Because phytoestrogens reduce receptor stimulation in a high endogenous estrogen environment but stimulate receptors in a low estrogen environment, they may be protective against breast cancer in premenopausal, but not postmenopausal, women. In addition to competing with endogenous estrogens, phytoestrogens inhibit the proliferative effect of environmental estrogens on human breast cancer cells. Xenoestrogens (e.g., pesticides) bind to both α- and β-estrogens. A-estrogen receptors are located in the kidneys, pituitary gland, and reproductive tract.
• Influencing sex hormone metabolism. Lignans and isoflavones reduce circulating estrogen levels by increasing levels of sex hormone-binding globulin. Results of in vitro studies also suggest that phytoestrogens inhibit aromatase, the enzyme that converts androgen to estrogen in adipose tissue.

Asian women have a lower risk of breast cancer. In addition to the 10 to 40 g of soy products they consume daily, Asian woman eat a low-fat diet. Hormonal changes are detected within 3 months of converting to a lower-fat diet. A low-fat diet is conducive to lower circulating levels of estrogen, estrone, and estradiol. Epidemiologic findings and animal studies both show a strong and consistent relationship between fat consumption and breast cancer incidence.[2] General explanations range from fat as a medium for transport of carcinogens to fat as an energy-dense source for free radical production.[3] The activity of individual fatty acids also has a profound effect. A case-control study demonstrated that the relative risk of breast cancer was greatest for women with lower adipose α-linolenic acid levels in their breast tissue.[4]

A high-fiber diet influences hormonal balance by increasing fecal excretion of endogenous estrogens and urinary lignan and isoflavone levels. Intestinal organisms deconjugate estrogen in bile and make it available for reabsorption.

LIFESTYLE CHANGES

A literature review revealed no solid evidence for secondary prevention or treatment of fibrocystic breast conditions through a dietary approach, including caffeine restriction and/or use of evening primrose oil, vitamin E, or pyridoxine.[5] Nonetheless, because fibrocystic breast disease remains, arguably, positively correlated with both caffeine and total methylxanthine (caffeine, theobromine, and theophylline) consumption, avoiding or limiting methylxanthine sources such as tea, coffee, chocolate, and cola drinks and drugs such as caffeine, certain analgesics, and theophylline may be helpful. Quitting smoking may also be protective, since nicotine stimulates cyst growth and formation. Furthermore, a low-fat (<21% energy), high-fiber (30 g/day), and soy isoflavone–rich diet does alter the intermediate markers for fibrocystic breast conditions.[5] Alcohol consumption has been associated with a non–dose-dependent reduction in the risk of benign proliferative epithelial disorders of the breast.[6] The same is not true of breast cancer.

A population-based, case-control study of women younger than 45 years suggests that recent consumption of alcohol in excess of 13 drinks per week has an adverse effect on breast tissue and may increase the risk of breast cancer.[7] Alcohol is postulated to have a weak causal dose-response relationship with breast cancer, with alcohol acting at a late stage in breast carcinogenesis. The increased risk of breast cancer associated with alcohol consumption in excess of 15 g per day may be reduced by adequate folate intake (>300 μg/day).[8] An alcohol-free diet, low in fat, with plenty of fresh fruits, vegetables, and soybeans is desirable.

Antioxidants, cruciferous vegetables, and soy are linked to a decreased risk of breast cancer,[3] as are white meat[9] and a daily fiber intake of 25 g that is rich in insoluble fiber, notably wheat bran.[10] Cruciferous vegetables, which appear to be particularly protective, are rich in the flavonoids and indoles that modify estrogen activity and phenols and isothiocyanates that induce various enzymes in phase II hepatic detoxification. High-adipose concentrations of lycopene have been associated with a reduced risk of breast cancer.[11] A human crossover trial showed that consumption of tomatoes containing 16.5 mg of lycopene for 21 days led to a 33% reduction in the amount of lymphocyte DNA damage sustained after exposure to hydrogen peroxide in vitro.[12] Lycopene has been shown to reduce the growth-stimulating effect of insulin-like growth factor on human breast cancer cells.[13] Data from the first National Health and Nutrition Examination Survey Epidemiologic Follow-up Study also support the hypothesis that sunlight and dietary vitamin D reduce the risk of breast cancer.[14]

Epidemiologic data comparing fat intake in the United States from 1950 to 1985 show a slight increase from 40% to 43.5%. Similar figures from Japan show an increase from 7.9% to 24.5%.[15] In 1985, the age-adjusted mortality rates for breast cancer per 100,000 people in the United States and Japan were 27 and 3.5, respectively.[2] Case-control and cohort studies suggest that an increased intake of 100 g of fat per day increases the cancer risk by approximately 25%. Fat intake should be limited and should favor the long-chain ω-3 fatty acids found in fish.

Red meat and coffee consumption appear unrelated to the risk of breast cancer.[16]

NUTRIENT THERAPY/DIETARY SUPPLEMENTS

Dietary behavior modification, rather than nutrient supplementation, seems appropriate, given the current state of knowledge about breast disease. Nonetheless, controlled clinical trials have demonstrated that iodine, vitamin E (100-600 IU twice daily), and evening primrose oil (1500 mg twice a day; 240 mg of γ-linolenic acid daily) administered from day 14 to day 28 of the menstrual cycle are all independently useful in the treatment of benign breast disease.[17] However, a literature review revealed that there was inadequate evidence to conclude that evening primrose oil or vitamin E is effective for relief of breast discomfort in fibrocystic conditions.[5] Other nutrient supplements with anecdotal support include vitamin A in toxic doses of 100,000 IU to 150,000 IU, beta-carotene (25-50 mg/day), choline (500 mg/day), and inositol (500 mg/day).

Nutrients may alter the progression of breast cancer. Metastasis of breast cancer cell lines to neighboring tissue requires aggregation and adhesion of the cancerous cells to tissue endothelium. Modified citrus pectin was shown to have anti-adhesive effects on breast carcinoma cell lines in vitro. Modified citrus pectin blocked the adhesion of malignant cells to blood vessel endothelium, thus inhibiting metastasis.[18]

Fish oil consumption is associated with protection against the promotional effects of animal fat in breast carcinogenesis.[19] Longer-chain ω-3 fatty acids appear to be particularly effective at suppressing breast carcinogenesis.[20] Results of a European study confirm that a relative ratio of ω-3 to ω-6 fatty acids favoring ω-3 fatty acids inhibits tumerogenesis.[21] On the other hand, diets rich in ω-6 polyunsaturated fatty acids (e.g., corn oil) stimulate the growth and metastasis of human breast cancer cells in athymic nude mice.[22] Greater tissue stores of trans-fatty acids also correlate with an increased risk of breast cancer.[21]

Despite laboratory data suggesting that several different vitamins may inhibit the growth of breast cancers, epidemiologic data on the relationship between vitamin supplement use and breast cancer are inconsistent, even within population groups. In a population-based, case-control study, investigators found a modest inverse association between breast cancer and use of multivitamins, vitamin C, and vitamin E among white women but not among black women.[23]

Recent studies also suggest an inverse association between folate intake and breast cancer among women who regularly consume alcohol.[24] A population-based, case-control study showed that dietary folate had a protective role in breast carcinogenesis.[25] The effect of folate may be enhanced by dietary intake of methionine, vitamin B_{12}, and vitamin B_6. Laboratory studies suggest that pyridoxal supplementation regulates breast cancer cell growth in vitro via a mechanism that appears to be steroid-independent.[26]

Although dietary factors are probably an important influence in breast cancer etiology, reductions in risk are more likely to be achieved through dietary modification rather than vitamin supplementation. Observational studies have suggested that vitamin E from dietary sources rich in the full spectrum of tocotrienols, rather than supplementation with α-tocopherol, may provide women with modest protection from breast cancer.[27] Eating carrots or spinach more than twice weekly reduces the risk of cancer.[28] A case-control study nested within a cohort provided evidence of an increase in the risk of breast cancer with decreasing beta-carotene, lutein, alpha-carotene, and β-cryptoxanthin levels.[29] A low intake of carotenoids may be associated with an increased risk of breast cancer. Owing to the complexity of nutrient interactions, further investigation of nutrient-nutrient and drug-nutrient interactions is recommended before confident predictions can be made regarding the use of nutrient supplementation in breast cancer cases.

HERBAL THERAPY

Herbs with hormonal effects have the potential to aggravate or suppress pathophysiologic processes in breast tissue. Chaste tree (*Vitex agnus-castus*), through its normalizing effect on ovarian function, is the herb most likely to favorably influence fibrocystic breast conditions.[30] Results of in vitro studies suggest that extracts of several estrogenic herbs, including hops, black cohosh, and chaste tree, and phytoestrogens such as genistein, daidzein, biochanin A, and coumestrol have potential in the prevention of breast cancer.[31]

Green tea is one interesting alternative treatment for breast cancer being investigated. Green tea, an antioxidant, enhances the activity of vitamins C and E and inhibits protein kinase C, lipid peroxidation, cell proliferation, and tumor-related activities. More than 10 cups of tea per day are required for cancer prevention effects.[32] Green tea contains large amounts of vitamin K, and therapeutic doses should be avoided by persons taking anticoagulants such as warfarin.

PRACTICE TIPS

- Avoiding coffee, colas, chocolate, and other sources of methylxanthines for more than 8 weeks may reduce breast tenderness in women with fibrocystic breast conditions.
- Tender, gritty breast tissue is likely to be due to fibroadenosis.
- A nontender, highly mobile, smooth lobulated mass is likely to be a fibroadenoma.
- Women who gain more than 10 kg as adults double their risk of developing breast cancer.
- Flaxseed is 75 times richer in lignans than other plant foods; 400 slices of whole-wheat bread provide a concentration of lignans similar to that in one cup of flaxseed.
- For optimum benefit, one to two heaping tablespoons of flaxseed should be eaten daily; it can be ground or used as flour and has a nutty flavor.

REFERENCES

1. Messina MJ, Loprinzi CL: Soy for breast cancer survivors: a critical review of the literature, *J Nutr* 131(suppl 11):3095S-3108S, 2001.
2. Weisburger JH: Dietary fat and risk of chronic disease: mechanistic insights from experimental studies, *J Am Dietetic Assoc* 97(suppl):S16-S23, 1997.
3. Kohlmeier L, Mendez M: Controversies surrounding diet and breast cancer, *Proc Nutr Soc* 56:369-82, 1997.
4. Klein V, Chajes V, Germain E, et al: Low alpha-linolenic acid content of adipose breast tissue is associated with an increased risk of breast cancer, *Eur J Cancer* 36:335-40, 2000.
5. Horner NK, Lampe JW: Potential mechanisms of diet therapy for fibrocystic breast conditions show inadequate evidence of effectiveness, *J Am Diet Assoc* 100:1368-80, 2000.
6. Rohan TE, Jain M, Miller AB: Alcohol consumption and risk of benign proliferative epithelial disorders of the breast: a case-cohort study, *Public Health Nutr* 1:139-45, 1998.
7. Swanson CA, Coates RJ, Malone KE, et al: Alcohol consumption and breast cancer risk among women under age 45 years, *Epidemiology* 8:231-7, 1997.

8. Zhang S, Hunter DJ, Hankinson SE, et al: A prospective study of folate intake and the risk of breast cancer, *JAMA* 281:1632-7, 1999.

9. Delfino RJ, Sinha R, Smith C, et al: Breast cancer, heterocyclic aromatic amines from meat and N-acetyltransferase 2 genotype, *Carcinogenesis* 21:607-15, 2000.

10. Wynder EL, Weisburger JH, Ng SK: Nutrition: the need to define 'optimal' intake as a basis for public policy decisions, *Am J Public Health* 82:346-50, 1992.

11. Zhang S, Tang G, Russell RM, et al: Measurement of retinoids and carotenoids in breast adipose tissue and a comparison of concentrations in breast cancer cases and control subjects, *Am J Clin Nutr* 66:626-32, 1997.

12. Riso P, Pinder A, Santangelo A, Porrini M: Does tomato consumption effectively increase the resistance of lymphocyte DNA to oxidative damage? *Am J Clin Nutr* 69:712-8, 1999.

13. Karas M, Amir H, Fishman D, et al: Lycopene interferes with cell cycle progression and insulin-like growth factor I signaling in mammary cancer cells, *Nutr Cancer* 36:101-11, 2000.

14. John EM, Schwartz GG, Dreon DM, Koo J: Vitamin D and breast cancer risk: the NHANES I Epidemiologic follow-up study, 1971-1975 to 1992. National Health and Nutrition Examination Survey, *Cancer Epidemiol Biomarkers Prev* 8:399-406, 1999.

15. Wynder El, Taioli E, Fujita Y: Ecologic study of lung cancer risk factors in the US and Japan with special reference to smoking and diet, *Jpn J Cancer Res* 83:418-23, 1992.

16. Tavani A, Pregnolato A, La Vecchia C, et al: Coffee consumption and the risk of breast cancer, *Eur J Cancer Prev* 7:77-82, 1998.

17. Werbach MR: *Textbook of nutritional medicine*, Tarzana, CA, 1999, Third Line Press.

18. Naik H, Pilat MJ, Donat T, et al: Inhibition of in vitro tumor cell-endothelial adhesion by modified citrus pectin: a pH modified natural complex carbohydrate, *Proc Am Assoc Cancer Res* 36: 377, 1995 (abstract 377).

19. Caygil CP, Charlett A, Hill MJ: Fat, fish, fish oil and cancer, *Br J Cancer* 74:159-64, 1996.

20. Rose DP, Connolly JM, Rayburn J, Coleman M: Influence of diets containing eicosapentaenoic or docosahexaenoic acid on growth and metastasis of breast cancer cells in nude mice, *J Natl Cancer Inst* 87:587-92, 1995.

21. Simonsen M, Strain J, van't Veer P, et al: Adipose tissue ω-3 fatty acids and breast cancer, in a population of European women, *Am J Epidemiol* 143S:153, 1996 (abstract).

22. Karmali RA, Adams L, Trout JR: Plant and marine ω-3 fatty acids inhibit experimental metastasis of rat mammary adenocarcinoma cells, *Prostaglandins Leukot Essent Fatty Acids* 48:309-14, 1993.

23. Moorman PG, Ricciuti MF, Millikan RC, Newman B: Vitamin supplement use and breast cancer in a North Carolina population, *Public Health Nutr* 4:821-7, 2001.

24. Eichholzer M, Luthy J, Moser U, Fowler B: Folate and the risk of colorectal, breast and cervix cancer: the epidemiological evidence, *Swiss Med Wkly* 131:539-49, 2001.

25. Shrubsole MJ, Jin F, Dai Q, et al: Dietary folate intake and breast cancer risk: results from the Shanghai Breast Cancer Study, *Cancer Res* 61:7136-41, 2001.

26. Davis BA, Cowing BE: Pyridoxal supplementation reduces cell proliferation and DNA synthesis in estrogen-dependent and -independent mammary carcinoma cell lines, *Nutr Cancer* 38:281-6, 2000.

27. Schwenke DC: Does lack of tocopherols and tocotrienols put women at increased risk of breast cancer? *J Nutr Biochem* 13:2-20, 2002.

28. Longnecker MP, Newcomb PA, Mittendorf R, et al: Intake of carrots, spinach, and supplements containing vitamin A in relation to risk of breast cancer, *Cancer Epidemiol Biomarkers Prev* 6:887-92, 1997.

29. Toniolo P, Van Kappel AL, Akhmedkhanov A, et al: Serum carotenoids and breast cancer, *Am J Epidemiol* 153:1142-7, 2001.

30. Mills S, Bone K: Principles and practice of phytotherapy, Edinburgh, 2000, Churchill Livingstone.

31. Dixon-Shanies D, Shaikh N: Growth inhibition of human breast cancer cells by herbs and phytoestrogens, *Oncol Rep* 6:1383-7, 1999.

32. Hinck G: The role of herbal products in the prevention of cancer, *Topics Clin Chiro* 6:54-62, 1999.

■ CHAPTER 15 ■

CANDIDIASIS

Candidiasis affects up to 75% of women. In 10% it is a recurrent problem. Patients may have localized candidal infection or fungal-type dysbiosis, a condition frequently associated with the overgrowth of *Candida albicans*. Oropharyngeal and vaginal candidiases are the most common local forms of mucosal fungal infections. Oral broad-spectrum antibiotics change bowel flora, favoring overgrowth and direct spread of *Candida* species from the bowel. Recurrent candidal vulvovaginitis may affect one in 10 women without any known predisposing factors. Decreases in salivary flow rates, secretion of antimicrobial proteins in saliva, and salivary neutrophil activity are risk factors for oral candidiasis.[1] Oral candidiasis is also associated with aging and systemic diseases.

Although most generalized infections occur in immunocompromised or debilitated patients, in some cases the condition is determined by the virulence of the *Candida* species itself. *Candida albicans* is a dimorphic fungus resident in the gastrointestinal tract. It uses at least two signal pathways to regulate its conversion from a commensal yeast form to an invasive filamentous hyphal form.[2] There is evidence that *C. albicans* infection of the mucous membranes depresses T-cell and natural killer cell function.

CLINICAL DIAGNOSIS

Oral candidiasis presents as thrush, whitish exudates on the oral mucous membrane, superficial glossitis with a beefy red tongue, and perlèche, fissuring, maceration, and crusting at the corners of the mouth. Genital candidiasis presents as intense erythema and pruritus of the vulvovaginal area, white patches on the vagina, and a thick white "cottage cheese" vaginal discharge. *Candida* infection is also prone to occur in warm, moist areas of the body and may cause erythematous skin lesions with minute superficial pustules in the axillary folds and submammary, groin, and intergluteal areas. Nail infections result in ridged, discolored nails with paronychia. Patients with fungal type dysbiosis tend to have diverse symptoms involving multiple organs. Common presentations include irritable bowel, chronic fatigue, and minimal psychoneurologic dysfunction (or "brain fog").[3] Predisposing factors include diabetes, use of oral contraceptives, systemic antibiotic therapy, pregnancy, immunosuppression, and old age.

THERAPEUTIC STRATEGY

Infection occurs because of an imbalance between the organism and host defenses. Virulence factors that contribute to pathogenesis of candidiasis include the ability to recognize and adhere to host cells with adhesins, reversibly change from yeast to hyphal growth forms, secrete aspartyl proteases and phospholipases, and undergo phenotypic switching in which antigen expression, colony morphology, and tissue affinity changes occur.[4] Phenotypic switching may provide cells with a flexibility that results in the adaptation of the organism to both the host's defenses and therapy.

C. *albicans* may both adhere to and enzymatically degrade mucins. Binding of *Candida* organisms to purified small intestinal mucin showed a close correlation with their hierarchy of virulence, with C. *dubliniensis*, C. *tropicalis*, and C. *albicans* being highly adherent.[5] The ability of *Candida* organisms to adhere to host tissue is considered essential in the early stages of colonization and tissue invasion. Adherence is achieved by a combination of specific, ligand-receptor interactions and nonspecific mechanisms such as electrostatic charge and van der Waals forces.[6] The yeast form of C. *albicans* is also able to adhere to a plethora of ligands. These include epithelial and bacterial cell-surface molecules, extracellular matrix proteins, and dental acrylic. In addition, saliva molecules, including basic proline-rich proteins, adsorbed to many oral surfaces promote C. *albicans* adherence. Adherence involves lectin, protein-protein, and hydrophobic interactions.[7]

As C. *albicans* organisms evade host defenses and colonize new environments by penetrating tissues, they are exposed to new adherence receptors and respond by expressing different adhesins. Prevention of adherence makes the organisms susceptible to removal by flushing.

Candidal vulvovaginitis occurs after a three-stage process of adhesion, blastopore germination, and epithelium invasion. Vaginal defense factors such as lactobacilli, cellular and humoral immunity, control and limit fungal growth.[8] Vaginal epithelial cells collected from healthy women with no history of vulvovaginal candidiasis exhibit a constant level of anticandidal activity, with no differences in activity at various stages of the menstrual cycle. Women with recurrent vulvovaginal candidiasis have reduced and fluctuating epithelial cell anticandidal activity.[9]

Local immunity is important in host defense against candidiasis. Cytokines and chemokines produced constitutively by vaginal and oral epithelial cells in response to C. *albicans* create a predominately proinflammatory state.[10] Production of interleukin-1α (IL-1α) and tumor necrosis factor α, but not IL-6, is increased on exposure to C. *albicans*. Recently, the potential of immunotherapy to control candidal vaginitis has included investigation of the use of antibodies against well-defined cell-surface adhesins or enzymes, the generation of yeast killer toxin–like candidacidal anti-idiotypic antibodies, and the generation of therapeutic vaccines and immunomodulators.[11]

LIFESTYLE CHANGES

Laboratory studies suggest that frequent consumption of carbohydrates, such as sucrose, glucose, maltose, or fructose, might represent a risk factor for oral candidiasis by enhancing adherence of *C. albicans* to epithelial cells.[12] However, although animal experiments indicated that refined dietary carbohydrate supplementation led to higher rates of candidal growth in the gastrointestinal tract and favored mucosal invasion, in human volunteers, adding a large amount of refined carbohydrates to the diet had only a limited influence on *Candida* species colonization.[13] Nonetheless, some restrictions on refined carbohydrates in susceptible persons may be worth trying because uncontrolled trials do suggest that avoidance of sugar minimizes growth.[14]

A yeast-free diet is advocated to avoid cross-sensitivity.[14] Such a diet excludes bread, rolls, and buns; beverages such as beer, wine, and cider; and condiments such as vinegar, soy sauce, and salad dressing. Smoked meats, dried fruit, and cheeses may also cause problems. Sourdough may be acceptable in certain patients, but cheeses such as gorgonzola are not.

Other potentially helpful measures are wearing cotton underwear, avoiding pantyhose, and using mild nonperfumed soap to minimize the risk of allergy.

NUTRIENT THERAPY/DIETARY SUPPLEMENTS

Clinical trials support eating 8 ounces of yogurt with live *Lactobacillus acidophilus* daily.[14] Strains of *Lactobacillus* isolated from dairy products and the genital tract competed with *C. albicans*. Inhibition was due to hydrogen peroxide and was trypsin-stable, heat-sensitive, and antagonized by catalase.[15] *Lactobacillus* organisms from "starters" showed antimicrobial activity against fungus isolated in a yogurt factory.[15] One of 21 *Lactobacillus* strains isolated from the vaginas of healthy women inhibited pathogenic bacteria by means of a bacteriocin-trypsin–sensitive, heat-stable compound. Growth of probiotics to restore gut flora is facilitated by prebiotics in the diet. Fructo-oligosacccharides encourage the growth of probiotic commensals.

Correction of iron and magnesium deficiency may also be helpful.[14] Two major responses to iron stress in fungi are a high-affinity ferric iron reductase and siderophore synthesis.[16] Iron uptake from siderophores occurs in *C. albicans* and is mediated by one or more high-affinity transport systems.[17] Serum exposure, which induces a morphogenic shift from yeast to the filamentous forms known to be required for virulence, also results in induction of iron transport from ferrichrome-type siderophores. In *C. albicans*, iron uptake from siderophores is regulated by iron availability. Iron deprivation induces uptake. Although correction of iron deficiency may be protective, excess iron supplementation may cause problems. In vitro, human milk showed a potent inhibitory effect on growth of *Candida* organisms.[18] Most, if not all, of this effect was caused by lactoferrin through its iron-binding capacity. The growth-inhibitory effect of human milk (i.e., mediated by lactoferrin) is fungistatic rather than fungicidal.

HERBAL THERAPY

Chamomile, chaste tree essential oils, bearberry extracts, and berberine sulfate have demonstrated in vitro activity against *Candida* organisms, and components of the essential oils of *Arnica* species have demonstrated potent activity against this yeast.[19] Citrus seed extract, rich in ascorbic and citric acid, is somewhat effective, particularly when used with amphotericin B. Ascorbic acid enhances the lethal effect of this drug.

PRACTICE TIPS

- Iron enhances the pathogenicity of *Candida* organisms and should only be given to correct iron deficiency.
- Garlic, vitamin C (2 g, twice daily), zinc, selenium, and a multivitamin/mineral supplement may be helpful.
- Cinnamon lozenges may be useful for thrush.

REFERENCES

1. Ueta E, Tanida T, Doi S, Osaki T: Regulation of *Candida albicans* growth and adhesion by saliva, *J Lab Clin Med* 136:66-73, 2000.
2. Calderone R, Suzuki S, Cannon R, et al: *Candida albicans*: adherence, signaling and virulence, *Med Mycol* 38(suppl 1):125-37, 2000.
3. Eaton K: Position statement on fungal-type dysbiosis, *J Nutr Env Med* 12:5-9, 2002.
4. Calderone RA, Fonzi WA: Virulence factors of *Candida albicans*, *Trends Microbiol* 9:327-35, 2001.
5. de Repentigny L, Aumont F, Bernard K, Belhumeur P: Characterization of binding of *Candida albicans* to small intestinal mucin and its role in adherence to mucosal epithelial cells, *Infect Immun* 68:3172-9, 2000.
6. Cotter G, Kavanagh K: Adherence mechanisms of *Candida albicans*, *Br J Biomed Sci* 57:241-9, 2000.
7. Cannon RD, Chaffin WL: Oral colonization by *Candida albicans*, *Crit Rev Oral Biol Med* 10:359-83, 1999.
8. Ferrer J: Vaginal candidosis: epidemiological and etiological factors, *Int J Gynaecol Obstet* 71(suppl 1):S21-S27, 2000.
9. Barousse MM, Steele C, Dunlap K, et al: Growth inhibition of *Candida albicans* by human vaginal epithelial cells, *J Infect Dis* 184:1489-93, 2001.

10. Steele C, Fidel PL: Cytokine and chemokine production by human oral and vaginal epithelial cells in response to *Candida albicans, Infect Immun* 70:577-83, 2002.

11. Magliani W, Conti S, Cassone A, et al: New immunotherapeutic strategies to control vaginal candidiasis, *Trends Mol Med* 8:121-6, 2002.

12. Pizzo G, Giuliana G, Milici ME, Giangreco R: Effect of dietary carbohydrates on the in vitro epithelial adhesion of *Candida albicans, Candida tropicalis,* and *Candida krusei, New Microbiol* 23:63-71, 2000.

13. Weig M, Werner E, Frosch M, Kasper H: Limited effect of refined carbohydrate dietary supplementation on colonization of the gastrointestinal tract of healthy subjects by Candida albicans, *Am J Clin Nutr* 69:1170-3, 1999.

14. Wernbach MR: *Textbook of nutritional medicine,* Tarzana, CA, 1999, Third Line Press.

15. Paraje MG, Albesa I, Eraso AJ: Conservation in probiotic preparations of *Lactobacillus* with inhibitory capacity on other species, *New Microbiol* 23:423-31, 2000.

16. Howard DH: Acquisition, transport, and storage of iron by pathogenic fungi, *Clin Microbiol Rev* 12:394-404, 1999.

17. Lesuisse E, Knight SA, Camadro JM, Dancis A: Siderophore uptake by *Candida albicans*: effect of serum treatment and comparison with *Saccharomyces cerevisiae, Yeast* 19:329-40, 2002.

18. Andersson Y, Lindquist S, Lagerqvist C, Hernell O: Lactoferrin is responsible for the fungistatic effect of human milk, *Early Hum Dev* 59:95-105, 2000.

19. Mills S, Bone K: *Principles and practice of phytotherapy,* Edinburgh, 2000, Churchill Livingstone.

■ CHAPTER 16 ■

CATARACTS

Age-related cataracts are the leading cause of visual disability. A cataract is a degenerative condition with loss of transparency of the lens. It presents as a gradual, painless loss of vision. Factors contributing to cataract formation include a family history, more than 22% body fat, central obesity, diabetes, dietary factors, and oxidative stress secondary to aging, smoking, and exposure to ultraviolet B light.[1]

Although cataract surgery is highly successful, prevention remains the preferred option.

CLINICAL DIAGNOSIS

Early visual changes suggesting cataract formation include changes in color perception, increased sensitivity to glare, blurred vision, monocular diplopia, and gradually progressive loss of vision. The extent of the visual loss depends on the size and location of the cataract. Cataracts are located in the posterior subcapsular area, the superficial cortex, and the center of the lens (nuclear cataract). Nuclear cataracts often cause myopia, and posterior subcapsular cataracts tend to be most noticeable in bright light. During ophthalmoscopy, small cataracts appear as dark defects against the red reflex. A large cataract may obliterate the red reflex.

THERAPEUTIC STRATEGY

One pathophysiologic explanation for senile cataract formation is deficient glutathione levels contributing to a faulty antioxidant defense system within the lens of the eye.[2] Insoluble protein is precipitated in the lens as a result of oxidative insults, electrolyte disturbances, and osmotic imbalance. Compared with normal lenses, cataracts contain less glutathione and high levels of hydrogen peroxide. Glutathione protects the lens by preventing oxidative damage from hydrogen peroxide and disulfide cross-linkage by maintaining sulfhydryl groups on proteins in their reduced form. By protecting sulfhydryl groups on proteins, which are important for active transport and membrane permeability, glutathione prevents increased permeability and protects the Na^+/K^+ adenosine triphosphatase–mediated active transport. The aim of intervention is to prevent oxidative damage to the lens.

Diabetic cataracts result when aldose reductase within the lens converts glucose to sorbitol or galactose to galactitol. These polyols cannot diffuse passively out of the lens and accumulate or are converted to fructose. The accumulation of polyols results in an osmotic gradient, which encourages diffusion of fluids from the aqueous humor. The water drags sodium with it, and swelling and electrolyte imbalance result in blurred vision. The reaction of lens proteins with sugars over time results in the formation of protein-bound advanced glycation end products.[3] The advanced glycation end products hypothesis proposes that accelerated chemical modification of proteins by glucose during hyperglycemia contributes to cataract formation. Glycoxidation products are formed from glucose by sequential glycation and auto-oxidation reactions. Flavonoids can bind to aldose reductase and inhibit polyol production; whereas avoidance of increased blood glucose, by reducing passive diffusion of glucose into the lens, can deplete the substrate for polyol production.

LIFESTYLE CHANGES

The lens, because of its exposure to light and ambient oxygen, is at high risk for photo-oxidative damage. Avoiding smoke and protecting eyes from UV light by wearing wraparound sunglasses is advisable. Epidemiologic evidence suggests that it is prudent to consume diets high in vitamins C and E and carotenoids, particularly the xanthophylls.[4] In fact, a high intake of fruits and vegetables seems protective.[5] One study showed that people who consumed less than three and a half servings of fruits and vegetables each day increased their risk of cataract formation by at least fivefold and possibly by 13-fold.[6] Significant inverse relationships between cataracts and consumption of meat, spinach, cheese, cruciferous vegetables, tomatoes, peppers, citrus fruits, and melon have been reported. Regular consumption of spinach, kale, and broccoli also decreases the risk of cataracts.

An increased risk of cataract formation was found in people with the highest intakes of butter, total fat, salt, and oil, with the exception of olive oil.[7]

NUTRIENT THERAPY/DIETARY SUPPLEMENTS

In a population-based study it was reported that compared with nonusers, persons who reported taking multivitamins or any supplement containing vitamin C or E for more than 10 years had a 60% lower 5-year risk for any cataract.[8] Vitamins C and E, beta-carotene, glutathione, and the enzymatic defense system of glutathione peroxidase, glutathione reductase, and superoxide dismutase protect the lens from oxidative damage. Lipoic acid (100 mg/day), selenium (200-400 µg/day), and vitamins E and C (400-500 IU/day) increase glutathione levels and activity.[9]

Vitamin C intake is inversely related to the prevalence of nuclear opacities; a statistically significant inverse trend between the prevalence of nuclear opacities and the duration of vitamin C use has been detected.[10,11] Women who use vitamin C supplements have a lower prevalence of cataracts than those who do not use the supplements, but only after they have taken vitamin C for 10 or more years.[12] A cohort study suggested that vitamin C diminished the risk of cortical cataracts in women younger than 60 years.[13] For each 1 mg/dL increase in the serum ascorbic acid level, a 26% decrease in cataract prevalence has been reported.[14] A daily dose of 300 mg may be adequate.

Carotenoids may reduce the risk of posterior subcapsular cataracts in women who have never smoked.[13] Prospective studies of the effect of carotenes and vitamin A on the risk of cataract formation indicated that persons consuming the most dietary vitamin A, lutein, and zeaxanthin had the lowest risk of cataracts.[15,16] Neither study demonstrated a decreased risk of cataract formation with intakes of other carotenoids (alpha-carotene, beta-carotene, lycopene, or β-cryptoxanthin). It is hypothesized that the protective effect of the carotenoids may be due to quenching of reactive oxygen species generated by exposure to UV light.[17] Vitamin A supplementation protects against nuclear cataracts.[18]

Animal and human studies suggest that vitamin E has a protective effect. Observational studies have shown that regular users of vitamin E supplements may halve the risk of cataracts.[19] The risk of developing cataracts appears lower in subjects with higher levels of vitamin E. In a longitudinal study researchers found that lens opacities were 30% less in regular users of a multiple vitamin, 57% less in regular users of supplemental vitamin E, and 42% less in those with higher plasma levels of vitamin E.[20] In a randomized, controlled trial, patients with early cataracts receiving 100 mg of vitamin E twice daily for 30 days had a significantly smaller increase in the size of their cortical cataracts than those receiving placebo. Reduced glutathione (GSH) levels were increased significantly only in those with cortical cataracts receiving vitamin E, and glutathione peroxidase levels were higher in the cortical cataract/vitamin E group than in the nuclear cataract/vitamin E group.[21] This study suggests that in the short term, vitamin E decreases oxidative stress in the cortex, and to a lesser extent, in the nucleus of cataractous lenses. This protective effect is attributable to enhanced GSH levels. A statistically significant relationship has been found between past vitamin E supplementation and prevention of cortical but not nuclear cataracts.[19] Until results from the Vitamin E and Cataract Prevention Study (a 4-year, prospective, randomized, controlled trial of vitamin E for cataract prevention) become available,[22] prolonged use of multivitamin supplements may be an effective alternative.[18]

Observational studies suggest that regular use of multivitamin supplements reduces the risk of nuclear opacification by one third.[19] Various B vitamins differentially modify the risk of nuclear and cortical cataracts.[18] Use of thiamin supplements is associated with reduced prevalence of nuclear and cortical cataracts. Riboflavin and niacin supplements exert a weaker protective influence on cortical cataracts. Riboflavin is a precursor of flavin adenine dinucleotide (FAD), a coenzyme for glutathione reductase. Folate appears to be protective against nuclear cataracts, whereas both folate and vitamin B_{12} supplements are strongly protective against cortical cataracts.

Despite data from experimental and observational studies suggesting that micronutrients with antioxidant capabilities may retard the development of age-related cataracts, overall, results of prospective trials have been disappointing. A randomized, double-blind clinical trial showed that daily supplementation with vitamin C (500 mg), vitamin E (400 IU), and beta-carotene (15 mg) had no apparent effect on the 7-year risk of development or progression of age-related lens opacities in a relatively well-nourished older adult cohort.[23] However, other studies demonstrate marginal benefit. An uncontrolled clinical trial suggested that up to 1 g of vitamin C daily combined with riboflavin, 15 to 25 mg/day, and zinc, 30 mg/day, decreased the risk of senile cataracts.[9] A multicenter, prospective, double-blind, randomized, placebo-controlled trial demonstrated that a mixture of oral antioxidant micronutrients (beta-carotene [18 mg/day], vitamin C [750 mg/day], and vitamin E [600 mg/day]) produced a small deceleration in progression of age-related cataracts after 3 years of daily supplementation.[24]

Patients with diabetes deserve special mention in view of the prevalence of cataracts in these patients. Diabetic cataracts are the result of prolonged sorbitol accumulation, oxidation and glycation. Flavonoids, particularly quercetin and its derivatives, are potent inhibitors of aldose reductase.[2] Theoretically, evening primrose oil may also reduce sorbitol accumulation resulting from inhibition of aldose reductase. Ascorbic acid also has potential as an aldose reductase inhibitor. Lipoic acid, with its potent antioxidant effect, may protect both vitamin C and E and reduce the risk of cataract formation in these patients.

HERBAL THERAPY

The active components of bilberry, flavonoid anthocyanosides, are potent antioxidants with a particular affinity for the eye and vascular tissues. A combination of bilberry, standardized to contain 25% anthocyanosides (180 mg twice daily), and vitamin E in the form of dl-tocopheryl acetate (100 mg twice daily), administered for 4 months, has been found to be somewhat effective in retarding the progression of cataracts.[25]

Other considerations include improving circulation with Ginkgo biloba (1000 mg twice daily) and taking grapeseed extract (100 mg twice daily) and flaxseed oil (1 tablespoon daily) for an antioxidant effect.

PRACTICE TIPS

- Avoid exposure to direct ultraviolet light and oxidizing agents such as cigarette smoke.
- A lifelong diet rich in antioxidants may be helpful.

REFERENCES

1. Schaumberg DA, Glynn RJ, Christen WG, et al: Relations of body fat distribution and height with cataract in men, *Am J Clin Nutr* 72:1495-502, 2000.
2. Head K: Natural therapies for ocular disorders. Part two: cataracts and glaucoma, *Altern Med Rev*6:141-66, 2001.
3. Lehman TD, Ortwerth BJ: Inhibitors of advanced glycation end product-associated protein cross-linking, *Biochim Biophys Acta* 1535:110-9, 2001.
4. Jacques PF: The potential preventive effects of vitamins for cataract and age-related macular degeneration, *Int J Vitam Nutr Res* 69:198-205, 1999.
5. Taylor A, Jacques PF, Epstein EM: Relations among aging, antioxidant status, and cataract, *Am J Clin Nutr* 62(suppl 6):1439S-1447S, 1995.
6. Jacques PF, Chylack LT Jr: Epidemiologic evidence of a role for the antioxidant vitamins and carotenoids in cataract prevention, *Am J Clin Nutr* 53(suppl 1): 352S-355S, 1991.
7. Tavani A, Negri E, La Vecchia C: Food and nutrient intake and risk of cataract, *Ann Epidemiol* 6:41-46, 1966.
8. Mares-Perlman JA, Lyle BJ, Klein R, et al: Vitamin supplement use and incident cataracts in a population-based study, *Arch Ophthalmol* 118:1556-63, 2000.
9. Werbach MR: *Textbook of nutritional medicine*, Tarzana, CA, 1999, Third Line Press.
10. Jacques PF, Chylack LT Jr, Hankinson SE, et al: Long-term nutrient intake and early age-related nuclear lens opacities, *Arch Ophthalmol* 119:1009-19, 2001.
11. Weber P, Bendich A, Schalch W: Vitamin C and human health—a review of recent data relevant to human requirements, *Int J Vitam Nutr Res* 66:19-30, 1996.
12. Jacques PF, Taylor A, Hankinson SE, et al: Long-term vitamin C supplement use and prevalence of early age-related lens opacities, *Am J Clin Nutr* 66:911-6, 1997.
13. Taylor A, Jacques PF, Chylack LT, et al: Long-term intake of vitamins and carotenoids and odds of early age-related cortical and posterior subcapsular lens opacities, *Am J Clin Nutr* 75:540-9, 2002.
14. Simon JA, Hudes ES: Serum ascorbic acid and other correlates of self-reported cataract among older Americans, *J Clin Epidemiol* 52:1207-11, 1999.
15. Chasen-Taber L, Willet WC, Seddon JM, et al: A prospective study of carotenoid and vitamin A intakes and risk of cataract extraction in US women, *Am J Clin Nutr* 70:509-16, 1999.
16. Brown L, Rimm EB, Seddon JM, et al: A prospective study of carotenoid intake and risk of cataract extraction in US men, *Am J Clin Nutr* 70:517-24, 1999.
17. Moeller SM, Jacques PF, Blumberg JB: The potential role of dietary xanthophylls in cataract and age-related macular degeneration, *J Am Coll Nutr* 19:522S-527S, 2000.
18. Kuzniarz M, Mitchell P, Cumming RG, Flood VM: Use of vitamin supplements and cataract: the Blue Mountains Eye Study, *Am J Ophthalmol* 132:19-26, 2001.
19. Leske MC, Chylack LT Jr, He Q, et al: Antioxidant vitamins and nuclear opacities: the longitudinal study of cataract, *Ophthalmology* 105:831-6, 1998.
20. Garrett SK, McNeil JJ, Silagy C, et al: Methodology of the VECAT study: vitamin E intervention in cataract and age-related maculopathy, *Ophthalmic Epidemiol* 6:195-208, 1999.
21. Nadalin G, Robman LD, McCarty CA, et al: The role of past intake of vitamin E in early cataract changes, *Ophthalmic Epidemiol* 6:105-12, 1999.

22. Seth RK, Kharb S: Protective function of alpha-tocopherol against the process of cataractogenesis in humans, *Ann Nutr Metab* 43:286-9, 1999.

23. Age-Related Eye Disease Study Research Group: A randomized, placebo-controlled, clinical trial of high-dose supplementation with vitamins C and E and beta carotene for age-related cataract and vision loss: AREDS report no. 9, *Arch Ophthalmol* 119:1439-52, 2001.

24. Chylack LT, Brown NP, Bron A, et al: The Roche European American Cataract Trial (REACT): A randomized clinical trial to investigate the efficacy of an oral antioxidant micronutrient mixture to slow progression of age-related cataract, *Ophthalmic Epidemiol* 9:49-80, 2002.

25. Bravetti G: Preventive medical treatment of senile cataract with vitamin E and anthocyanosides: clinical evaluation, *Ann Ophthalmol Clin Ocul* 115:109, 1989.

■ CHAPTER 17 ■

CARPAL TUNNEL SYNDROME

Carpal tunnel syndrome results from entrapment of the median nerve at the level of the wrist.

CLINICAL DIAGNOSIS

Patients complain of a pins-and-needles sensation in the pulps of the thumb and index and middle fingers and in half of the ring finger. Patients wake from sleep at night with tingling, which subsides on shaking the hand. Sensory deficits may develop in the palmar aspect of the first three digits.

THERAPEUTIC STRATEGY

Intervention depends on the cause. Nutritional intervention is sometimes tried in idiopathic cases.

NUTRIENT THERAPY/DIETARY SUPPLEMENTS

When carpal tunnel syndrome is the result of high doses of lithium or deficiency of vitamin B_6 and/or vitamin B_2, nutrient intervention is more likely to help.[1] Because vitamin B_2 is required for conversion of pyridoxal into the active metabolite pyridoxal-5-phosphate, combined supplementation may be useful.[2] A significant inverse association between plasma pyridoxal-5-phosphate concentration and the prevalence of pain, the frequency of tingling, and nocturnal awakening has been detected.[3]

In contrast, there is little convincing evidence for use of pyridoxine as the sole treatment for patients with idiopathic carpal tunnel syndrome.[4] Nonetheless, it may be of some value as an adjunct in conservative therapy by altering pain perception and increasing the pain threshold.

HERBAL THERAPY

Horse chestnut seed (*Aesculus hippocastanum*), through its antiedemic action, may be helpful.[5]

PRACTICE TIPS

- Taking pyridoxine in doses of 100 mg daily or more over long periods may cause sensory neuropathy.
- Turmeric (300 mg), like Boswellia (300 mg), reduces inflammation by blocking eicosanoid production.

REFERENCES

1. Werbach MR: *Textbook of nutritional medicine*, Tarzana, CA, 1999, Third Line Press.
2. Folkers K, Ellis J: Successful therapy with vitamin B_6 and vitamin B_2 of the carpal tunnel syndrome and need for determination of the RDAs for vitamin B_6 and B_2 for disease states, *Ann N Y Acad Sci* 585:295-301, 1990.
3. Keniston RC, Nathan PA, Leklem JE, et al: Vitamin B_6, vitamin C, and carpal tunnel syndrome. A cross-sectional study of 441 adults, *J Occup Environ Med* 39:949-59, 1997.
4. Jacobson MD, Plancher KD, Kleinman WB: Vitamin B_6 (pyridoxine) therapy for carpal tunnel syndrome, *Hand Clin* 12:253-7, 1996.
5. Mills S, Bone K: *Principles and practice of phytotherapy*, Edinburgh, 2000, Churchill Livingstone.

■ CHAPTER 18 ■

CERVICAL CANCER

Invasive cervical cancer accounts for more than 10% of all cancers world-wide. It is the second most common cancer among women. Infection with oncogenic type human papilloma viruses is associated with most cases of cervical cancer; however, it is believed that nutritional status may be linked with cervical dysplasia and progression to cancer.

Possible primary preventive strategies include reducing risky sexual behaviors and using dietary supplements, vaccines, and other chemopreventive agents.[1,2]

CLINICAL DIAGNOSIS

Diagnosis of dysplasia is made by means of a routine Papanicolaou test. Cervical cancer should be suspected in women with an offensive, watery, brown, or clear vaginal discharge; dyspareunia; or postcoital or any other abnormal vaginal blood loss.

THERAPEUTIC STRATEGY

From a nutritional perspective, studies have shown that lower levels of antioxidants coexisting with low levels of folic acid increase the risk for carcinoma in situ.[3] Although it has yet to be shown that nutritional adequacy prevents a problem, maintaining satisfactory levels of these nutrients seems reasonable.

LIFESTYLE CHANGES

A diet rich in fresh fruits and vegetables is desirable. Clinical evidence suggests that women deficient in folic acid, beta-carotene, selenium, and/or vitamins A, C, or E may have an increased risk for cervical dysplasia. Although the relationship with vitamin E status is less consistent, low vitamin C and carotenoid levels are associated fairly consistently with both cervical dysplasia and cancer.[4] Although epidemiologic evidence remains uncertain about the role of folate in cervical cancer prevention,[5] folate depletion is particularly believed to be a risk factor for human papillomavirus infection and cervical dysplasia.[6] A case-control study indicated that low erythrocyte folate levels enhance the effect of other risk factors for cervical dysplasia, in particular, human papilloma virus 16 infection.[7] Because the effect of folate status may be restricted to early preneoplastic cervical lesions,[4] it is suggested that regular consumption of folic acid–rich foods may be prudent.

NUTRIENT THERAPY/DIETARY SUPPLEMENTS

A population-based, case-control study suggested that dietary selenium and vitamins A, C, and E had a protective effect.[8] Evidence from controlled clinical trials suggests that selenium and folic acid deficiencies increase the risk of cervical dysplasia; however, it is more difficult to establish whether supplementation with selenium (200 μg daily) and folic acid (5 mg twice daily) is protective.[9]

Although folic acid (10 mg daily) lowers the total plasma homocysteine level,[10] results of a case-control study did not support the hypothesis that folate, homocysteine, and vitamin B_{12} are markers for cervical dysplasia.[11] Results from phase III folic acid and beta-carotene chemoprevention trials have also been disappointing.[12] Beta-carotene (30 mg daily) did not enhance the regression of high-grade cervical intraepithelial neoplasia over a 2-year period.[13]

The possibility that vitamin A or related retinoids could be administered either systemically or locally, early in the neoplastic process, to inhibit the progress of cervical cancer deserves serious consideration.[14] Epidemiologic studies have shown an inverse relationship between dietary intake or serum levels of vitamin A and the development of cervical dysplasia and cancer. A prospective study showed that the rate of progression of carcinoma in situ or invasive cervical cancer was 4.5 times higher in women with low serum retinol levels than in those with high serum retinol levels.[15] Results of controlled clinical trials support the use of a cervical sponge with beta-trans-retinoic acid in the treatment of cervical dysplasia.[9] Results of a randomized phase III trial confirmed that cervical caps with sponges containing 1.0 mL of 0.372% beta-trans-retinoic acid, inserted daily for 4 days and then every 2 days for 3 and 6 months thereafter, reversed cervical intrepithelial neoplasia, but not more advanced dysplasia.[16]

HERBAL THERAPY

Topical application of meadowsweet (*Filipendula ulmaria*), an herb rich in flavonoids (particularly rutin and quercetin), phenolic glycosides, and essential oils with various salicylates, may be useful.[17]

PRACTICE TIPS

- There is speculation that indole-3-carbinol, found in cabbage, broccoli, and cauliflower, may have a protective effect.
- Women with low intakes of vitamin A and beta-carotene are at higher risk for cervical dysplasia and carcinoma in situ than those with a high intake of these nutrients.
- Some patients with cervical dysplasia may respond to various combinations of nutrients in a regimen that includes one or more of: folic acid (5 mg) and vitamin E (250 IU) given twice daily; sodium selenite (200-300 µg), beta-carotene (25-50 mg), vitamin C (2-4 g), pyridoxine (50-150 mg), and zinc (25 mg) given once daily; and/or vitamin A (25,000 IU twice daily for 3 months).

REFERENCES

1. Rock CL, Michael CW, Reynolds RK, et al: Prevention of cervix cancer, *Crit Rev Oncol Hematol* 33:169-85, 2000.
2. Giuliano AR: The role of nutrients in the prevention of cervical dysplasia and cancer, *Nutrition* 16:570-3, 2000.
3. Kwasniewska A, Tukendorf A, Semczuk M: Folate deficiency and cervical intraepithelial neoplasia, *Eur J Gynaecol Oncol* 18:526-30, 1997.
4. Potischman N, Brinton LA: Nutrition and cervical neoplasia, *Cancer Causes Control* 7:113-26, 1996.
5. Eichholzer M, Luthy J, Moser U, et al: Folate and the risk of colorectal, breast and cervix cancer: the epidemiological evidence, *Swiss Med Wkly* 131:539-49, 2001.
6. Harper JM, Levine AJ, Rosenthal DL, et al: Erythrocyte folate levels, oral contraceptive use and abnormal cervical cytology, *Acta Cytol* 38:324-30, 1994.
7. Butterworth CE Jr, Hatch KD, Macaluso M, et al: Folate deficiency and cervical dysplasia, *JAMA* 267:528-33, 1992.
8. Slattery ML, Abbott TM, Overall JC, et al: Dietary vitamins A, C, and E and selenium as risk factors for cervical cancer, *Epidemiology* 1:8-15, 1990.
9. Wernbach MR: *Textbook of nutritional medicine*, Tarzana, CA, 1999, Third Line Press.
10. Thomson SW, Heimburger DC, Cornwell PE, et al: Correlates of total plasma homocysteine: folic acid, copper, and cervical dysplasia, *Nutrition* 16:411-6, 2000.
11. Goodman MT, McDuffie K, Hernandez B, et al: Case-control study of plasma folate, homocysteine, vitamin B_{12}, and cysteine as markers of cervical dysplasia, *Cancer* 89:376-82, 2000.
12. Giuliano AR, Gapstur S: Can cervical dysplasia and cancer be prevented with nutrients? *Nutr Rev* 56:9-16, 1998.
13. Keefe KA, Schell MJ, Brewer C, et al: A randomized, double blind, phase III trial using oral beta-carotene supplementation for women with high-grade cervical intraepithelial neoplasia, *Cancer Epidemiol Biomarkers Prev* 10:1029-35, 2001.

14. Eckert RL, Agarwal C, Hembree JR, et al: Human cervical cancer. Retinoids, interferon and human papillomavirus, *Adv Exp Med Biol* 375:31-44, 1995.

15. Nagata C, Shimizu H, Higashiiwai H, et al: Serum retinol level and risk of subsequent cervical cancer in cases with cervical dysplasia, *Cancer Invest* 17: 253-8, 1999.

16. Meyskens FL, Surwit E, Moon TE, et al: Enhancement of regression of cervical intraepithelial neoplasia II (moderate dysplasia) with topically applied all-trans-retinoic acid: a randomized trial, *J Natl Cancer Inst* 86:539-43, 1994.

17. Mills S, Bone K: *Principles and practice of phytotherapy*, Edinburgh, 2000, Churchill Livingstone.

■ CHAPTER 19 ■

CHRONIC FATIGUE SYNDROME

The cause of chronic fatigue syndrome (CFS) remains disputed. Postulates range from a psychosomatic disorder to immune dysfunction following various triggers including viral infection, food, and chemical sensitivity.[1] Homeostatic systems may become deranged and held in that state by minor stressors. A review of the literature on CFS shows relationships between CFS and hyperresponsiveness and hyporesponsiveness in immune function, several hypothalamo-pituitary axes, and the sympathetic nervous system.[2] Intervention is problematic.

CLINICAL DIAGNOSIS

CFS is characterized by the recent or distinct onset of unexplained persisting or relapsing generalized fatigue that lasts more than 6 months, is exacerbated by minor exercise, and leads to a significant reduction in previous levels of daily activity. Rest does not substantially relieve the fatigue. Concentration is impaired and short-term memory is poor. Patients are often depressed. Vague complaints of myalgia, migratory arthralgia, sore throat, postexertional malaise, unrefreshing sleep, sleep disturbance, mild fever, and lymphadenopathy are common.

THERAPEUTIC STRATEGY

A review of 44 studies concluded that there was insufficient evidence to ascertain the effectiveness of supplements or drugs in the treatment of CFS, although behavioral interventions such as graded exercise therapy and cognitive behavioral therapy showed positive results.[3] Nonetheless, nutritional intervention attempts can target stressors and symptoms. In the case of the former, detection of food sensitivity and elimination of suspected problem foods may be helpful. In the case of the latter, intervention may focus on correcting nutritional deficiencies and improving the efficiency of cellular energy generation. In both cases enhanced oxidation may contribute to the clinical picture. Food intolerance may amplify oxidation via cytokine induction.

LIFESTYLE CHANGES

Awareness of food sensitivity and avoidance of problem foods may help a small group of patients. Fatigue has been linked to sensitivity to sugar and grains such as wheat, corn, and rice. Elimination diets for sensitive patients and correction of gut dysbiosis with lactobacilli and bifidobacilli deserve consideration.

NUTRIENT THERAPY/DIETARY SUPPLEMENTS

Controlled clinical trials report benefit from evening primrose oil and fish oil, L-carnitine supplementation, and correction of magnesium deficiency.[4,5] Uncontrolled trials suggest that beta-carotene, coenzyme Q10, malic acid, vitamin B_{12}, and vitamin C may each be beneficial in some patients.

CFS is characterized by a lack of energy. Levels of nutrients involved in energy metabolism are often reduced in patients with CFS. Supplementation with at least 300 mg of magnesium and 1200 to 2400 mg of malate daily produces variable results.[6] Malate plays an important role in mitochondrial energy generation. In one group of patients, after 3 months of taking 100 mg of coenzyme Q10, daily exercise tolerance improved and clinical symptoms and postexercise fatigue decreased.[6] Coenzyme Q10 facilitates cellular respiration, and levels are progressively reduced in these patients after mild exercise and normal daytime activity. Clinical trials of oral L-carnitine (up to 1 g three to four times daily) had mixed results, but in one study statistically significant improvement in a number of clinical parameters was observed between 4 and 8 weeks of treatment.[7] However, a recent study demonstrated that serum carnitine deficiency did not contribute to or cause symptoms in many patients with CFS.[8] A possible explanation is that only some patients are carnitine responders. Carnitine, an amino acid derivative, facilitates oxidation of fatty acids.

Several nutrient deficiencies have been detected in patients with CFS. In fact, a detailed review of the literature suggests that marginal deficiencies of folate, vitamin B_{12}, vitamin C, magnesium, sodium, zinc, L-tryptophan, L-carnitine, coenzyme Q10, and/or essential fatty acids may contribute to CFS.[5] Although these nutrient deficiencies are believed to reflect the illness process rather than an inadequate diet, they may nonetheless contribute to the patient's symptoms. A pilot study provided preliminary evidence of reduced functional B vitamin status, particularly of pyridoxine, in these patients.[9] This is consistent with anecdotal reports from some patients with CFS who benefit from vitamin supplementation. Supplementation with vitamin B_{12} in doses ranging from 3000 µg four times weekly to 9000 µg daily induces well-being,[10] even in a substantial proportion of individuals with normal serum levels. Fatigue and depression are prominent symptoms in patients with folate and/or vitamin C deficiency. Furthermore, fatigue, lassitude, and depression may respond to vitamin C supplementation. On the other hand, treatment with some deficient nutrients, for example, essential fatty acids, has more unpredictable results.[11] Nonetheless, a case series of patients with CFS did suggest improvement after 3 months of essential fatty acid supplementation.[2] The authors hypothesized that changes in essential fatty acid metabolite ratios are a normal physiologic response to stressors, but when stressors are excessive or prolonged, receptor downregulation and substrate depletion lead to unpredictable outcomes.

HERBAL THERAPY

Given that oxidative stress may be involved in the pathogenesis of CFS, supplementation with glutathione, N-acetylcysteine, α-lipoic acid, oligomeric proanthocyanidins, *Ginkgo biloba*, and *Vaccinium myrtillus* (bilberry) may be beneficial.[12]

Adaptogens help the body cope with stress. Herbs that are tonics help to revitalize the patient and correct immune function (e.g., astragalus and Siberian ginseng may be useful). Extracts of *Echinacea purpurea* and *Panax ginseng* have been shown to enhance cellular immune function of peripheral blood mononuclear cells from both healthy individuals and patients with depressed cellular immunity as in CFS.[13] Goldenseal, echinacea, pau d'arco, and astragalus may be used in rotation to stimulate the immune system.[14]

Licorice, by stimulating the adrenal glands, may provide benefit. No studies to support the use of ginseng, astragalus, licorice, echinacea, or St. John's wort in the treatment of CFS have been published.[15]

PRACTICE TIPS

• Magnesium is particularly helpful for patients in whom myalgia dominates.
• Reduced nicotinamide adenine dinucleotide, in doses of 5 mg given twice daily, may benefit patients with CFS.

REFERENCES

1. Graham J: Chronic fatigue syndrome—a review, *J Aust Coll Nutr Env Med* 20: 19-28, 2001.
2. Gray JB, Martinovic AM: Eicosanoids and essential fatty acid modulation in chronic disease and the chronic fatigue syndrome, *Med Hypotheses* 43:31-42, 1994.
3. Whiting P, Bagnall AM, Sowden AJ, et al: Interventions for the treatment and management of chronic fatigue syndrome: a systematic review, *JAMA* 286:1378-9, 2001.
4. Werbach MR: *Textbook of nutritional medicine*, Tarzana, CA, 1999, Third Line Press.

5. Chilton SA: Cognitive behaviour therapy for the chronic fatigue syndrome. Evening primrose oil and magnesium have been shown to be effective, *BMJ* 312:1096, 1996.

6. Werbach MR: Nutritional strategies for treating chronic fatigue syndrome, *Altern Med Rev* 5:93-108, 2000.

7. Plioplys AV, Plioplys S: Amantadine and L-carnitine treatment of chronic fatigue syndrome, *Neuropsychobiology* 35:16-23, 1997.

8. Soetekouw PM, Wevers RA, Vreken P, et al: Normal carnitine levels in patients with chronic fatigue syndrome, *Neth J Med* 57:20-4, 2000.

9. Heap LC, Peters TJ, Wessely S: Vitamin B status in patients with chronic fatigue syndrome, *J R Soc Med* 92:183-5, 1999.

10. Newbold HL: Vitamin B_{12}: placebo or neglected therapeutic tool? *Med Hypotheses* 28:155-64, 1989.

11. Warren G, McKendrick M, Peet M: A case-controlled study of red-cell membrane essential fatty acids (EFA) and a placebo-controlled CFS treatment study with high dose of EFA, *Acta Neurol Scand* 99:112-6, 1999.

12. Logan AC, Wong C: Chronic fatigue syndrome: oxidative stress and dietary modifications, *Altern Med Rev* 6:450-9, 2001.

13. See DM, Broumand N, Sahl L, et al: In vitro effects of echinacea and ginseng on natural killer and antibody-dependent cell cytotoxicity in healthy subjects and chronic fatigue syndrome or acquired immunodeficiency syndrome patients, *Immunopharmacology* 35:229-35, 1997.

14. Diefendorf D, Healey J, Kalyn W, editors: *The healing power of vitamins, minerals and herbs*, Surry Hills, Australia, 2000, Readers Digest.

15. Pinn G: Herbal therapy in rheumatology, *Aust Fam Physician* 30:878-83, 2001.

■ CHAPTER 20 ■

COLON CANCER

Survival is closely related to the clinical and pathologic stage at which colon cancer is diagnosed and treated. Developed Western nations have a higher incidence of colon cancer than Eastern and underdeveloped countries. This difference has been related to dietary habits. The Western diet is associated with higher levels of fecal cholesterol, bile acids, and peroxidized fats.

CLINICAL DIAGNOSIS

Colorectal cancer should be investigated in persons older than 40 years who complain of a persistent change in bowel habits and vague abdominal discomfort, often precipitated by eating and relieved by defecation. In colon cancer, constipation predominates, pain is colicky in nature, and patients often have anemia caused by occult blood loss. In rectal cancer, diarrhea is more common, tenesmus is prevalent, and the stool is often blood-stained.

THERAPEUTIC STRATEGY

Bowel cancer may be prevented by avoiding carcinogens in the diet, creating a bowel environment unfavorable to carcinogen production, and reducing bowel transit time. Consumption of fiber may reduce the risk of colon cancer because it has all of these effects.

LIFESTYLE CHANGES

Diet is related to colon cancer, but the relationship is complex and requires clarification.[1] Sugar, salt, and alcohol increase the risk; whereas a diet low in fat (particularly animal fat), limited in protein, and rich in complex carbohydrates and fiber is protective.[2] Men with diets rich in meat, fish, poultry, and eggs have an increased risk, and women who consume the largest percentage of their food items in the form of plant foods have a reduced risk of colon cancer.[3] With respect to particular food items, tomatoes,[4] whole grains,[5] and the *Brassica* vegetables (including cabbage, kale, broccoli, brussels sprouts, and cauliflower) are particularly beneficial.[6] Two hundred grams of raw carrot, eaten at breakfast each day for 3 weeks, increased fecal bile acid and fat excretion by 50%, and stool weight by 25%.[7] These changes to stool composition suggest an associated change in bacterial flora or metabolism.

A high-fat diet is associated with an increased risk of colon cancer. Although no increased risk has been identified for the cis-form of the fatty acids, results of a case-control study confirmed that trans-fatty acids are carcinogenic.[8] Furthermore, among women who consume high levels of trans-fatty acids, those who are estrogen-negative (i.e., postmenopausal and not taking hormone replace therapy) double their risk of colon cancer. The level of trans-fatty acids consumed had no influence on the risk of colon cancer in women who were estrogen-positive. Laboratory studies suggest that the enhancement of colon cell proliferation and carcinogenesis by a high-fat diet may be mediated through elevated serum leptin levels.[9]

A high intake of red meat has been associated with a heightened risk of colon cancer. Although this may be linked to an intake of animal fat, it may also be explained by the fact that red meat is a rich source of heme. Animal experiments showed that dietary heme increased colonic mucosal exposure to luminal irritants and enhanced proliferation of colonic epithelium.[10] Dietary calcium phosphate inhibited the cytolytic and hyperproliferative effects of dietary heme. Although high levels of physical activity had the strongest inverse relationship, in a study that confirmed different lifestyle patterns have age-specific and tumor site–specific associations, a high intake of calcium was found to reduce the risk of colon cancer.[11] A randomized, single-blind, controlled study demonstrated that the proliferative activity of colonic epithelial cells was decreased and the markers of normal cellular differentiation were restored when the daily intake of calcium was increased to 1200 mg through consumption of low-fat dairy food by subjects at risk for colonic neoplasia.[12]

A high-fiber diet provides protection by changing the bowel flora and intestinal metabolic end products; increasing stool size and diluting the concentration of carcinogens present; irreversibly adsorbing carcinogens; altering hormonal balance; and influencing bile acid production.[13] The crude fiber fraction and phytic acid, a constituent of wheat bran, have an independent cancer-protective potential; wheat bran alone or combined with psyllium appears to most effectively inhibit the earlier phases of carcinogenesis.[14] Despite strong evidence from epidemiologic studies, recent investigators have questioned the ability of high-fiber and low-fat diets to protect against colorectal cancer.[15]

NUTRIENT THERAPY/DIETARY SUPPLEMENTS

Epidemiologic and animal studies suggest an inverse relationship between calcium consumption and colon cancer. Daily calcium supplementation in doses of at least 1.5 g may suppress colonic cell transformation at an early stage of carcinogenesis.[2] Studies generally have shown a beneficial effect, when in addition to a regular diet, calcium intake is increased by 1.2 to 2 g daily for periods of at least 2 months.[16] Although results of epidemiologic studies on calcium, vitamin D, and colon cancer have been inconsistent, because experimental studies regularly show a protective effect and data from a large case-control study were confirmatory, the inverse relationship between calcium intake and the risk of colon cancer is increasingly being accepted.[17]

Epidemiologic evidence supports the notion that a high folate intake is protective against colon cancer.[18] The increased risk of colon cancer associated with folate deficiency is probably attributable to extensive incorporation of uracil into human DNA, leading to chromosomal breaks.[19] Vitamin B_{12} and B_6 deficiencies similarly increase uracil incorporation and chromosomal breaks. In fact, a deficiency of any micronutrient—including folic acid, vitamins B_{12}, B_6, B_3, C, and E, iron, and zinc—mimics radiation damage of DNA, causing single- and double-strand breaks, oxidative lesions, or both.[19] Although there is substantial variability among individuals, a significant decrease in the antioxidant capacity of colorectal mucosa in patients affected by colorectal cancer has been reported.[20] A randomized, controlled trial of beta-carotene (20 mg) and α-tocopherol (50 mg) indicated that beta-carotene treatment did not decrease the prevalence of colon cancer, but the vitamin E group had fewer new colorectal cancers.[21] However, a prospective study over 14 years did not demonstrate any substantial effect of vitamin E or C supplementation on overall colorectal cancer mortality.[22] Nonetheless, a significant reduction in adenoma recurrence after polypectomy was found in patients randomly assigned to receive vitamin A, C, and E supplementation.[23]

A diet low in animal fat and trans-fatty acids may be protective; so may a diet rich in ω-3 fatty acids. A randomized study of patients with stage 1 or stage 2 colon cancer or adenomatous polyps suggested that 9 g of ω-3 fatty acid daily may be a useful chemopreventive agent in some cases.[24] In fact, a low plasma phospholipid ω-6/ω-3 fatty acid ratio may serve as a nutritional marker of colonic epithelial cell hyperproliferation, colon tumor growth, and metastasis.

HERBAL THERAPY

In vivo screening assays suggest, among others, that Korean red ginseng powder, green tea catechins, curcumin, compounds from garlic and onion, and resveratrol from red grapes may have a cytostatic effect, inhibiting progression of established aberrant crypt foci.[25] For example, curcumin has been shown to possess anti-inflammatory and anticancer activities.

Cyclooxygenase (COX)-2 plays an important role in colon carcinogenesis. Colon tumors have been shown to highly express COX-2 protein. Curcumin markedly inhibits the messenger RNA and protein expression of COX-2, but not COX-1.[26] In vitro studies showed that berberine, an isoquinoline alkaloid with anti-inflammatory and antitumor-promoting effects, also effectively inhibited COX-2 transcriptional activity in colon cancer cells in a dose- and time-dependent manner at concentrations higher than 0.3 µmol/L.[27] Given that many nonsteroidal anti-inflammatory drugs also suppress COX-1, it is tempting to speculate that herbal products that inhibit one or both forms of the COX enzyme will be effective agents for the prevention of cancer in humans.

PRACTICE TIPS

- An adequate total dietary fiber intake appears to be one that prevents constipation and yields stool of 200 to 250 g, passed once or twice a day.
- A high sugar intake increases bowel transit time.
- A diet that is high in fiber derived from vegetables, grains, and fruits, low in fat, and rich in calcium is protective.
- Eating whole-meal grain bread with fried meat may be protective because heterocyclic amine carcinogens, such as those found in fried meat, may adsorb to insoluble fiber.
- Garlic and onions have a protective effect.
- Regularly taking nonsteroidal anti-inflammatory drugs (NSAIDs) appears to reduce the risk of colon cancer. Persons who do not take NSAIDs may increase by 50% their risk of developing colon cancer.

REFERENCES

1. Willett WC: Diet and cancer, *Oncologist* 5:393-404, 2000.
2. Wernbach MR: Dietary protection against colon cancer, *J Aust Coll Nutr Env Med* 17:27, 1998.
3. Slattery ML, Berry TD, Potter J, et al: Diet diversity, diet composition, and risk of colon cancer (United States), *Cancer Causes Control* 8:872-82, 1997.
4. La Vecchia C: Mediterranean epidemiological evidence on tomatoes and the prevention of digestive-tract cancers. *Proc Soc Exp Biol Med* 218:125-8, 1998.
5. Jacobs DR, Slavin J, Marquart L: Whole grain intake and cancer: a review of the literature, *Nutr Cancer* 24:221-9, 1995.
6. van Poppel G, Verhoeven DT, Verhagen H, et al: Brassica vegetables and cancer prevention. Epidemiology and mechanisms, *Adv Exp Med Biol* 472:159-68, 1999.
7. Robertson J, Brydon WG, Tadesse K, et al: The effect of raw carrot on serum lipids and colon function, *Am J Clin Nutr* 32:1889-92, 1979.
8. Slattery ML, Benson J, Ma KN, et al: Trans-fatty acids and colon cancer, *Nutr Cancer* 39:170-5, 2001.
9. Liu Z, Uesaka T, Watanabe H, et al: High fat diet enhances colonic cell proliferation and carcinogenesis in rats by elevating serum leptin, *Int J Oncol* 19:1009-14, 2001.
10. Sesink AL, Termont DS, Kleibeuker JH, et al: Red meat and colon cancer: dietary haem-induced colonic cytotoxicity and epithelial hyperproliferation are inhibited by calcium, *Carcinogenesis* 22:1653-9, 2001.

11. Slattery ML, Edwards SL, Boucher KM, et al: Lifestyle and colon cancer: an assessment of factors associated with risk, *Am J Epidemiol* 150:869-77, 1999.

12. Holt PR, Atillasoy EO, Gilman J, et al: Modulation of abnormal colonic epithelial cell proliferation and differentiation by low-fat dairy foods: a randomized controlled trial, *JAMA* 280:1074-9, 1998.

13. Weisburger JH, Reddy BS, Rose DP, et al: Protective mechanisms of dietary fibers in nutritional carcinogenesis. In Bronzetti G, Hayatsu H, De Flora S, et al, editors: *Antimutagenesis and anticarcinogenesis mechanisms III*, New York, 1993, Plenum Press.

14. Slavin JL, Martini MC, Jacobs DR, et al: Plausible mechanisms for the protectiveness of whole grains, *Am J Clin Nutr* 70(suppl 3):459S-463S, 1999.

15. Schatzkin A, Lanza E, Corle D, et al: Lack of effect of a low-fat, high-fiber diet on the recurrence of colorectal adenomas, *N Engl J Med* 342:1149-55, 2000.

16. Holt PR: Studies of calcium in food supplements in humans, *Ann N Y Acad Sci* 889:128-37, 1999.

17. Kampman E, Slattery ML, Caan B, et al: Calcium, vitamin D, sunshine exposure, dairy products and colon cancer risk (United States), *Cancer Causes Control* 11:459-66, 2000.

18. Prinz-Langenohl R, Fohr I, Pietrzik K: Beneficial role for folate in the prevention of colorectal and breast cancer, *Eur J Nutr* 40:98-105, 2001.

19. Ames BN: DNA damage from micronutrient deficiencies is likely to be a major cause of cancer, *Mutat Res* 475:7-20, 2001.

20. Pappalardo G, Guadalaxara A, Maiani G, et al: Antioxidant agents and colorectal carcinogenesis: role of beta-carotene, vitamin E and vitamin C, *Tumori* 82:6-11, 1996.

21. Albanes D, Heinonen OP, Huttunen JK, et al: Effects of alpha-tocopherol and beta-carotene supplements on cancer incidence in the Alpha-Tocopherol Beta-Carotene Cancer Prevention Study, *Am J Clin Nutr* 62(suppl 6):1427S-1430S, 1995.

22. Jacobs EJ, Connell CJ, Patel AV, et al: Vitamin C and vitamin E supplement use and colorectal cancer mortality in a large American Cancer Society cohort, *Cancer Epidemiol Biomarkers Prev* 10:17-23, 2001.

23. Biasco G, Paganelli GM: European trials on dietary supplementation for cancer prevention, *Ann N Y Acad Sci* 889:152-6, 1999.

24. Huang YC, Jessup JM, Forse RA, et al: N-3 fatty acids decrease colonic epithelial cell proliferation in high-risk bowel mucosa, *Lipids* 31(suppl):S313-S317, 1996.

25. Wargovich MJ: Colon cancer chemoprevention with ginseng and other botanicals, *J Korean Med Sci* 16(suppl):S81-S86, 2001.

26. Goel A, Boland CR, Chauhan DP: Specific inhibition of cyclooxygenase-2 (COX-2) expression by dietary curcumin in HT-29 human colon cancer cells, *Cancer Lett* 172:111-8, 2001.

27. Fukuda K, Hibiya Y, Mutoh M, et al: Inhibition by berberine of cyclooxygenase-2 transcriptional activity in human colon cancer cells, *J Ethnopharmacol* 66:227-33, 1999.

▪ CHAPTER 21 ▪

CORYZA

The cost of coryza, or the common cold, exceeds $3.5 billion per year in the United States.

CLINICAL DIAGNOSIS

The common cold presents as a clear watery nasal discharge that becomes mucopurulent in a day or two; sneezing, nasal obstruction, and a mild sore throat are common. Hoarseness, a cough, lethargy, headaches, and tearing may also be present.

THERAPEUTIC STRATEGY

There is some evidence that the progression of coryza can be retarded or even prevented when the host's immune status is enhanced at the first suggestion of symptoms. Vigorous early intervention appears to be the key.

LIFESTYLE CHANGES

Droplets spread the virus. Overcrowded areas should be avoided.

NUTRIENT THERAPY/DIETARY SUPPLEMENTS

The use of vitamin C as a panacea for the common cold has long been debated. Analysis of a cohort of smokers from the Alpha-Tocopherol Beta-Carotene Cancer Prevention Study showed that neither administration of dietary vitamins C and E and beta-carotene nor supplementation with vitamin E (50 mg/day) and beta-carotene (20 mg/day) had any meaningful association with the incidence of the common cold.[1] However, the doses used were therapeutically unrealistic. Analysis of 23 studies suggested that vitamin C in daily doses of two or more grams was effective in managing the common cold.[2] A review of 30 clinical trials confirmed that the duration of cold symptoms was moderately reduced by relatively high doses of this vitamin.[3] Although vitamin C has not been found to provide prophylaxis, large doses can have an anticholinergic effect and dry nasal secretions.[4]

Trials of zinc supplementation for treatment of colds have been going on for more than a decade, with contradictory results. A randomized, double-blind, placebo-controlled trial demonstrated that zinc lozenges reduced the duration and severity of cold symptoms, especially cough.[5] However, two clinical trials suggested that zinc lozenges had no effect on symptom severity, although it was suggested that zinc gluconate lozenges containing 13.3 mg of zinc had some impact on duration.[6] The authors concluded that zinc compounds had little utility for treatment of the common cold. However, another randomized, double-blind, placebo-controlled clinical trial suggested that zinc gluconate lozenges reduced the duration of symptoms by 42%.[7] In a review of eight double-blind, placebo-controlled trials, Garland and Hagmeyer[8] found that four trials suggested that treatment of the common cold with zinc gluconate lozenges, containing adequate doses of elemental zinc, may be effective in reducing the duration and severity of cold symptoms.[8] Common adverse effects include an unpleasant taste, mouth irritation, and nausea. Successful therapy seemed most likely when the intervention was started within 48 hours and lozenges were sucked every 2 hours while subjects were awake. The minimum effective dose appeared to be 13.3 mg of elemental zinc per lozenge. Perhaps the situation is best summarized by the Cochrane Project systematic review in which it was concluded that evidence of the effect of zinc lozenges for treating the common cold remains inconclusive.[9] Variations in the therapeutic effect of zinc in treating the common cold may result from binding of free zinc (e.g., by citric acid, sorbitol, or mannitol) or from failure to take an adequate dose. Eighty milligrams daily has been suggested as an adequate dose.

HERBAL THERAPY

A review of 17 clinical studies suggested that echinacea is probably a safe, efficacious treatment for the common cold; however, the results were unclear because of inherent flaws in study design.[10] A problem in interpreting the efficacy of echinacea is the high variation of bioactive compound present in different preparations.[11] Favorable studies suggest that echinacea effectively reduces the frequency, duration, and severity of symptoms. Furthermore, existing literature suggests that echinacea should be used as a treatment for illness, not as a means of prevention.[12] Studies suggest that the plant and its active components affect phagocytosis, but not the specific immune system. However, only certain preparations of echinacea are effective.[13,14] Herbal combinations that include echinacea are available.[15]

A combination of echinacea to enhance immunity and fresh garlic for its antimicrobial effect is another option. A randomized, controlled trial showed that volunteers taking an allicin-containing garlic supplement (one capsule daily) were less likely to contract a cold and recovered faster if they were infected.[16]

Herbal treatment for coryza and influenza is similar, although more vigorous in the case of influenza.[17] In addition to echinacea and garlic, recommended herbs include fresh grated ginger and cinnamon in hot water for mucosal symptoms and goldenseal for catarrh and associated sinusitis. For a sore throat, topical kava for its anesthetic effect and licorice for its soothing anti-inflammatory effect are useful. St. John's wort is used for its antiviral effect in cases of influenza.

PRACTICE TIPS

- There appears to be no advantage in taking nutrients or herbs prophylactically.

REFERENCES

1. Hemila H, Kaprio J, Albanes D, et al: Vitamin C, vitamin E, and beta-carotene in relation to common cold incidence in male smokers, *Epidemiology* 13:32-7, 2002.
2. Hemila H: Vitamin C supplementation and common cold symptoms: factors affecting the magnitude of the benefit, *Med Hypotheses* 52:171-8, 1999.
3. Douglas RM, Chalker EB, Treacy B: Vitamin C for preventing and treating the common cold, *Cochrane Database Syst Rev* 2:CD000980, 2000.
4. Turner RB, Schaffner W, Young MG: Will anything work for the common cold? *Patient Care* Nov;15-24, 2000.
5. Prasad AS, Fitzgerald JT, Bao B, et al: Duration of symptoms and plasma cytokine levels in patients with the common cold treated with zinc acetate. A randomized, double-blind, placebo-controlled trial, *Ann Intern Med* 133:245-52, 2000.
6. Turner RB, Cetnarowski WE: Effect of treatment with zinc gluconate or zinc acetate on experimental and natural colds, *Clin Infect Dis* 31:1202-8, 2000.
7. Zinc lozenges reduce the duration of common cold symptoms, *Nutr Rev* 55:82-5, 1997.
8. Garland ML, Hagmeyer KO: The role of zinc lozenges in treatment of the common cold, *Ann Pharmacother* 32:63-9, 1998.
9. Marshall I: Zinc for the common cold, *Cochrane Database Syst Rev* 2:CD001364, 2000.
10. Giles JT, Palat CT, Chien SH, et al: Evaluation of echinacea for treatment of the common cold, *Pharmacotherapy* 20:690-7, 2000.
11. Linde K, ter Riet G, Hondras M, et al: Systematic reviews of complementary therapies—an annotated bibliography. Part 2: herbal medicine, *BMC Complement Altern Med* 1:5, 2001.
12. Percival SS: Use of echinacea in medicine, *Biochem Pharmacol* 60:155-8, 2000.
13. Turner RB, Riker DK, Gangemi JD: Ineffectiveness of echinacea for prevention of experimental rhinovirus colds, *Antimicrob Agents Chemother* 44:1708-9, 2000.
14. Grimm W, Muller HH: A randomized controlled trial of the effect of fluid extract of *Echinacea purpurea* on the incidence and severity of colds and respiratory infections, *Am J Med* 106:138-43, 1999.

15. Henneicke-von Zepelin H, Hentschel C, Schnitker J, et al: Efficacy and safety of a fixed combination phytomedicine in the treatment of the common cold (acute viral respiratory tract infection): results of a randomised, double blind, placebo controlled, multicentre study, *Curr Med Res Opin* 15:214-27, 1999.
16. Josling P: Preventing the common cold with a garlic supplement: a double-blind, placebo-controlled survey, *Adv Ther* 18:189-93, 2001.
17. Mills S, Bone K: *Principles and practice of phytotherapy*, Edinburgh, 2000, Churchill Livingstone.

▪ CHAPTER 22 ▪

DEPRESSION

Late-life depression is significantly underdiagnosed and undertreated, despite an overall prevalence of depression of 5% to 8%, increasing to 15% by 65 years of age.[1]

Depression affects more than 17 million adults in the United States each year, costing the nation $44 billion in treatment, disability, and lost productivity.[2] A comprehensive treatment of late-life depression, which includes social and psychologic support, has a response rate of 80% to 90%.[1]

A serious consequence is premature death from fatal myocardial infarction, stroke, or suicide.

CLINICAL DIAGNOSIS

Depression has emotional, physical, and social repercussions. It is characterized by despondency, a lack of motivation, poor self-esteem, sleep disturbance, and mental and physical slowness. Masked depression presents as flatness of mood, loss of interest, avoidance of people, lethargy, an inability to cope with stress, and pervasive anxiety. Results of laboratory tests are normal.

THERAPEUTIC STRATEGY

Depression has been linked to a low level of monoamines. Increasing the cerebral level of serotonin and/or norepinephrine has an antidepressant effect. β-Adrenergic blocking drugs, which produce a condition in the brain that is functionally similar to monoamine depletion, produce depression. Effective antidepressants, such as the tricyclics and monoamine oxidase inhibitors, raise the concentration of the amines at the postsynaptic level.[3] Evidence suggests that precursors of norepinephrine and serotonin might be useful in treating patients with mild or moderate depression.[4]

In addition to the biogenic amine theory of depression, a perturbation of the normal hypothalamic-pituitary-adrenal axis deserves consideration. A frequent finding in endogenous depression is suppression of the normal hypothalamic-pituitary-adrenal axis characterized by hypersecretion of corticotropin-releasing hormone, hypersensitivity of the adrenal cortex to corticotropin, and increased cortisol levels.[5,6] A sequela of prolonged cortisol increase is a reduction in serotonin synthesis. Excess cortisol activates the enzyme tryptophan pyrrolase, shunting tryptophan away from the serotonin pathway into niacin production.[7] Depression, a frequent feature of medical conditions, may be mediated by inflammatory cytokines through this mechanism. Interleukin-1 (IL)-1 and IL-6 are potent activators of the hypothalamic-pituitary-adrenal axis through stimulation of corticotropin-releasing hormone. Cytokines such as IL-1, IL-6, and tumor necrosis factor may act as neuromodulators in depression.

LIFESTYLE CHANGES

Exercise is a natural antidepressant. A low-fat, high–complex-carbohydrate diet favors a robust emotional state. Turkey, salmon, and milk are rich sources of tryptophan and may lighten depression. Some people who have started a caffeine-free and sugar-free diet report feeling less depressed, moody, and tired.

Borderline nutrient deficiencies may predispose individuals to depression. In fact, depression may be one of the earliest signs of an incipient mineral deficiency. Correction of a selenium, zinc, or magnesium deficiency improves mood. Depression is also associated with iron deficiency anemia and may take months to resolve after the anemia has been corrected.

Vitamin deficiencies may be associated with depression. Depression is the first symptom of experimental scurvy, and deficiency of vitamin B_5 results in depression accompanied by fatigue and "burning feet."

NUTRIENT THERAPY/DIETARY SUPPLEMENTS

Controlled clinical trials have demonstrated that any one of the following nutrients elevates mood in depressed patients: L-5-hydroxytryptophan, 25 to 75 mg daily; L-tryptophan, 2 to 3 g daily; phenylalanine, 200 to 2000 mg; L-tyrosine, 2 g; calcium, 10 mg twice daily; acetyl-L-carnitine, 500 mg four times daily; inositiol, 12 g daily; lithium, 400 µg; phosphatidylserine, 300 mg daily; S-adenosylmethionine, 80 mg twice daily; thiamine, 50 mg daily; vitamin C, 1000 mg daily; and vitamin B_{12} injections. Correction of deficiency of vitamin C (500 mg daily), selenium (200 µg daily), iron (300 mg ferrous sulfate three times daily), or folic acid (800 µg daily) has also been shown to be effective in clinical trials.[8] Although evidence for the use of vitamins and amino acids as sole agents for treatment of psychiatric symptoms is not strong, there is intriguing preliminary evidence for the use of tryptophan, phenylalanine, and folate as adjuncts to enhance the effectiveness of conventional antidepressants.[9]

Tryptophan and 5-hydroxytryptophan are serotonin precursors, and phenylananine and tyrosine are norepinephrine precursors. Cerebral serotonin synthesis is dependent on the availability of L-tryptophan and its immediate metabolite 5-hydroxytryptophan (5-HTP). Therapeutic use of 5-HTP bypasses the conversion of L-tryptophan into 5-HTP by the enzyme tryptophan hydroxylase, the rate-limiting step in the synthesis of serotonin or 5-hydroxytryptamine.[10] 5-HTP easily crosses the blood-brain barrier. A number of studies have demonstrated that 5-HTP reduces symptoms of depression. Various studies have indicated that more than 50% of patients with depression respond to 5-HTP in doses ranging from 200 to 3000 mg daily, and some studies indicate that 5-HTP, in a dose as low as 200 mg/day, is more effective than placebo and almost as effective as various tricyclic antidepressants.[4] After 2 weeks at doses of 50 to 300 mg daily, 5-HTP seems to reduce symptoms of major depression in a substantial number of patients. In another reasonably large study of outpatients with mild or moderate depression, investigators found that L-tryptophan was associated with a significantly better outcome than placebo.[11] This study is noteworthy because the responses of the subjects were monitored for a relatively long period (i.e., 3 months). 5-HTP, with its relatively low degree of side effects and low cost, deserves consideration in the treatment of depression.

The production and transport of L-tryptophan from the blood stream into the central nervous system can be compromised by several factors, including vitamin B_6 deficiency. Vitamin B_6, 40 mg daily, helps to alleviate depression in women taking oral contraceptives. It has also been suggested that chromium may have an antidepressant effect by enhancing insulin utilization and increasing tryptophan availability in the central nervous system.[12] Several single-blind trials have suggested specificity of response to chromium. Side effects were rare and mild, and most commonly included enhanced dreaming and mild psychomotor activation. Chromium may also have an effect on norepinephrine release.

In addition to the findings on tryptophan, there is intriguing preliminary evidence that folate and phenylalanine may enhance the effectiveness of conventional antidepressants, that S-adenosylmethionine may have antidepressant effects, and that ω-3 polyunsaturated fatty acids, particularly docosahexaenoic acid, may have mood elevating and stabilising effects.[9] W-3 poly unsaturated fatty acids may have mood elevating and stabilising effects.

However, of the natural remedies for depression, it is an herb that enjoys greatest scientific support.

HERBAL THERAPY

A recent study showed that β-adrenergic receptors were downregulated and 5-HTP2 receptors were upregulated by *Hypericum perforatum* (St. John's wort).[13] Effective antidepressant drugs (e.g., the tricyclic antidepressant, imipramine), downregulate both 5-HTP2 receptors and β-adrenergic receptors. In addition to acting at the level of neuroreceptors, *H. perforatum* may influence the hypothalamic-pituitary-adrenal axis. Results of laboratory tests in depressed patients and control subjects show marked inhibition of IL-6 release with *H. perforatum*.[14] Therefore it is not surprising that animal and clinical studies support the use of *H. perforatum* in the treatment of depression. Animal studies suggest that *H. perforatum* effectively inhibits the synaptic reuptake of serotonin, noradrenaline, and dopamine. However, although clinical trials confirm that *H. perforatum* is more effective than placebo, some question its efficacy compared with that of standard antidepressants in the treatment of mild-to-moderate depression.[15,16]

A recent, randomized, controlled, double-blind review of eight cases of generally good methodological quality suggested that St. John's wort is 23% to 55% more effective than placebo but is 6% to 18% less effective than tricyclic antidepressants in the treatment of mild to moderate depression.[17] Another study confirmed its superiority to placebo, and four studies showed no differences in effectiveness when compared with antidepressant drugs.[18] In a recent review, investigators concluded that St. John's wort is an effective antidepressant for mild to moderate depression and causes fewer side effects, although further trials are needed to establish long-term efficacy and safety.[19]

Given that *H. perforatum* appears comparable to numerous routinely prescribed antidepressant drugs, its ability to achieve equivalent results with fewer side effects in mild to moderate depression deserves particular attention.[5] Its low incidence of side effects may indeed make it particularly useful in the elderly.[20] A possible therapeutic regimen, with a standardized preparation providing 0.3% hypericin, is an initial dose of 300 to 400 mg daily with increases in the dose to 600 to 900 mg over the next 2 to 4 weeks as needed.[21] Maximal benefits may only be noted in 4 to 6 weeks.

A cautionary note is that *H. perforatum* appears to have little or no therapeutic value for severe depression. In a randomized, double-blind, placebo-controlled clinical trial of 900 mg given daily for 4 to 8 weeks, with increases to 1200 mg daily in the absence of an adequate response, Shelton et al[22] concluded that St. John's wort was not effective for treatment of major depression. This may be cause for concern because an American study indicated that complementary and alternative therapies were used more than conventional therapies by people with self-defined severe depression.[23] Furthermore, responses to a small telephone survey indicated that most subjects took St. John's wort for depression, and 74% did not seek medical advice.[24] Dosage ranged from 300 to 1200 mg daily, and the mean duration of therapy was around 7 weeks, with 84% reporting improvement and 47% reporting side effects.

It should be noted that although many of the herbal agents said to benefit depressed patients appear to be safe, serious neuropsychiatric side effects and interactions have been reported for several over-the-counter "antidepressants."[25] Stricter oversight by regulating agents is required.

PRACTICE TIPS

- Depression, insomnia, and food cravings may result when brain serotonin levels are depleted.
- Low levels of vitamin B_6, folate, or selenium may reduce cerebral serotonin levels.
- A mild serotonin syndrome may be precipitated in patients who mix St. John's wort with serotonin reuptake inhibitors.
- Patients taking antidepressants, including Prozac, should be cautioned against taking herbs, particularly ephedra and ginseng.
- Depressed patients may have an increased risk for infection; and community-dwelling older adults with chronic, mild depressive symptoms have poorer T-cell responses than persons who are not depressed.[26]

A CASE HISTORY BY PAUL HOLMAN

Don is a 48-year-old architect who presented with a 9-month history suggestive of depression. His symptoms included lowered mood, reduced energy and motivation, poor sleep (initial insomnia and early morning wakening), poor appetite, and weight loss of 6 kg. He was still able to work and found that his spirits would rally if he were involved in an interesting project. He was not suicidal, but his self-confidence was quite low. His general health was good except for a several-year history of chronic nasal congestion and poor digestion (recurrent bloating, pain, and erratic bowel habits).

The history revealed that Don had divorced 18 months previously. He and his wife now had little contact, and there were no children. His mother, to whom he was close, had died 6 months after the divorce, and it was at that time that he had felt his energy and mood slipping. Don's brother lives abroad, and his father had died several years earlier, leaving few other close relationships or social supports in Don's life. The family history revealed that a paternal uncle had had bipolar disorder and that a maternal great-aunt had been treated for a thyroid condition.

Don's lifestyle left much to be desired. On the dietary front, he had no breakfast and usually had a salad sandwich for lunch. Dinner, formerly a cooked meal at home, had now become an erratic affair with take-away fried rice and dim sums as staples. He found that coffee tended to pick him up, as did alcohol, which he was now consuming at a level exceeding 30 standard drinks per week. In his youth he had been a competitive swimmer, but he had not engaged in regular exercise for years.

There were no obvious nutritional deficiency symptoms or signs. Don presented himself as a moderately depressed intelligent man with little to say for himself. He had the build of a mesomorphic endomorph. Closer questioning revealed that he had always felt on the low energy side and that eating fatty foods made this worse. Skipping breakfast and even lunch had been a lifelong habit, and he seldom felt very hungry before evening. He was aware that desserts or light meals such as fish and salad tended to improve his mental clarity, but he had never undertaken systematic dietary change. His former wife had noticed that cheese or cream made his nasal stuffiness worse, and he therefore avoided heavy milk products.

A provisional formulation is included in Table 22-1.

Because he clearly satisfied the criteria for major depression, an antidepressant would normally be the first choice of treatment. However, Don had been influenced by his mother to distrust medication and was seeking a more natural alternative. The fact that he was not suicidal, still coping with work, and able to muster a reserve of enthusiasm for his profession persuaded me that we had some leeway for further investigation and "enlightened experimentation" with diet and lifestyle.

Since men are often difficult to retain in treatment, it was important to make effective progress as quickly as possible. Don was advised to try eating a regular lunch with a substantial protein content and to have a lower-fat, higher-protein evening meal, to reduce consumption of alcohol, and to engage in some exercise.

Don began receiving the following:

- Tyrosine, 500 mg in the morning
- Tryptophan, 500 mg at night
- Multivitamin supplement for slow oxidizers supplying vitamins B_1, B_2, and B_6 (10 mg); niacin (25 mg); folate (0.5 mg); vitamin C (200 mg); and below recommended daily allowance quantities of potassium, magnesium, iron, zinc, copper, manganese, and chromium
- Added vitamin B_1, 50 mg in the morning
- Magnesium, 100 mg at night

The following investigations were initiated: B_1 (EKT stimulation test); determination of erythrocyte folate, serum B_{12}, and calcium, erythrocyte magnesium, fasting amino acid, and plasma essential fatty acid levels; complete blood count; liver function tests; iron studies; thyroid function tests; and hair mineral analysis. All tests were to be done before use of supplements was started.

At the time of the first follow-up visit, Don was sleeping a little better, but his mood was largely unaltered. He managed to reduce his alcohol consumption by 50%. Abnormal results from the investigations were mild ery-

TABLE 22-1 ■ **Don's Provisional Formulation**

PREDISPOSING FACTORS	PRECIPITATING FACTORS	PERPETUATING FACTORS
Family History of Depression	Divorce	Social isolation
Depression	Death of parent	Poor diet
Social isolation	Alcohol	Lack of exercise
Slow oxidizer		Alcohol
? Food sensitivity		? Low thyroid status

throcyte macrocytosis, mildly raised γ-glutamyl transferase level, a low erythrocyte folate level, marginally low magnesium level, low level of branched-chain amino acids methionine and tyrosine, and low-normal thyroid hormone levels (thyroxine, 11.0 pmol/L; thyroid-stimulating hormone, 2.5 mIU/L). Hair mineral analysis showed a generally flat low pattern with a raised calcium/phosphorus ratio supporting the slow oxidizer diagnosis, raised calcium/magnesium ratio, raised calcium/potassium ratio (reduced thyroid hormone function), and increased sodium/potassium and sodium/magnesium ratios, implying stress. Most of our initial hypotheses concerning the paucity of nutrient intake and Don's metabolic type seemed confirmed by test results. Don was clearly low in a range of nutrients, and his diet was also clearly inappropriate for a slow oxidizer. He had experienced no side effects from supplementation, and so we increased tyrosine to 1000 mg and tryptophan to 1000 mg and added folate to make a total of 2.5 mg per day.

We discussed further the possibility of a more nutrient-dense whole food diet with fatty fish twice weekly.

Over the next 3 months, Don was able to implement some major lifestyle changes with improvement in diet, reduction (but not elimination) of alcohol intake, and a dramatic increase in exercise. His mood improved consistently. Had it not, we could have tried a course of vitamin B_{12} injections (even though the B_{12} level was greater than 300 pmol/L) and further increased the amino acid doses (e.g., tyrosine, 1500 mg; tryptophan, 2000 mg). If he had not managed to improve his diet substantially, it might have been appropriate to add an amino acid mixture or nondairy protein supplement together with essential fatty acids.

Support and encouragement were major therapeutic factors. Results of his thyroid function tests were considerably improved at the 6-month mark. Long-term considerations include looking at food sensitivity issues and examination of gastrointestinal function. On the psychologic front, the crucial issue of social isolation would be the main concern because this is an important risk factor for suicide in middle-aged men with depression.

REFERENCES

1. Gottfries CG: Late life depression, *Eur Arch Psychiatry Clin Neurosci* 251(suppl 2):II57-61, 2001.
2. National Institute of Mental Health website: http://www.nimh.gov.
3. Cameron OG: Psychopharmacology, *Psychosom Med* 61:585-90, 1999.
4. Meyers S: Use of neurotransmitter precursors for treatment of depression, *Altern Med Rev* 5:64-71, 2000.
5. Miller AL: St. John's wort (*Hypericum perforatum*): clinical effects on depression and other conditions, *Altern Med Rev* 3:18-26, 1998.
6. van Praag HM: Faulty cortisol/serotonin interplay. Psychopathological and biological characterization of a new, hypothetical depression subtype (SeCA depression), *Psychiatry Res* 65:143-57, 1996.

7. Linde K, Ramirez G, Mulrow C, et al: St. John's wort for depression: an overview and meta-analysis of randomised clinical trials, *Br Med J* 313:253-8, 1996.

8. Werbach MR: *Textbook of nutritional medicine*, Tarzana, CA, 1999, Third Line Press.

9. Stoll A: *The Omega 3 Connection*, New York, 2001, Simon and Schuster.

10. Birdsall TC: 5-Hydroxytryptophan: a clinically-effective serotonin precursor, *Altern Med Rev* 3:271-80, 1998.

11. Poldinger W, Calanchini B, Schwarz W: A functional-dimensional approach to depression: serotonin deficiency as a target syndrome in a comparison of 5-hydroxytryptophan and fluvoxamine, *Psychopathology* 24:53-81, 1991.

12. McLeod MN, Golden RN: Chromium treatment of depression, *Int J Neuropsychopharmacol* 3:311-4, 2000.

13. Thiele B, Brink I, Ploch M: Modulation of cytokine expression by Hypericum extract. *J Geriatr Psychiatry Neurol* 7:S60-S62, 1994.

14. Müller WEG, Rolli M, Schäfer, et al: Effects of Hypericum extract (LI 160) in biochemical models of antidepressant activity, *Pharmacopsychiatry* 30:S102-S107, 1997.

15. Nathan P: The experimental and clinical pharmacology of St John's wort (*Hypericum perforatum* L.), *Mol Psychiatry* 4:333-8, 1999.

16. Linde K, Mulrow CD: St John's wort for depression, *Cochrane Database Syst Rev* 2:CD000448, 2000.

17. Gaster B, Holroyd J: St John's wort for depression: a systematic review, *Arch Intern Med* 160:152-6, 2000.

18. Beaubrun G, Gray GE: A review of herbal medicines for psychiatric disorders, *Psychiatr Serv* 51:1130-4, 2000.

19. Linde K, ter Riet G, Hondras M, et al: Systematic reviews of complementary therapies—an annotated bibliography. Part 2: Herbal medicine, *BMC Complement Altern Med* 1:5, 2001. 20.

20. Vorbach EU, Arnoldt KH, Wolpert E: St John's wort: a potential therapy for elderly depressed patients? *Drugs Aging* 16:189-97, 2000.

21. Glisson J, Crawford R, Street S: The clinical applications of *Ginkgo biloba*, St. John's wort, saw palmetto, and soy, *Nurse Practitioner* 24:30-49, 1999.

22. Shelton RC, Keller MB, Gelenberg A, et al: Effectiveness of St John's wort in major depression: a randomized controlled trial, *JAMA* 285:1978-86, 2001.

23. Kessler RC, Soukup J, Davis RB, et al: The use of complementary and alternative therapies to treat anxiety and depression in the United States, *Am J Psychiatry* 158:289-94, 2001.

24. Beckman SE, Sommi RW, Switzer J: Consumer use of St. John's wort: a survey on effectiveness, safety, and tolerability, *Pharmacotherapy* 20:568-74, 2000.

25. Pies R: Adverse neuropsychiatric reactions to herbal and over-the-counter "antidepressants," *J Clin Psychiatry* 61:815-20, 2000.

26. McGuire L, Kiecolt-Glaser JK, Glaser R: Depressive symptoms and lymphocyte proliferation in older adults, *J Abnorm Psychol* 111:192-7, 2002.

▪ CHAPTER 23 ▪

DIABETES MELLITUS

The World Health Organization has predicted that between 1997 and 2025, the number of patients with diabetes will double to reach about 300 million. The leading cause of death and morbidity in patients with diabetes is cardiovascular disease caused by macrovascular and microvascular degeneration.

Diabetes mellitus is the most common genetic disease in the Western world today. It is the phenotype for more than 150 genotypes. Each of these genotypes is characterized by impaired glucose tolerance and impaired control of intermediary metabolism. The two most important modifiable factors contributing to the development of type 2 diabetes mellitus are obesity and physical inactivity. Nonetheless, a survey of patients with diabetes revealed that 78% were taking prescribed medication for their diabetes, 44% were taking over-the-counter supplements, and 31% were taking alternative medications.[1]

CLINICAL DIAGNOSIS

There are two distinct types of diabetes from a clinical perspective. Type 1, or juvenile-onset, diabetes is common in lean individuals, usually younger than 30 years, who present with thirst, polyuria, and weight loss. Management requires insulin. Type 2, or noninsulin-dependent, diabetes is usually found in older individuals with a family history of diabetes. Patients with type 2 diabetes are often overweight and complain of increasing fatigue and nocturia. They are susceptible to infections and vascular disease. Management focuses on lifestyle intervention to reduce insulin resistance.

Because the complications of type 2 diabetes progress while the individual is asymptomatic, screening is recommended. Blood sugar assessment is indicated in everyone older than 65 years and in persons with at least two risk factors. Risk factors include a family history, obesity, hypertension, gestational diabetes, hyperlipidemia, and being older than 40 years. A definitive diagnosis is made when an increased blood glucose level is found on two separate occasions in an asymptomatic individual. A random blood glucose level in excess of 11 mmol/L or a fasting venous plasma glucose level equal to or exceeding 7.8 mmol/L is considered diagnostic. High blood glucose levels and oxidative stress produce advanced glycation end products, a complex and heterogeneous group of compounds that have been implicated in diabetes-related complications.[2]

THERAPEUTIC STRATEGY

Although current therapies for type 2 diabetes mellitus focus primarily on weight reduction, an alternate approach to control is to arrest the progress of the disease.[3] The aim is to keep the fasting blood sugar level between 4.4 and 6.1 mmol/L and prevent postprandial blood sugar levels exceeding 8.0 mmol/L. The aim of dietary intervention is to prevent excessive fluctuation and peaks in blood glucose levels. Good blood glucose control prevents complications. The blood glycemic index has been shown to be independently related to glycosylated hemoglobin (HbA_{1c}), and a lower dietary glycemic index is related to lower HbA_{1c} concentrations, independently of fiber intake.[4] In patients with diabetes, an HbA_{1c} level below 7.0% can be treated by diet and exercise, regardless of the blood glucose levels.

Patients with diabetes are prone to both small- and large-vessel disease. Epidemiologic studies suggest that dietary glycemic load is positively associated with risk of type 2 diabetes and coronary artery disease. Clinical data support the physiologic relevance of the dietary glycemic load as a potential risk factor for coronary artery disease in free-living women, particularly those prone to insulin resistance.[5] High-density lipoprotein (HDL) cholesterol is protective, and the HDL concentration drops by 0.06 mmol/L for every 15-unit increase in the glycemic index.[6] A high dietary glycemic index and high glycemic load are associated with a lower concentration of plasma HDL. In addition, a high glycemic index increases the risk of small-vessel disease, predisposing patients to neuropathy, nephropathy, and cataracts. Oxidative damage caused by dysregulation of glucose metabolism is thought to be an important mechanism in the pathogenesis of this condition. Glutathione, coenzyme Q10, and lipoic acid appear to have therapeutic potential.[7]

Mineral and amino acid supplements are also used in an attempt to reduce diabetic complications. Minerals such as magnesium, calcium, potassium, zinc, chromium, and vanadium appear to be associated with insulin resistance; whereas amino acids, including L-carnitine, taurine, and L-arginine, might help to reverse insulin resistance.[7]

LIFESTYLE CHANGES

A controlled prospective study showed that type 2 diabetes can be prevented by changes in diet and exercise of high-risk subjects.[8] These lifestyle changes even reduce the risk of diabetes in individuals who are not overweight. The ideal diet for enhancing insulin sensitivity reduces body weight by decreasing fat while sparing muscle tissue. Research suggests that a diet low in total fat and cholesterol, relatively rich in monounsaturated fats, and high in complex carbohydrates, particularly soluble fiber (up to 40 g/day), with a low glycemic index may improve insulin resistance in the long term.[3]

A lower dietary glycemic index is related to a lower HbA_{1c} concentration.[9] The glycemic index compares the increase in blood glucose after ingestion of a food with the amount blood glucose would rise after ingestion of an equivalent amount of glucose (see Figure 23-1). Whole foods, particularly those rich in soluble fiber, are absorbed more slowly and produce lower blood glucose levels. Foods with a glycemic index of less than 55 are desirable. Good choices are apples, grapefruit, beans, lentils, dense grainy bread, and bran cereals. Oats and guar gum deserve particular attention.

Soluble fiber forms a gel in the intestine, slowing absorption, effectively lowering the glycemic index, and with prolonged use, decreasing serum cholesterol levels. Foods rich in soluble fiber (per 100 g of edible portion) are peanuts (6.4 g), whole wheat bread (6 g), kidney and white beans (5.7 g), fresh pears (5 g), peas (4.5 g), cooked corn (4.3 g), potatoes with skin (2.5 g), carrots (2.2 g), green beans (1.9 g), peaches (1.5 g), and bananas (1.1 g).

In addition to eating a diet rich in fruits and vegetables, choosing low-fat dairy products reduced in saturated fat, total fat, and cholesterol (DASH diet) results in a better lipid profile.[10] Controlled clinical trials confirm the benefit of a vegetarian diet rich in monounsaturated fats and low in carbohydrates. Trans-fatty acids increase and polyunsaturated fatty acids decrease the risk of type 2 diabetes.[11] Frequent small meals, moderate protein restriction, and alcohol avoidance are also advocated. However, data from the Health Professionals' Follow-up Study indicate that moderate alcohol consumption is associated with lower risk of ischemic heart disease in men with type 2 diabetes.[12] The benefits of moderate consumption did not statistically differ by beverage type.

It has been suggested that a diet rich in whole grains, cereal fiber, and dietary magnesium may reduce the risk of diabetes. A large prospective cohort study of older women demonstrated that total grain, whole-grain,

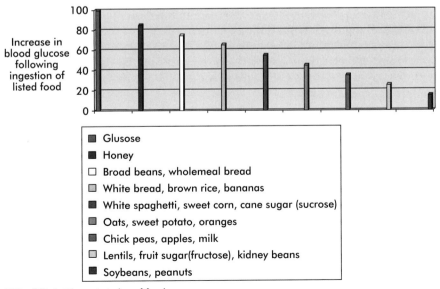

FIG. 23-1 Glycemic index of foods.

total dietary fiber, cereal fiber, and dietary magnesium intakes had strong inverse associations with the incidence of diabetes.[13] It has been postulated that the ability of fiber-rich cereal products to decrease diabetes risk may be mediated primarily by their superior magnesium content.[14] Magnesium depletion provokes insulin resistance, and high-magnesium diets have a preventive, although not curative, effect in certain animal models of diabetes. Magnesium repletion was associated with a decrease in atherogenic lipid fractions and a reduced insulin-stimulated glucose uptake in magnesium-deficient persons with type 1 diabetes.[15]

Many culinary plants have been shown to enhance glucose oxidation.[16] Their clinical importance has yet to be demonstrated.

NUTRIENT THERAPY/DIETARY SUPPLEMENTS

It is postulated that specific nutritional supplements may be used to target key dysfunctions that contribute to maintaining hyperglycemia in type 2 diabetes,[17] for example:

- Bioactive chromium may moderate skeletal muscle insulin resistance.
- Conjugated linoleic acid may temper adipocyte insulin resistance.
- High-dose biotin may restrain excessive hepatic glucose output.
- Coenzyme Q10 may moderate beta cell failure.

Hydroxycitrate, carnitine, or pyruvate may disinhibit hepatic fatty acid oxidation with a subsequent decrease in serum free fatty acids in the short term and regression of visceral obesity in the longer term.

Nutrients that have been found, in clinical trials, to improve the glycemic response include the following[18]: biotin (9-16 mg daily) pyridoxine α-ketoglutarate (600 mg three times daily), vitamin C (0.5-1.0 g twice daily), calcium (1 g/day), magnesium (400 mg/day), or zinc (220 mg twice daily). Patients with type 2 diabetes demonstrated less oxidative stress when supplemented with 30 mg zinc daily as zinc gluconate or 400 μg daily of chromium as chromium pidolate or both.[19]

Although the impact of chromium on insulin resistance remains equivocal,[7] persons with type 2 diabetes have been shown to benefit from glucose tolerance factor supplementation, such as 9 mg of brewers' yeast daily. Furthermore, a double-blind crossover trial in patients with type 2 diabetes showed that chromium supplementation, either as brewers' yeast (23.3 μg chromium/day) or trivalent chromium chloride (CrCl3) (200 μg chromium/day), resulted in better control of glucose and lipid variables with decreasing drug dosages.[20]

Vitamin E has emerged as of particular interest to patients with diabetes. It dampens inflammation. RRR-α-tocopherol supplementation (1200 IU/day) significantly lowered levels of C-reactive protein and monocyte interleukin-6 in activated monocytes.[21] Vitamin E is beneficial in both large- and small-vessel disease. A double-blind, placebo-controlled, randomized study showed that vitamin E supplementation (1000 IU for 3 months) improved endothelial vasodilator function in patients with type 1 diabetes.[22] Impaired endothelial vasodilator function is related to low-density lipoprotein (LDL) vitamin E content in young diabetics. A double-blind study showed that patients with type 1 diabetes receiving 250 IU (168 mg) RRR-α-tocopherol three times a day had decreased lipoprotein oxidation.[23] Lipid oxidation increased when vitamin E supplementation was stopped. Compared with the control group, patients with type 2 diabetes who received vitamin E, 600 mg daily, for 4 months showed improvement in the indices of oxidative stress.[24] Glycosylated hemoglobin, plasma insulin, norepinephrine, and epinephrine levels were also lower.

Clinical trials have also demonstrated that various supplements, including vitamin E, may prevent or minimize diabetic complications such as the following[18]:

- Neuropathy. Supplements that are sometimes helpful include the following: acetyl-L-carnitine (1-3 g daily), α-lipoic acid (600-1200 mg), evening primrose oil (6 g/day), sodium selenite (100 μg), vitamin B_{12} (500 μg three times daily), and vitamin E (1200-1600 IU). Results from 15 clinical trials suggest that short-term daily treatment (for 3 weeks) with 600 mg α-lipoic acid (thioctic acid) intravenously or 1800 mg orally reduces the chief symptoms of diabetic polyneuropathy and improves neuropathic deficits.[25] Oral treatment with α-lipoic acid for 4 to 7 months tends to reduce neuropathic deficits; α-lipoic acid also improves cardiac autonomic neuropathy and may provide long-term improvement in motor and sensory nerve conduction in the lower limbs over 2 years. Vitamin E improves the ratio of cardiac sympathetic to parasympathetic tone.[24] Anecdotal evidence suggests that topical cayenne may be helpful for the pain of diabetic neuropathy.
- Platelet hyperaggregability. Platelet stickiness may be reduced by administration of 500 mg of taurine three times daily or 1200 to 1600 IU vitamin E. The high risk of vascular occlusion may be reduced by supplements. (Refer to the sections on ischemic heart and peripheral vascular disease.)
- Albuminuria. Elevated levels of urinary albumin excretion predict a high risk for progression to end-stage renal disease. In fact, microalbuminuria, an established risk factor for renal disease progression in type 1 diabetes, is the earliest clinical sign of diabetic nephropathy. A double-blind, randomized, crossover trial demonstrated that daily administration of vitamin C (1250 mg) and vitamin E (680 IU) for 4 weeks lowered albumin excretion in patients with type 2 diabetes and microalbuminuria or macroalbuminuria.[26] The clinical relevance of the finding requires clarification.

HERBAL THERAPY

Metformin, a useful biguanide pharmaceutical, was developed from an herb.[27] Insulin requirements may be altered by *Panax ginseng* and Siberian ginseng. Ginseng is hypothesized to play a role in carbohydrate metabolism. A short-term clinical study demonstrated that American ginseng (*Panax quinquefolius* L) attenuated postprandial glycemia in both diabetic and non-diabetic subjects, provided it was taken 40 minutes before the glucose challenge.[28] For nondiabetic subjects, it may be important for American ginseng to be taken with a meal to prevent unintended hypoglycemia.

Garlic and onion may stimulate insulin production, and guar gum and aloe vera may slow sugar absorption.[27] A literature review located 10 studies that suggested oral aloe vera might be a useful adjunct for lowering blood glucose levels in patients with diabetes and for reducing blood lipid levels in patients with hyperlipidemia. However, despite promising results, the clinical effectiveness of oral aloe vera is not sufficiently defined at present.[29]

Dandelion may enhance the hypoglycemic effect of drugs used to treat diabetes[30]; and culinary herbs such as cinnamon, witch hazel, green and black teas, allspice, bay leaves, nutmeg, cloves, mushrooms, brewers' yeast, Korean ginseng, flaxseed meal, and basil may modify blood glucose levels.[16]

Ginkgo biloba also has an effect. Ingestion of 120 mg of *Ginkgo biloba* extract (EGb 761) daily for 3 months by healthy glucose-tolerant individuals caused a significant increase in pancreatic beta-cell insulin and C-peptide response; in patients with noninsulin-dependent diabetes it may increase the hepatic metabolic clearance rate of both insulin and hypoglycemic agents.[31] The result is reduced insulin-mediated glucose metabolism and an elevated blood glucose level.

PRACTICE TIPS

- Avocados and beans are good food sources for patients with diabetes.
- Patients with diabetes benefit from a diet rich in whole fresh foods; three to five servings of vegetables, two to four servings of fruit, and six to eleven servings of breads, cereal, pasta, and rice per day are recommended.
- Life-long supplementation with vitamin E deserves consideration in patients with type 1 diabetes.
- Long-term administration of nicotinamide in doses up to 1 g daily may benefit insulin secretion by prediabetic subjects.
- Diabetic control may be improved by combining 100 mg of niacin daily with chromium supplementation.

REFERENCES

1. Ryan EA, Pick ME, Marceau C: Use of alternative medicines in diabetes mellitus, *Diabet Med* 18:242-5, 2001.
2. Singh R, Barden A, Mori T, Beilin L: Advanced glycation end-products: a review, *Diabetologia* 44:129-46, 2001.

3. Ruhe RC, McDonald RB: Use of antioxidant nutrients in the prevention and treatment of type 2 diabetes, *J Am Coll Nutr* 20(suppl 5):363S-369S, 2001.
4. Buyken AE, Toeller M, Heitkamp G, et al: Eurodiab IDDM Complications Study Group. Glycemic index in the diet of European outpatients with type 1 diabetes: relations to glycated hemoglobin and serum lipids, *Am J Clin Nutr* 73:574-81, 2001.
5. Liu S, Manson JE, Stampfer MJ, et al: Dietary glycemic load assessed by food-frequency questionnaire in relation to plasma high-density-lipoprotein cholesterol and fasting plasma triacylglycerols in postmenopausal women, *Am J Clin Nutr* 73:560-6, 2001.
6. Ford ES, Liu S: Glycemic index and serum high-density lipoprotein cholesterol concentration among us adults, *Arch Intern Med* 161:572-6, 2001.
7. Kelly GS: Insulin resistance: lifestyle and nutritional interventions, *Altern Med Rev* 5:109-132, 2000.
8. Tuomilehto J, Lindstrom J, Eriksson JG, et al: Finnish Diabetes Prevention Study Group. Prevention of type 2 diabetes mellitus by changes in lifestyle among subjects with impaired glucose tolerance, *N Engl J Med* 344:1343-50, 2001.
9. Buyken AE, Toeller M, Heitkamp G, et al: Glycemic index in the diet of European outpatients with type 1 diabetes: relations to glycated hemoglobin and serum lipids, *Am J Clin Nutr* 73:574-81, 2001.
10. Obarzanek E, Sacks FM, Vollmer WM, et al: DASH Research Group. Effects on blood lipids of a blood pressure-lowering diet: the Dietary Approaches to Stop Hypertension (DASH) Trial, *Am J Clin Nutr* 74:80-9, 2001.
11. Salmeron J, Hu FB, Manson JE, et al: Dietary fat intake and risk of type 2 diabetes in women, *Am J Clin Nutr* 73:1019-26, 2001.
12. Tanasescu M, Hu FB, Willett WC, et al: Alcohol consumption and risk of coronary heart disease among men with type 2 diabetes mellitus, *J Am Coll Cardiol* 38:1836-42, 2001.
13. Meyer KA, Kushi LH, Jacobs DR Jr, et al: Carbohydrates, dietary fiber, and incident type 2 diabetes in older women, *Am J Clin Nutr* 71:921-30, 2000.
14. McCarty MF: Toward practical prevention of type 2 diabetes, *Med Hypotheses* 54:786-93, 2000.
15. Djurhuus MS, Klitgaard NA, Pedersen KK, et al: Magnesium reduces insulin-stimulated glucose uptake and serum lipid concentrations in type 1 diabetes, *Metabolism* 50:1409-17, 2001.
16. Broadhurst CL, Polansky MM, Anderson RA: Insulin-like biological activity of culinary and medicinal plant aqueous extracts in vitro, *J Agric Food Chem* 48:849-52, 2000.
17. McCarty MF: Toward a wholly nutritional therapy for type 2 diabetes, *Med Hypotheses* 54:483-7, 2000.
18. Werbach MR: *Textbook of nutritional medicine*, Tarzana, CA, 1999, Third Line Press.
19. Anderson RA, Roussel AM, Zouari N, et al: Potential antioxidant effects of zinc and chromium supplementation in people with type 2 diabetes mellitus, *J Am Coll Nutr* 20:212-8, 2001.
20. Bahijiri SM, Mira SA, Mufti AM, et al: The effects of inorganic chromium and brewer's yeast supplementation on glucose tolerance, serum lipids and drug dosage in individuals with type 2 diabetes, *Saudi Med J* 21:831-7, 2000.
21. Devaraj S, Jialal I: Alpha tocopherol supplementation decreases serum C-reactive protein and monocyte interleukin-6 levels in normal volunteers and type 2 diabetic patients, *Free Radic Biol Med* 29:790-2, 2000.

22. Skyrme-Jones RA, O'Brien RC, Berry KL, et al: Vitamin E supplementation improves endothelial function in type I diabetes mellitus: a randomized, placebo-controlled study, *J Am Coll Cardiol* 36:94-102, 2000.

23. Engelen W, Keenoy BM, Vertommen J, et al: Effects of long-term supplementation with moderate pharmacologic doses of vitamin E are saturable and reversible in patients with type 1 diabetes, *Am J Clin Nutr* 72:1142-9, 2000.

24. Manzella D, Barbieri M, Ragno E, et al: Chronic administration of pharmacologic doses of vitamin E improves the cardiac autonomic nervous system in patients with type 2 diabetes, *Am J Clin Nutr* 73:1052-7, 2001.

25. Ziegler D, Reljanovic M, Mehnert H, et al: Alpha-lipoic acid in the treatment of diabetic polyneuropathy in Germany: current evidence from clinical trials, *Exp Clin Endocrinol Diabetes* 107:421-30, 1999.

26. Gaede P, Poulsen HE, Parving HH, et al: Double-blind, randomised study of the effect of combined treatment with vitamin C and E on albuminuria in type 2 diabetic patients, *Diabet Med* 18:756-60, 2001.

27. Pinn G: Herbs and metabolic/endocrine disease, *Aust Fam Physician* 30:146-50, 2000.

28. Vuksan V, Sievenpiper JL, Koo VY, et al: American ginseng (*Panax quinquefolius* L) reduces postprandial glycemia in nondiabetic subjects and subjects with type 2 diabetes mellitus, *Arch Intern Med* 160:1009-13, 2000.

29. Vogler BK, Ernst E: Aloe vera: a systematic review of its clinical effectiveness, *Br J Gen Pract* 49:823-8, 1999.

30. Diefendorf D, Healey J, Kalyn W, editors: *The healing power of vitamins, minerals and herbs*, Surry Hills, Australia, 2000, Readers Digest.

31. Kudolo GB: The effect of 3-month ingestion of *Ginkgo biloba* extract (EGb 761) on pancreatic beta-cell function in response to glucose loading in individuals with non-insulin-dependent diabetes mellitus, *J Clin Pharmacol* 41:600-11, 2001.

CHAPTER 24

ECZEMA/ATOPIC DERMATITIS

Eczema, a chronic, recurrent skin disease, is the most common inflammatory skin disease of childhood. Patients experience intractable itching, skin damage, soreness, sleep loss, and the social stigma of visible skin lesions.

Although a genetic predisposition and a combination of allergic and non-allergic factors appear to be important in determining disease expression, the cause remains unknown. Eczema often occurs in families with hay fever and/or asthma.

CLINICAL DIAGNOSIS

Eczema, or atopic dermatitis, has been described as an "itch that rashes." In infants, eczema presents as red skin with small vesicles and oozing cracks. Lesions are frequently found on the face and wrists, in flexures, and in a diaper distribution around the buttocks. During childhood, eczema presents as papules and skin thickening in the flexures. In adulthood, eczema presents as papules and crusted thickened lesions that may weep as a result of scratching. Lesions are found in flexures; on the neck, face, legs, feet, and backs of the hands; and in the ano-genital region.

THERAPEUTIC STRATEGY

In a review of randomized, controlled, clinical trials Hoare et al[1] concluded that although there is evidence to support the use of oral cyclosporine, topical corticosteroids, psychologic approaches, and ultraviolet light in the treatment of atopic eczema, there is insufficient evidence to make recommendations on, among others, maternal allergen avoidance, dietary restriction, Chinese herbs, and evening primrose oil. Nonetheless, defects in the metabolism of γ-linolenic acid (GLA) are thought to play a major role in the pathogenesis of atopic eczema.

GLA is a product of linoleic acid and a precursor of the prostaglandin 1 series and arachidonic acid (AA). Typical Western diets contain almost 10 times more linoleic acid (18:2 ω-6) than α-linolenic acid (18:3 ω-3). This dietary balance exacerbates any underlying problem with GLA production favoring AA-derived eicosanoids and shifting the T-helper type 1/type 2 cell ratio in favor of immunoglobulin E (IgE) production. IgE is the principal antibody produced in the allergic response. IgE triggers release of vasoactive amines from mast cells. When ω-3 fatty acids replace AA in cell membranes, atopic individuals benefit from the following:

- Reduced availability of AA. Low levels of cyclic adenosine monophosphate in atopic individuals are perceived to impair the negative feedback mechanism that prevents release of AA from cell membranes.[2]
- Reduced production of proinflammatory prostaglandin (PGE_2) from AA and consequently decreased IgE production.
- Decreased production of highly inflammatory leukotrienes.

The aims of intervention in atopic dermatitis are to avoid exposure to factors that trigger an attack and to create a cellular environment that favors a less inflammatory response.

LIFESTYLE CHANGES

Breast-feeding of infants at high risk, supplemented by extensively hydrolyzed formula during the first 6 months of life and delayed introduction of solid foods (particularly eggs, nuts, wheat, and fish), may reduce the development of food allergy.[3] Although popular, maternal allergen avoidance or dietary restriction during breast-feeding is controversial. There is currently insufficient evidence to recommend it in cases of established atopic eczema,[1] and the evidence also fails to suggest that maternal antigen avoidance prevents the development of atopic eczema during the first 12 to 18 months of life.[4] In fact, prescription of an antigen avoidance diet to a high-risk woman during pregnancy is not only unlikely to substantially reduce her risk of giving birth to an atopic child, but such a diet may have an adverse effect on other aspects of maternal and fetal nutrition.

Despite popular belief, general avoidance of allergic triggers has had little success in preventing initiation of infantile or adult eczema. Nonetheless, targeted dietary restrictions may be helpful. A randomized, controlled trial showed that children sensitive to eggs benefit from exclusion of eggs from their diets as part of the overall management of atopic eczema.[5] Analyses, based on the International Study of Asthma and Allergies in Childhood, revealed a consistent pattern of reduced symptoms with increased consumption of cereal, rice, nuts, starch, and vegetables.[6] In a study of adults, only a small subgroup responded to oral provocation with food additives.[7] Milk, eggs, shellfish, wheat, chocolate, nuts, and strawberries are foods that are popularly linked with eczema.

NUTRIENT THERAPY/DIETARY SUPPLEMENTS

Novel, unconventional approaches have failed to provide unequivocal, convincing evidence of efficacy when stringent scientific criteria are applied.[8]

Nonetheless, Horrobin[9] claims that in most, although not all, studies of atopic eczema, administration of GLA resulted in clinical improvement, reducing skin roughness and lowering elevated blood catecholamine concentrations. Certainly, infants receiving 3 g of GLA a day for 28 days, although not they did not completely recover, did demonstrate some gradual improvement in erythema, excoriations, lichenification, and itching.[10] However, no effect on the serum concentrations of dihomo-γ-linolenic acid and AA or biosynthesis of prostaglandins E_1 and E_2 could be demonstrated on administration of GLA to healthy volunteers.[11]

In addition to the conflicting results found for polyunsaturated fatty acids, one clinical trial has shown that vitamin C, 50 to 75 mg/kg, is beneficial[12]; and a clinical study indicated that 9-cis-retinoic acid was a valuable drug when it was given at low doses to patients with chronic hand eczema.[13] Supplementation with specific nutrients, particularly calcium, iodine, vitamin C, and ω-3 fatty acids, has also been proposed.[14] This recommendation resulted from a prospective study in which patients with symptomatic atopic dermatitis were found to have significantly lower intakes of dairy products, fish, egg, pork, oranges, nonspecified fruits, apples, kiwis, green or red peppers, peanuts, and hazelnuts.

HERBAL THERAPY

A traditional Chinese herbal therapy (Zemaphyte), containing a mixture of 10 herbs, has been shown to be effective in two double-blind crossover trials for the treatment of atopic eczema.[15] Witch hazel cream may help some patients, and *Calendula officinalis* (pot marigold) soothes skin and heals ulcers but should be avoided by those allergic to daisy-like flowers.

PRACTICE TIPS

- Oatmeal baths reduce itching.
- Licorice cream reduces the burning or itching side effects of cortisone creams.
- Flaxseed oil and fish are good sources of ω-3 fatty acids.
- Further skin dryness can be avoided by bathing in warm, never hot, water and applying a moisturizer within 3 minutes of bathing.
- Herbal creams and ointments work best on dry patches, whereas liquids or lotions are better suited to oozing lesions.
- Popular treatment protocols include vitamins A and B_6, zinc and selenium, biotin, evening primrose oil, and lecithin.

REFERENCES

1. Hoare C, Li Wan Po A, Williams H: Systematic review of treatments for atopic eczema. *Health Technol Assess (Rockv)* 4:1-19, 2000.
2. Kankaanpaa P, Sutas Y, Salminen S, et al: Dietary fatty acids and allergy, *Ann Med* 31:282-7, 1999.
3. Arshad SH: Food allergen avoidance in primary prevention of food allergy, *Allergy* 56(suppl 67):113-6, 2001.
4. Kramer MS: Maternal antigen avoidance during pregnancy for preventing atopic disease in infants of women at high risk, *Cochrane Database Syst Rev* (2):CD000133, 2000.
5. Lever R, MacDonald C, Waugh P, Aitchison T: Randomised controlled trial of advice on an egg exclusion diet in young children with atopic eczema and sensitivity to eggs, *Pediatr Allergy Immunol* 9(1):13-9, 1998.
6. Ellwood P, Asher MI, Bjorksten B, et al: Diet and asthma, allergic rhinoconjunctivitis and atopic eczema symptom prevalence: an ecological analysis of the International Study of Asthma and Allergies in Childhood (ISAAC) data. ISAAC Phase One Study Group, *Eur Respir J* 17(3):436-43, 2001.
7. Worm M, Ehlers I, Sterry W, Zuberbier T: Clinical relevance of food additives in adult patients with atopic dermatitis, *Clin Exp Allergy* 30(3):407-14, 2000.
8. Worm M, Henz BM: Novel unconventional therapeutic approaches to atopic eczema, *Dermatology* 201(3):191-5, 2000.
9. Horrobin DF: Essential fatty acid metabolism and its modification in atopic eczema, *Am J Clin Nutr* 71:367S-72S, 2000.
10. Fiocchi A, Sala M, Signoroni P, et al: The efficacy and safety of gamma-linolenic acid in the treatment of infantile atopic dermatitis, *J Int Med Res* 22:24-32, 1994.
11. Martens-Lobenhoffer J, Meyer FP: Pharmacokinetic data of gamma-linolenic acid in healthy volunteers after the administration of evening primrose oil (Epogam), *Int J Clin Pharmacol Ther* 36:363-6, 1998.
12. Werbach MR: *Textbook of nutritional medicine*, Tarzana, CA, 1999, Third Line Press.
13. Bollag W, Ott F: Successful treatment of chronic hand eczema with oral 9-cis-retinoic acid, *Dermatology* 199:308-12, 1999.
14. Barth GA, Weigl L, Boeing H, et al: Food intake of patients with atopic dermatitis, *Eur J Dermatol* 11:199-202, 2001.
15. Latchman Y, Whittle B, Rustin M, et al: The efficacy of traditional Chinese herbal therapy in atopic eczema, *Int Arch Allergy Immunol* 104:222-6, 1994.

■ CHAPTER 25 ■

FIBROMYALGIA

Fibromyalgia presents as widespread chronic musculoskeletal pain and tenderness, often accompanied by sleep disturbance and fatigue. The central features of the condition are a distressing body sensation and tender points. Absence of a disturbance in muscle, fascia, and other soft tissues coupled with the inadequate response to anti-inflammatory agents support the postulate that fibromyalgia results from dysfunction of the pain modulation system. Patients appear to neither perceive nor respond normally to physical or psychologic stresses.[1] The cause of fibromyalgia is disputed.

Fibromyalgia is characterized by a lowered pain threshold. Exercise raises the pain threshold, whereas increased psychologic stress, insomnia, and anxiety reduce it. Lifestyle modifications and pharmacologic interventions meant to relieve pain, improve sleep quality, and treat mood disorders are often ineffective or have only short-term effectiveness.[2]

CLINICAL DIAGNOSIS

Diffuse generalized or localized pain, in the absence of local causes, that has persisted for at least 3 months and more than five tender points are the core diagnostic features of fibromyalgia. A tender point is painful to palpation when digital pressure of no more than 4 kg is applied. The pain response over tender areas exceeds that anticipated from the pressure exerted. Pain is not referred. Muscle tightness, skin hyperalgesia on pinching, reduced grip strength, and a dermal red reflex response or flare exceeding that anticipated by scratch intensity are all characteristic. There is an increased incidence of depressive symptoms.

Fatigue, sleep disturbances, and short-term morning stiffness are common. Results of laboratory tests are normal.

THERAPEUTIC STRATEGY

Like multiple chemical sensitivity and posttraumatic stress disorder, fibromyalgia often appears to be induced by relatively short-term stress, followed by a chronic pathologic condition. Stress, it is hypothesized, may induce a self-perpetuating vicious cycle. One such cycle may result from elevated levels of nitric oxide and its potent oxidant product, peroxynitrite[3];

another may result from hyperactivity of cortisol releasing hormone (CRH), altering the set point of other hormonal axes.[4] Another postulate suggests that fibromyalgia may result from a sympathetically maintained pain syndrome in which ongoing sympathetic hyperactivity sensitizes primary nociceptors and induces widespread pain and allodynia.[5] Recent research with heart rate variability analysis demonstrated that patients with fibromyalgia have changes consistent with relentless circadian sympathetic hyperactivity. On the other hand, a subset of patients may be predisposed to fibromyalgia caused by excess use of excitatory neurotransmitters (excitotoxins, e.g., monosodium glutamate [MSG] and aspartate), leading to neurotoxicity.[6] Other small studies have implicated the following:

- Levels of certain cytokines are elevated in fibromyalgia.[7,8] Interleukin 8 (IL-8) promotes sympathetic pain.[7] IL-6 induces hyperalgesia, fatigue, and depression.[8]
- A relative deficiency in the branched-chain amino acids. They supply energy to the muscle and regulate protein synthesis in the muscles.[9]
- A high level of plasma serotonin in relation to serum level, which is associated with pain, discomfort, and increased anxiety.[10]

Whatever the mechanism, of the many complementary and alternative medicine therapies used, research data support only the use of mind-body, acupuncture, and manipulative therapies.[11] Despite dubious efficacy, supplements may nonetheless be taken with a view to attempting to modulate the changed pain perception, abnormal sleep patterns, muscle energy metabolism and microcirculation characteristic of fibromyalgia.

LIFESTYLE CHANGES

Along with physical measures such as hot baths/showers and massage, some patients may benefit from a reduced intake of caffeine, alcohol, and sugar. An observational study demonstrated that a mostly raw vegetarian diet significantly improved fibromyalgia symptoms.[12] An open, randomized, controlled trial concluded that a vegetarian diet, although a poor option compared with amitriptyline, did significantly decrease pain in patients with fibromyalgia.[13] Like patients with other rheumatoid conditions, patients with fibromyalgia may subjectively and objectively benefit from an uncooked vegan diet.[14] Berries, fruits, vegetables and roots, nuts, germinated seeds, and sprouts are rich sources of carotenoids, vitamins C and E, polyphenolic compounds, and fiber substrates of lignan production.[14]

NUTRIENT THERAPY/DIETARY SUPPLEMENTS

Nutrient management of fibromyalgia lacks clarity and is characterized by hope rather than conviction. Various controlled clinical trials suggest that L-5-hydroxytryptophan (100 mg three times daily), S-adenosyl-L-methionine, vitamin E (20-100 mg daily), malic acid (2400 mg daily), correction of selenium deficiency (90-200 µg daily) and/or magnesium (600 mg/day) may benefit some patients.[15] All of these supplements have achieved a measure of symptomatic success in some patients. A number of studies support the use of tryptophan, both to improve sleep patterns and symptoms such as tender points, fatigue, and morning stiffness. However, intravenous S-adenosyl-L-methionine improved subjective perceptions of pain and overall well-being but not tender points.[16]

Selenium and magnesium deficiency are individually associated with muscle pain. Magnesium deficiency is associated with fatigue, sleep disturbance, and anxiety. An open trial over 8 weeks found 200-600 mg magnesium and 1,200-2,400 mg malate daily significantly decreased the mean tender point index.[17] Supplementation of magnesium with malic acid would theoretically enhance ATP production by a sluggish respiratory chain. Supplementing a combination of calcium and magnesium to fibromyalgia subjects also reduces the number of tender points detected by digital palpation. It has been suggested that fibromyalgia patients with high hair calcium and magnesium levels may benefit from calcium and magnesium supplementation.[18] Other supplements on trial are anthocyanidins and melatonin. A recent, small, double-blind, randomized, crossover trial found anthocyanidins had a small but statistically significant benefit at a dose of 80 mg daily.[19] A minimum of 3 months treatment with anthocyanins is recommended. In an open trial patients had less pain and were sleeping better after 30 days of administration of melatonin, 3 g daily.[20]

HERBAL THERAPY

Herbal therapy is no less perplexing. Nonetheless, recent successes have been reported using a proprietary herbal preparations containing chlorella.[21] A blend of ascorbigen and broccoli powder has also been reported to reduce pain sensitivity.[22] In addition, a nonspecific approach may be implemented using St. John's wort 300 mg tds to reduce depression and improve pain tolerance.[23] Valerian or chamomile may improve sleep.[23]

PRACTICE TIPS

- Correction of magnesium deficiency (400 mg daily) may normalize a reduced pain threshold.
- Patients of professions unable to prescribe selenium may benefit from vitamin E supplementation.
- Ascorbic acid appears to exert a substantial analgesic effect in pharmacological dosages.
- Caffeine enhances the potency of peripherally acting analgesics.
- L-carnitine 3 grams daily relieves muscle pain from excess exercise.

REFERENCES

1. Clauw DJ: Elusive syndromes: treating the biologic basis of fibromyalgia and related syndromes, *Cleve Clin J Med* 68(10):830, 832-4, 2001.
2. Crofford LJ, Appleton BE: Complementary and alternative therapies for fibromyalgia, *Curr Rheumatol Rep* 3(2):147-56, 2001.
3. Pall ML: Common etiology of posttraumatic stress disorder, fibromyalgia, chronic fatigue syndrome and multiple chemical sensitivity via elevated nitric oxide/peroxynitrite, *Med Hypotheses* 57(2):139-45, 2001.
4. Neeck G, Crofford LJ: Neuroendocrine perturbations in fibromyalgia and chronic fatigue syndrome, *Rheum Dis Clin North Am* 26(4):989-1002, 2000.
5. Martinez-Lavin M: Is fibromyalgia a generalized reflex sympathetic dystrophy? *Clin Exp Rheumatol* 19(1):1-3, 2001.
6. Smith JD, Terpening CM, Schmidt SO, Gums JG: Relief of fibromyalgia symptoms following discontinuation of dietary excitotoxins, *Ann Pharmacother* 35(6):702-6, 2001.
7. Gur A, Karakoc M, Nas K, et al: Cytokines and depression in cases with fibromyalgia, *J Rheumatol* 29(2):358-61, 2002.
8. Wallace DJ, Linker-Israeli M, Hallegua D, et al: Cytokines play an aetiopathogenetic role in fibromyalgia: a hypothesis and pilot study, *Rheumatology* (Oxford) 40(7):743-9, 2001.
9. Maes M, Verkerk R, Delmeire L, et al: Serotonergic markers and lowered plasma branched-chain-amino acid concentrations in fibromyalgia, *Psychiatry Res* 97(1):11-20, 2000.
10. Ernberg M, Voog U, Alstergren P, et al: Plasma and serum serotonin levels and their relationship to orofacial pain and anxiety in fibromyalgia, *J Orofac Pain* 14(1):37-46, 2000.
11. Berman BM, Swyers JP: Complementary medicine treatments for fibromyalgia syndrome, *Baillieres Best Pract Res Clin Rheumatol* 13(3):487-92, 1999.
12. Donaldson MS, Speight N, Loomis S: Fibromyalgia syndrome improved using a mostly raw vegetarian diet: An observational study, *BMC Complement Altern Med* 1(1):7, 2001.
13. Azad KA, Alam MN, Haq SA, et al: Vegetarian diet in the treatment of fibromyalgia, *Bangladesh Med Res Counc Bull* 26(2):41-7, 2000.
14. Hanninen, Kaartinen K, Rauma AL, et al: Antioxidants in vegan diet and rheumatic disorders, *Toxicology* 155(1-3):45-53, 2000.
15. Werbach MR, Moss J: *Textbook of nutritional medicine*, Tarzana, CA, 1999, Third Line Press.
16. Volkmann H, Norregaard J, Jacobsen S, et al: Double-blind, placebo-controlled cross-over study of intravenous S-adenosyl-L-methionine in patients with fibromyalgia, *Scand J Rheumatol* 26(3):206-11, 1997.
17. Russell IJ, Michalek JE, Flechas JD, Abraham GE: Treatment of fibromyalgia syndrome with Super Malic: a randomized, double blind, placebo controlled, crossover pilot study, *J Rheumatol* 22:953-8, 1995.
18. Ng SY: Hair calcium and magnesium levels in patients with fibromyalgia: a case center study, *J Manipulative Physiol Ther* 22(9):586-93, 1999.
19. Edwards AM, Blackburn L, Christie S, et al: Food supplements in the treatment of primary fibromyalgia: a double-blind, crossover trial of anthocyanidins and placebo, *J Nutr Environ Med* 10:189-99, 2000.

20. Citera G, Arias MA, Maldonado-Cocco JA, et al: The effect of melatonin in patients with fibromyalgia: a pilot study, *Clin Rheumatol* 19(1):9-13, 2000.
21. Merchant RE, Andre CA: A review of recent clinical trials of the nutritional supplement Chlorella pyrenoidosa in the treatment of fibromyalgia, hypertension, and ulcerative colitis, *Altern Ther Health Med* 7(3):79-91, 2001.
22. Bramwell B, Ferguson S, Scarlett N, Macintosh A: The use of ascorbigen in the treatment of fibromyalgia patients: a preliminary trial, *Altern Med Rev* 5(5):455-62, 2000.
23. Cauffield JS, Forbes HJ: Dietary supplements used in the treatment of depression, anxiety, and sleep disorders, *Lippincotts Prim Care Pract* 3(3):290-304, 1999.

■ CHAPTER 26 ■

FOOD INTOLERANCE

Although humans eat approximately two or three tons of food in a lifetime, the prevalence of adverse food reactions, confirmed by history and challenges, is between 2% to 8% in young infants and less than 2% in adults.[1] In view of the serious repercussions of a very few of these reactions, it has even been suggested that future food labeling include information on specific allergens, provided that it is warranted by population prevalence of the adverse reaction and threshold levels of the allergen.[2]

CLINICAL DIAGNOSIS

Food-induced reactions are responsible for a variety of symptoms involving the skin, gastrointestinal tract, and respiratory tract.[3] At worst, immunoglobulin E (IgE)–mediated food allergy, occurring within minutes or hours of eating the offending food, may precipitate cardiovascular symptoms including hypotension, shock, cardiac dysrhythmias, and death.[4] Any symptom—including dizziness, hot flushes, myalgia, arthralgia, depression, irritability, fatigue, and bloating—may be a manifestation of food intolerance. Chronic disorders suspected to sometimes be associated with food intolerance include irritable bowel syndrome, arthritis, asthma, and even schizophrenia.

THERAPEUTIC STRATEGY

Mechanisms underlying food intolerance or adverse food reactions include immunologic reactions (e.g., food allergy), enzyme defects, irritant effects, and toxic reactions.[5] Immunologic reactions to food allergens or food components, resulting in either immediate-in-time mediated reactions (IgE, mast cells, and basophils) or delayed-in-time reactions that cause conditions such as food-induced enterocolitis,[6] may carry the most serious consequences. IgE is produced in response to naturally occurring food components such as glycoproteins.

Regardless of the severity of the reaction or the mechanism involved, the strategy for treatment of food allergies depends on identification and subsequent avoidance of the food substance inducing the reaction.

LIFESTYLE CHANGES

Dietary change may be implemented by means of an empirical diet, a simple food exclusion diet, an oligoantigenic elimination diet, or a rotation diet.

In instances in which a food trigger has not been identified, an empirical diet may be used. This involves excluding foods most commonly associated with adverse food reactions. The vast majority of food-induced allergic reactions are attributable to cow's milk, egg white, wheat, soy, peanuts, fish, and tree nuts in children and peanuts, tree nuts, fish, and shellfish in adults.[3,4] For example, the foods most often involved in skin reactions (e.g., hives, eczema, or pruritus) in children are egg, peanut, cows' milk, soy, fish, and wheat; the most common causes of skin reactions in adults are egg, peanuts, and cows' milk.[7] The food that often needs to be excluded is one that is usually eaten frequently and in large amounts. Unfortunately, new food allergens appear to be emerging and include tropical fruits, sesame seeds, psyllium, spices, and condiments.[4] Instead of blindly eliminating high-risk foods, an alternate approach to the simple food exclusion diet involves identifying the problem food by using a checklist and monitoring symptoms. Although these approaches are easy to implement and do not put the individual at nutritional risk, they are only effective when a single food is involved.

In contrast to diets in which only minor modifications are implemented, the oligoantigenic elimination and rotation diets involve a total dietary change. In both instances these options, when used in identifying food triggers, have proved difficult. In the case of the former, a simple low-allergen diet consisting of one meat (e.g., lamb), one carbohydrate (e.g., white rice), one vegetable (e.g., potatoes), one fruit (e.g., pears), and one type of fat (e.g., sunflower oil) is introduced. Less restrictive dietary options are also available. This basic diet, which should be maintained for no less than 2 and no longer than 4 weeks, creates an opportunity for the patient to become asymptomatic. Foods are than gradually and sequentially reintroduced as the patient is monitored for untoward reactions. Any foods that trigger symptoms are immediately eliminated. A maintenance diet is slowly developed in response to successive food challenges. Oral challenge is the definitive method of demonstrating sensitivity or tolerance to a food. With careful incremental dosing and a low starting dose, oral challenges for the determination of food hypersensitivity have an excellent safety record.

In the case of the rotation diet, instead of severely restricting the number of foods eaten, emphasis is placed on food groups. Foods from particular food groups are rotated over a 5-day period. During any 5-day period, not more than one food from a food group may be eaten. Each day, it is particularly important to avoid foods that share common allergens. Consequently, on any one day, persons on the rotation diet are not permitted to select beans with soybeans, lentils, peas, or peanuts. They are also not permitted on any one day to eat rye with barley, corn, millet, rice, or oats. Hidden allergens may prove to be a problem. Persons susceptible to corn may unknowingly risk a food reaction by licking an envelope adhesive; taking vitamin tablets; eating peanut butter or pickles; drinking beer, wine, or liqueurs; or even brushing their teeth with certain brands of toothpaste. The rotation diet is particularly useful in cases in which cross-sensitivity within food groups has occurred. It also provides a better nutritional balance than that obtained with the oligoantigenic elimination diet.

Total avoidance of known food allergens remains the safest approach for susceptible persons, particularly because the concentrations of allergens in foods can vary; the concentration of three of four tomato allergens increases during ripening.[8] In any event, the threshold dose for provocation of allergic food reactions has yet to be determined.[9] It is also worth noting that in food-allergic individuals, glycoproteins and other natural food allergens usually retain their allergenicity after heating or proteolysis. Food exclusion methods for managing food intolerance can be successfully used in the primary care setting.[10]

NUTRIENT THERAPY/DIETARY SUPPLEMENTS

Because gut permeability may enhance the risk of food allergy, it is good practice to take probiotics after antibiotics have been administered to encourage restoration of a normal bowel flora. Potential dietary deficiency resulting from an elimination diet may also be minimized or prevented by dietary supplementation.

HERBAL THERAPY

The herbal approach to adverse food reactions is to enhance digestion with bitter or aromatic herbs, encourage bowel healing with meadowsweet or chamomile, and enhance immunity with echinacea.[11] Antiallergic herbs such as scullcap and anti-inflammatory herbs such as *Matricaria recutita* (chamomile) may also be used.

PRACTICE TIPS

- Despite common fears about food additives and food processing and the obsession with so-called natural foods, the greatest dangers come from naturally occurring foods and food ingredients.[5]
- Citrus fruits and tomatoes are foods commonly linked to migraine.
- Dairy products and gluten are commonly linked to gastrointestinal and/or respiratory problems.
- Gluten is found in wheat, rye, oats, and barley.
- A clinical study has suggested that a mild intolerance of cow's protein may present as chronic refractory constipation in children.[12]

• Skin prick tests are of little value in the evaluation of adverse food reactions not mediated by IgE.

REFERENCES

1. Spergel JM, Pawlowski NA: Food allergy. Mechanisms, diagnosis, and management in children, *Pediatr Clin North Am* 49:73-96, 2002.
2. Yeung JM, Applebaum RS, Hildwine R: Criteria to determine food allergen priority, *J Food Prot* 63:982-6, 2000.
3. Sampson HA: Food allergy. Part 1: immunopathogenesis and clinical disorders, *J Allergy Clin Immunol* 103:717-28, 1999.
4. Ebo DG, Stevens WJ: IgE-mediated food allergy—extensive review of the literature, *Acta Clin Belg* 56:234-47, 2001.
5. David TJ: Adverse reactions and intolerance to foods, *Br Med Bull* 56:34-50, 2000.
6. Metcalfe DD: Food allergy, *Prim Care* 5:819-29, 1998.
7. Martin BL: Skin manifestations of food allergies, *J Am Osteopath Assoc* 99(suppl 3):S15-16, 1999.
8. Kondo Y, Urisu A, Tokuda R: Identification and characterization of the allergens in the tomato fruit by immunoblotting, *Int Arch Allergy Immunol* 126:294-9, 2001.
9. Taylor SL, Hefle SL, Bindslev-Jensen C, et al: Factors affecting the determination of threshold doses for allergenic foods: how much is too much? *J Allergy Clin Immunol* 109:24-30, 2002.
10. Biddle J, Anderson J: Report on a 12 month trial of food exclusion methods in a primary care setting, *J Nutr Env Med* 12:11-7, 2002.
11. Mills S, Bone K: *Principles and practice of phytotherapy*, Edinburgh, 2000, Churchill Livingstone.
12. Daher S, Tahan S, Sole D, et al: Cow's milk protein intolerance and chronic constipation in children, *Pediatr Allergy Immunol* 12:339-42, 2001.

■ CHAPTER 27 ■

GOUT

Gout is a group of heterogeneous conditions characterized by increased serum urate and crystal deposition, resulting in arthritis, tophi, and renal damage. Gout is more commonly encountered in middle-aged men who present with intense pain affecting one or two large joints. Recurrent acute attacks occur at intervals varying from 2 to 21 days.

CLINICAL DIAGNOSIS

Gout typically affects large joints, which become red, swollen, warm, and exquisitely tender. The metatarsophalangeal joint of the big toe is most commonly the first site affected. Tophi, nodular deposits of urate crystals, may rarely be seen in the ear cartilage, bursae, or tendon sheaths. Nephrolithiasis may impair renal function.

THERAPEUTIC STRATEGY

Uric acid is formed by oxidation of the purine bases found in nucleic acid. Uric acid, when not excreted in the urine (70%) and stool, may be deposited in tissue. Urate deposits trigger an inflammatory response with release, among others, of tumor necrosis factor and various interleukins (e.g., interleukins 1, 6, and 8). The goals of intervention are to reduce production of urates, increase uric acid excretion, and decrease inflammation.

Production of uric acid can be reduced by blocking xanthine oxidase.[1] This enzyme catalyzes the oxidative hydroxylation of purine substrates with generation of reactive oxygen species and the formation of uric acid. Allopurinol is a clinically useful xanthine oxidase inhibitor routinely used in the treatment of gout. Renal excretion of uric acid can be increased to prevent tubular resorption of uric acid by using high doses of salicylates (5 g). It should be noted that only high doses of salicylates have a uricosuric effect. In doses of less than 2 g, salicylates have the reverse effect, inhibiting tubular secretion. Another approach is to dampen the inflammatory response. Both nonsteroidal anti-inflammatory drugs and colchicine have an anti-inflammatory effect.

LIFESTYLE CHANGES

A low-purine diet is a generally accepted approach. Foods high in purines such as organ meats, anchovies, and caviar should be avoided; and foods with moderate purine content such as seafood, legumes, spinach, and meat should be restricted. Overall, the acid-ash content of the diet should be decreased by avoiding excess consumption of cheese, meat, legumes, grains, plums, and cranberries. Increasing the intake of milk products, most vegetables, and fruit will increase the alkaline-ash content of the diet. Alcohol, particularly beer, should be restricted. A high fluid intake is also recommended.

NUTRIENT THERAPY/DIETARY SUPPLEMENTS

Uncontrolled trials suggest that taking 800 µg of folic acid daily or 0.5 g of vitamin C twice a day may be beneficial.[2] Although a mild uricosuric agent, vitamin C administration should be started slowly and gradually increased over 4 to 8 weeks as it may precipitate an attack if rapid reduction in tissue uric acid is induced.

HERBAL THERAPY

Claims have been made that celery, nettle, and birch help to eliminate uric acid.[3] Globe artichoke has also traditionally been used in the treatment of gout. Apart from colchicine, no herbal remedies compare with orthodox medical treatment for acute attacks.[4] Colchicine, an alkaloid derivative of *Colchicum autumnale*, suppresses release of inflammatory mediators from neutrophils. Side effects limit its usefulness. Colchicine is also present in commercially available *Ginkgo biloba*. In fact, significant levels of colchicine (49-763 µg /L) were found in placental blood of patients using nonprescription herbal dietary supplements during pregnancy.[5] A number of traditional Chinese medicinal plants, selected according to the clinical efficacy and prescription frequency for the treatment of gout, have demonstrated xanthine oxidase inhibitory activity.[6]

Herbs rich in antioxidants such as turmeric and grapeseed extract may be helpful.

PRACTICE TIPS

- Certain people experience some symptomatic relief as a result of eating around 250 g of cherries daily.
- Aspirin and niacin can precipitate an attack of gout.
- Natural therapies do not offer a viable alternative to conventional drug intervention.

REFERENCES

1. Borges F, Fernandes E, Roleira F: Progress towards the discovery of xanthine oxidase inhibitors, *Curr Med Chem* 9:195-217, 2002.
2. Werbach MR: *Textbook of nutritional medicine*, Tarzana, CA, 1999, Third Line Press.
3. Mills S, Bone K: *Principles and practice of phytotherapy*, Edinburgh, 2000, Churchill Livingstone.
4. Pinn G: Herbs and metabolic/endocrine disease, *Aust Fam Physician* 30:146-50, 2000.
5. Petty HR, Fernando M, Kindzelskii AL, et al: Identification of colchicine in placental blood from patients using herbal medicines, *Chem Res Toxicol* 14:1254-8, 2001.
6. Kong LD, Cai Y, Huang WW, et al: Inhibition of xanthine oxidase by some Chinese medicinal plants used to treat gout, *J Ethnopharmacol* 73:199-207, 2000.

■ CHAPTER 28 ■

HERPES INFECTION

Herpes results from infection with a DNA virus. In many, but not all, cases, herpes virus infection produces a subclinical primary infection. The virus persists in a latent form and manifests as clinical disease if reactivated by triggers as diverse as sun exposure or suppression of cell-mediated immunity by a viral infection or stress. It has been postulated that specific signal molecules, including epinephrine, interleukin 6, cyclic adenosine monophosphate, glucocorticoids, and prostaglandins that are upregulated during episodes of acute and chronic stress reactivate latent herpes simplex virus and cause recurrent disease.[1]

CLINICAL DIAGNOSIS

After an incubation period of 2 to 7 days, herpes presents as localized areas of paresthesia. After 1 to 3 days, red macules appear, followed by vesicles around day 4. Ulceration results in painful superficial ulcers with sharp edges and dry crusts. Lesions are most commonly found on the lips (herpes labialis), genitalia (genital herpes), or trunk (herpes zoster).

THERAPEUTIC STRATEGY

Intervention is focused on avoiding factors that trigger reactivation of the virus, maintaining good cell-mediated immunity, and suppressing viral replication. Supplements may have an impact at each of these levels. Animal studies suggest that deficiencies of selenium and vitamin E can activate latent viruses, including herpes. Nutrients and herbs influence the immune system, and immune control of primary and recurrent genital herpes appears to be effected largely by CD4 and CD8 lymphocytes, T-helper 1 cytokines, and interferon.[2] Certain herbs and amino acids influence viral replication.

LIFESTYLE CHANGES

Because lysine inhibits and arginine enhances viral replication, a diet rich in lysine and low in arginine should be eaten. Half a large loin chop, a cup of baked beans, or a serving of two eggs each contains almost 1 g of lysine. Chocolate, peas, nuts, and beer should be avoided.

NUTRIENT THERAPY/DIETARY SUPPLEMENTS

Lysine supplementation is an option for the management of herpes.[3] It has long been recognized that daily oral supplements of 1000 mg of L-lysine may reduce the risk of outbreaks of recurrent herpes simplex labialis.[4] A good regimen appears to be L-lycine, 1 to 3 g daily, between meals until lesions have healed, then 500 mg daily to prevent recurrences.

Controlled clinical trials have shown that in addition to lysine, lithium, vitamin C (200 mg daily), and flavonoids (200 mg three times daily) are helpful.[5] A double-blind, placebo-controlled, randomized clinical trial demonstrated that application of a zinc oxide/glycine cream every 2 hours within 24 hours of onset of symptoms significantly shortened the duration of cold sore lesions with less blistering, soreness, itching, and tingling.[6]

HERBAL THERAPY

Anecdotal and animal studies suggest that echinacea, licorice, St. John's wort, garlic, and clove are all beneficial. An extract of *Echinacea purpurea* (Echinaforce), shown to have immunomodulating properties, has been advocated in the lay press for the treatment of genital herpes. However, a single-center, prospective, double-blind, placebo-controlled crossover trial over a 1-year period involving 50 patients demonstrated no statistically significant benefit.[7] Goldenseal (125 mg) may be used in rotation with or as an alternative to echinacea in the early treatment of herpes infections.[8]

Laboratory investigation has suggested that a number of Chinese herbs may alter replication of the herpes virus,[9] and certain herbal extracts also appear to shorten the duration of attacks.[10] Further investigation is required.

PRACTICE TIPS

- Topical application of vitamin C or E, lithium, and zinc may aid healing.
- Repeated application of milk to labial lesions is reported to provide some relief.
- Aloe vera is considered an effective adjunct in the treatment of herpes.

REFERENCES

1. Sainz B, Loutsch JM, Marquart ME, et al: Stress-associated immunomodulation and herpes simplex virus infections, *Med Hypotheses* 56:348-56, 2001.

2. Cunningham AL, Mikloska Z: The holy grail: immune control of human herpes simplex virus infection and disease, *Herpes* 8(suppl 1):6A-9A, 2001.
3. Tomblin FA, Lucas KH: Lysine for management of herpes labialis, *Am J Health Syst Pharm* 58:298-300, 304, 2001.
4. Thein DJ, Hurt WC: Lysine as a prophylactic agent in the treatment of recurrent herpes simplex labialis, *Oral Surg Oral Med Oral Pathol* 58:659-66, 1984.
5. Werbach MR: *Textbook of nutritional medicine*, Tarzana, CA, 1999, Third Line Press.
6. Godfrey HR, Godfrey NJ, Godfrey JC, et al: A randomized clinical trial on the treatment of oral herpes with topical zinc oxide/glycine, *Altern Ther Health Med* 7:49-56, 2001.
7. Vonau B, Chard S, Mandalia S, et al: Does the extract of the plant *Echinacea purpurea* influence the clinical course of recurrent genital herpes? *Int J STD AIDS* 12:154-8, 2001.
8. Diefendorf D, Healey J, Kalyn W, editors: *The healing power of vitamins, minerals and herbs*, Surry Hills, Australia, 2000, Readers Digest.
9. Kuo YC, Chen CC, Tsai WJ, et al: Regulation of herpes simplex virus type 1 replication in Vero cells by Psychotria serpens: relationship to gene expression, DNA replication, and protein synthesis, *Antiviral Res* 51:95-109, 2001.
10. Hijikata Y, Tsukamoto Y: Effect of herbal therapy on herpes labialis and herpes genitalis, *Biotherapy* 11:235-40, 1998.

▪ CHAPTER 29 ▪

HYPERTENSION

Systemic hypertension affects more than 50 million adults and is one of the most common risk factors for cardiovascular morbidity and death. There is a linear increase in mortality when systolic pressure rises above 110 mm Hg and/or diastolic pressure rises above 70 mm Hg. In fact, mild hypertension is responsible for more than 50% of the excess mortality attributable to hypertension.

The cause of essential hypertension remains obscure, but psychologic stress is a recognized risk factor. A recent study of university students confirmed that mild real-life stress does indeed increase arterial pressure and impair cardiovascular homeostasis.[1] Furthermore, the perceived stress of ambulatory surgery in geriatric patients is associated with a clinical hypertensive response that is ameliorated by self-selected perioperative music.[2] Musical intervention reduces heart rate, blood pressure, myocardial oxygen consumption, gastrointestinal motility, anxiety, and pain.[3] Other natural therapies that may contribute to reducing high blood pressure include diet, exercise, stress management, supplements, and herbs.[4]

CLINICAL DIAGNOSIS

Hypertension is diagnosed when the diastolic blood pressure exceeds 90 mm Hg and/or the systolic pressure exceeds 160 mm Hg. Borderline hypertension is diagnosed within the systolic pressure range of 140 to 159 mm Hg and/or diastolic pressures of 90 to 94 mm Hg. Because intervention depends on accurate diagnosis, it is important that the protocol for determining blood pressure be meticulously followed.[5]

THERAPEUTIC STRATEGY

The main factors regulating blood pressure are cardiac output and peripheral resistance. Vascular tone, blood volume, and viscosity are all important. The diameter of the arterioles is influenced by the elasticity of arterial walls, the autonomic nervous system, and local factors. Decreasing peripheral resistance and preventing fluid overload may reduce blood pressure.

LIFESTYLE CHANGES

Weight loss and controlled alcohol and sodium consumption are generally accepted measures for managing hypertension. Of the nutritional measures, losing excess weight and reducing excess alcohol intake result in the greatest quantitative reduction in hypertension, followed by reducing sodium and increasing potassium intake.[6] Most randomized, controlled studies confirm that even a modest weight loss of less than 10% is associated with a significant reduction in systolic and diastolic blood pressure of roughly 3 mm Hg in overweight people.[7] With respect to cardiovascular risk, the optimal body mass index is 22.6 kg/m^2 in men and 21.1 kg/m^2 in women.[8]

Regular consumption of 30 to 40 g of alcohol daily has a pressor effect. In fact, there is an increased prevalence of hypertension among women consuming 15 or more units weekly.[9] One unit, or 10 g, of absolute alcohol is equivalent to a half a pint of beer, one measure of spirits, or a glass of sherry or wine. However, drinking no more than 20 g daily does appear to benefit cardiovascular health. Such benefits may be due to phytochemicals rather than alcohol itself. Short-term oral administration of red wine polyphenolic compounds to normotensive rats decreased blood pressure.[10] This hemodynamic effect was associated with enhanced endothelium-dependent relaxation and induction of gene expression of inducible nitric oxide synthase and cyclooxygenase-2 within the arterial wall.

Sodium is another factor in the complex of interacting systems regulating blood pressure. Although sodium has been clearly linked to higher blood pressure levels in the general population, its optimal intake in any one individual is difficult to ascertain. The current U.S. dietary guideline of 2.4 g or 100 mmol of sodium, or 6 g of salt (sodium chloride), daily is debatably an acceptable target.[11,12] A little more than one teaspoon of salt provides the recommended intake of sodium.

Blood pressure is successfully reduced by the Dietary Approaches to Stop Hypertension (DASH) diet, which requires doubling of the average daily serving of fruit, vegetables, and dairy products and reduction of fats and oils by half, red meat by two thirds, and snacks and sweets by three quarters.[13] Fruits and vegetables are good sources of potassium, and potassium is as effective as exercise in reducing blood pressure.[6] Sodium reduction to levels below the currently recommended 100 mmol daily further reduces blood pressure in persons on this diet.[14] The success of the DASH diet may be attributable to the combined impact of its swing toward eating lower-calorie foods, its relatively high potassium to sodium ratio, and its high intake of dairy products.

Results of many studies have linked increased consumption of milk and milk products with lower blood pressure and a reduced risk of hypertension.[15] According to a recent review, evidence from animal, clinical, and epidemiologic studies indicates that high blood pressure is associated with abnormalities of calcium metabolism, leading to increased calcium loss, secondary activation of the parathyroid gland, increased movement of calcium from bone, and increased risk of urinary tract stones.[16] A review of clinical and biochemical evidence supports the hypothesis that dairy products may lower blood pressure and the risk of stroke by reducing blood pressure, platelet aggregation, and insulin resistance.[17] Calcium, bioactive peptides produced during digestion of milk proteins, and as yet unidentified components in whole milk may protect against hypertension.[18] Low-fat milk remains the preferred option because milk fat is rich in palmitic acid, a fatty acid that further elevates cholesterol in persons with hypercholesterolemia. Hypercholesterolemia, like smoking, reduces nitric oxide, the primary compound responsible for vasodilation in arteries.[19]

NUTRIENT THERAPY/DIETARY SUPPLEMENTS

Professionally supervised therapeutic interventions range from medically supervised, water-only fasting to intravenous infusion of L-arginine. Water-only fasting is a safe and effective means of normalizing blood pressure as a prelude to behavioral change,[20] and systemic infusion of L-arginine (1 g/min; total, 30 g) produces a drop in mean arterial pressure of 5 mm Hg, a fall only matched by hydralazine infusion.[21] Short-term L-arginine infusion appears to facilitate vagal control of heart rate in healthy humans, probably by means of increased nitric oxide synthesis.

Less heroic natural interventions are also available. Controlled clinical trials have shown that correction of calcium or potassium deficiency lowers raised blood pressure as does supplementation with a daily dose of coenzyme Q10 (100 mg), taurine (6 g), L-tryptophan (3 g), or vitamin C (1g in divided doses).[22] A 12-week randomized, double-blind, placebo-controlled trial showed that twice-daily administration of 60 mg of oral coenzyme Q10 achieved a mean reduction in systolic blood pressure of 17.8 ± 7.3 mm Hg.[23] None of the patients exhibited orthostatic blood pressure changes.

Dietary intervention remains the mainstay of nutritional intervention.

HERBAL THERAPY

Most herbs used in the treatment of essential hypertension act as peripheral vasodilators. Herbs to be considered include the following[24]:

- Hawthorn, particularly the leaves. Hawthorn reduces raised blood pressure and has a cardiotrophic effect. In a pilot study, after 10 weeks of administration of hawthorn extract (500 mg daily), a promising reduction in resting diastolic blood pressure was observed.[25]
- Valerian. Valerian has a calming effect and reduces vascular resistance. Its vasodilator effect may be central or peripheral. Stress management to treat hypertension is a clinically recognized approach, supported by findings from randomized trials.[26]
- Dandelion leaves. Dandelion acts as a diuretic.

• Garlic. Garlic lowers blood pressure and has other cardiovascular benefits. Long-term ingestion of 300 to 900 mg of garlic powder has been found to attenuate age-related increases in aortic stiffness.[27] These data support the hypothesis that garlic intake has a protective effect on the elastic properties of the aorta in aging humans. Animal studies suggest that the blood pressure–lowering effects of garlic might be partially attributable to a reduction in the synthesis of vasoconstrictor prostanoids.[28] The overall effect of garlic on blood pressure may be insignificant.[29]

Other herbs that lower blood pressure include olive leaves, yarrow, cramp bark, and mistletoe. Results of animal experiments suggest that Korean red ginseng has a hypotensive effect.[30] An extract of ginkgo leaves may regulate hypertension and protect cerebral microcirculatory function.[31]

The effect of antihypertensive medication may be enhanced by black cohosh, ephedra, garlic, ginseng, or hawthorn.[32]

PRACTICE TIPS

• A diet low in fat and rich in fruits, vegetables, cereals, and low-fat dairy products is beneficial.
• Guavas are an excellent choice.
• Patients taking medication for hypertension should avoid eating licorice, which may neutralize the effect of antihypertensive drugs.

REFERENCES

1. Lucini D, Norbiato G, Clerici M, et al: Hemodynamic and autonomic adjustments to real life stress conditions in humans, *Hypertension* 39:184-8, 2002.
2. Allen K, Golden LH, Izzo JL, et al: Normalization of hypertensive responses during ambulatory surgical stress by perioperative music, *Psychosom Med* 63:487-92, 2001.
3. White JM: Music as intervention: a notable endeavor to improve patient outcomes, *Nurs Clin North Am* 36:83-92, 2001.
4. Khosh F, Khosh M: Natural approach to hypertension, *Altern Med Rev* 6:580-9, 2001.
5. Jamison JR: *Differential diagnosis for primary practice*, Edinburgh, 1999, Churchill Livingstone.
6. Morgan TO: Hypertension, *Med Today* 1:51-5, 2000.
7. Hermansen K: Diet, blood pressure and hypertension, *Br J Nutr* 83(suppl 1):S113-S119, 2000.
8. Kannel WB, D'Agostino RB, Cobb JL: Effect of weight on cardiovascular disease, *Am J Clin Nutr* 63:419S-422S, 1996.
9. Nanchahal K, Ashton WD, Wood DA: Alcohol consumption, metabolic cardiovascular risk factors and hypertension in women, *Int J Epidemiol* 29:57-64, 2000.

10. Diebolt M, Bucher B, Andriantsitohaina R: Wine polyphenols decrease blood pressure, improve NO vasodilatation, and induce gene expression, *Hypertension* 38:159-65, 2001.

11. McCarron DA: The dietary guideline for sodium: should we shake it up? Yes! *Am J Clin Nutr* 71:1013-9, 2000.

12. Kaplan NM: The dietary guideline for sodium: should we shake it up? No, *Am J Clin Nutr* 71:1020-6, 2000.

13. Blackburn GL: The public health implications of the dietary approaches to stop hypertension trial, *Am J Clin Nutr* 74:1-2, 2001.

14. Sacks FM, Svetkey LP, Vollmer WM, et al: DASH-Sodium Collaborative Research Group. Effects on blood pressure of reduced dietary sodium and the Dietary Approaches to Stop Hypertension (DASH) diet. DASH-Sodium Collaborative Research Group, *N Engl J Med* 344:3-10, 2001.

15. Groziak SM, Miller GD: Natural bioactive substances in milk and colostrum: effects on the arterial blood pressure system, *Br J Nutr* 84(suppl 1):S119-S125, 2000.

16. Cappuccio FP, Kalaitzidis R, Duneclift S, et al: Unraveling the links between calcium excretion, salt intake, hypertension, kidney stones and bone metabolism, *J Nephrol* 13:169-77, 2000.

17. Massey LK: Dairy food consumption, blood pressure and stroke, *J Nutr* 131:1875-8, 2001.

18. Pfeuffer M, Schrezenmeir J: Bioactive substances in milk with properties decreasing risk of cardiovascular diseases, *Br J Nutr* 84(suppl 1):S155-S159, 2000.

19. Brown AA, Hu FB: Dietary modulation of endothelial function: implications for cardiovascular disease, *Am J Clin Nutr* 73:673-86, 2001.

20. Goldhamer A, Lisle D, Parpia B, et al: Medically supervised water-only fasting in the treatment of hypertension, *J Manipulative Physiol Ther* 24:335-9, 2001.

21. Chowdhary S, Nuttall SL, Coote JH, et al: L-arginine augments cardiac vagal control in healthy human subjects, *Hypertension* 39:51-6, 2002.

22. Wernbach MR: *Textbook of nutritional medicine*, Tarzana, CA, 1999, Third Line Press.

23. Burke BE, Neuenschwander R, Olson RD: Randomized, double-blind, placebo-controlled trial of coenzyme Q10 in isolated systolic hypertension, *South Med J* 94:1112-7, 2001.

24. Mills S, Bone K: *Principles and practice of phytotherapy*, Edinburgh, 2000, Churchill Livingstone.

25. Walker AF, Marakis G, Morris AP, et al: Promising hypotensive effect of hawthorn extract: a randomized double-blind pilot study of mild, essential hypertension, *Phytother Res* 16:48-54, 2002.

26. Kondwani KA, Lollis CM: Is there a role for stress management in reducing hypertension in African Americans? *Ethn Dis* 11:788-92, 2001.

27. Breithaupt-Grogler K, Ling M, Boudoulas H, et al: Protective effect of chronic garlic intake on elastic properties of aorta in the elderly, *Circulation* 96:2649-55, 1997.

28. Al-Qattan KK, Khan I, Alnaqeeb MA, et al: Thromboxane-B2, prostaglandin-E2 and hypertension in the rat 2-kidney 1-clip model: a possible mechanism of the garlic induced hypotension, *Prostaglandins Leukot Essent Fatty Acids* 64:5-10, 2001.

29. Ackermann RT, Mulrow CD, Ramirez G, et al: Garlic shows promise for improving some cardiovascular risk factors, *Arch Intern Med* 161:813-24, 2001.

30. Jeon BH, Kim CS, Park KS, et al: Effect of Korea red ginseng on the blood pressure in conscious hypertensive rats, *Gen Pharmacol* 35:135-41, 2000.

31. Zhang J, Fu S, Liu S, et al: The therapeutic effect of *Ginkgo biloba* extract in SHR rats and its possible mechanisms based on cerebral microvascular flow and vasomotion, *Clin Hemorheol Microcirc* 23:133-8, 2000.

32. Diefendorf D, Healey J, Kalyn W, editors: *The healing power of vitamins, minerals and herbs*, Surry Hills, Australia, 2000, Readers Digest.

■ CHAPTER 30 ■

IRRITABLE BOWEL SYNDROME

Irritable bowel syndrome (IBS) is the most common functional gastrointestinal syndrome encountered in primary practice. It is estimated that one in 10 persons has the condition, and the prevalence in females is double that in males.

Postprandial symptoms are common in patients with IBS. Gas problems and abdominal pain are the most frequent complaints.[1] Foods rich in carbohydrates, as well as fatty foods, coffee, alcohol, and hot spices most frequently cause symptoms.

CLINICAL DIAGNOSIS

IBS is the preferred working diagnosis in any patient complaining of chronic or recurrent abdominal pain, bloating, chronic diarrhea, or constipation.[2] IBS manifests as any combination of abdominal pain and distention; increased frequency of bowel movements and relief of pain with bowel movements; constipation; mucus in the stool; symptoms of indigestion such as flatulence, nausea, or anorexia; and varying degrees of anxiety or depression. On physical examination, the abdomen may feel tense and be tender to touch.

THERAPEUTIC STRATEGY

The precise etiology of IBS is unknown, but the problem has been postulated to either result from local (i.e., bowel) or central (i.e., psychologic) dysfunction.[3] One hypothesis is that motor abnormalities in the smooth muscle of the bowel cause either hypercontractility with spastic colon and diarrhea or slowed contractility with constipation and distention. Another hyposthesis is that the disorder arises from the patient's inappropriate response to healthy bowel activity. Pharmacologic approaches are consistent with both these postulates. Smooth-muscle relaxants, bulking agents, and prokinetic agents target the bowel; and psychotropic agents are used to treat any associated anxiety or depression.[4] Management of IBS with natural medicine focuses on relieving symptoms.

LIFESTYLE CHANGES

Dietary changes may relieve symptoms through elimination of food triggers or modulation of disturbed motor function. Food sensitivity may induce the development of IBS. Avoidance of trigger foods reduces symptoms.[5] The more common culprits are dairy products, onions, wheat, chocolate, coffee, eggs, nuts, citrus fruits, tea, rye, potatoes, barley, oats, corn, garlic, and soy. Patients with grain sensitivities may benefit from an increase in pectin-based fiber found in citrus fruits, apples, and other fruits and vegetables.

Dietary changes may target alleviation of particular symptoms. Gas symptoms may be relieved by reducing the intake of beans, cabbage, lentils, legumes, apples, grapes, and raisins. Fiber may help to overcome colonic motor dysfunction; however, doses of at least 12 g per day may be required for patients with constipation-predominant disease.[6] However, bran may exacerbate symptoms. Therefore when bulking approaches are used, a combination of soluble and insoluble fiber-containing foods and supplements should be added gradually. Psyllium seed and ispaghula are more readily tolerated bulking agents than wheat bran. A deficiency in short-chain fatty acids may exacerbate colonic symptoms. Short-chain fatty acids are produced by bacterial metabolism of soluble fiber. Asparagus and Jerusalem artichokes, apple and citrus pectins, guar gum, and legumes are particularly good sources of soluble fiber and short-chain fatty acids.

NUTRIENT THERAPY/DIETARY SUPPLEMENTS

Avoidance of food sensitivity triggers and a low-fat, a high-fiber diet may provide a beneficial outcome by modifying the bacterial flora and metabolism within the bowel lumen.[7] A study showed that administration of *Lactobacillus plantarum*, a probiotic, decreased pain and flatulence in patients with IBS.[8] Probiotics such as *Lactobacillus acidophilus* and *Bifidobacterium bifidum* are helpful in certain cases of IBS.[9] Prebiotics are nondigestible food ingredients that benefit the host by selectively stimulating certain colonic bacteria. Oligosaccharides are prebiotics that serve as a substrate for probiotics. A diet rich in fructooligosaccharides and soybean oligosaccharides bolsters the bifidobacteria in the large bowel and may benefit patients with IBS.[10] However, because oligosaccharides are largely indigestible, large amounts in the colon may provoke gastrointestinal symptoms similar to symptoms of IBS. A clinical study demonstrated that although symptoms worsened in patients with IBS at the onset of treatment, continuous treatment for 12 weeks with 20 g of fructooligosaccharides daily did not exacerbate symptoms.[11]

Aberrant small bowel motor function may be ameliorated by reduction of dietary lactose, sorbitol, and fructose. Also, pancreatic supplements reduce postprandial symptoms in healthy subjects and are likely to be beneficial in IBS.[12]

HERBAL THERAPY

Various herbs may successfully relieve particular symptoms.[12] Peppermint or chamomile may reduce abdominal pain in patients with colic. Peppermint oil capsules, taken 15 to 30 minutes before a meal, are reported to relieve the pain, bloating, and flatulence associated with IBS.[13] Three trials over 2 to 4 weeks indicated that taking capsules containing 0.2 to 0.4 mg of peppermint oil, three times a day, provided significant benefit.[14] Only subjects taking capsules benefited. Enteric-coated capsules allow menthol, the active antispasmodic, to be delivered directly to the large intestine and prevent its absorption by the stomach.[15] Absorption of menthol may explain the conflicting clinical outcomes reported in a review of research on the efficacy of peppermint in this condition. Menthol relaxes the muscles in the small intestine by reducing calcium reflux. One in five patients experienced a side effect such as heartburn, nausea, vomiting, blurred vision, or a burning sensation in the anal area.

Other spasmolytic herbs, chamomile (*Matricaria chamomilla*), and cramp bark (*Viburnum opulus*) may reduce the cramping pain associated with IBS. Chamomile also has a mild sedative effect.

Sedative herbs such as valerian (*Valeriana officinalis*) and scullcap (*Scutellaria lateriflora*) have both relaxing and antispasmodic properties and are therefore particularly useful for patients who also have insomnia and/or anxiety.[16]

Slippery elm may be used as a stool softener, and dandelion root can be used as a gentle laxative in patients complaining of constipation. A number of other herbs may also be considered.[17]

PRACTICE TIPS

- Coffee, alcohol, and low-fiber, high-sugar, and high-fat foods should be avoided.
- Sipping two or three cups of basil tea between meals may ease flatulence. Tea can be prepared by pouring boiling water (125 mL) over one to two teaspoons of dried basil and brewing for 15 minutes.
- Eating sugar-free products that contain artificial sweeteners such as sorbitol, xylitol, or mannitol may exacerbate gas.
- Constipation can be relieved by a high-fiber, high-fluid diet.
- Prunes stimulate peristalsis directly through dihydroxphenyl isatin and indirectly through their high fiber and sorbitol content.
- Corn may trigger a flare of symptoms in susceptible persons.
- Licorice root, peppermint, and psyllium may relieve symptoms.
- If beans cause problems, they can be soaked in water, but the water should be thrown away before the beans are cooked.

REFERENCES

1. Simren M, Mansson A, Langkilde AM, et al: Food-related gastrointestinal symptoms in the irritable bowel syndrome, *Digestion* 63:108-15, 2001.
2. Talley NJ: Irritable bowel syndrome. Practical management, *Aust Fam Physician* 29:823-8, 2000.
3. Starbuck J: Irritable bowel syndrome: a gut reaction, *Nutr Sci News* 5:127-32, 2000.
4. Jailwala J, Imperiale TF, Kroenke K: Pharmacologic treatment of the irritable bowel syndrome: a systematic review of randomized, controlled trials, *Ann Intern Med* 133:136-47, 2000.
5. Gaby A: The role of hidden food allergy/intolerance in chronic disease, *Altern Med Rev* 3:90-100, 1998.
6. Camilleri M: Therapeutic approach to the patient with irritable bowel syndrome, *Am J Med* 107:27S-32S, 1999.
7. Werbach MR: *Textbook of nutritional medicine*, Tarzana, CA, 1999, Third Line Press.
8. Nobaek S, Johansson ML, Molin G, et al: Alteration of intestinal microflora is associated with reduction in abdominal bloating and pain in patients with irritable bowel syndrome, *Am J Gastroenterol* 95:1231-8, 2000.
9. Duffy LC, Leavens A, Griffiths E, et al: Perspectives on bifidobacteria as biotherapeutic agents in gastrointestinal health, *Dig Dis Sci* 44:1499-505, 1999.
10. Schrezenmeir J, de Vrese M: Probiotics, prebiotics and synbiotics—approaching a definition, *Am J Clin Nutr* 73:361S-364S, 2001.
11. Olesen M, Gudmand-Hoyer E: Efficacy, safety, and tolerability of fructooligosaccharides in the treatment of irritable bowel syndrome, *Am J Clin Nutr* 72:1570-5, 2000.
12. Suarez F, Levitt MD, Adshead J, et al: Pancreatic supplements reduce symptomatic response of healthy subjects to a high fat meal, *Dig Dis Sci* 44:1317-21, 1999.
13. Mills S, Bone K: *Principles and practice of phytotherapy*, Edinburgh, 2000, Churchill Livingstone.
14. Diefendorf D, Healey J, Kalyn W, editors: *The healing power of vitamins, minerals and herbs*, Surry Hills, Australia, 2000, Readers Digest.
15. Castleman M: Herbal healthwatch: minty relief for irritable bowel syndrome, *Herb Q* 86:8-9, 2000.
16. Pittler M, Ernst E: Peppermint of for irritable bowel syndrome: a critical review and meta-analysis, *Am J Gastroenterol* 93:1131-5, 1998.
17. Bone K: Phytotherapy and irritable bowel syndrome, *Br J Phytother* 4:190-8, 1998.
18. Khosh F: A natural approach to irritable bowel syndrome, *Townsend Lett Doc Pat* 204:62-4, 2000.

CHAPTER 31

Inflammatory Bowel Disease

Ulcerative colitis and Crohn's disease are prevalent examples of inflammatory bowel disease (IBD). Patients have dysentery and abdominal pain. Extraintestinal manifestations include arthritis, skin rashes, ocular disorders, and anemia. IBD is characterized by exacerbations and remissions. In an attempt to avoid side effects from prescribed medicines, as a result of unsatisfactory outcomes, or in search of a cure, patients may try complementary medicine alternatives. Studies suggest that around four in 10 patients have tried alternative health therapies for their gastrointestinal problems.[1,2] In one survey, 19% of respondents reported use of megavitamin therapy, 17% reported use of dietary supplements, and 14% reported use of herbal medicine.[2]

CLINICAL DIAGNOSIS

The clinical picture of IBD includes attacks of dysentery; urgency; the presence of mucus in the stool; nocturnal diarrhea; cramping lower abdominal pain; and constitutional findings such as fever, malaise, and weight loss. The major complication of Crohn's disease is bowel stricture. Colorectal cancer is a serious complication of ulcerative colitis.

THERAPEUTIC STRATEGY

The etiology of IBD is unknown, but postulates range from an autoimmune disorder to psychosomatic dysfunction. One possible explanation is an immune-based inflammatory response of bowel mucosa to neurotransmitters and neurohumoral peptides. Because inflammation is fundamental to the pathogenesis of both ulcerative colitis and Crohn's disease, the aims of intervention are to dampen the inflammatory response and improve nutrition of the epithelial lining.

Nitric oxide is a weak radical produced from L-arginine by the enzyme nitric oxide synthase (NOS). NOS exists in three distinct isoforms—constitutively expressed neuronal NOS1 and endothelial NOS3, plus an inducible isoform, NOS2. Constitutively expressed NOS has been shown to be critical to normal physiology, and inhibition of NOS1 or NOS3 causes damage. NOS2 is capable of production of large amounts of nitric oxide during inflammation, which results in injury, perhaps through the generation of potent radicals such as peroxynitrite.[3] Nitric oxide diminishes acetyl coenzyme A (CoA) metabolism in colonocytes; and nitric oxide, in combination with peroxide and sulfide, impairs oxidation of substrates in colonocytes, causing acute injury.[4] The aims of treatment are to reduce nitric oxide, peroxide, and sulfide generation in the colon. Plasma levels of antioxidant vitamins (ascorbic acid, alpha-and beta-carotene, lycopene, and β-cryptoxanthin) are all significantly lower in patients with Crohn's disease than in control subjects.[5] Patients with Crohn's disease are oxidatively stressed.[6]

Dietary fats influence inflammatory responses. Fats rich in ω-6 polyunsaturated fatty acids enhance interleukin 1 (IL-1) production and tissue responsiveness to cytokines; fats rich in ω-3 polyunsaturated fatty acids have the opposite effect. Monounsaturated fatty acids decrease tissue responsiveness to cytokines, and IL-6 production is enhanced by the total unsaturated fatty acid intake. Feeding linoleic acid to animals increases prostaglandin E$_2$ production, influences tumor necrosis factor–induced IL-1 and IL-6 production in a positive curvilinear fashion, and enhances leukotriene B$_4$ production in moderate doses but suppresses it in high doses.[7]

The aims of intervention are to restore and maintain the bowel as a competent mucosal barrier. Supplementation with ω-3 fatty acids and antioxidants may dampen the inflammatory response, and dietary choice and bowel microflora can affect production of butyrate, the preferred fuel for colonic epithelium.

LIFESTYLE CHANGES

Elimination of food triggers, such as dairy products, and the introduction of a high-fiber, low–refined-carbohydrate diet deserve consideration in the management of IBD.

Short-chain fatty acids, produced by colonic bacterial fermentation of dietary fiber, play a pivotal role in the integrity and metabolism of colonic mucosa. Butyric acid, the preferred fuel for colonic epithelial cells, has a trophic effect on colonic epithelium. Because oxidation of ω-butyrate governs the epithelial barrier function of colonocytes, the functional activity of short-chain acyl-CoA dehydrogenase may be critical in maintaining colonic mucosal integrity.[8]

Ulcerative colitis is associated with a block in beta-oxidation of short-chain fatty acids in colonic epithelial cells. Sulfides inhibit short-chain acyl-CoA dehydrogenase. Sulfur is essential for ω-butyrate formation, and its production aids in the disposal of hydrogen produced by colonic bacteria. Patients with ulcerative colitis have enhanced sulfate metabolism, and removal of foods rich in sulfur amino acids—such as milk, eggs, and cheese—has therapeutic benefits.[9] Clinical and endoscopic evidence of improvement was observed in patients with ulcerative colitis within 4 weeks of beginning daily administration of 30 g of germinated barley foodstuff that contained glutamine-rich protein and the hemicellulose-rich fiber made from brewers'spent grain by milling and sieving.[10] Studies have shown that the fiber fraction supports maintenance of epithelial cell populations, facilitates epithelial repair, and increases production of short-chain fatty acids, especially butyrate. In controlled clinical trials, butyric acid enemas have been found to be beneficial in the treatment of ulcerative colitis.[11] 5-Aminosalicylic acid, which reduces fermentative production of hydrogen sulfide by colonic bacteria, and aminoglycosides, which inhibit sulfate-reducing bacteria, are also of therapeutic benefit in active cases.[9]

NUTRIENT THERAPY/DIETARY SUPPLEMENTS

Research is focused on emerging biologic therapies that target tumor necrosis factor, promote anti-inflammatory cytokines, disrupt immune cell trafficking, or reduce oxidation and on nonconventional treatments, including diet therapies, prebiotics, and probiotics.[12] Supplements that enhance the competence of the bowel mucosa tend to normalize bowel permeability.

Supplementation with ω-3 fatty acids plus antioxidants significantly changes the eicosanoid precursor profile and may lead to the production of eicosanoids with attenuated proinflammatory activity.[13] Omega-3 polyunsaturated fatty acids, eicosapentaenoic acid (3.2 g), and docosahexaenoic acid (2.4 g) specifically inhibit natural cytotoxicity and may achieve clinical improvement in ulcerative colitis.[14] Epidemiologic studies have demonstrated a low incidence of IBD in Eskimos, and some patients specifically cite use of fish oil for IBD[1]; however, the efficacy of ω-3 fatty acids in IBD remains controversial.[15] Discrepancies between studies may have resulted from different study designs and the use of various formulations and dosages. Other possibly useful supplements include glycosaminoglycans, vitamin E (α-tocopherol, 40 IU/kg daily), and correction of any deficiency of magnesium (400 mg daily), zinc (220 mg three times daily), or vitamin K.[11]

In Crohn's disease, controlled clinical trials have indicated that correction of zinc deficiency (220 mg twice daily plus 2 mg of copper daily) is helpful.[11] Permeability of the small intestine is often increased in patients with Crohn's disease and may be pathogenic for clinical relapses. Results of a 12-month study suggested that 8 weeks of zinc supplementation (110 mg of zinc sulfate three times daily) could resolve altered bowel permeability in patients with Crohn's disease in remission.[16] Improving intestinal barrier function may help reduce the risk of relapses.

HERBAL THERAPY

Laboratory studies showed that slippery elm, fenugreek, devil's claw, tormentil, and wei tong ning have antioxidant effects and merit formal evaluation as novel therapies for IBD.[17] With the exception of fenugreek, all these herbs, like 5-aminosalicylates, scavenge superoxide in a dose-dependent fashion.

Chamomile and meadowsweet may be useful in patients with mucus in the stool, which suggests underlying inflammation.[18] Administration of licorice before meals also deserves consideration.

Small nonrandomized studies suggest that *Boswellia serrata* may be effective in the treatment of ulcerative colitis.[19]

PRACTICE TIPS

- Colorectal cancer must be ruled out in patients with a long history of IBD, especially those with ulcerative colitis.
- A daily intake of 1500 mg of calcium reduces the risk of colon cancer in patients with IBD.

REFERENCES

1. Giese LA: A study of alternative health care use for gastrointestinal disorders, *Gastroenterol Nurs* 23:19-27, 2000.
2. Heuschkel R, Afzal N, Wuerth A, et al: Complementary medicine use in children and young adults with inflammatory bowel disease, *Am J Gastroenterol* 97:382-8, 2002.
3. Kubes P, McCafferty DM: Nitric oxide and intestinal inflammation, *Am J Med* 109:150-8, 2000.
4. Roediger WE, Babidge WJ: Nitric oxide effect on colonocyte metabolism: co-action of sulfides and peroxide, *Mol Cell Biochem* 206:159-67, 2000.
5. Wendland BE, Aghdassi E, Tam C, et al: Lipid peroxidation and plasma antioxidant micronutrients in Crohn disease, *Am J Clin Nutr* 74:259-64, 2001.
6. Geerling BJ, v Houwelingen AC, Badart-Smook A, et al: The relation between antioxidant status and alterations in fatty acid profile in patients with Crohn disease and controls, *Scand J Gastroenterol* 34:1108-16, 1999.
7. Grimble RF, Tappia PS: Modulation of pro-inflammatory cytokine biology by unsaturated fatty acids, *Z Ernahrungswiss* 37(suppl 1):57-65, 1998.
8. Babidge W, Millard S, Roediger W: Sulfides impair short chain fatty acid beta-oxidation at acyl-CoA dehydrogenase level in colonocytes: implications for ulcerative colitis, *Mol Cell Biochem* 181:117-24, 1998.
9. Roediger WE, Moore J, Babidge W: Colonic sulfide in pathogenesis and treatment of ulcerative colitis, *Dig Dis Sci* 42:1571-9, 1997.
10. Kanauchi O, Iwanaga T, Mitsuyama K: Germinated barley foodstuff feeding. A novel neutraceutical therapeutic strategy for ulcerative colitis, *Digestion* 63:S60-S677, 2001.
11. Werbach MR: *Textbook of nutritional medicine*, Tarzana, CA, 1999, Third Line Press.
12. Mutlu EA, Farhadi A, Keshavarzian A: New developments in the treatment of inflammatory bowel disease, *Expert Opin Investig Drugs* 11:365-85, 2002.

13. Geerling BJ, Badart-Smook A, van Deursen C, et al: Nutritional supplementation with N-3 fatty acids and antioxidants in patients with Crohn's disease in remission: effects on antioxidant status and fatty acid profile, *Inflamm Bowel Dis* 6:77-84, 2000.

14. Almallah YZ, El-Tahir A, Heys SD, et al: Distal procto-colitis and n-3 polyunsaturated fatty acids: the mechanism(s) of natural cytotoxicity inhibition, *Eur J Clin Invest* 30:58-65, 2000.

15. Belluzzi A, Boschi S, Brignola C, et al: Polyunsaturated fatty acids and inflammatory bowel disease, *Am J Clin Nutr* 71:339S-342S, 2000.

16. Sturniolo GC, Di Leo V, Ferronato A, et al: Zinc supplementation tightens "leaky gut" in Crohn's disease, *Inflamm Bowel Dis* 7:94-8, 2001.

17. Langmead L, Dawson C, Hawkins C, et al: Antioxidant effects of herbal therapies used by patients with inflammatory bowel disease: an in vitro study, *Aliment Pharmacol Ther* 16:197-205, 2002.

18. Mills S, Bone K: *Principles and practice of phytotherapy*, Edinburgh, 2000, Churchill Livingstone.

19. Pinn G: The herbal basis of some gastroenterology therapies, *Aust Fam Physician* 30:254-8, 2001.

■ CHAPTER 32 ■

INSOMNIA

Approximately one in three adults experiences insomnia in any one year. More than one in 20 persons experience chronic and/or severe insomnia. Treatment can be problematic because the recommended duration for hypnotic drug use is 4 weeks. The time limitation advocated for hypnotic drug use has been set to prevent habituation and the withdrawal symptoms after long-term use.[1]

Insomnia may be associated with anxiety and depression.

CLINICAL DIAGNOSIS

Insomnia often presents as delayed sleep onset, poor sleep maintenance, and/or early-morning waking with an inability to return to sleep. Persons with insomnia have difficulty getting to sleep and staying asleep, and they wake unrefreshed.

THERAPEUTIC STRATEGY

Most adults sleep around 6.5 to 8 hours daily. Acute stress and environmental disturbances are the most common causes of transient and short-term insomnia. Chronic insomnia is often associated with medical conditions, psychiatric problems such as depression, or persistent psychophysiologic disorders such as inadequate sleep hygiene. Learned insomnia is linked to acute or persistent anxiety. The aim of intervention is to eliminate or control barriers to sleep. This involves creating external and internal environments that are conducive to sleep.[2]

Two internal variables influencing sleep and arousal, the daily circadian rhythm and central neurotransmitters, are amenable to nutritional intervention. Except for a physiologic mid-afternoon dip in alertness, the circadian rhythm of sleepiness and alertness promotes a daily cycle of nighttime sleep and daytime alertness. The major sleep-regulating neurotransmitter in the central nervous system (CNS) is serotonin. In contrast to many prescription and over-the-counter medications, interventions that increase CNS serotonin levels and restore a normal circadian rhythm do not cause daytime drowsiness, reduce sleep quality, or alter the normal sleep pattern.

Normal sleep consists of four to six behaviorally and electroencephalographically defined cycles. There are two distinct types of sleep, nonrapid eye movement (NREM) sleep and rapid eye movement (REM) sleep. NREM sleep has four stages. Stage 1 NREM sleep is very light, and during this stage, sleepers are easily aroused. The majority of a typical night's sleep is spent in stage 2 NREM sleep, which is characterized by steep spindles on electroencapholograms. Stages 3 and 4 of NREM sleep are often referred to collectively as *delta sleep* or *slow-wave sleep*. REM sleep is characterized by a low level of muscle tone, episodic rapid eye movements, and relatively low-voltage, mixed-frequency EEG activity, somewhat similar to stage 1 REM sleep or wakefulness.

LIFESTYLE CHANGES

Caffeine, nicotine, and alcohol should be limited because each can impair both falling asleep and staying asleep. Alcohol promotes fragmentation of normal sleep. It initially reduces sleep latency and decreases arousals but then causes increased waking in the second half of the night. Nicotine can disrupt sleep and reduce the total sleep time. Younger smokers are most prone to daytime sleepiness and minor accidents. Caffeine may reduce sleep latency, but it fragments sleep, causing sleep disruption in the latter part of the night.[3] Because it has a half-life of 3 to 7 hours, caffeine consumed during the day may be an important cause of restlessness at night.

Milk is a rich source of tryptophan and nicotinic acid, one of the B group of vitamins that influences the conversion of tryptophan to serotonin. The belief that drinking a warm glass of milk before going to bed will help one sleep is biochemically plausible.

NUTRIENT THERAPY/DIETARY SUPPLEMENTS

Melatonin, a hormone secreted by the pineal gland, regulates the sleep-wakefulness cycle.[4] The body produces melatonin in response to the absence of light. Production starts around dusk and peaks between 2:00 and 4:00 AM. Single low doses of melatonin, provided that they mimic the nocturnal physiologic concentration of this hormone, exert immediate sleep-inducing effects. Significant decreases in sleep latency occurred when melatonin was administered to young healthy volunteers between 6:00 and 8:00 PM, but not at 9:00 PM.[5] Around bedtime, 1 to 3 mg of melatonin is helpful for insomnia, with 3 to 5 mg required for schedule changes that disrupt the circadian schedule such as jet lag or shift work.[6] Adverse effects of melatonin most commonly reported in clinical trials included sedation, headache, depression, tachycardia, and pruritus.

L-Tryptophan is the amino acid precursor to serotonin, the neurotransmitter thought to induce sleep. A dose of 1 to 2 g of L-tryptophan has been reported to halve sleep latency and decrease waking time. Up to 5 g may be taken. The sleep patterns of insomniacs taking tryptophan more closely resemble those of normal sleepers than those of untreated insomniacs or persons taking sleeping tablets. In fact, the only change noted in the architecture of tryptophan-assisted sleep is an increase in duration of the third and fourth stages of slow-wave sleep. Unlike other hypnotics, tryptophan appears to reduce wakefulness without decreasing the periods of REM sleep. REM suppression and rebound are not a problem. The immediate precursor of serotonin, 5-hydroxytryptophan (10 mg), is currently being used as a sleep aid, a treatment for depression, and a weight loss aid.[7] The Food and Drug Administration recalled the product when contaminated L-tryptophan was found to be responsible for eosinophilia-myalgia syndrome. It is currently available by prescription. When tryptophan is taken with vitamin B_6 (50 mg) and niacinamide (500 mg), the conversion of tryptophan to serotonin is favored.

Controlled clinical trials suggest that deficiency of potassium or thiamine may contribute to insomnia.[8]

HERBAL THERAPY

Herbs considered for use in sleep disorders include valerian, catnip, chamomile, gotu kola, hops, lavender, passionflower, and scullcap.[9] Of these herbs, valerian (*Valeriana officinalis*) has been most consistently shown to have sleep-inducing, anxiolytic, and tranquilizing effects in in vivo animal studies and clinical trials.[7] The efficacy of valerian may be attributable to its diverse constituents. The major constituents include the monoterpene bornyl acetate and the sesquiterpene valerenic acid, and some of these constituents have a sedative effect through direct action on the amygdaloid body of the brain and/or inhibition of enzyme-induced breakdown of cerebral γ-aminobutyric acid (GABA). The nonvolatile monoterpenes (valepotriates) possess sedative activity, and aqueous extracts of the roots contain appreciable amounts of GABA, which, if bioavailable, could directly cause sedation. A lignan, hydroxypinoresinol, with the ability to bind to benzodiazepine receptors is also present. The considerable variation in the composition and content of valerian and the instability of some of its constituents pose serious problems for standardization, but the range of components that contribute to its overall activity suggest that it may correct a variety of underlying conditions that benefit from a general sedative or tranquilizing effect.[10] The rhizome and roots of valerian are used as a hypnotic and daytime sedative or anxiolytic.

Results of clinical trials indicate that 400 to 900 mg of valerian extract taken at bedtime improves sleep quality, decreases sleep latency, and reduces the number of night awakenings.[7,11] Valerian tends to normalize the sleep profile, reducing periods of wakefulness and enhancing the efficacy of sleep periods. A randomized, double-blind, placebo-controlled, crossover study with multiple dosages of valerian demonstrated that slow-wave sleep latency was reduced after administration of valerian over several days.[11] The effect was dose related; a single dose was not effective, but valerian taken over a number of days improved both the sleep structure and sleep perception of insomniacs. The researchers concluded that valerian could be recommended for the treatment of patients with mild psychophysiologic insomnia. Another randomized, controlled, double-blind trial indicated that neither single nor repeated evening administration of 600 mg of native valerian root extract had any relevant adverse effect on reaction time, alertness, and concentration the morning after.[12] In contrast to these encouraging reports, in a sleep laboratory study researchers found that the effects of 900 mg of valerian were not significantly different from those of placebo.[13] Valerian is classified as a safe herb. When taken in combination with St. Johns wort, valerian is particularly useful for insomniacs with depression or anxiety.[14]

Because anxiety is often the underlying cause of insomnia, kava kava deserves consideration in certain cases.[15] Animal studies have shown that kava extracts and kava lactones induce sleep and muscle relaxation. Kava may act on GABA and benzodiazepine-binding sites in the brain. In a pilot study that included 24 patients with stress-induced insomnia treated for 6 weeks, valerian and kava were compared for efficacy.[16]

Kava, 120 mg, or valerian, 600 mg, administered daily for 6 weeks achieved an equally significant reduction in total stress levels and improved volunteers' sleep patterns. Most patients have no side effects, and the most common effects are vivid dreams with valerian (16%) and dizziness with kava (12%). Several relatively short-term clinical studies have provided favorable evidence that kava is effective in treating anxiety and insomnia. A dose of 180 to 210 mg of kava lactones daily is recommended as a sleep aid.[17]

Panax ginseng (Korean or Asian ginseng), *Panax quinquefolius* (American ginseng), and *Panax vietnamensis* (Vietnamese ginseng) are reported to have sleep-modulating effects.[18] Results of several studies indicate that the effect of ginseng may be, at least in part, related to maintaining normal sleep and wakefulness. In some people this herb may stimulate rather than sedate. Ginseng has an inhibitory effect on the CNS and may modulate neurotransmission. Known as an adaptogen capable of normalizing physiologic disturbances, ginseng may depress the CNS by regulation of GABAergic neurotransmission. The recommended daily dosage is 1 to 2 g of the crude root, or 200 to 600 mg of extract.[19] Since the possibility of hormone-like or hormone-inducing effects cannot be ruled out, some authors suggest limiting treatment to 3 months.

Although current data suggest that the use of some herbal treatments in insomnia may be efficacious, further laboratory and clinical studies are required to validate their safety and efficacy.[20]

PRACTICE TIPS

- Although passion flower, *Passiflora incarnata* (4-8 g), and hops, *Humulus lupulus* (0.5 g dried herb), may be taken as tea, neither is recommended for pregnant women.

- It is important to note that ethanol and other CNS depressants can potentiate the effects of kava.
- Chromium supplementation may impair sleep in certain persons.
- Patients whose sleep is disturbed because of restless leg syndrome may benefit from 400 µg of folic acid and 400 IU of vitamin E nightly.
- Magnesium, 250 mg, and vitamin B_6, 50 mg, enhance conversion of tryptophan to serotonin.
- Some people find as little as 0.3 mg of melatonin nightly helpful.

REFERENCES

1. Eddy M, Walbroehl GS: Insomnia, *Am Fam Physician* 59:1911-6, 1999.
2. Jamison JR: *Maintaining health in primary care*, Edinburgh, 2001, Churchill Livingstone.
3. Recognizing problem sleepiness in your patients. National Center on Sleep Disorders Research Working Group, *Am Fam Physician* 59:937-44, 1999.
4. Diefendorf D, Healey J, Kalyn W, editors: *The healing power of vitamins, minerals and herbs*, Surry Hills, Australia, 2000, Readers Digest.
5. Pires ML, Benedito-Silva AA, Pinto L, et al: Acute effects of low doses of melatonin on the sleep of young healthy subjects, *J Pineal Res* 31:326-32, 2001.
6. Chase JE, Gidal BE: Melatonin: therapeutic use in sleep disorders, *Ann Pharmacother* 31:1218-26, 1997.
7. Attele AS, Xie JT, Yuan CS: Treatment of insomnia: an alternative approach, *Altern Med Rev* 5:249-59, 2000.
8. Wernbach MR: *Textbook of nutritional medicine*, Tarzana, CA, 1999, Third Line Press.
9. Cauffield JS, Forbes HJ: Dietary supplements used in the treatment of depression, anxiety, and sleep disorders, *Lippincotts Prim Care Pract* 3:290-304, 1999.
10. Houghton PJ: The scientific basis for the reputed activity of valerian, *J Pharm Pharmacol* 51:505-12, 1999.
11. Donath F, Quispe S, Diefenbach K, et al: Critical evaluation of the effect of valerian extract on sleep structure and sleep quality, *Pharmacopsychiatry* 33:47-53, 2000.
12. Kuhlmann J, Berger W, Podzuweit H, et al: The influence of valerian treatment on "reaction time, alertness and concentration" in volunteers, *Pharmacopsychiatry* 32:235-41, 1999.
13. Kohnen R, Oswald WD: The effects of valerian, propranolol, and their combination on activation, performance, and mood of healthy volunteers under social stress conditions, *Pharmacopsychiatry* 21:447-8, 1988.
14. Mills S, Bone K: *Principles and practice of phytotherapy*, Edinburgh, 2000, Churchill Livingstone.
15. Miller LG, Murrey WJ: Herbal medications, nutraceuticals, and anxiety and depression. In Miller LG, Murrey WJ, Wallace WJ, *Herbal medicine: a clinician's guide*, New York, 1998, Pharmaceutical Products Press.
16. Wheatley D: Kava and valerian in the treatment of stress-induced insomnia, *Phytother Res* 15:549-51, 2001.

17. Robbers JE, Tyler VE: Nervous system disorders. In *Tyler's herbs of choice*, New York, 1999, Haworth Press, Inc.
18. Attele AS, Wu JA, Yuan CS: Ginseng pharmacology: multiple constituents and multiple actions, *Biochem Pharmacol* 58:1685-93, 1999.
19. Schulz V, Hansel R, Tyler VE: Rational phytotherapy. In *Agents that increase resistance to diseases*, New York, 1998, Springer-Verlag.
20. Wing YK: Herbal treatment of insomnia, *Hong Kong Med J* 7:392-402, 2001.

■ CHAPTER 33 ■

ISCHEMIC HEART DISEASE

Ischemic heart disease (IHD) remains a major cause of death in both men and women. In fact in 1990, the two leading causes of death were IHD (6.3 million deaths) and cerebrovascular accidents (4.4 million deaths).[1]

The best current approach to IHD is prevention through lifestyle choices. This includes being a nonsmoker, maintaining a blood pressure under 140/90 mm Hg and a body mass index (BMI) of 25 or less, walking for more than 20 minutes at least three times a week, taking a daily aspirin tablet, and managing blood lipid levels by diet, exercise, and, if necessary, medication. Because the benefit of estrogen replacement is dubious at best,[2] a preventive approach is strongly advocated for both women and men.

CLINICAL DIAGNOSIS

Primary prevention is achieved by screening and minimizing risk factors in healthy people. In addition to clues provided by a family history and increasing age, major risk factors are smoking, hypertension, and hypercholesterolemia. Low vitamin E, high fibrinogen, and high plasma total homocysteine levels, and the even more sensitive plasma S-adenosylhomocysteine level, have emerged as important predictors of coronary artery disease.[3,4] Although elevated plasma-free fatty acid concentrations are associated with an increased risk of heart disease, a single fasting measurement of plasma-free fatty acid levels does not improve the ability to predict the onset of IHD.[5]

Secondary prevention depends on early recognition of symptoms. Angina, experienced as constricting substernal tightness that lasts a few seconds to 15 minutes, is an early warning sign of cardiac ischemia in men. The pain, relieved by sublingual nitroglycerine or rest, may radiate to the angle of the jaw, neck, back, left shoulder, or inner aspect of either arm. In persons with stable angina, pain predictably occurs on exertion. Compared with persons with stable angina, those with unstable and spasm angina are at greater risk for infarction. In persons with unstable angina, the pain lasts longer, occurs more frequently, and may occur at rest. In persons with spasm angina, pain is unpredictable and arrhythmia is more likely.

Cardiac ischemia in women is often precipitated by coronary artery spasm, and heart attacks in one in three women are believed to go unreported. In women, chest tightness, nausea, and dizziness are common indicators of myocardial ischemia. Cardiac ischemia should be ruled out in women who complain of breathlessness, perspiration, a sensation of fluttering in the heart, and chest tightness.

THERAPEUTIC STRATEGY

The targets of intervention are both the inflammatory process underlying atherosclerosis and the occlusive critical event. Intervention is focused on factors predisposing to plaque formation and on prevention of vascular occlusion through clot formation or spasm. Endothelial function is fundamental to prevention.[6]

The main functions of the endothelium are to maintain blood circulation and fluidity, regulate vascular tone, and modulate platelet and leukocyte adhesion and leukocyte transmigration. Inflammatory stimuli such as oxidized low-density lipoprotein (LDL), free radicals, lipopolysaccharide, or cytokines (e.g., tumor necrosis factor) activate the endothelium. The activated endothelium upregulates cell adhesion and cytokine release, creating an environment conducive to atherosclerosis.

Local mechanical factors (e.g., flow stress in hypertension) or metabolic changes (e.g., hypoxia) stimulate release of chemicals that mediate vascular tone. Major endothelium vasoconstrictors are thromboxane A_2, prostaglandin H_2, and endothelin 1. Major endothelium-derived vasodilators include nitric oxide and prostacyclin. Nitric oxide is derived from L-arginine in the presence of nitric oxide synthase (NOS). Constitutively expressed NOS has been shown to be critical to normal physiology. Inhibition of endothelium NOS causes damage. Endothelium-derived NOS, in addition to having a pivotal role in regulating vascular tone by relaxing smooth muscles and causing vasodilation, has a potent antiatherogenic effect by inhibiting leukocyte-endothelium interactions, smooth muscle cell proliferation, and platelet aggregation.[7] Acute cardiac events are associated with decreased platelet-derived nitric oxide release. Smoking and hypercholesterolemia decrease nitric oxide levels.

Smoking, hypercholesterolemia, hyperhomocysteinemia, hypertension, and diabetes mellitus each adversely affect endothelial function. Physical exercise, hormone replacement therapy, and high-density lipoprotein (HDL) cholesterol improve endothelial function. HDL cholesterol inhibits endothelium-induced cytokines and enhances vasodilatation.

LIFESTYLE CHANGES

A dietary pattern of greater intake of red meats, high-fat dairy products, and refined grains shows a significant positive correlation with insulin, C-peptide, leptin, and homocysteine concentrations and an inverse correlation with the plasma folate concentration.[8] The Western dietary pattern appears to have a positive correlation with cardiovascular risk biomarkers. In contrast, a prudent dietary pattern with higher intakes of fruit, vegetables, whole grains, fish, and poultry has a positive correlation with plasma folate concentration and an inverse correlation with insulin and homocysteine concentrations and is predictive of a lower risk of IHD.[9] This diet is rich in ω-3 fatty acids, antioxidant vitamins (especially vitamins E and C), folic acid, and L-arginine—all dietary factors that are emerging as important modulators of endothelial function.[6]

A diet rich in fruits, vegetables, low-fat dairy products, fiber, and minerals—particularly calcium, potassium, and magnesium—has a potent antihypertensive effect. This diet promotes a favorable mineral intake. Although limiting sodium chloride affects blood pressure in older persons and patients with diabetes and hypertension, recent meta-analyses suggest that an adequate intake of minerals, certainly potassium and probably calcium, rather than restriction of sodium, should be the focus of dietary recommendations.[10] A plant-based diet also provides phytoestrogens. Genistein, a phytoestrogen found in soybeans, influences endothelium-dependent vasodilation with potency similar to that of estradiol. Genistein, like estradiol, causes L-arginine/nitric oxide–dependent vasodilation.[11] Box 33-1 provides a template for cardiovascular health.[12-14]

NUTRIENT THERAPY/DIETARY SUPPLEMENTS

In addition to prudent dietary choices, nutrients that deserve particular attention are ω-3 fatty acids, folate, and antioxidants, especially vitamin E.

■ Box 33-1 ■

LIFESTYLE CHOICES FOR A HEALTHY HEART

Behavior targets:
Be a nonsmoker.
Have a body mass index less than 25.
Drink alcohol but limit daily intake to 10 g (e.g., one glass of wine per day).
Perform moderate to vigorous physical activity for 30 or more minutes daily.

Select a diet characterized by:
A high cereal fiber content.
Marine ω-3 fatty acids. Eat oily fish (e.g., sardines, salmon, tuna).
Rich folate content.
A high ratio of polyunsaturated to saturated fat. Avoid red meat and high-fat dairy products.
Low in transfatty acids. Use cold processed oils (e.g., olive oil) in preference to margarine.
A low glycemic load.
Rich in antioxidants. Eat a plant-based diet; drink tea.

Omega-3 fatty acids favorably affect the lipid profile, platelet aggregation, and arrhythmia. Docosahexaenoic acid decreases vascular adhesion, and eicosapentaenoic acid increases nitric oxide production. Despite inconsistent clinical results, around 4 g of ω-3 fatty acids daily does appear to improve endothelium function, especially in patients with diabetes. Evidence from a clinical trial suggests that dietary supplementation with ω-3 polyunsaturated fatty acids (900 mg daily) over 3.5 years led to a clinically important and statistically significant cardiovascular benefit.[15] Persons taking ω-3 fatty acids may be expected to benefit from good antioxidant cover with vitamin E; however, results of clinical trials performed to assess the impact of vitamin E and other antioxidants have been somewhat discouraging.

In a placebo-controlled, randomized trial in which a combined daily antioxidant supplement of vitamin E (600 mg), vitamin C (250 mg), and carotene (20 mg) was taken for an average of 5 years, no benefits were detected with respect to either vascular or nonvascular mortality and major vascular events.[16] Overall, it appears that results of clinical trials with beta-carotene supplements have been disappointing, and clinical trials of vitamins C and E have produced scanty data and discrepant results.[17] Despite good epidemiologic support for the potency of vitamin E, the Alpha-Tocopherol, Beta-Carotene Cancer Prevention Study with a low-dose vitamin E supplementation (50 mg/day) and the Cambridge Heart Antioxidant Study (400-800 mg/day) failed to live up to expectations.[17] In fact, the results of the GISSI-Prevenzione[15] (300 mg/day) and HOPE (400 mg/day) trials[17] suggested that vitamin E had no clinically relevant effect on the risk of cardiovascular events. Furthermore, a small randomized prospective trial showed that the protective increase in HDL2 resulting from simvastatin plus niacin was attenuated by concurrent therapy with antioxidants.[18] The authors did not explain the finding. However, taking an antioxidant vitamin cocktail over 5 years, although not deemed beneficial, was regarded as "doing no harm."[19]

In contrast to the neutral or negative findings reported in some studies, a controlled trial on the primary preventive effect of daily supplementation with 50 mg (75 IU) of α-tocopherol did demonstrate a marginal reduction in the incidence of fatal coronary heart disease in male smokers with no history of myocardial infarction.[20] Certainly, vitamin E in doses varying from 300 to 1000 IU, administered over a number of months, does improve endothelial function, as does vitamin C in doses of 1 to 3 g daily. Furthermore, epidemiologic and experimental data suggest that a molar vitamin C/vitamin E plasma ratio of less than 0.8 is associated with an increased risk of heart disease and a ratio in excess of 1.3 may be desirable.[21] Although antioxidants cannot be construed as providing a viable preventive or therapeutic option, difficulty in establishing an appropriate dose and selecting the appropriate supplement and nutrient interactions make it premature to disregard any potential contribution.

Folic acid is a primary determinant of plasma homocysteine levels. Homocysteine is an intermediate produced in the conversion of methionine (an essential sulfur-containing amino acid) to cysteine. Cysteine is required for production of glutathione, a compound involved in oxidation-reduction reactions. Homocysteine may promote atherogenesis through endothelial dysfunction and oxidative stress. In five to 10 times its normal concentration, homocysteine is likely to directly damage endothelium, promote proliferation of vascular smooth muscle cells, exhibit procoagulant activity, and increase collagen synthesis.[22]

Despite conflicting clinical reports,[22] some clinical studies have shown that hyperhomocysteinemia is associated with an increased risk of occlusive arterial disease and venous thromboembolism.[23] A double-blind, placebo-controlled, randomized trial showed that folic acid supplementation significantly improved endothelial dysfunction in patients with coronary atherosclerosis.[24] A controlled clinical trial indicated that a daily intake of 400 μg or more of folic acid significantly lowered homocysteine levels.[25] Although further clinical trials are required to determine whether folic acid supplementation may reduce cardiovascular events, it would seem that persons younger than 60 years with coronary disease and no known risk factors may benefit from taking at least 500 μg of folate daily.[22] Supplementation or consumption of fortified food is advocated to achieve a daily target of 926 μg folic acid.

Other nutrients of potential benefit in the treatment of IHD according to at least one controlled clinical trial are listed in Box 33-2.[26] L-Arginine, the substrate for NOS, in doses of 14 g daily may improve endothelial function. However, the dose may be critical and further investigation is required. Glutamine has recently been added to the list of hopefuls. Results of animal studies and of a trial in which a single oral dose of glutamine (80 mg/kg) was administered to patients with chronic stable angina suggest that glutamine may be cardioprotective in patients with coronary heart disease.[27]

■ Box 33-2 ■

ISCHEMIC HEART DISEASE: EVIDENCE-BASED NUTRIENT INTERVENTION

Vitamin E (800 IU daily)
Vitamin C (1000 mg daily)
Omega-3 fatty acids (MaxEPA capsules, 10-20 g daily)
L-Arginine (7 g three times daily)
N-acetylcysteine (several grams daily)*
Glycosaminoglycans, natural heparin-like substances (100-200 mg daily)
Glutamine (80 mg/kg)

---

* Reduces elevated homocysteine levels, but oxidation may be enhanced in healthy persons.

HERBAL THERAPY

Hawthorn, garlic, ginger, turmeric, and cayenne may be particularly useful in the treatment of IHD.[28] Hawthorn reduces myocardial oxygen demand; it is an antioxidant, it causes coronary vasodilation, and it may help control benign arrhythmia. Clinical trials suggest that an effective dose is 180 mg of 5:1 hawthorn extract daily.

Antiplatelet herbs include turmeric, garlic, and ginger. Turmeric, unlike ginger, is thought to inhibit thromboxane without reducing prostacyclin activity. Turmeric extract in doses equivalent to 20 mg of curcumin daily may be effective. Garlic, taken as a fresh clove or 80 mg of garlic powder daily, reduces coagulation. Garlic inhibits platelet aggregation and enhances fibrinolysis. *Capsicum frutescens* (cayenne) also has fibrinolytic activity. Endothelial function is believed to be improved by antioxidants. Turmeric, garlic, tea, and wine all have an antioxidant effect. Turmeric is most effective against hydroxyl radicals and, although weaker than vitamin C, appears more potent than vitamin E. Its hypolipidemic and antioxidant effects need further clinical validation. The flavonoids in tea are thought to be responsible for reversing endothelial vasomotor dysfunction in patients with IHD. This effect is detected 2 hours after consumption of 450 mL of tea and was also observed in subjects who drank 900 mL of tea daily for 4 weeks.[29] Oral caffeine had no short-term effect on flow-mediated dilation.

Red wine and purple grape juice contain flavonoids with antioxidant and antiplatelet properties believed to be protective against cardiovascular events. Grapeseed extract (100 mg) daily and one glass (10 g) of red wine daily provide a similar cardiovascular benefit. Both in vitro incubation and oral supplementation with purple grape juice decrease platelet aggregation, increase platelet-derived nitric oxide release, and decrease superoxide production.[30] These findings may be a result of antioxidant-sparing and/or a direct effect of select flavonoids found in purple grape juice. The suppression of platelet-mediated thrombosis represents a potential mechanism for the beneficial effects of purple grape products, independent of alcohol consumption, in cardiovascular disease. Whatever the mechanism, a recent study of more than 25,000 male smokers, 50 to 69 years of age, with no previous myocardial infarction, indicated that the intake of flavonols and flavones was inversely associated with nonfatal myocardial infarction.[31] The association between flavonoid intake and coronary death was weaker.

PRACTICE TIPS

- Eating 35 g or more of cold-deep-water fish daily is cardioprotective.
- Nuts are a rich source of arginine.
- Myocardial oxygenation may be improved by L-carnitine, 750 mg, three times daily and/or coenzyme Q10, 150 mg daily.
- Magnesium deficiency increases the risk of coronary artery spasm.

- A daily intake of at least 130 mg of vitamin C and 67 mg of vitamin E may be required for cardiovascular health.[21]
- Optimal intake levels for protection against cardiovascular disease may be 20 mg of beta-carotene, 800 IU of vitamin E, and 750 mg of vitamin C.
- A very high relative cardiovascular risk seems to be associated with vitamin C/vitamin E ratios of 0.5 to 0.7 or less; a lower risk has been linked to ratios of around 1.3 to 1.5.

REFERENCES

1. Murray CJ, Lopez AD: Mortality by cause for eight regions of the world: Global Burden of Disease Study, *Lancet* 349:1269-76, 1997.
2. Giardina EG: Heart disease in women, *Int J Fertil Womens Med* 45:350-7, 2000.
3. Malinow MR: Plasma concentrations of total homocysteine predict mortality risk, *Am J Clin Nutr* 74:3, 2001.
4. Kerins DM, Koury MJ, Capdevila A, et al: Plasma S-adenosylhomocysteine is a more sensitive indicator of cardiovascular disease than plasma homocysteine, *Am J Clin Nutr* 74:723-9, 2001.
5. Pirro M, Maurie'ge P, Tchernof A, et al: Plasma free fatty acid levels and the risk of ischemic heart disease in men: prospective results from the Que'bec Cardiovascular Study, *Atherosclerosis* 160:377-84, 2002.
6. Brown AA, Hu FB: Dietary modulation of endothelial function: implications for cardiovascular disease, *Am J Clin Nutr* 73:673-86, 2001.
7. Carr M, Frei B: The role of natural antioxidants in preserving the biological activity of endothelium-derived nitric oxide, *Free Radic Biol* 28:1806-14, 2000.
8. Fung TT, Rimm EB, Spiegelman D, et al: Association between dietary patterns and plasma biomarkers of obesity and cardiovascular disease risk, *Am J Clin Nutr* 73:61-7, 2001.
9. Hu FB, Rimm EB, Stampfer MJ, et al: Prospective study of major dietary patterns and risk of coronary heart disease in men, *Am J Clin Nutr* 72:912-21, 2000.
10. Hermansen K: Diet, blood pressure and hypertension, *Br J Nutr* 83(suppl 1): S113-S119, 2000.
11. Walker HA, Dean TS, Sanders TA, et al: The phytoestrogen genistein produces acute nitric oxide-dependent dilation of human forearm vasculature with similar potency to 17ss-estradiol, *Circulation* 103:258-62, 2001.
12. Stampfer MJ, Hu FB, Manson JE, et al: Primary prevention of coronary heart disease in women through diet and lifestyle, *N Engl J Med* 343:16-22, 2000.
13. Hu FB, Stampfer MJ, Manson JE, et al: Dietary saturated fats and their food sources in relation to the risk of coronary heart disease in women, *Am J Clin Nutr* 70:1001-8, 1999.
14. Joshipura KJ, Hu FB, Manson JE, et al: The effect of fruit and vegetable intake on risk for coronary heart disease, *Ann Intern Med* 134:1106-14, 2001.
15. Dietary supplementation with n-3 polyunsaturated fatty acids and vitamin E after myocardial infarction: results of the GISSI-Prevenzione trial. Gruppo Italiano per lo Studio della Sopravvivenza nell'Infarto miocardico, *Lancet* 354:447-55, 1999.

16. Heart Protection Study Collaborative Group. MRC/BHF Heart Protection Study of antioxidant supplementation in 20,536 high risk individuals: a randomized placebo-controlled trial, *Lancet* 360:23-33, 2002.

17. Marchioli R, Schweiger C, Levantesi G, et al: Antioxidant vitamins and prevention of cardiovascular disease: epidemiological and clinical trial data, *Lipids* 36(suppl):S53-S63, 2001.

18. Brown BG, Zhao XQ, Chait A, et al: Simvastatin and niacin, antioxidant vitamins, or the combination for the prevention of coronary disease, *N Engl J Med* 345:1583-92, 2001.

19. Collins R, Peto R, Armitage J: The MRC/BHF Heart Protection Study: preliminary results, *Int J Clin Pract* 56:53-6, 2002.

20. Virtamo J, Rapola JM, Ripatti S, et al: Effect of vitamin E and beta carotene on the incidence of primary nonfatal myocardial infarction and fatal coronary heart disease, *Arch Intern Med* 158:668-75, 1998.

21. Gey KF: Vitamin E plus C an interacting conutrients required for optimal health. A critical constructive review of epidemiology and supplementation data regarding cardiovascular disease and cancer, *Biofactors* 7:113-74, 1998.

22. Pearce KA, Boosalis MG, Yeager B: Update on vitamin supplements for the prevention of coronary disease and stroke, *Am Fam Physician* 62:1359-66, 2000.

23. Cattaneo M: Hyperhomocysteinaemia and atherothrombosis, *Ann Med* 32(suppl 1):46-52, 2000.

24. Title LM, Cummings PM, Giddens K: Effect of folic acid and antioxidant vitamins on endothelial dysfunction in patients with coronary artery disease, *J Am Coll Cardiol* 36:758-65, 2000.

25. Rydlewicz A, Simpson JA, Taylor RJ, et al: The effect of folic acid supplementation on plasma homocysteine in an elderly population, *QJM* 95: 27-35, 2002.

26. Werbach MR: *Textbook of nutritional medicine*, Tarzana, CA, 1999, Third Line Press.

27. Khogali SE, Pringle SD, Weryk BV, et al: Is glutamine beneficial in ischemic heart disease? *Nutrition* 18:123-6, 2002.

28. Mills S, Bone K: *Principles and practice of phytotherapy*, Edinburgh, 2000, Churchill Livingstone.

29. Duffy SJ, Keaney JF Jr, Holbrook M, et al: Short-and long-term black tea consumption reverses endothelial dysfunction in patients with coronary artery disease, *Circulation* 104:151-6, 2001.

30. Freedman JE, Parker C, Li L, et al: Select flavonoids and whole juice from purple grapes inhibit platelet function and enhance nitric oxide release, *Circulation* 103:2792-8, 2001.

31. Hirvonen T, Pietinen P, Virtanen M, et al: Intake of flavonols and flavones and risk of coronary heart disease in male smokers, *Epidemiology* 12:62-7, 2001.

■ CHAPTER 34 ■

MENOPAUSE

Menopause is a physiologic stage during which women adjust to estrogen deprivation. The nature and intensity of menopausal symptoms vary among women and are related to estrogen fluctuations. Hot flashes and sleep disturbances are common complaints. Estrogen replacement therapy relieves vasomotor and urogenital symptoms, may improve mood and cognition, and may delay the onset of Alzheimer's disease. For maximum benefit, hormone replacement therapy should be initiated shortly after the start of menopause.[1]

There is insufficient evidence to recommend for or against hormone therapy for postmenopausal women. Because hormone replacement therapy carries distinct advantages and disadvantages, the decision to take synthetic estrogens, phytoestrogens, or neither is a personal choice.

CLINICAL DIAGNOSIS

Although menopausal women have many different symptoms, the impact of the symptoms varies. Menopause presents with missed menstrual periods, vasomotor instability, urogenital atrophy, and psychologic changes. Vasomotor instability results in hot flashes, night sweats, palpitations, insomnia, and dizziness. Urogenital atrophy causes vaginal dryness, dyspareunia, vulvovaginal itching, dysuria, urinary frequency and urgency, and a predisposition to incontinence. Symptoms that appear to be specifically related to hormonal changes of menopausal transition are vasomotor symptoms, vaginal dryness, and breast tenderness.[2]

Withdrawal of estrogen is associated with an increased risk of osteoporosis and cardiovascular disease.

THERAPEUTIC STRATEGY

The goal of intervention is to minimize the impact of estrogen deprivation. Several phytonutrients have estrogen-like activity. Although isoflavones, indoles, isothiocyanates, and lignans dampen the effect of endogenous estrogens in premenopausal women, they have an agonist effect in menopausal women. Phyoestrogens bind to estrogen receptors and have a weak estrogenic effect. Phytoestrogens are less potent than hormone replacement but have greater tissue selectivity.[3] However, it has recently been suggested that although treatment with phytoestrogens is fashionable, there is remarkably little evidence of benefit.[4] A recent small study demonstrated that 50 g of textured soy protein containing 60 mg of total isoflavones daily, taken for 10 to 14 days, did not affect mean baseline or peak luteinizing hormone concentrations in premenopausal or postmenopausal women, indicating a lack of estrogen-like effect at the level of the pituitary.[5] However, in postmenopausal subjects, mean luteinizing hormone secretion decreased after soy was discontinued, suggesting a residual estrogenic effect.

LIFESTYLE CHANGES

For those seeking general support in menopause, dietary choices that enhance phytoestrogen consumption may be helpful. Particularly good sources of isoflavones are chickpeas and soybeans. In one study, after subjects followed a soy-rich diet for 6 months, lipid profiles showed a favorable outcome, similar to that observed in subjects receiving hormone replacement therapy. Subject compliance with the soy-rich diet was however low.[6] Cruciferous vegetables are a good source of indoles and isocyanates. Flaxseed is a good source of lignans, and phenolic compounds are ubiquitous phytonutrients found in cereals, fruits, and vegetables.

NUTRIENT THERAPY

Clinical trials support the use of phytoestrogens and vitamin E supplements in menopause.[7] The North American Menopause Society concurs, observing that although the health effects in humans cannot be clearly attributed to isoflavones alone, foods or supplements that contain isoflavones have some physiologic effects.[8] As little as 60 to 140 mg of soybeans daily may decrease the frequency of hot flashes.[9] A review on the efficacy of phytoestrogens in reducing the symptoms of menopause indicated that a diet rich in isoflavones (average dose of 50 mg of genistein daily) was associated with a reduced incidence of vasomotor symptoms.[10] Although some data seem to support the efficacy of isoflavones in reducing the incidence and severity of hot flashes, the most convincing health effects have been attributed to the actions of isoflavones on lipids.[8]

Epidemiologic studies suggest that hormone replacement raises high-density lipoprotein cholesterol and triglyceride levels and lowers low-density lipoprotein cholesterol and lipoprotein(a) levels, possibly achieving a 50% reduction in postmenopausal cardiovascular risk.[3] In a cross-sectional study, intakes of genistein, daidzein, and total isoflavones were each positively associated with high-density lipoprotein cholesterol levels and inversely associated with postchallenge insulin levels in postmenopausal women.[11] A role for dietary soy in protection against cardiovascular disease was postulated. However, estrogen deprivation is only one intervention target. Adiposity is an independent risk factor for cardiovascular disease in postmenopausal women. Weight loss may reduce C-reactive protein levels and mediate a measure of cardioprotection in obese, postmenopausal women.[12] An integrated approach is required.

Although genetic factors are more important, the most important single nongenetic factor determining the risk of osteoporosis in postmenopausal women is estrogen deficiency.[13] Bone mineral densities, adjusted for weight and years since menopause, are significantly different in persons with high and low intakes of soy isoflavones.[14] In the early but not the late postmenopausal group, significant differences were also found with respect to backache between the high and low intake categories of soy isoflavones.[15] Taking 40 g of soy protein daily, with an isoflavone content of 2.25 mg or more per gram of protein, is protective against both spinal bone loss and cardiovascular disease.[15]

HERBAL THERAPY

A study, in which the most common dietary supplements were soy (29%), *Ginkgo biloba* (16%), and black cohosh (10%), showed that perceived quality of life and overall control of menopausal symptoms were highest among women using dietary supplements.[16] Those who added supplements to hormone replacement therapy also reported reduction in vaginal dryness and improvement in libido and mood. Nonetheless, herbs should only be taken with caution. When dong quai, ginseng, black cohosh, and licorice root—all herbs frequently included in menopausal remedies—were tested in vitro, it was found that dong quai and ginseng both significantly induced the growth of MCF-7 cells, a human breast cancer cell line.[17] Black cohosh and licorice root did not.

Black cohosh and wild yam (*Dioscorea villosa*) are saponin-containing herbs that may help adaptation to new hormone levels.[18] Black cohosh root extract has a good safety profile and has demonstrated efficacy in relieving menopausal symptoms.[19] A number of clinical studies of Remifemin, a standardized extract of black cohosh, have demonstrated efficacy for the alleviation of menopausal complaints such as hot flashes, anxiety, and depression.[20] However, in a randomized clinical trial among patients with breast cancer, investigators found that black cohosh was not significantly more efficacious than placebo in relieving most menopausal symptoms, including the number and intensity of hot flashes.[21] Black cohosh has low toxicity and is well tolerated with few or mild side effects.

Wild yam root has also been found to affect estrogenic activity.[22] Extracts of wild yam (*Dioscorea villosa*) containing steroidal saponins, including diosgenin, are thought to influence endogenous steroidogenesis when applied topically in the form of a cream. In a double-blind, placebo-controlled crossover study, healthy women with menopausal symptoms, after 3 months of treatment with wild yam cream, reported little benefit and no significant side effects.[23]

Herbs may also be used for specific menopausal symptoms. Substantial improvement in psychologic and psychosomatic symptoms were noted after 12 weeks of treatment with St. John's wort, one tablet three times daily (900 mg of *Hypericum perforatum* [Kira]).[24] Kava, in conjunction with hormone replacement therapy, is effective against menopausal anxiety.[25] A randomized, multicenter, double-blind, parallel-group study showed that ginseng reduced depression and enhanced well-being in postmenopausal women.[26] Sage (*Salvia officinalis*) and hawthorn may help to relieve hot flashes.[18]

PRACTICE TIPS

- Hot flashes may be relieved by drinking tea, made by steeping in boiling water one teaspoon of crushed anise seeds or one to two teaspoons of fennel seeds, or more cautiously, one half teaspoon of licorice root.
- *Panax ginseng* has some estrogenic activity but may exacerbate irritability and insomnia.
- Chamomile and grapeseed extracts have weak estrogenic activity.

REFERENCES

1. Shaywitz SE, Shaywitz BA, Pugh KR, et al: Effect of estrogen on brain activation patterns in postmenopausal women during working memory tasks, *JAMA* 281:1197-202, 1999.
2. Dennerstein L, Dudley EC, Hopper JL, et al: A prospective population-based study of menopausal symptoms, *Obstet Gynecol* 96:351-8, 2000.
3. Ariyo AA, Villablanca AC: Estrogens and lipids. Can HRT designer estrogens, and phytoestrogens reduce cardiovascular risk markers after menopause? *Postgrad Med* 111:23-30, 2002.
4. Pinn G: Herbs used in obstetrics and gynaecology, *Aust Fam Physician* 30:351-4, 356, 2001.
5. Nicholls J, Lasley BL, Nakajima ST, et al: Effects of soy consumption on gonadotropin secretion and acute pituitary responses to gonadotropin-releasing hormone in women, *J Nutr* 132:708-14, 2002.
6. Chiechi LM, Secreto G, Vimercati A, et al: The effects of a soy rich diet on serum lipids: the Menfis randomized trial, *Maturitas* 41:97-104, 2002.
7. Werbach MR: *Textbook of nutritional medicine*, Tarzana, CA, 1999, Third Line Press.
8. The role of isoflavones in menopausal health: consensus opinion of The North American Menopause Society, *Menopause* 7:215-29, 2000.
9. Glisson J, Crawford R, Street S: The clinical applications of *Ginkgo biloba*, St. John's wort, saw palmetto, and soy, *Nurse Practitioner* 24:28-49, 1999.
10. Arena S, Rappa C, Del Frate E, et al: A natural alternative to menopausal hormone replacement therapy. Phytoestrogens, *Minerva Ginecol* 54:53-7, 2002.

11. Goodman-Gruen D, Kritz-Silverstein D: Usual dietary isoflavone intake is associated with cardiovascular disease risk factors in postmenopausal women, *J Nutr* 131:1202-6, 2001.

12. Tchernof A, Nolan A, Sites CK, et al: Weight loss reduces C-reactive protein levels in obese postmenopausal women, *Circulation* 105:564-9, 2002.

13. Cohen AJ, Roe FJ: Review of risk factors for osteoporosis with particular reference to a possible aetiological role of dietary salt, *Food Chem Toxicol* 38: 237-53, 2000.

14. Somekawa Y, Chiguchi M, Ishibashi T, et al: Soy intake related to menopausal symptoms, serum lipids, and bone mineral density in postmenopausal Japanese women, *Obstet Gynecol* 97:109-15, 2001.

15. Potter SM, Baum JA, Teng H, et al: Soy protein and isoflavones: their effects on blood lipids and bone density in postmenopausal women, *Am J Clin Nutr* 68(suppl 6):1375S-1379S, 1998.

16. Kam IW, Dennehy CE, Tsourounis C: Dietary supplement use among menopausal women attending a San Francisco health conference, *Menopause* 9:72-8, 2002.

17. Amato P, Christophe S, Mellon PL: Estrogenic activity of herbs commonly used as remedies for menopausal symptoms, *Menopause* 9:145-50, 2002.

18. Mills S, Bone K: *Principles and practice of phytotherapy*, Edinburgh, 2000, Churchill Livingstone.

19. Hardy ML: Herbs of special interest to women, *J Am Pharm Assoc (Wash)* 40: 234-42, 2000.

20. McKenna DJ, Jones K, Humphrey S, et al: Black cohosh: efficacy, safety, and use in clinical and preclinical applications, *Altern Ther Health Med* 7:93-100, 2001.

21. Jacobson JS, Troxel AB, Evans J, et al: Randomized trial of black cohosh for the treatment of hot flashes among women with a history of breast cancer, *J Clin Oncol* 19:2739-45, 2001.

22. Rosenberg Z and RS, Jenkins DJ, Diamandis EP: Effects of natural products and nutraceuticals on steroid hormone-regulated gene expression, *Clin Chim Acta* 312:213-9, 2001.

23. Komesaroff PA, Black CV, Cable V, et al: Effects of wild yam extract on menopausal symptoms, lipids and sex hormones in healthy menopausal women, *Climacteric* 4:144-50, 2001.

24. Grube B, Walper A, Wheatley D: St. John's wort extract: efficacy for menopausal symptoms of psychological origin, *Adv Ther* 16:177-86, 1999.

25. De Leo V, la Marca A, Morgante G, et al: Evaluation of combining kava extract with hormone replacement therapy in the treatment of postmenopausal anxiety, *Maturitas* 39:185-8, 2001.

26. Wiklund IK, Mattsson LA, Lindgren R, et al: Effects of a standardized ginseng extract on quality of life and physiological parameters in symptomatic postmenopausal women: a double-blind, placebo-controlled trial, *Int J Clin Pharmacol Res* 19:89-99, 1999.

■ CHAPTER 35 ■

MIGRAINE

Migraine is a common vascular headache. It is especially prevalent in women. Patients with migraine are believed to have an inherent vasomotor instability. Headaches are characterized by initial intracranial arterial vasoconstriction, followed by a period of extracranial vasodilation. A spreading neuronal depression across the occipital lobe and cerebral cortex appears to be preceded by an excitatory wave. Various inflammatory vasoactive chemicals and neurotransmitters are postulated to be released in response to diverse stressors. Migraine triggers include red wine, hunger, lack of sleep, glare, perfume, and periods of letdown. It is estimated that 20% of migraines are caused by food sensitivities.

Sleep, pregnancy, and exhilaration can deactivate migraine. Many over-the-counter,[1] nutritional, botanical, and dietary supplements are used with varying success to treat and prevent migraine headaches.[2]

CLINICAL DIAGNOSIS

Migraines are moderately severe, unilateral, or generalized throbbing headaches associated with nausea, vomiting, and photophobia. The headache usually persists for 4 to 72 hours. Migraines fall into two general categories: migraines without aura and migraines with aura. Migraines without aura are often associated with hemianopic field defects and scotomata. Migraines with aura are preceded by a 15- to 20-minute episode of visual or sensory experience, often associated with paresthesia affecting the arm and face.

THERAPEUTIC STRATEGY

One approach to migraine management consists of attempts to reset biologic and environmental homeostasis. The postulate is that migraine is a response to pineal circadian irregularity. The pineal gland is perceived as the connection between migraine headaches and environmental triggers. Melatonin is believed to enable resynchronization of biologic rhythms. Synthesized from serotonin by the enzyme N-acetyltransferase, melatonin is released centrally in a circadian cycle, subsequently relieving migraine and other headaches. A number of studies have demonstrated that melatonin levels are lower in patients with migraine than in control subjects; this is particularly true in women.[3]

Another more pedestrian and generally accepted approach is to dampen inflammatory mediators and untoward neurotransmission. The aim of many nutritional and botanical therapies is to alleviate migraine by decreasing platelet aggregation, preventing the release of vasoactive neurotransmitters, and avoiding food triggers.

LIFESTYLE CHANGES

Lifestyle changes involve avoiding trigger foods. Certain foods containing vasoactive amines, such as tyramine and phenylalanine, can cause migraines in sensitive patients. Examples include aged cheeses, red wine, beer, chocolate, and yogurt. Food additives such as monosodium glutamate, aspartame, and sodium nitrate are also recognized migraine triggers.

One study showed that patients with migraine, by limiting their fat intake to no more than 20 g daily, could achieve statistically significant decreases in headache frequency, intensity, and duration and medication intake.[4]

NUTRIENT THERAPY/DIETARY SUPPLEMENTS

There is some clinical support for melatonin in the management of migraine.[3] A small, open trial showed that melatonin infusion provided delayed relief in patients with migraine.[5] In a double-blind, placebo-controlled crossover study, 5 mg of melatonin was found to be particularly useful for patients with headache and disturbed sleep phase syndrome.[6]

With respect to interventions that dampen inflammation and neuroexcitation, fish oil and magnesium, possibly in the form of magnesium taurine, deserve consideration.[7] Clinical trials have shown that headaches may be relieved by daily administration of fish oil containing 2.7 g of eicosapentaenoic acid and 1.8 g of docosahexaenoic acid or 600 mg of magnesium.[8] Increased levels of extracellular magnesium, like increased tissue levels of taurine, could be expected to dampen neuronal hyperexcitation, counteract vasospasm, increase tolerance to focal hypoxia, and stabilize platelets. Current evidence suggests that up to 50% of patients with migraine have lowered levels of ionized magnesium during an acute migraine attack.[9] Magnesium might conceivably establish the threshold for an attack through its abilities to stabilize cell membranes, counteract vasospasm, and inhibit platelet aggregation. By the 12th week of a controlled trial, patients with migraine taking 600 mg of magnesium orally as trimagnesium citrate had less frequent attacks and fewer headache days than control subjects.[10]

In clinical trials, improvements have also been reported with use of 400 mg of riboflavin daily, 83 μg of chromium orotate daily, or 500 mg of vitamin

C twice daily.[8] Several studies have shown high-dose riboflavin, a coenzyme in the electron-transport chain, to be effective in migraine prophylaxis.[2] In a randomized trial of 3 months' duration, 400 mg of riboflavin reduced both migraine attack frequency and headache days in 59% of participants.[11]

A shotgun approach with a combination of agents known to influence serotonin blood level, vascular tone, and inflammatory reactions has been tried. Taking low doses of tryptophan, niacin, calcium, caffeine, and acetylsalicylic acid soon after the onset of migraine symptoms provided significant benefit to patients in a small preliminary study.[12] Taking 500 mg of L-tryptophan every 6 hours significantly reduces the frequency of migraine.[2]

HERBAL THERAPY

Herbal intervention focuses on inhibiting inflammatory neurotransmitters. Feverfew is a popular herbal remedy for preventing migraine. Vogler et al[13] noted that feverfew appears to be more effective than placebo, but in a systematic review, they concluded that feverfew's clinical effectiveness in the prevention of migraine has yet to be established. Differences in clinical outcome may be linked to parthenolide, one of feverfew's several active constituents. In one double-blind, crossover study, feverfew in doses of at least 125 mg of dried feverfew leaf standardized to 0.2% parthenolide content, used continuously for at least 4 to 6 weeks, was found to reduce the mean number and severity of attacks and the degree of nausea and vomiting.[2] No serious side effects have been reported, but no long-term toxicity studies have been performed.

Other herbs that may be useful are *Ginkgo biloba* extract, with its three specific platelet-activating factor antagonists, and ginger, with its gingerols and shogaols that inhibit arachidonate-induced platelet aggregation. The recommended dosage of ginkgo, standardized to 24% ginkgo heterosides, is 40 mg three times per day; the recommended dosage of ginger is 1 g of dried herb daily.[2] A randomized, parallel-group, placebo-controlled, double-blind clinical study showed that patients with migraine can benefit from prophylactic treatment with a special extract of *Petasites hybridus* (50 mg twice daily).[14]

A meta-analysis of English-language, randomized, placebo-controlled trials revealed that antidepressants were effective as prophylaxis for chronic headache.[15] A number of herbs have an antidepressant effect.

PRACTICE TIPS

- Patients with migraine may need to avoid foods that undergo fermentation during processing including red wine, beer, meat extracts, pickled herring, chicken livers, yogurt, and aged cheese.
- Potentially problematic fresh foods rich in vasoactive amines include overripe bananas, avocados, red plums, oranges, and tomatoes.

- Patients with migraine should be wary of chocolate, peanuts, cured meats, and caffeine.
- Chewing 300 to 500 mg of niacin may alleviate the intensity of migraine if done at the appearance of the aura.

REFERENCES

1. Freitag FG: Do over-the-counter medications help the physician manage migraine headache? *Curr Pain Headache Rep* 6:156-61, 2002.
2. Sinclair S: Migraine headaches: nutritional, botanical and other alternative approaches, *Altern Med Rev* 4:86-95, 1999.
3. Gagnier JJ: The therapeutic potential of melatonin in migraines and other headache types, *Altern Med Rev* 6:383-9, 2001.
4. Bic Z, Blix GG, Hopp HP, et al: The influence of a low-fat diet on incidence and severity of migraine headaches, *J Womens Health Gend Based Med* 8:623-30, 1999.
5. Claustrat B, Brun J, Geoffriau M, et al: Nocturnal plasma melatonin profile and melatonin kinetics during infusion in status migrainosus, *Cephalalgia* 17:511-7, 1997.
6. Nagtegaal JE, Smits MG, Swart AC, et al: Melatonin-responsive headache in delayed sleep phase syndrome: preliminary observations, *Headache* 38:303-7, 1998.
7. McCarty MF: Magnesium taurate and fish oil for prevention of migraine, *Med Hypotheses* 47:461-6, 1996.
8. Werbach MR: *Textbook of nutritional medicine*, Tarzana, CA, 1999, Third Line Press.
9. Mauskop A, Altura BM: Role of magnesium in the pathogenesis and treatment of migraine, *Clin Neurosci* 5:24-7, 1998.
10. Peikert A, Wilimzig C, Kohne-Volland R: Prophylaxis of migraine with oral magnesium: results from a prospective, multi-center, placebo-controlled and double blind randomized study, *Cephalalgia* 16:257-63, 1996.
11. Schoenen J, Lenaerts M, Bastings E: High dose riboflavin as a prophylactic treatment of migraine: results of an open pilot study, *Cephalalgia* 14:328-9, 1994.
12. Gedye A: Hypothesized treatment for migraines using low doses of tryptophan, niacin, calcium, caffeine, and acetylsalicylic acid, *Med Hypotheses* 56:91-4, 2001.
13. Vogler BK, Pittler MH, Ernst E: Feverfew as a preventive treatment for migraine: a systematic review, *Cephalalgia* 18:704-8, 1998.
14. Grossmann W, Schmidramsl H: An extract of *Petasites hybridus* is effective in the prophylaxis of migraine, *Altern Med Rev* 6:303-10, 2001.
15. Tomkins GE, Jackson JL, O'Malley PG, et al: Treatment of chronic headache with antidepressants: a meta-analysis, *Am J Med* 111:54-63, 2001.

■ CHAPTER 36 ■

OSTEOARTHRITIS

Degenerative joint disease represents joint failure. It is the clinical manifestation of a net loss of articular cartilage. The amount of articular cartilage matrix represents the balance between the synthesis and catabolism of proteoglycans, collagen, and hyaluronic acid. Osteoarthritis develops when there is disproportion between the load applied to the articular cartilage and the quality of the cartilaginous matrix. In addition to mechanical stress, varying degrees of inflammation may exacerbate osteoarthritis. In certain patients, interleukin-1 (IL-1) and other products of inflammation activate gelatinase, a metalloenzyme that contributes to cartilage degradation.

Along with a genetic predisposition, obesity, excessive use, aging, and previous trauma are associated with osteoarthritis. Risk factors for osteoarthritis range from those that cause mechanical damage to local joint geometry and structure to metabolic factors such as antioxidant status.[1] As many as 1 in 10 adults may show radiologic evidence of osteoarthritis.

CLINICAL DIAGNOSIS

Osteoarthritis is gradual in onset, and clinical manifestations vary from patient to patient. The disease is often asymmetric. The first metacarpophalangeal joint, knees, hips and lumbar and cervical spine are frequently involved. Classic signs and symptoms of osteoarthritis are as follows:

• Stiffness that is mild in the early morning and recurs after periods of rest
• Pain that worsens with prolonged joint use and is relieved by rest
• Loss of function

Prevalent findings on examination include local tenderness, soft tissue swelling, joint crepitus, and bony swelling, often unassociated with joint deformity. Mobility is restricted. An inflammatory variant is likely in patients with pain during rest and/or nocturnal pain, warm, tender joints, and/or joint effusion.

Osteoarthritic joints show irregular loss of cartilage, sclerosis of subchondral bone, subchondral cysts, marginal osteophytes, and variable degrees of synovial inflammation.

THERAPEUTIC STRATEGY

Osteoarthritis appears to be a mechanically driven but chemically mediated disease process characterized by imperfect or aberrant cartilage repair. The prime objectives of management are reduction of pain, preservation of function, and prevention of further damage. The intervention strategy is to minimize cartilage breakdown, encourage cartilage replenishment, and limit cartilage damage caused by mechanical trauma or secondary synovitis.

Nitric oxide, under certain conditions (e.g., septic arthritis), may have a protective anabolic effect on cartilage; however, in osteoarthritis, nitric oxide is consistently produced and associated with matrix degradation and chondrocyte apoptosis.[2] Although nitric oxide does not appear to be the initiating signal for apoptosis in chondrocytes, in vivo nitric oxidase synthase inhibitors may be useful in the treatment of osteoarthritis because they block the catabolic activities of nitric oxide.[3] Niacinamide and other inhibitors of adenosine diphosphate ribosylation have been shown to suppress cytokine-mediated induction of nitric oxide synthase in several types of cells.[4] Adequate selenium nutrition may also downregulate cytokine signaling, and ample intake of fish oil can be expected to decrease synovial IL-1 production. Synovium-generated IL-1, by inducing nitric oxide synthase and thereby inhibiting chondrocyte synthesis of aggrecan and type II collagen, may be crucial to the pathogenesis of osteoarthritis.

Management in osteoarthritis is problematic and continually being reviewed.[5,6]

LIFESTYLE CHANGES

Maintaining an ideal body weight reduces the risk of joint damage. An energy-balanced diet rich in vegetables, fruits, and whole grains and low in fat is recommended. By losing 5 kg (2 body mass index units), women and men with a body mass index greater than 25 kg/m^2 reduce their likelihood of knee osteoarthritis by 50% and 25%, respectively.[7] Wearing soft-soled shoes or foam rubber innersoles and walking rather than jogging also reduce mechanical stress. The articular joint surface is avascular, and movement improves nutrient diffusion; therefore, regular exercise is advocated. Exposure to sunlight, resulting in adequate vitamin D synthesis, may also be protective.

Avoidance of allergenic foods is reported to relieve symptoms such as pain and stiffness in some cases.[8] The family Solanaceae is a rich source of glycoalkaloids, have been incriminated with tomato, potato, eggplant, peppers, and tobacco as possible triggering agents. It may take months of following a glycoalkaloid-free diet before improvement is noted.

NUTRIENT THERAPY/DIETARY SUPPLEMENTS

Alternatives to traditional nonsteroidal anti-inflammatory drugs (NSAIDs) with fewer side effects are being sought.[9,10] Nutrient therapy of osteoarthritis has a two-pronged focus. Some nutrients reduce inflammation and cartilage destruction (e.g., cyclooxygenase-2 inhibitors)[9]; others enhance cartilage synthesis and repair (e.g., glucosamine).[10] In view of the documented efficacy of glucosamine in relieving pain, improving function, and possibly inhibiting structural progression,[11] some suggest that glucosamine should be considered a potential first-line agent in patients with knee osteoarthritis and mild to moderate pain.[10] However, others maintain that there is little or no scientific evidence for the effects of this and other nutrients in patients with knee, hip, or hand osteoarthritis.[12] Despite reservations, there is scientific support for serious consideration of nutrients in the treatment of patients with osteoarthritis.

The postulate that glucosamine and chondroitin sulfates halt or reverse joint degeneration by stimulating synthesis and inhibiting degradation of proteoglycans enjoys biologic and some clinical support.[13] Joint cartilage consists of cells embedded in a matrix of fibrous collagen within a concentrated water-proteoglycan gel. Proteoglycans stabilize cell membranes and increase intracellular ground substance. They enhance flexibility and provide resistance to compression, which counteracts physical stress. Depletion of sulfated proteoglycans is an early manifestation of osteoarthritis. Both chondroitin and glucosamine sulfates serve as substrates for proteoglycan synthesis.

The glucosamine component of glucosamine sulfate is quickly and almost completely absorbed from the gastrointestinal tract and is rapidly incorporated into articular cartilage. Articular cartilage concentrates glucosamine. Glucosamine acts as a substrate for glycosaminoglycans and hyaluronic acid, essential components of proteoglycans. Hyaluronic acid, in addition to contributing to the matrix of cartilage, suppresses the anti-catabolic effect of IL-1 in chondrocyte cell cultures. Most individuals taking glucosamine sulfate achieve a 50% to 70% reduction in articular pain, joint tenderness, and swelling.[14] Approximately 95% of patients with osteoarthritis of the knee respond well to glucosamine sulfate, and in 60%, improvement is reputed to be excellent. Preliminary evidence suggests that patients with arthritis of the shoulder or elbow also respond well. The typical oral dose of glucosamine sulfate is 500 mg three times daily for a minimum of 6 weeks. Most individuals benefit from repeated courses. Improvement persists for 6 to 12 weeks after cessation of a 6-week course of treatment. In a review of 16 randomized, controlled trials Towheed et al[15] concluded that glucosamine was both effective and safe for managing osteoarthritis.[15] In addition, in a randomized, double-blind placebo-controlled trial of patients with knee osteoarthritis who took 1500 mg of glucosamine sulfate daily for 3 years, long-term combined structure-modifying and symptom-modifying effects were detected.[16]

Glucosamine sulfate may be a disease-modifying agent in osteoarthritis. Since it is safe for long-term administration, continuous administration is appropriate. Glucosamine sulfate does cause mild side effects in 6% to 12% of cases. Gastrointestinal disturbances, drowsiness, headaches, and skin reactions have been reported. Individuals with active peptic ulcers and individuals taking diuretics tend to have an increased incidence of side effects.

Although glucosamine has been described as effective when used alone, it is probably reasonable to use it in combination with chondroitin sulfate, pending further studies.[17] In a meta-analysis of 13 double-blind placebo-controlled trials of more than 4 weeks' duration, McAlindon et al[18] concluded that oral or parenteral glucosamine or chondroitin for treatment of hip or knee osteoarthritis provided moderate to significant benefits. The majority of physiologic benefits from chondroitin sulfates appear to result from increased availability of the monosaccharide building blocks, glucuronic acid and N-acetylgalactosamine. Chondroitin sulfates are well tolerated after oral administration, although 3% of individuals report slight dyspepsia. The typical oral dosage is 400 mg twice daily; however, a single dose of 800 mg per day appears to be equally effective according to pharmacokinetic data. Repeated cycles of administration are needed to produce the best results.

Various combination therapy options are available. A 16-week randomized, double-blind, placebo-controlled crossover trial showed that glucosamine hydrochloride (1500 mg/day), chondroitin sulfate (1200 mg/day), and manganese ascorbate (228 mg/day) relieved symptoms of knee osteoarthritis.[19] Although clinical findings suggest that glucosamine sulfate (1500 mg) and chondroitin sulfate (1200 mg) are an effective and safe alternative to NSAIDs for alleviation of symptoms,[20] glucosamine sulfate does not inhibit cyclooxygenase and proteolytic enzymes involved in inflammation. Low doses of NSAIDs may be added to this combination for treatment of patients with inflammatory osteoarthritis.

Despite growing enthusiasm, it must be noted that unanimous agreement on use of these supplements is lacking. There are those who believe there is no reliable scientific evidence that either chondroitin sulfate or glucosamine sulfate have structure-modifying actions with respect to prohibiting or healing lesions or restoring cartilage synthesis.[12] Furthermore, these agents have not been evaluated by the Food and Drug Administration or recommended for the treatment of osteoarthritis but are available as health food supplements.

In addition to promotion of cartilage synthesis, management of osteoarthritis may be achieved by reducing cartilage destruction. Nutrients that may help in the maintenance and regeneration of cartilage are boron and vitamin D. Boron appears to participate in hydroxylation reactions influencing the synthesis of steroid hormones and vitamin D. A trial indicated that boron supplementation, 6 mg per day as sodium tetraborate decahydrate for 8 weeks, benefited 50% of individuals with osteoarthritis whose diets are likely to be low in boron.[21]

Vitamin D plays a role in the normal turnover of articular cartilage. Studies suggest that vitamin D (400-1600 IU) may slow the progression of and possibly help prevent the development of osteoarthritis. Certainly, osteoarthritis is three times more likely in persons with low serum and dietary levels of vitamin D.[22]

S-adenosylmethionine, another proven therapy for osteoarthritis, functions as a methyl donor and upregulates the proteoglycan synthesis of chondrocytes.[8] In vitro studies have shown that S-adenosylmethionine stimulates the synthesis of proteoglycans by human articular chondrocytes. Human studies suggest that S-adenosylmethionine, in doses of 1200 mg per day, may be as effective as NSAIDs.[8] Such intervention is particularly important in patients with inflammatory osteoarthritis.

IL-1 targets synovial cells and liberates prostaglandin E_2, proteases, collagenases, and glycosidases. It appears to decrease S-adenosylmethionine levels in chondrocytes, a situation that may be reversed by supplementation with S-adenosylmethionine.

Synovium-generated IL-1 induces nitric oxide synthase, thereby inhibiting chondrocyte synthesis of aggrecan and type II collagen. Aspirin, steroids, and niacinamide can suppress nitric oxide synthase and may blunt the antianabolic impact of IL-1 on chondrocytes. Clinical studies have shown that treatment with niacinamide, 900 to 4000 mg per day, usually increases joint mobility and decreases joint discomfort, inflammation, and pain after 3 to 4 weeks of treatment.[4,8] Progressive improvement occurs for up to 3 years if niacinamide administration is continued. Patients who stop taking niacinamide gradually revert to their pretreatment state. Niacinamide was most effective when taken in frequent, divided doses. It is generally well tolerated and appears to be relatively safe for long-term use. Patients taking large amounts of this vitamin (e.g., 1500 mg/day or more) should have periodic tests to monitor liver function.

Although not believed to initiate the process, oxidative stress is believed to contribute to the progression of osteoarthritis. Vitamins A, C, and E may influence osteoarthritis by protecting against oxidative damage and modulating the inflammatory response.[8] High intakes of antioxidants, especially vitamin C, may reduce the risk of cartilage loss and disease progression in osteoarthritis.[23] Because the antioxidant efficiency of vitamin C does not increase linearly with its serum concentration and because efficiency for scavenging free radicals declines as the concentration of ascorbate increases, the optimal intake may be 150 mg daily.[24] In addition to its antioxidant effect, vitamin C may promote cartilage health. Vitamin C deficiency may reduce mechanical integrity of cartilage, since vitamin C is involved in electron donation in the synthesis of type II collagen, hydroxylation of proline to hydroxyproline in collagen synthesis, and glycosaminoglycan synthesis as a sulfate carrier.

Like vitamin C, vitamin E is a free radical scavenger. Vitamin E, in doses of 600 IU three times daily, reduced pain in a 10-day trial.[25] Its antiinflammatory activity may be mediated by inhibiting prostaglandin synthesis and stabilizing lysosomal membranes. In vitro studies suggest that normal plasma levels of vitamin E enhance lipoxygenation of arachidonic acid and that higher concentrations have a suppressive effect.[26] The efficacy of nutrient supplementation in suppressing inflammation varies, depending on the degree of inflammation involved. This may partially explain the apparent failure of trace element, vitamin combination of selenium-ACE, in a controlled double-blind trial, to demonstrate any significant efficacy at 3 or 6 months in the treatment of osteoarthritis.[27] Selenium may downregulate cytokine signaling.

Clinical trials have demonstrated individual benefit from sodium selenite (140 μg daily), superoxide dismutase, cartilage extract, and molybdenum.[28] Results of an animal study confirmed that a diet supplemented with vitamins and selenium might be useful in prevention or therapy of mechanically induced osteoarthritis.[29] There are at least four mechanisms, ranging from oxidative stress to cellular differentiation, by which the nutrient vitamins A, C, D, and E may be related to the processes that impede or give rise to osteoarthritis[30]; and recent data indicate that low intake of these micronutrients may adversely influence the progression of knee osteoarthritis and the incidence of hip osteoarthritis.[31]

A controlled, double-blind, crossover study has also demonstrated that folate and cobalamin supplementation provide benefit.[32]

HERBAL THERAPY

A review of herbal therapy for osteoarthritis indicated that avocado-soybean unsaponifiables were effective.[33] Symptomatic pain relief and improvement of functional disability were reported with the use of avocado-soybean extracts. An avocado-soybean extract and Ayurvedic preparation (Articulin-F), an herbal remedy that contains (per capsule) 450 mg of *Withania somnifera* root, 100 mg of *Boswellia serrata* stem, 50 mg of *Curcuma longa* rhizome, and 50 mg of a zinc complex have been reported to be beneficial.[8]

Other herbs that appear to have some therapeutic usefulness include devil's claw, willow bark, and nettle. A number of studies suggest that *Harpagophytum procumbens* extract (devil's claw) has a beneficial effect.[34] Although *H. procumbens* has no demonstrable anti-inflammatory effect, it does appear to have an analgesic effect. In a randomized, double-blind study over 4 weeks, two daily doses of oral *H. procumbens* extract (600 and 1200, respectively, containing 50 and 100 mg of the marker harpagoside) were found to reduce low back pain with no evidence of side effects, except possibly mild and infrequent gastrointestinal symptoms.[35]

White willow bark contains salicin, which acts more slowly than aspirin, lasts longer, and has fewer side effects. A 4-week blinded trial showed that oral administration of willow bark (*Salix* spp.) extract resulted in dose-dependent pain relief.[36] Doses of 120 mg and 240 mg of salicin were used. In doses of 60 to 120 mg a day, salicin is used to treat musculoskeletal pain and headaches.

A randomized, controlled, double-blind, crossover study of patients with osteoarthritic pain at the base of the thumb or index finger indicated that stinging nettle leaf (*Urtica dioica*), applied locally each day for 1 week, reduced pain and disability.[37] Other nutriceuticals, including ginger extracts, require more extensive investigation.[11]

PRACTICE TIPS

- Cayenne (*Capsicum* spp.) may be helpful in osteoarthritis but not rheumatoid arthritis.
- Capsaicin, an effective pain killer when applied in a thin layer to the skin over the affected area and rubbed in well at least four times daily, is available in cream or ointment form.
- Analgesia from acetaminophen (paracetamol) in doses up to 1.0 g six times per day may be prescribed.
- Aspirin may inhibit proteoglycan synthesis and should be avoided by patients with osteoarthritis.
- In inflammatory osteoarthritis, NSAIDs may be protective by inhibiting synovial production of IL-1, which induces synthesis and release of matrix-degrading proteinases from chondrocytes.
- Glucosamine use is reputed to halve the effective dose of NSAIDs required.
- Boron may induce remission in some patients with osteoarthritis.
- Niacinamide, 500 to 1000 mg three times daily, may benefit patients with osteoarthritis.

REFERENCES

1. Sowers M: Epidemiology of risk factors for osteoarthritis: systemic factors, *Curr Opin Rheumatol* 13:447-51, 2001.
2. Lotz M: The role of nitric oxide in articular cartilage damage, *Rheum Dis North Am* 25:269-82, 1999.
3. Greisberg J, Bliss M, Terek R: The prevalence of nitric oxide in apoptotic chondrocytes of osteoarthritis, *Osteoarthritis Cartilage* 10:207-11, 2002.
4. McCarty MF, Russell AL: Niacinamide therapy for osteoarthritis—does it inhibit nitric oxide synthase induction by interleukin 1 in chondrocytes? *Med Hypotheses* 53:350-60, 1999.
5. Rollins G: Updated guidelines include new drugs and therapies for the treatment of osteoarthritis, *Rep Med Guidel Outcomes Res* 11:1-2, 5, 2000.
6. McKinney RH, Ling SM: Osteoarthritis: no cure, but many options for symptom relief, *Cleve Clin J Med* 67:665-71, 2000.
7. Meisler JG, St Jeor S: Foreword, *Am J Clin Nutr* 63(suppl 3):409S-411S, 1996.
8. Gaby AR: Natural treatments for osteoarthritis, *Altern Med Rev* 4:330-41, 1999.
9. Wildy KS, Wasko MC: Current concepts regarding pharmacologic treatment of rheumatoid and osteoarthritis, *Hand Clin* 17:321-38, xi, 2001.

10. Hochberg MC: What a difference a year makes: reflections on the ACR recommendations for the medical management of osteoarthritis, *Curr Rheumatol Rep* 3:473-8, 2001.

11. Reginster JY, Gillot V, Bruyere O, Henrotin Y: Evidence of nutriceutical effectiveness in the treatment of osteoarthritis, *Curr Rheumatol Rep* 2:472-7, 2000.

12. Hauselmann HJ: Nutripharmaceuticals for osteoarthritis, *Best Pract Res Clin Rheumatol* 15:595-607, 2001.

13. Kelly GS: The role of glucosamine sulfate and chondroitin sulfates in the treatment of degenerative joint disease, *Altern Med Rev* 3:27-39, 1998.

14. Glucosamine sulfate, *Altern Med Rev* 4:193-5, 1999.

15. Towheed TE, Anastassiades TP, Shea B, et al: Glucosamine therapy for treating osteoarthritis (Cochrane Review), *Cochrane Database Syst Rev* 1:CD002946, 2001.

16. Reginster JY, Deroisy R, Rovati LC, et al: Long-term effects of glucosamine sulphate on osteoarthritis progression: a randomised, placebo-controlled clinical trial, *Lancet* 357:251-60, 2001.

17. Deal CL, Moskowitz RW: Nutraceuticals as therapeutic agents in osteoarthritis. The role of glucosamine, chondroitin sulfate, and collagen hydrolysate, *Rheum Dis Clin North Am* 25:379-95, 1999.

18. McAlindon TE, LaValley MP, Gulin JP, et al: Glucosamine and chondroitin for treatment of osteoarthritis: a systematic quality assessment and meta-analysis, *JAMA* 283:1469-75, 2000.

19. Leffler CT, Philippi AF, Leffler SG, et al: Glucosamine, chondroitin, and manganese ascorbate for degenerative joint disease of the knee or low back: a randomized, double-blind, placebo-controlled pilot study, *Mil Med* 164:85-91, 1999.

20. de los Reyes GC, Koda RT, Lien EJ: Glucosamine and chondroitin sulfates in the treatment of osteoarthritis: a survey, *Prog Drug Res* 55:81-103, 2000.

21. Newnham RE: Essentiality of boron for healthy bones and joints, *Environ Health Perspect* 102(suppl 7): 83-5, 1994.

22. McAlindon T, Felson DT, Zhang Y, et al: Relation of dietary intake and serum levels of vitamin D to progression of osteoarthritis of the knee among participants in the Framingham study, *Ann Intern Med* 125:353-9, 1996.

23. McAlindon P, Jacques P, Zhang Y et al: Do antioxidant micronutrients protect against the development and progression of knee osteoarthritis? *Arthritis Rheum* 39:648-56, 1996.

24. Frei B, England L, Ames BN: Ascorbate is an outstanding antioxidant in human blood plasma, *Proc Natl Acad Sci U S A* 86:6377-81, 1989.

25. Machtey I, Ouaknine L: Tocopherol in osteoarthritis. A controlled pilot study, *J Am Geriat Soc* 26:328-30, 1978.

26. Goetzl EJ: Vitamin E modulates lipoxygenation of arachidonic acid in leukocytes, *Nature* 288:183-5, 1980.

27. Hill J, Bird HA: Failure of selenium-ace to improve osteoarthritis, *Br J Rheumatol* 29:211-3, 1990.

28. Werbach MR: *Textbook of nutritional medicine*, Tarzana, CA, 1999, Third Line Press.

29. Kurz B, Jost B, Schunke M: Dietary vitamins and selenium diminish the development of mechanically induced osteoarthritis and increase the expression of antioxidative enzymes in the knee joint of STR/1N mice, *Osteoarthritis Cartilage* 10:119-26, 2002.

30. Sowers M, Lachance L: Vitamins and arthritis. The roles of vitamins A, C, D, and E, *Rheum Dis Clin North Am* 25:315-32, 1999.
31. Perkins PJ, Doherty M: Nonpharmacologic therapy of osteoarthritis, *Curr Rheumatol Rep* 1:48-53, 1999.
32. Flynn MA, Irvin W, Krause G: The effect of folate and cobalamin on osteoarthritic hands, *J Am Coll Nutr* 13:351-6, 1994.
33. Little CV, Parsons T: Herbal therapy for treating osteoarthritis (Cochrane Review), *Cochrane Database Syst Rev* 1:CD002947, 2001.
34. Ernst E, Chrubasik S: Phyto-anti-inflammatories. A systematic review of randomized, placebo-controlled, double-blind trials, *Rheum Dis Clin North Am* 26:13-27, vii, 2000.
35. Chrubasik S, Junck H, Breitschwerdt H, et al: Effectiveness of harpagophytum extract WS 1531 in the treatment of exacerbation of low back pain: a randomized, placebo-controlled, double-blind study, *Eur J Anaesthesiol* 16: 118-29, 1999.
36. Chrubasik S, Eisenberg E, Balan E, et al: Treatment of low back pain exacerbations with willow bark extract: a randomized double-blind study, *Am J Med* 109:9-14, 2000.
37. Randall C, Randall H, Dobbs F, et al: Randomized controlled trial of nettle sting for treatment of base-of-thumb pain, *J R Soc Med* 93:305-9, 2000.

■ CHAPTER 37 ■

OSTEOPOROSIS

One in two women has an osteoporosis-related fracture in her lifetime. Major risk factors for osteoporosis are genotype, age, menopausal status, and lifestyle. However, genetic factors appear to be far more important than the combination of nutritional, hormonal, environmental, and lifestyle factors in the pathogenesis of osteoporosis.[1] In osteoporosis, an imbalance between bone resorption and bone formation results in decreased bone mass. Remodeling of bone takes place throughout adult life, with osteoclasts resorbing old bone and osteoblasts creating new bone; 3% of cortical and 25% of trabecular bone are remodeled each year. During the first 5 to 10 years after menopause, 2% to 4% of bone tissue is lost annually.

Management is initially focused on natural measures. A balanced diet including adequate calcium and vitamin D intake, appropriate exercise, smoking cessation, avoidance of excessive alcohol intake, and injury prevention are all important.[2] Nonpharmacologic management and the potential of nutraceuticals and functional foods to influence the course of osteoporosis have recently been reviewed.[3]

CLINICAL DIAGNOSIS

Osteoporosis is asymptomatic until a significant amount of bone mass has been lost. Two common clinical presentations are (1) loss of height with development of a dowager's hump and backache and (2) fractures after no or minor trauma. An imbalance of markers of bone formation (i.e., alkaline phosphatase and serum osteocalcin) and bone resorption (i.e., hydroxyproline, urinary calcium, and N-telopeptides) is present. Results of other laboratory tests are normal. Reduced bone mass can be detected by using dual-photon absorptiometry or computed tomography.

THERAPEUTIC STRATEGY

Bone is subject to continual remodeling; the efficacy of remodeling is affected by the nutrient environment. Bone is renewed through resorption of old bone by osteoclasts and formation of new bone by osteoblasts. Osteoclastic activity is stimulated by parathyroid hormone (PTH) when serum calcium levels are low. Conversely, calcitonin is secreted from the thyroid gland in response to hypercalcemia and antagonizes the bone-resorptive effects of PTH. Interaction between osteoclasts and osteoblasts is a coupled process. Bone formation is encouraged by sodium fluoride, anabolic fragments of PTH, and insulin-like growth factor. Primarily antiresorptive treatments include estrogen, calcium, bisphosphonates, and calcitonin. Estrogens enhance calcium absorption in postmenopausal women. Studies of early intervention in a cohort of postmenopausal women showed that calcium supplementation and alcohol use were significantly associated with reduced levels of urinary type I collagen cross-linked N-telopeptides (markers for bone resorption) and lower mean serum levels of osteocalcin (a marker of bone formation).[4] Calcium appears to dampen bone remodeling. Smoking was only associated with lower osteocalcin levels, and physical activity was not significantly associated with a change in either of the markers.[4]

Depressed bone formation plays a causal role in osteoporosis. Cytokine-induced nitric oxide production has been shown to inhibit osteoblast growth and differentiation in vitro. Results of an animal study confirmed that inducible nitric oxide synthetase–mediated osteoblast apoptosis and depressed bone formation are important in the pathogenesis of inflammation-mediated osteoporosis.[5] Three inflammatory cytokines—interleukin-1 (IL-1), interleukin-6 (IL-6), and tumor necrosis factor α (TNF-α)—increase osteoclast formation, activity, and lifespan.[6] Feedback interactions of the cytokines result in a small increase in IL-1 and TNF-α formation, leading to a significant increase in levels of all three cytokines, whereas lack of any one of these cytokines decreases the levels of the others.[7] The rapid rate of postmenopausal bone loss is mediated by these three inflammatory cytokines. Estrogen may reduce bone resorption by inhibiting the release of cytokines and removing the cytokine stimulus for osteoclast formation and bone loss. Osteoblasts have progesterone, not estrogen, receptors. Progesterone is the significant hormone at the level of bone synthesis.

The aim of intervention is to create an environment unfavorable to bone resorption or, at best, favorable to deposition. Adequate nutrition, coupled with modulation of inflammatory cytokines, is one intervention option. Nutrition is important for bone health at all ages.[8-10]

LIFESTYLE CHANGES

Skeletal health requires an adequate supply of nutrients. Calcium and vitamin D are essential for adequate bone mineral density; magnesium contributes to diverse processes that support bone remodeling; and fluorine and strontium have bone-forming effects, but in excess they may compromise bone strength.[8] Calcium and vitamin D are fundamental to nutritional preventive strategies. Inadequate calcium intake results in a predisposition to low peak bone mass and an increased risk of osteoporosis. Fractional calcium absorption ranges from 17% to 58% and is positively associated with body mass index, dietary fat, and serum 1,25 dihydroxyvitamin D and PTH concentrations.[11] It is inversely associated with total calcium intake, dietary fiber intake, alcohol consumption, physical activity, and symptoms of constipation. Dietary fat, dietary fiber, serum 1,25 dihydroxyvitamin D concentration, and alcohol consumption are independent predictors of calcium absorption, explaining 21% of the observed variation.

Dairy foods are a major source of dietary calcium. However, a review of the effects of dairy foods on bone health indicated that 53% of these effects were not significant and 5% were unfavorable.[12] The authors concluded that milk and yogurt are likely to be beneficial, but cottage cheese may adversely affect bone health. Women younger than 30 years are most likely to benefit. Researchers in the United States have reported that symptoms from lactose maldigestion are not a major impediment to the ingestion of a dairy-rich diet supplying approximately 1500 mg of calcium day, the amount required to reduce the severity of osteoporosis, according to a National Institutes of Health consensus conference.[13]

Soybeans provide a nondairy option. Soybeans contain around 138 mg of calcium per 90-g serving (one-half cup boiled soybeans), and bioavailability is largely equivalent to that in milk.[14] Human studies also show that soy protein consumption is associated with less excretion of calcium in the urine than consumption of equivalent amounts of whey or mixed animal protein.[15] For every gram of protein consumed, around 1 mg of calcium is lost in the urine. Sodium has a similar effect. For each gram of sodium ingested, the urinary calcium content increases by around 15 mg. However, it has recently been suggested that a reduction in salt intake from 9 g to 6 g per day cannot be considered an intervention measure in the prevention of osteoporosis.[1] In addition to calcium, soybeans contain flavonoids, which favor bone strength.

Tea is another source of flavonoids. Compared with persons who do not drink tea, tea drinkers were found to have significantly greater mean bone mineral density measurements at the lumbar spine and greater trochanter, but not at the femoral neck.[16] Tea drinking may protect against osteoporosis in older women, in contrast to coffee drinking, which is regarded as a risk factor for reduced bone mineral density. Results of a 3-month study suggest that prunes, 100 g daily, may exert positive effects on bone in postmenopausal women.[17] Animal studies have previously suggested that prunes, a rich source of flavonoids and phenolic compounds, are highly effective in modulating bone mass in an ovarian hormone–deficient rat model of osteoporosis.

Smoking is a risk factor for osteoporosis. A cross-sectional study of postmenopausal women showed that the impaired calcium absorption in smokers appeared to be due almost entirely to suppression of the PTH-calcitriol endocrine axis.[18] Impairment of calcium absorption could lead to accelerated bone loss and limit the usefulness of dietary calcium supplementation in smokers.

NUTRIENT THERAPY/DIETARY SUPPLEMENTS

Controlled clinical trials have indicated that, in addition to drinking milk regularly and eating soybeans, daily supplementation with ω-3 fatty acids (eicosapentaenoic acid, 1800-3600 mg, and docosahexaenoic acid, 1200-2400 mg) and correction of any deficiency of calcium, magnesium zinc, copper, or vitamins D and K may prevent or reverse osteoporosis.[19] A lack of consensus about different criteria used as a basis for estimating average requirements and population reference values has resulted in considerable variation in dietary recommendations for calcium and vitamin D.[20] Slow calcium turnover makes it difficult to conclusively determine the effects of deprivation or replenishment. Consequently, national recommendations vary: 700 mg/day in the United Kingdom and European Union, 800 mg/day in Australia, and 1000 mg/day in North America.[21] Calcium supplementation, beyond the recommended daily allowance, as a means of decreasing the risk of osteoporosis, is only effective in about half the population. Bone mineral density and turnover in adults are related to the vitamin D receptor gene. Only 50% of people have the heterozygous vitamin D receptor gene that is associated with a slowed rate of bone density loss during calcium supplementation.[22] Furthermore, although a placebo-controlled trial demonstrated that calcium citrate (400 mg twice daily) averted bone loss and stabilized bone density in the spine, femoral neck, and radial shaft in women relatively soon after menopause,[23] a calcium intake of 1 to 1.5 g daily plus vitamin D, 400 IU or more daily, is widely recommended for maintaining bone health in this group.[24]

In addition to some perplexity regarding the appropriate dose of calcium, there is some confusion regarding when to take the supplement. One study demonstrated that calcium loads up to 1000 mg had no significant effect on the markers of bone formation and resorption, although even small calcium doses (200 mg) decreased serum PTH levels and rapidly increased serum ionized calcium concentrations. This effect was similar whether calcium was taken in the morning or in the evening.[25] Another study of early postmenopausal women suggested that bone resorption fluctuates and peaks at night, reflecting the circadian rhythm of serum PTH. The authors of this study found that 1000 mg of calcium administered at 11:00 PM reduced bone resorption markers overnight and 500 mg of calcium administered in the morning had a similar effect during the day.[26] Calcium supplementation (625 mg of calcium carbonate three times daily) with a meal or combined calcium supplementation and estrogen therapy is not associated with a significant increased risk of calcium oxalate stone formation in the majority of postmenopausal patients with osteoporosis.[27]

Although calcium is the dominant mineral, other minerals are important. Animal experiments suggest that magnesium supplementation, despite apparently reducing calcium absorption, promotes bone formation, prevents bone resorption, and increases the dynamic strength of bone.[28] Boron is especially effective in cases of magnesium, potassium, and vitamin D deficiency.[4]

Vitamin D deficiency not only causes osteomalacia; it can also exacerbate osteoporosis. Certainly, evidence supports routine daily supplementation with 700 to 800 mg of calcium and 400 to 800 IU of vitamin D for elderly persons at risk for osteoporosis.[29] A population-based study of young women at 38° south latitude indicated that dietary intake of vitamin D was important for metabolism in winter but insignificant during summer.[30] The need for vitamin D supplementation varies with sun exposure. Furthermore, combined administration of vitamin D_3 (0.75 µg/day) and vitamin K_2 (45 mg/day) provided postmenopausal women with osteoporosis better protection against lumbar bone loss than calcium or either vitamin alone.[31] Vitamin K is essential for the activation of osteocalcin. Epidemiologic studies have shown that undercarboxylation of osteocalcin and the presence of an *apo epsilon4* allele are associated with an increased risk of fractures and reduced bone mineral density. Laboratory studies have shown that heparan sulfate proteoglycans on the cell surface and apolipoprotein E in the lipoprotein particles contribute to lipoprotein–vitamin K1 uptake by osteoblasts.[10] This mechanism clarifies the role of vitamin K in γ-carboxylation of γ-linolenic acid (GLA)–containing bone proteins such as osteocalcin and explains how suboptimal vitamin K status is linked to osteoporosis.

Another vitamin that benefits bone is vitamin C. Vitamin C is an important stimulus for osteoblast-derived proteins. A community-based cohort study demonstrated that vitamin C supplementation appeared to enhance bone mineral density, especially among postmenopausal women receiving concurrent estrogen therapy and calcium supplements.[32] Vitamin C appears to benefit bone health though diverse mechanisms including antioxidant protection, stimulation of osteoblast-derived proteins, and modulation of inflammatory cytokines. In humans, cytokine concentrations of TNF-α, IL-6, and IL-1 are significantly elevated immediately after participation in a marathon. Vitamin C supplementation at 1500 mg/day for 7 days before and 2 days after the race attenuated these increases.[33] A prospective study suggested that although an insufficient dietary intake of vitamins C and E may substantially increase the risk of hip fracture in current smokers, a more adequate intake seemed to be protective.[34]

In contrast to the protective effects of vitamins D, K, and C, vitamin A is a potential risk factor. In a cross-sectional, nested case-control study, retinol intake was found to be negatively associated with bone mineral density.[35] For every 1-mg increase in daily retinol intake, the risk for hip fracture was increased by 68%. For daily intakes greater than 1.5 mg, compared with intakes of less than 0.5 mg, bone mineral density was reduced by 6% for the total body, by 14% at the lumbar spine, and by 10% at the femoral neck with double the risk for a hip fracture.

In addition to minerals and vitamins, phytochemicals affect bone health. Bone mineral density in postmenopausal women, especially in the cortex of the radius and ulna, rose by approximately 4% during daily supplementation with a 57-mg isoflavone extract.[36] Isoflavones offer a range of possibilities. Ipriflavone, an isoflavone synthesized from the soy isoflavone daidzein, effectively inhibits bone resorption and enhances bone formation.[37] Ipriflavone's primary antiresorptive mechanisms involve inhibiting PTH-, vitamin D-, prostaglandin E_2-, and IL-1β–stimulated bone resorption. It also stimulates alkaline phosphatase activity, which is an indicator of new bone formation. Ipriflavone enhances the effect of low-dose estrogen on bone preservation and appears to exert its bone-protective effects by inhibiting osteoclastic activity and enhancing osteoblastic activity. It enhances estrogen's effect without possessing intrinsic estrogenic activity. Animal studies suggest that the protective effect of this synthetic isoflavone may be partly due to its ability to enhance calcium absorption.[38] Ipriflavone restrains bone loss in postmenopausal women and elderly men.

Isoflavones can also be obtained from soy protein isolates. In a study of perimenopausal women consuming isoflavones (80.4 mg daily) in soy protein isolates, bone loss from the lumbar spine was attenuated over a 24-week period.[39] A parallel-group, double-blind trial showed that soy protein, 40 g daily containing 2.25 mg isoflavones per gram of protein, significantly increased bone mineral content and density in the lumbar spine but not elsewhere.[40] Animal studies suggest that soy is more protective of trabecular bone than cortical bone. Despite conflicting results, health benefits are likely to be derived from consumption of 10 g of isoflavone-rich soy protein daily, an amount typical of the Asian diet and equivalent to 15% of the protein intake in the American diet.[41]

The risk-benefit profile of various treatments for osteoporosis—including calcium supplements, fluoride, and calcitriol—has recently been reviewed and compared.[42]

HERBAL THERAPY

A combined treatment regimen of a symptom-oriented herbal blend plus a high-potency vitamin/mineral was unsuccessful in protecting women against the predictable acceleration of bone mineral loss associated with the early postmenopausal period.[43] Nonetheless, two herbs, evening primrose oil and red clover, warrant mention. A red clover isoflavone preparation containing genistein, daidzein, formononetin, and biochanin increased the bone mineral density of the proximal radius and ulna by 4.1% over 6 months at a dosage of 57 mg/day and by 3.0% at a dosage of 85.5 mg/day.[37] The response, when 28.5 mg of isoflavones was administered daily, was not significant.

Evening primrose oil is an important source of GLA. Animal studies suggest that ω-3 and ω-6 essential fatty acid (GLA) supplementation may have a role in reducing the age-related decline in calcium absorption.[44] Dietary supplementation with flaxseed, flaxseed oil, and fish oil (eicosapentaenoic acid) significantly reduces cytokine production while increasing calcium absorption, bone calcium content, and bone density.[45] Supplementation with ω-3 fatty acids, such as flaxseed or fish oil, decreases the production of IL-1,

IL-6, and TNF-α in cell cultures. However, in a review of human studies there was no conclusive support for increasing the level of ω-3 fatty acids or manipulating the ratio of GLA to eicosapentaenoic acid in the diet to slow the rapid bone loss of menopause.[45]

PRACTICE TIPS

- Supplements used to reduce the risk of osteoporosis should include, at least, calcium, magnesium, and vitamin D.
- Calcium and vitamin D supplements can act as an adjunct to regular therapy.
- Bone density measurement is the best indicator of osteoporotic fracture risk; up to 50% of trabecular bone must be lost before this is detectable on plain x-ray films.
- Consumption of up to two cups of coffee daily is not a risk factor for osteoporosis, provided a glass of milk is consumed daily throughout adulthood.
- Girls accrue 50% of their total bone mass during puberty, compared with boys who accrue 22% during this period.

REFERENCES

1. Cohen AJ, Roe FJ: Review of risk factors for osteoporosis with particular reference to a possible aetiological role of dietary salt, *Food Chem Toxicol* 38: 237-53, 2000.
2. Management of postmenopausal osteoporosis: position statement of the North American Menopause Society, *Menopause* 9:84-101, 2002.
3. Mundy GR: Osteoporosis: pathophysiology and non-pharmacological management, *Best Pract Res Clin Rheumatol* 15:727-45, 2001.
4. Hla MM, Davis JW, Ross PD, et al: The relation between lifestyle factors and biochemical markers of bone turnover among early postmenopausal women, *Calcif Tissue Int* 68:291-6, 2001.
5. Armour KJ, Armour KE, van't Hof RJ, et al: Activation of the inducible nitric oxide synthase pathway contributes to inflammation-induced osteoporosis by suppressing bone formation and causing osteoblast apoptosis, *Arthritis Rheum* 44:2790-6, 2001.
6. Grimble RF: Nutritional modulation of cytokine biology, *Nutrition* 14:634-40, 1998.
7. Jilka RL: Cytokines, bone remodeling and estrogen deficiency: a 1998 update, *Bone* 23:75-81, 1998.
8. Schaafsma A, de Vries PJ, Saris WH: Delay of natural bone loss by higher intakes of specific minerals and vitamins, *Crit Rev Food Sci Nutr* 41:225-49, 2001.
9. Branca F, Vatuena S: Calcium, physical activity and bone health—building bones for a stronger future, *Public Health Nutr* 4:117-23, 2001.
10. Newman P, Bonello F, Wierzbicki AS, et al: The uptake of lipoprotein-borne phylloquinone (vitamin K1) by osteoblasts and osteoblast-like cells: role of

heparan sulfate proteoglycans and apolipoprotein E, *J Bone Miner Res* 17:426-33, 2002.

11. Wolf RL, Cauley JA, Baker CE, et al: Factors associated with calcium absorption efficiency in pre- and perimenopausal women, *Am J Clin Nutr* 72:466-71, 2000.

12. Weinsier RL, Krumdieck CL: Dairy foods and bone health: examination of the evidence, *Am J Clin Nutr* 72:681-9, 2000.

13. Suarez FL, Adshead J, Furne JK, Levitt MD: Lactose maldigestion is not an impediment to the intake of 1500 mg calcium daily as dairy products, *Am J Clin Nutr* 68:1118-22, 1998.

14. Weaver CM, Plawecki KL: Dietary calcium: adequacy of a vegetarian diet, *Am J Clin Nutr* 59(suppl 5):1238S-1241S, 1994.

15. Messina MJ: Legumes and soybeans: overview of their nutritional profiles and health effects, *Am J Clin Nutr* 70(suppl 3):439S-450S, 1999.

16. Hegarty VM, May HM, Khaw KT: Tea drinking and bone mineral density in older women, *Am J Clin Nutr* 71:1003-7, 2000.

17. Arjmandi BH, Khalil DA, Lucas EA, et al: Dried plums improve indices of bone formation in postmenopausal women, *J Womens Health Gend Based Med* 11:61-8, 2002.

18. Need AG, Kemp A, Giles N, et al: Relationships between intestinal calcium absorption, serum vitamin D metabolites and smoking in postmenopausal women, *Osteoporos Int* 13:83-8, 2002.

19. Wernbach MR: *Textbook of nutritional medicine*, Tarzana, CA, 1999, Third Line Press.

20. Prentice A: What are the dietary requirements for calcium and vitamin D? *Calcif Tissue Int* 70:83-8, 2002.

21. Nordin BC: Calcium requirement is a sliding scale, *Am J Clin Nutr* 71:1381-3, 2000.

22. Ferrari S, Rizzoli R, Chevalley T, et al: Vitamin-D-receptor-gene polymorphisms and change in lumbar-spine bone mineral density, *Lancet* 345:423-4, 1995.

23. Ruml LA, Sakhaee K, Peterson R, et al: The effect of calcium citrate on bone density in the early and mid-postmenopausal period: a randomized placebo-controlled study, *Am J Ther* 6:303-11, 1999.

24. Holick MF: Vitamin D and bone health, *J Nutr* 126(suppl 4):1159S-1164S, 1996.

25. Karkkainen MU, Lamberg-Allardt CJ, Ahonen S, et al: Does it make a difference how and when you take your calcium? The acute effects of calcium on calcium and bone metabolism, *Am J Clin Nutr* 74:335-42, 2001.

26. Scopacasa F, Need AG, Horowitz M, et al: Effects of dose and timing of calcium supplementation on bone resorption in early menopausal women, *Horm Metab Res* 34:44-7, 2002.

27. Domrongkitchaiporn S, Ongphiphadhanakul B, Stitchantrakul W, et al: Risk of calcium oxalate nephrolithiasis in postmenopausal women supplemented with calcium or combined calcium and estrogen, *Maturitas* 41:149-56, 2002.

28. Toba Y, Kajita Y, Masuyama R, et al: Dietary magnesium supplementation affects bone metabolism and dynamic strength of bone in ovariectomized rats, *J Nutr* 130:216-20, 2000.

29. Gennari C: Calcium and vitamin D nutrition and bone disease of the elderly, *Public Health Nutr* 4:547-59, 2001.

30. Pasco JA, Henry MJ, Nicholson GC, et al: Vitamin D status of women in the Geelong Osteoporosis Study: association with diet and casual exposure to sunlight, *Med J Aust* 175:401-5, 2001.

31. Iwamoto J, Takeda T, Ichimura S: Effect of combined administration of vitamin D$_3$ and vitamin K$_2$ on bone mineral density of the lumbar spine in postmenopausal women with osteoporosis, *J Orthop Sci* 5:546-51, 2000.

32. Morton DJ, Barrett-Connor EL, Schneider DL: Vitamin C supplement use and bone mineral density in postmenopausal women, *J Bone Miner Res* 16:135-40, 2001.

33. Nieman DC, Peters EM, Henson DA, et al: Influence of vitamin C supplementation on cytokine changes following an ultramarathon, *J Interferon Cytokine Res* 20:1029-35, 2000.

34. Melhus H, Michaelsson K, Holmberg L, et al: Smoking, antioxidant vitamins, and the risk of hip fracture, *J Bone Miner Res* 14:129-35, 1999.

35. Melhus H, Michaelsson K, Kindmark A, et al: Excessive dietary intake of vitamin A is associated with reduced bone mineral density and increased risk for hip fracture, *Ann Intern Med* 129:770-8, 1998.

36. Clifton-Bligh PB, Baber RJ, Fulcher GR, et al: The effect of isoflavones extracted from red clover (Rimostil) on lipid and bone metabolism, *Menopause* 8:259-65, 2001.

37. Head KA: Ipriflavone: an important bone-building isoflavone, *Altern Med Rev* 4:10-22, 1999.

38. Arjmandi BH, Khalil DA, Hollis BW: Ipriflavone, a synthetic phytoestrogen, enhances intestinal calcium transport in vitro, *Calcif Tissue Int* 67:225-9, 2000.

39. Alekel DL, Germain AS, Peterson CT, et al: Isoflavone-rich soy protein isolate attenuates bone loss in the lumbar spine of perimenopausal women, *Am J Clin Nutr* 72:844-52, 2000.

40. Potter SM, Baum JA, Teng H, et al: Soy protein and isoflavones: their effects on blood lipids and bone density in postmenopausal women, *Am J Clin Nutr* 68(suppl 6): 1375S-1379S, 1998.

41. Messina M, Gardner C, Barnes S: Gaining insight into the health effects of soy but a long way still to go: commentary on the fourth international symposium on the role of soy in preventing and treating chronic disease, *J Nutr* 132:547S-551S, 2002.

42. Kleerekoper M, Schein JR: Comparative safety of bone remodeling agents with a focus on osteoporosis therapies, *J Clin Pharmacol* 41:239-50, 2001.

43. Cook A, Pennington G: Phytoestrogen and multiple vitamin/mineral effects on bone mineral density in early postmenopausal women: a pilot study, *J Womens Health Gend Based Med* 11:53-60, 2002.

44. Claassen N, Coetzer H, Steinmann CM, et al: The effect of different n-6/n-3 essential fatty acid ratios on calcium balance and bone in rats, *Prostaglandins Leukot Essent Fatty Acids* 53:13-9, 1995.

45. Kettler DB: Can manipulation of the ratios of essential fatty acids slow the rapid rate of postmenopausal bone loss? *Altern Med Rev* 6:61-77, 2001.

■ CHAPTER 38 ■

PEPTIC ULCER SYNDROME

Peptic ulcer syndrome is a spectrum of conditions ranging from mild ulcer dyspepsia to gastric or duodenal ulceration. Although more patients have functional dyspepsia, those with ulceration are at risk of serious complications. Gastric cancer is a complication of gastric ulcers, and duodenal ulcers may hemorrhage or cause intestinal strictures. Psychologic predisposition, chemical exposure including cigarette smoking, ingestion of aspirin and nonsteroidal anti-inflammatory drugs (NSAIDs), and *Helicobacter pylori* infection are predisposing factors.

CLINICAL DIAGNOSIS

The typical presentation of peptic ulcer syndrome includes symptom periodicity, abdominal pain, and a relationship between pain and eating. The pain may be well localized in the epigastric area or be present as a gnawing ache in the right hypochondrium. Dyspeptic symptoms include heartburn, water brash, and flatulence.

THERAPEUTIC STRATEGY

In a literature review, it was estimated that psychosocial factors contribute to 30% to 65% of ulcers, whether related to NSAIDs, *H. pylori*, or neither.[1] Psychophysiologically stressed, ambitious, hardworking persons appear to be at increased risk. Health risk behaviors—including smoking, poor sleep habits, irregular meals, heavy drinking, and use of NSAIDs—are postulated to increase the duodenal acid load, alter blood flow, and impair gastroduodenal mucosal defenses, possibly by means of hypothalamic-pituitary-adrenal axis activation. The resistance of the gastric mucosa to injury is attributable to a series of factors collectively known as *mucosal defense*. Many components of mucosal defense are regulated by prostaglandins and nitric oxide.[2] Animal experiments showed leptin accelerates ulcer healing by mechanisms involving the upregulation of transforming growth factor α and increased production of nitric oxide caused by upregulation of constitutive nitric oxide synthase and inducible nitric oxide synthase in the area of the ulcer.[3] Impaired production of these mediators predisposes the stomach to injury.

NSAIDs are known to alter prostaglandin metabolism. *H. pylori* stimulates cytokine production by epithelial cells that recruit and activate immune and inflammatory cells in the underlying lamina propria, causing chronic, active gastritis. Although *H. pylori* alone may not be sufficient cause for peptic ulcer disease, both it and NSAIDs are independent causes of gastric and duodenal damage. Therefore it has been suggested that patients taking NSAIDs who are found to have gastric or duodenal ulcers should be tested for the bacterium and specifically treated.[4] Oxidative stress can be reduced by bacterial eradication in the first stages of mild gastritis.[5]

Strategies for the management of peptic ulcer syndrome focus on eradication of *H. pylori*, modifying the immune/inflammatory response, and enhancing host repair mechanisms.

LIFESTYLE CHANGES

Dietary intervention, which has tended to emphasize a bland diet and avoidance of alcohol and spices, has been largely unsatisfactory. Nonetheless, diet continues to be considered an important environmental factor contributing to peptic ulcer syndrome. In a review of 30 years of research Misciagna et al[6] concluded that soluble fiber from fruit and vegetables seems to be protective against duodenal ulcer, but refined sugars are a risk factor. Another cross-sectional population study indicated that subjects with a verified peptic ulcer had lower intakes of vegetables and fermented milk products.[7] Eating one cup of yogurt, especially a brand with viable bifidobacteria and lactobacilli, two or three times a day soothes an active ulcer. The intake of milk, meat, bread, and total fat—including saturated, monounsaturated fatty acids, and linolenic acid—was higher in the ulcer group.[7] On the other hand, particular fats may be beneficial.

Alarcon de las Lastra et al[8] have suggested that olive oil, with its elevated content of antioxidant agents, may alter gastric secretion in response to food; they report that a diet rich in olive oil was associated with a high percentage of gastric ulcer healing and afforded greater resistance to NSAID-induced gastric ulcerogenesis. Animal peptic ulcer models have shown that the lipid fraction in certain foodstuffs has a protective effect.[9] Jayaraj et al[9] speculate that *H. pylori* infection might be explained by the presence or absence of protective lipids or ulcerogenic factors in the staple human diet. Lipid obtained from stored polished rice or rice bran is ulcerogenic in animal models.

Some clinical and laboratory evidence supports the use of cabbage, rhubarb, and licorice for peptic ulcer disease.[10] Although cabbage is often avoided by ulcer-prone patients, controlled trials have shown that 1 L of raw cabbage juice daily protects against ulcer recurrence.[11] Animal studies suggest this may be due to its *S*-methylmethionine and glutamine content. Half a head of cabbage in the form of juice or eaten raw may help alleviate an ulcer flare-up.

NUTRIENT THERAPY/DIETARY SUPPLEMENTS

The efficacy of aluminum, bismuth, and magnesium in treating peptic ulcers is generally accepted. Controlled clinical trials have demonstrated that calcium carbonate, 1000 mg, 60 to 180 minutes before meals and at bedtime serves as a potent antacid, and ω-3 fatty acids, zinc (zinc sulfate, 220 mg three times daily), and vitamin C (1 g daily) have each been shown to offer a degree of protection against aspirin- or NSAID-induced ulceration.[11] Short-term administration of 50,000 IU of vitamin A daily improves ulcer healing, as does use of 200 mg of D,L-cysteine four times daily. Several other nutrients are also believed to promote healing.[11]

Nutritional attempts to eradicate or at least control *H. pylori* include the use of cranberry juice and probiotics in the form of lactobacilli. A high molecular mass constituent derived from cranberry juice inhibits the sialic acid–specific adhesion of *H. pylori* to human gastric mucus and erythrocytes.[12] Human *Lactobacillus acidophilus* strain LB secretes an antibacterial substance(s) that disadvantages *H. pylori*.[13] Resolution of intestinal metaplasia of the gastric mucosa after eradication of *H. pylori* is promoted by administration of 500 mg of ascorbic acid after the midday meal.[14] Because *H. pylori* infection increases the risk of gastric cancer, it is noteworthy that results of a randomized trial confirmed that dietary supplementation with vitamin C and beta-carotene may interfere with the precancerous process.[15]

HERBAL THERAPY

Various herbs may be used. Administration of licorice and mucilaginous herbs some 30 minutes before eating in the case of duodenal ulcers and just before eating in the case of gastric ulcers may enhance healing and protect gastric mucosa.[16] Licorice enhances gastric mucoprotection and pancreatic bicarbonate secretion in the duodenum. Licorice root can safely be used for treating duodenal and gastric ulcers, but in excess doses can cause hypokalemia, hypertension, and heart failure.[17]

Meadowsweet (*Filipendula ulmaria*), used as a gentle astringent, normalizes stomach acid even in patients taking salicylates. Mucilages such as slippery elm (*Ulmus fulva*) may benefit patients with hyperacidity and inflammation when taken before meals for gastric problems and after meals for reflux esophagitis. Peppermint oil may benefit nonulcer dyspepsia, provided a preexisting reflux problem is not worsened by relaxation of the cardiac sphincter.[10] Bitter herbs such as dandelion (*Taraxacum officinale*) or gentian (*Gentiana lutea*) may enhance the tone of the gastroesophageal sphincter and improve gastric emptying; however, bitter herbs do increase gastric acidity.[16]

Chamomile (*Matricaria recutita*) is taken for its anti-inflammatory effect to interrupt the tissue destruction cycle and provide symptomatic relief through its spasmolytic and carminative activities. Raw crushed garlic[18] and goldenseal (500-mg tablet) can be taken for their antibacterial effects. Echinacea may also enhance immunity and reduce the risk of *H. pylori* establishing itself in the ulcer crater. Anxious patients may benefit from valerian.

PRACTICE TIPS

- Bananas and one teaspoon of fresh ginger or one-half teaspoon of powdered ginger in a cup of boiling water may be used for relief of dyspepsia.
- Heartburn may be precipitated by consumption of chocolate, peppermint, or spicy or fatty foods.
- Cranberry juice increases vitamin B_{12} absorption in patients receiving omeprazole, a proton pump inhibitor.
- Ginger, by increasing gastric secretion, may decrease the effectiveness of antacids.
- Manuka honey may help to relieve ulcers; however, the honey must be unpasteurized. Therefore the label should read "active manuka honey." One tablespoon, to be taken on an empty stomach at night, is recommended for patients with ulcers.
- Chronic heartburn may be eased with 1000 mg of pantothenic acid administered twice daily plus 500 mg of choline administered as lecithin three times daily.

REFERENCES

1. Levenstein S: The very model of a modern etiology: a biopsychosocial view of peptic ulcer, *Psychosom Med* 62:176-85, 2000.
2. Wallace JL: Nonsteroidal anti-inflammatory drugs and the gastrointestinal tract. mechanisms of protection and healing: current knowledge and future research, *Am J Med* 110(1A):19S-23S, 2001.
3. Konturek PC, Brzozowski T, Sulekova Z, et al: Role of leptin in ulcer healing, *Eur J Pharmacol* 414:87-97, 2001.
4. Lazzaroni M, Porro GB: Review article: *Helicobacter pylori* and NSAID gastropathy, *Aliment Pharmacol Ther* 15(suppl 1):22-7, 2001.
5. Pignatelli B, Bancel B, Plummer M, et al: *Helicobacter pylori* eradication attenuates oxidative stress in human gastric mucosa, *Am J Gastroenterol* 96:1758-66, 2001.
6. Misciagna G, Cisternino AM, Freudenheim J: Diet and duodenal ulcer, *Dig Liver Dis* 32:468-72, 2000.
7. Elmstahl S, Svensson U, Berglund G: Fermented milk products are associated to ulcer disease. Results from a cross-sectional population study, *Eur J Clin Nutr* 52:668-74, 1998.
8. Alarcon de la Lastra C, Barranco MD, Motilva V, et al: Mediterranean diet and health: biological importance of olive oil, *Curr Pharm Des* 7:933-50, 2001.
9. Jayaraj AP, Tovey FI, Lewin MR, et al: Duodenal ulcer prevalence: experimental evidence for the possible role of dietary lipids, *J Gastroenterol Hepatol* 15:610-6, 2000.

10. Pinn G: The herbal basis of some gastroenterology therapies, *Aust Fam Phys* 30:254-8, 2001.
11. Werbach MR: *Textbook of nutritional medicine*, Tarzana, CA, 1999, Third Line Press.
12. Burger O, Ofek I, Tabak M, et al: A high molecular mass constituent of cranberry juice inhibits *Helicobacter pylori* adhesion to human gastric mucus, *FEMS Immunol Med Microbiol* 29:295-301, 2000.
13. Coconnier MH, Lievin V, Hemery E, et al: Antagonistic activity against *Helicobacter* infection in vitro and in vivo by the human *Lactobacillus acidophilus* strain LB, *Appl Environ Microbiol* 64:4573-80, 1998.
14. Zullo A, Rinaldi V, Hassan C, et al: Ascorbic acid and intestinal metaplasia in the stomach: a prospective, randomized study, *Aliment Pharmacol Ther* 14:1303-9, 2000.
15. Correa P, Fontham ET, Bravo JC, et al: Chemoprevention of gastric dysplasia: randomized trial of antioxidant supplements and anti-*Helicobacter pylori* therapy, *J Natl Cancer Inst* 92:1881-8, 2000.
16. Mills S, Bone K: *Principles and practice of phytotherapy*, Edinburgh, 2000, Churchill Livingstone.
17. Craig WJ: Health-promoting properties of common herbs, *Am J Clin Nutr* 70(suppl 3):491S-499S, 1999.
18. Cellini L, Di Campli E, Masulli M, et al: Inhibition of *Helicobacter pylori* by garlic extract (*Allium sativum*), *FEMS Immunol Med Microbiol* 13:273-7, 1996.

■ CHAPTER 39 ■

PERIPHERAL ARTERIAL DISEASE

Over 8 million people in the United States have peripheral arterial disease; up to one half of these individuals are symptomatic. Furthermore, subjects with evidence of peripheral vascular or cardiac disease have, on average, a significant reduction in cognitive function equivalent to about 4 or 5 years of additional age.[1] Because underlying atherosclerosis is an important factor in peripheral vascular disease, it is common practice to routinely implement conservative strategies to reduce the risk of ischemia (see chapter 33). Despite consensus to treat risk factors for peripheral arterial disease and use exercise rehabilitation for patients with claudication, only antiplatelet therapy and possibly angiotensin-converting enzyme inhibitors for the prevention of ischemic events are conclusively supported by results of placebo-controlled trials that specifically investigated peripheral arterial disease.[2]

CLINICAL DIAGNOSIS

The extent of occlusion, the collateral circulation, and the functional demands of the area determine the clinical presentation of occlusive arterial disease. Intermittent claudication and absent distal pulses are indicative of impaired limb perfusion. Muscle ischemia presents as pain in the calves, buttocks, thigh, or feet. The pain is exacerbated by exercise. The distance a patient can walk without needing to stop and rest is used as an indication of the severity of the disease. Ischemia produces a pale limb, possibly with patchy cyanotic discoloration. In chronic cases, nails are deformed and slow growing; muscles are atrophied; and the skin is shiny, atrophic, and hairless. Ischemic neuritis may cause shooting pains and paresthesia.

THERAPEUTIC STRATEGY

The focus of treatment for peripheral arterial disease is to improve limb viability and modify risk factors that predispose to and exacerbate the condition. Impaired limb perfusion causes metabolic imbalance. Metabolic derangements, including impaired oxygen delivery and/or extraction, reduced nitric oxide synthesis, reduced glucose oxidation, accumulation of toxic metabolites, and reduced carnitine availability all correlate with disease severity.[3] Interventions to maintain and improve perfusion of the ischemic limb are designed to both prevent further occlusion of the compromised artery and to enhance dilation and growth of collateral vessels. When successful, these measures substantially improve the patient's quality of life by reducing the severity of claudication.

Strong independent modifiable risk factors associated with the pathogenesis of peripheral arterial disease are cigarette smoking, diabetes mellitus, an increased fibrinogen level, and/or increased systolic blood pressure.[4] High plasma concentrations of homocysteine and low plasma concentrations of folate have also been identified as significant independent risk factors in older people.[5] One study suggests that, of all the variables that increase the risk of atherosclerosis, diabetes and cigarette smoking pose the greatest risk[6]; another identifies the ratio of total cholesterol to high-density lipoprotein cholesterol and the C-reactive protein level as the strongest independent predictors.[7] Certainly, the serum C-reactive protein level, independently of previous ischemic heart disease, is a strong predictor of myocardial infarction in patients with peripheral vascular disease who require revascularization.[8] These risk factors are evidence of, or suggest a predisposition to, chronic inflammation, an important process in the pathogenesis of atherothrombosis.

LIFESTYLE CHANGES

Two lifestyle choices that benefit patients with overt or incipient peripheral arterial disease are exercise and being a nonsmoker. Nicotine and other products of cigarette smoke adversely affect lipids, blood coagulation, and vascular stability.[9] The proatherogenic effects of smoking that injure the endothelium are observed, to a lesser extent, in passive smokers. Smoking and smokers should be avoided.

Regular aerobic exercise stimulates vessel wall relaxation and development of a collateral circulation. Meta-analysis shows that patients with claudication who persisted with an exercise program for 6 or more months can increase their pain-free walking time by 180% and their maximal walking time by 120%.[10] Walking three or more times per week for at least 30 minutes (or until pain cannot be tolerated) is recommended. Another study showed that 12 weeks of treadmill walking for 1 hour a day on 3 days of the week increased pain-free walking time and decreased the resting plasma short-chain acylcarnitine concentration. The reduced acylcarnitine levels correlated with improvement in peak walking time.[11] Reduced pain and a transient increase in urinary nitrite/nitrate excretion resulting from exercise suggest that the underlying mechanism may involve nitric oxide.[12] All persons with peripheral arterial disease should exercise regularly.

NUTRIENT THERAPY/DIETARY SUPPLEMENTS

Controlled clinical trials have demonstrated that patients with arterial insufficiency benefit from any one of the following: L-carnitine, 2 g daily; vitamin E, 300 to 1600 IU daily; inositol hexanicotinate, 1 to 2 g daily; ω-6 fatty acids, 4 g daily; and vitamin C, 500 mg three times daily.[13] Uncontrolled trials suggest that flavonoids, folic acid, glycosaminoglycans, vitamin B_6, and correction of magnesium deficiency are beneficial.

Carnitine plays a major role in energy production at the mitochondrial level through stimulation of fatty acid metabolism. It improves glucose disposal, may reduce insulin resistance, and is important in energy production in muscle. Carnitine and its derivative, propionyl-L-carnitine, are endogenous cofactors that enhance carbohydrate metabolism and reduce the intracellular accumulation of toxic metabolites in hypoxic conditions. A randomized, double-blind, placebo-controlled trial demonstrated that propionyl-L-carnitine, in doses of 2 g daily taken over a 6-month period, increased peak walking time and delayed the onset of pain.[14] In addition to walking performance, preliminary data have suggested that 4 or more weeks of supplementation increased muscle strength in these patients.[15] Another study in which a similar daily dose was used indicated that although propionyl-L-carnitine benefited patients with severe claudication with maximal walking distance of 250 meters or less, it did not benefit those with mild functional impairment.[16] At these therapeutic doses, only minor side effects (e.g., nausea) have been reported.

In addition to targeting energy production in an effort to limit anoxic damage, another therapeutic approach is to enhance perfusion. Interventions to reduce further vascular occlusion may represent attempts to dampen inflammation by using antioxidants and ω-3 fatty acids. Three months of administration of 40 g of extra-virgin olive oil and 16 g of fish oil daily favors a less atherogenic plasma-lipid profile in patients with peripheral vascular disease.[17]

Vitamins may have beneficial effects. Vitamin C in doses of 500 mg three times daily is occasionally recommended. The vitamin C concentration is lower in patients with higher C-reactive protein levels and more severe peripheral arterial disease.[18]

Vitamin E, a lipid-soluble vitamin, is a potent antioxidant and, at high doses, may inhibit platelet aggregation. However, long-term supplementation with α-tocopherol (50 mg/day) and beta-carotene (20 mg/day) produced no symptomatic benefit in smokers,[19] and no preventive effect was apparent from the ingestion of 50 mg (75 IU) of vitamin E per day.[20] Nonetheless, clinical trials assessing vitamin E in the treatment of peripheral vascular disease are flawed and vitamin E remains a possible option. Vitamin E in doses of 300 to 1600 IU daily is frequently used. A more effective therapeutic choice may be α-tocopheryl nicotinate (200 mg three times daily).

Niacin is vital to cellular metabolism, principally through its role in the coenzymes nicotinamide adenine dinucleotide and nicotinamide adenine dinucleotide phosphate, in oxidation-reduction reactions. It also improves the lipid profile. Niacin supplementation decreases low-density lipoprotein cholesterol and plasma fibrinogen levels in subjects with peripheral vascular disease.[21,22] Although the recommended dosage range is 1.5 to 4 g daily, taken in two or three doses, niacin in doses of 100 to 300 mg daily causes flushing and provides temporary pain relief. Significant improvement in patients with peripheral vascular disease has also been reported with administration of 2 g of inositol nicotinate twice daily for at least 3 months.[23] Inositol nicotinate contains six molecules of niacin. Although arterial dilation may be a factor, it has been postulated that reduction in fibrinogen level, improvement in blood viscosity, and resultant improvement in oxygen transport all contribute to its therapeutic efficacy. Although high-dose niacin is reported to induce unwanted reactions including flushing, pruritus, gastrointestinal complaints, and impaired glucose tolerance, no adverse effects have been reported in response to inositol hexaniacinate in doses of 4 g daily.

L-Arginine has been found to be effective in a few patients with peripheral vascular disease.[3] It is a safe, semi-essential amino acid that increases nitric oxide production and improves endothelial function.[24] Endothelium-derived nitric oxide favors vasodilation, inhibits platelet aggregation, modulates leukocyte adherence, and inhibits proliferation of smooth muscle cells.[25]

HERBAL THERAPY

Herbs that may improve vascular perfusion include ginkgo and garlic. In a meta-analysis of eight randomized, placebo-controlled, double-blind trials, Pittler and Ernst[26] concluded that *Ginkgo biloba* extract was superior to placebo in the symptomatic treatment of intermittent claudication. Although ginkgo extracts are significantly more effective than placebo in increasing walking distance, the magnitude of the overall treatment effect is modest and of uncertain clinical relevance.[27] Nonetheless, a dose of 60 mg two or three times a day is suggested.[28]

Garlic enhances relaxation of blood vessel walls, inhibits platelet aggregation, tends to normalize plasma lipid levels, enhances fibrinolytic activity, and reduces blood pressure and glucose levels.[29] The therapeutic dose and nature of garlic supplementation are unclear. Fresh garlic is most effective if consumed raw.[30] Aged garlic extract has moderate cholesterol-lowering, blood pressure–reducing, selective platelet aggregation, and adhesion-inhibiting effects at doses of 2.4 to 7.2 g/day.[31] Taking garlic in doses of 800 mg (powdered) each day over 5 or more weeks increases the pain-free walking distance in patients with intermittent claudication.[32] In a review of randomized trials of garlic therapy in patients with lower limb atherosclerosis, Jepson et al[33] found only one small trial of short duration that reported no positive effect on walking distance. The safety of garlic as a long-term treatment for intermittent claudication is uncertain.

PRACTICE TIPS

- L-Carnitine, 3 g daily, eases muscle pain caused by overexercise.
- Magnesium, 400 mg daily, will benefit patients with peripheral vascular disease who are magnesium-deficient.
- Aspirin in doses of 150 mg/day decreases platelet aggregation but increases the risk of bleeding peptic ulcers.
- Garlic, 800 mg/day, decreases platelet aggregation and can be used synergistically with vitamin E, 400 IU daily, to decrease platelet adhesiveness.
- Popular belief suggests that use of vitamin E, 500 IU daily for 1 month, may relieve muscle cramps.
- Anecdotal evidence suggests that 4.8 g of calcium gluconate at bedtime reduces muscle cramps.

REFERENCES

1. Elwood PC, Pickering J, Bayer A, et al: Vascular disease and cognitive function in older men in the Caerphilly cohort, *Age Ageing* 31:43-8, 2002.
2. Regensteiner JG, Hiatt WR: Current medical therapies for patients with peripheral arterial disease: a critical review, *Am J Med* 112:49-57, 2002.
3. Brevetti G, Corrado S, Martone VD, et al: Microcirculation and tissue metabolism in peripheral arterial disease, *Clin Hemorheol Microcirc* 21:245-54, 1999.
4. Meijer WT, Grobbee DE, Hunink MG, et al: Determinants of peripheral arterial disease in the elderly: the Rotterdam study, *Arch Intern Med* 160:2934-8, 2000.
5. Aronow WS, Ahn C: Association between plasma homocysteine and peripheral arterial disease in older persons, *Coron Artery Dis* 9:49-50, 1998.
6. Creager MA: Medical management of peripheral arterial disease, *Cardiol Rev* 9:238-45, 2001.
7. Ridker PM, Stampfer MJ, Rifai N: Novel risk factors for systemic atherosclerosis: a comparison of C-reactive protein, fibrinogen, homocysteine, lipoprotein(a), and standard cholesterol screening as predictors of peripheral arterial disease, *JAMA* 285:2481-5, 2001.
8. Rossi E, Biasucci LM, Citterio F, et al: Risk of myocardial infarction and angina in patients with severe peripheral vascular disease: predictive role of C-reactive protein, *Circulation* 105:800-3, 2002.
9. Powell JT: Vascular damage from smoking: disease mechanisms at the arterial wall, *Vasc Med* 3:21-8, 1998.
10. Regensteiner JG: Exercise in the treatment of claudication: assessment and treatment of functional impairment, *Vasc Med* 2:238-42, 1997.
11. Hiatt WR, Regensteiner JG, Hargarten ME, et al: Benefit of exercise conditioning for patients with peripheral arterial disease, *Circulation* 81:602-9, 1990.

12. Arosio E, Cuzzolin L, De Marchi S, et al: Increased endogenous nitric oxide production induced by physical exercise in peripheral arterial occlusive disease patients, *Life Sci* 65:2815-22, 1999.

13. Werbach MR: *Textbook of nutritional medicine*, Tarzana, CA, 1999, Third Line Press.

14. Hiatt WR, Regensteiner JG, Creager MA, et al: Propionyl-L-carnitine improves exercise performance and functional status in patients with claudication, *Am J Med* 110:616-22, 2001.

15. Barker GA, Green S, Askew CD, et al: Effect of propionyl-L-carnitine on exercise performance in peripheral arterial disease, *Med Sci Sports Exerc* 33: 1415-22, 2001.

16. Brevetti G, Diehm C, Lambert D: European multicenter study on propionyl-L-carnitine in intermittent claudication, *J Am Coll Cardiol* 34:1618-24, 1999.

17. Ramirez-Tortosa MC, Suarez A, Gomez MC, et al: Effect of extra-virgin olive oil and fish-oil supplementation on plasma lipids and susceptibility of low-density lipoprotein to oxidative alteration in free-living Spanish male patients with peripheral vascular disease, *Clin Nutr* 18:167-74, 1999.

18. Langlois M, Duprez D, Delanghe J, et al: Serum vitamin C concentration is low in peripheral arterial disease and is associated with inflammation and severity of atherosclerosis, *Circulation* 103:1863-8, 2001.

19. Tornwall ME, Virtamo J, Haukka JK, et al: The effect of alpha-tocopherol and beta-carotene supplementation on symptoms and progression of intermittent claudication in a controlled trial, *Atherosclerosis* 147:193-7, 1999.

20. Swain RA, Kaplan-Machlis B: Therapeutic uses of vitamin E in prevention of atherosclerosis, *Altern Med Rev* 4:414-23, 1999.

21. Philipp CS, Cisar LA, Saidi P, et al: Effect of niacin supplementation on fibrinogen levels in patients with peripheral vascular disease, *Am J Cardiol* 82:697-9, A9, 1998.

22. Chesney CM, Elam MB, Herd JA, et al: Effect of niacin, warfarin, and antioxidant therapy on coagulation parameters in patients with peripheral arterial disease in the Arterial Disease Multiple Intervention Trial (ADMIT), *Am Heart J* 140:631-6, 2000.

23. Inositol hexaniacinate, *Altern Med Rev* 3:222-3, 1998.

24. Lerman A, Suwaidi JA, Velianou JL: L-Arginine: a novel therapy for coronary artery disease? *Expert Opin Investig Drugs* 8:1785-93, 1999.

25. Brown AA, Hu FB: Dietary modulation of endothelial function: implications for cardiovascular disease, *Am J Clin Nutr* 73:673-86, 2001.

26. Pittler MH, Ernst E: *Ginkgo biloba* extract for the treatment of intermittent claudication: a meta-analysis of randomized trials, *Am J Med* 108:276-81, 2000.

27. Linde K, ter Riet G, Hondras M, et al: Systematic reviews of complementary therapies—an annotated bibliography. Part 2: herbal medicine, *BMC Complement Altern Med* 1:5, 2001.

28. Glisson J, Crawford R, Street S: The clinical applications of *Ginkgo biloba*, St. John's wort, saw palmetto, and soy, *Nurse Pract* 24:28, 31, 35-36, 1999.

29. Rahman K: Historical perspective on garlic and cardiovascular disease, *J Nutr* 131(3s):977S-979S, 2001.

30. Ali M, Bordia T, Mustafa T: Effect of raw versus boiled aqueous extract of garlic and onion on platelet aggregation, *Prostaglandins Leukot Essent Fatty Acids* 60: 43-7, 1999.

31. Steiner M, Li W: Aged garlic extract, a modulator of cardiovascular risk factors: a dose-finding study on the effects of AGE on platelet functions, *J Nutr* 131(3s):980S-984S, 2001.
32. Kieswetter H, Jung F, Jung EM, et al: Effects of garlic coated tablets in peripheral arterial occlusive disease, *Clin Investig* 7:383-6, 1993.
33. Jepson RG, Kleijnen J, Leng GC: Garlic for peripheral arterial occlusive disease, *Cochrane Database Syst Rev* 2:CD000095, 2000.

■ CHAPTER 40 ■

PREMENSTRUAL SYNDROME

Premenstrual syndrome (PMS) refers to a group of menstruation-related disorders that are estimated to affect up to 40% of women of childbearing age. PMS, sometimes referred to as *premenstrual tension (PMT)*, is a constellation of psychologic, behavioral, and somatic symptoms that occur in most cycles and remit after menstruation. True PMS only occurs during the luteal phase of the menstrual cycle, with a symptom-free period during the follicular phase.[1]

Despite overlaps, a number of dominant clinical presentations have been described, and a discrete pathogenesis has been postulated.[2] PMT-A is attributed to hormonal imbalance with a relative estrogen excess and progesterone deficiency; PMT-C, to prostaglandin E_1 deficiency and increased carbohydrate tolerance with functional hypoglycemia; PMT-D, to low estrogen levels; PMT-H, to aldosterone excess; and PMT-P, to prostaglandin imbalance.[3] Approximately 5% of women with PMS have PMT-D, one of the more disabling and severe forms of PMS.[4]

CLINICAL DIAGNOSIS

Major clinical findings include mood lability, irritability, fatigue, and breast swelling and tenderness. PMT-A is characterized by psychologic symptoms such as anxiety, irritability, mood swings, and tension. Sugar craving and an increased appetite, headaches, fatigue, dizziness, and palpitations dominate the clinical picture of PMT-C. Patients with PMT-D complain of depression, forgetfulness, confusion, and insomnia. Fluid retention, breast tenderness, and abdominal bloating trouble patients with PMT-H; and their weight may fluctuate by more than 3 kg in each cycle. Patients with PMT-P have a reduced pain threshold and complain of dysmenorrhea.

THERAPEUTIC STRATEGY

Although various natural approaches have been advocated for the reduction of certain symptoms of PMS, the efficacy of nutritional and herbal interventions is disputed. A review of seven trials of herbal medicine and 13 trials of dietary supplements revealed no compelling evidence for using these therapies in the management of PMS.[5] However, most trials did have various methodological limitations, including failure to discriminate among the various symptom patterns. Because each clinical pattern is associated with a particular hormonal or metabolic imbalance, the dominant clinical presentation, or type of PMS, can be easily identified. Therapy is focused on appropriate symptomatic intervention.

LIFESTYLE CHANGES

Nutrient analysis of the diet diaries of women with PMS showed a significant increase in total energy and all macronutrients before menstruation when compared with nutrient intake after menstruation.[6] When adjusted for energy, the diets of women with PMS showed a significant premenstrual increase in fat, carbohydrate, and simple sugars compared with the diets of women without PMS. Anecdotal evidence suggests that women on a diet rich in fruits, vegetables, and soy products and low in dairy products and saturated fat before menstruation often experience fewer premenstrual symptoms. Despite inadequate scientific validation, nutritional modification has not been rejected as a therapeutic option, particularly for women with certain symptom patterns.

A crossover study of women showed that a low-fat vegetarian diet was associated with an increased serum sex hormone binding globulin concentration and reductions in body weight, duration and intensity of dysmenorrhea, and duration of premenstrual symptoms.[7] A high intake of complex carbohydrates rich in flavonoids is postulated to modulate human estrogen levels. Dietary avoidance of animal products in favor of plant products may modify gut bacteria and recirculation of glucuronide-linked estrogen. Restriction of animal fats, including dairy products, and trans fatty acids influences estrogen levels. Such dietary changes, particularly when combined with a low salt (<3 g/day) intake, may benefit patients with PMT-H. A diet rich in complex carbohydrates, fiber, and seeds and the use of cold-pressed oils may have a general benefit; and limiting the intake of alcohol, tea, coffee, chocolate, and sugar to less than 6 tablespoons daily may be particularly helpful for patients with PMT-D.

NUTRIENT THERAPY/DIETARY SUPPLEMENTS

Although many types of dietary supplements have been advocated for symptomatic relief of premenstrual syndrome, only calcium was demonstrated to have significant benefit in a large, rigorous, double-blind, placebo-controlled trial.[8] Calcium reduces emotional, behavioral, and physical symptoms of PMS. It has been hypothesized that women with symptoms during the luteal phase have an underlying calcium dysregulation with secondary hyperparathyroidism and vitamin D deficiency. PMS is postulated to be a clinical manifestation of a calcium deficiency state unmasked after the rise in ovarian steroid hormone concentrations during the menstrual cycle. Estrogen regulates calcium metabolism, intestinal calcium absorption, and parathyroid hormone gene expression and secretion. Alterations in calcium homeostasis have long been associated with many affective disturbances such as those encountered in PMS in general and in PMT-A in particular. Symptoms of PMS and hypocalcemia are similar, and clinical trials in women with PMS have demonstrated that calcium supplementation effectively alleviates the majority of mood and somatic symptoms.[9] A prospective, randomized, double-blind, placebo-controlled, parallel-group, multicenter, clinical trial demonstrated that 1200 mg of elemental calcium, administered daily in the form of calcium carbonate, reduced luteal-phase symptoms in women with PMS.[10] In a literature review, Ward and Holimon[11] concluded that calcium supplementation of 1200 to 1600 mg/day, unless contraindicated, should be considered a sound treatment option for women who experience PMS. The supplemental dose of calcium can be adjusted downward in the few patients who routinely consume large quantities of calcium in their diet.

Preliminary trials have suggested potential efficacy of tryptophan in the treatment of PMS.[12] A randomized, controlled, clinical trial indicated that patients with premenstrual dysphoric disorder characteristic of PMT-A benefited from treatment with 6 g of L-tryptophan administered daily over three consecutive cycles.[13] Results suggested that increasing serotonin synthesis during the late luteal phase of the menstrual cycle was therapeutic.

Results of some clinical trials also support the use of vitamins in PMS. In a randomized, double-blind study in which 400 IU of d-α-tocopherol was administered over three cycles, significant improvement in certain affective and physical symptoms was observed.[14] Vitamin E has been successfully used to decrease mastalgia, headaches, fatigue, depression, and insomnia. In daily doses of 300 to 400 IU, vitamin E reduces symptoms in patients with PMT-A and PMT-D.

A review of randomized, placebo-controlled trials of the effectiveness of vitamin B_6 in the management of PMS indicated that doses of vitamin B_6 up to 100 mg daily are likely to reduce premenstrual symptoms and premenstrual depression.[15] Administration of vitamin B_6 in doses of 40 to 100 mg, starting 3 days before the onset of symptoms and continuing until menstruation, appears to have some success in relieving headaches, fatigue, irritability, and edema. In a randomized, double-blind, placebo-controlled, crossover trial that investigated daily dietary supplementation with 50 mg of vitamin B_6 and 200 mg of magnesium (as magnesium oxide), this combination was found to be particularly useful for reducing PMT-A symptoms.[16] Vitamin B_6 increases cell membrane transfer and utilization of magnesium. Even magnesium in doses of 4.5 mg daily for 9 days, starting 7 days before menstruation, may be effective in patients with mastalgia, weight gain, and nervous tension.

It has also been suggested that administration of vitamin A (100,000 IU), twice a day from day 15 to the onset of menses for two to six cycles, may reduce edema and mastodynia and provide some relief of dysmenorrhea and backache.

HERBAL THERAPY

Evening primrose oil and chaste tree berry appear to be the most helpful botanical options for some patients with PMS.[16] Chaste tree modulates pituitary-ovarian stimulation. Chaste berry, prescribed as 2 mL of 1:2 extract taken with water, may be taken each morning on a long-term basis to correct hormonal imbalance.[17] It takes 3 months to achieve the full benefit of therapy.

Some women believe that wild yam combined with chaste tree (225 mg with 0.5% agnoside) helps reduce irritability, bloating, and depression in PMS. Wild yam contains diosgenin, a substance that can be converted into progesterone in the laboratory but not in the human body. Its beneficial effects are probably related to alkaloids that are muscle relaxants and steroidal saponins that may alleviate muscle strain and pain.

In doses of 3 to 4 g daily, evening primrose oil may help women with PMT-C associated with prostaglandin deficiency.[17] However, analysis of seven placebo-controlled trials, five of which were randomized, suggested that evening primrose oil was of little value in the management of PMS.[18] Nonetheless, some practitioners believe that administration of evening primrose oil (Efamol), two tablets twice daily 3 days before the onset of symptoms until the start of menses, reduces mastodynia and symptoms of fibrocystic breast disease.

Although further investigation is required, other herbs may offer symptomatic relief.[17] Gingko taken throughout the menstrual cycle eases breast discomfort, dandelion acts as a diuretic, and willow bark acts as an analgesic. Siberian ginseng may be used as an adaptogen to counter the adverse effects of stress. Valerian may relieve anxiety and insomnia, and St. John's wort (*Hypericum perforatum*) can relieve symptoms of depression. Results of a pilot study suggest that *H. perforatum* (300 mg) may reduce psychologic symptoms in PMS.[19]

Combined nutrient and herbal prescriptions that may be helpful are as follows[20]:

- Vitamin B$_6$ (100 mg), magnesium (200 mg), valerian, and foods rich in phytoestrogens for patients with PMT-A (for patients with PMT-H, vitamin E should be added)
- A reduced intake of fat and simple sugars and supplementation with magnesium (200 mg), vitamin E (100 IU), and evening primrose oil (3 g midcycle) for patients with PMT-C
- Phytoestrogens, *H. perforatum*, black cohosh, and magnesium for patients with PMT-D
- Magnesium (100-800 mg) and feverfew for patients with PMT-P

PRACTICE TIPS

- Premenstrual bloating may be reduced by nibbling parsley in the days before menstruation, because parsley compounds have a diuretic effect.
- In some women, premenstrual bloating may be reduced by consumption of rice or millet and avoidance of wheat products.
- Women with premenstrual tension may benefit from drinking decaffeinated coffee and caffeine-free colas and eating carob instead of chocolate.
- Soy protein–containing isoflavone glycosides increase the length of the follicular phase of the menstrual cycle, whereas miso with isoflavone aglycones does not.

REFERENCES

1. Stearns S: PMS and PMDD in the domain of mental health nursing, *J Psychosoc Nurs Ment Health Serv* 39:16-27, 2001.
2. Abraham GE: Nutritional factors in the etiology of premenstrual syndromes, *J Reprod Med* 28:446-64, 1983.
3. Tricky R: *Women, hormones and the menstrual cycle: herbal and medical solutions from adolescence to menopause*, Sydney, Australia, 1998, Allen & Unwin.
4. Frackiewicz EJ, Shiovitz TM: Evaluation and management of premenstrual syndrome and premenstrual dysphoric disorder, *J Am Pharm Assoc (Wash)* 41:437-47, 2001.
5. Stevinson C, Ernst E: Complementary/alternative therapies for premenstrual syndrome: a systematic review of randomized controlled trials, *Am J Obstet Gynecol* 185:227-35, 2001.
6. Cross GB, Marley J, Miles H, et al: Changes in nutrient intake during the menstrual cycle of overweight women with premenstrual syndrome, *Br J Nutr* 85:475-82, 2001.
7. Barnard ND, Scialli AR, Hurlock D, et al: Diet and sex-hormone binding globulin, dysmenorrhea, and premenstrual symptoms, *Obstet Gynecol* 95:245-50, 2000.
8. Bendich A: The potential for dietary supplements to reduce premenstrual syndrome (PMS) symptoms, *J Am Coll Nutr* 19:3-12, 2000.
9. Thys-Jacobs S: Micronutrients and the premenstrual syndrome: the case for calcium, *J Am Coll Nutr* 19:220-7, 2000.
10. Thys-Jacobs S, Starkey P, Bernstein D, et al: Calcium carbonate and the premenstrual syndrome: effects on premenstrual and menstrual symptoms. Premenstrual Syndrome Study Group, *Am J Obstet Gynecol* 179:444-52, 1998.
11. Ward MW, Holimon TD: Calcium treatment for premenstrual syndrome, *Ann Pharmacother* 33:1356-8, 1999.
12. Pearlstein T, Steiner M: Non-antidepressant treatment of premenstrual syndrome, *J Clin Psychiatry* 61(suppl 12):22-7, 2000.
13. Steinberg S, Annable L, Young SN, et al: A placebo-controlled study of the effects of L-tryptophan in patients with premenstrual dysphoria, *Adv Exp Med Biol* 467:85-8, 1999.

14. London RS, Murphy L, Kitlowski KE, et al: Efficacy of alpha-tocopherol in the treatment of the premenstrual syndrome, *J Reprod Med* 32:400-4, 1987.
15. Wyatt KM, Dimmock PW, Jones PW, et al: Efficacy of vitamin B_6 in the treatment of premenstrual syndrome: systematic review, *BMJ* 318:1375-81, 1999.
16. De Souza MC, Walker AF, Robinson PA, et al: A synergistic effect of a daily supplement for 1 month of 200 mg magnesium plus 50 mg vitamin B_6 for the relief of anxiety-related premenstrual symptoms: a randomized, double-blind, crossover study, *J Womens Health Gend Based Med* 9:131-9, 2000.
16. Hardy ML: Herbs of special interest to women, *J Am Pharm Assoc (Wash)* 40: 234-42, 2000.
17. Mills S, Bone K: *Principles and practice of phytotherapy*, Edinburgh, 2000, Churchill Livingstone.
18. Budeiri D, Li Wan Po A, Dornan JC: Is evening primrose oil of value in the treatment of premenstrual syndrome? *Control Clin Trials* 17:60-8, 1996.
19. Stevinson C, Ernst E: A pilot study of *Hypericum perforatum* for the treatment of premenstrual syndrome, *BJOG* 107:870-6, 2000.
20. Werbach MR: *Textbook of nutritional medicine*, Tarzana, CA, 1999, Third Line Press.

■ CHAPTER 41 ■

PROSTATE CANCER

Prostate cancer, the most common malignancy in males, is a disease of older men. Delaying the onset of prostate cancer by a few years may prevent death from this disease.

Scientific evidence suggests that dietary differences may partially explain the variability in prostate cancer rates around the world.[1] Although a case-control study demonstrated a positive association between total energy intake and preclinical prostate cancer,[2] links between prostate cancer and specific dietary factors remain obscure.[3] In fact, despite supportive epidemiologic and laboratory evidence, the suggestion that nutritional factors— especially reduced fat intake and consumption of soy proteins, vitamin E derivatives, and selenium—may have a protective effect against prostate cancer remains hypothetical.[4]

Nonetheless, specific features of prostate cancer, including its high prevalence, long latency, and significant mortality and morbidity, do provide opportunities for chemoprevention.

CLINICAL DIAGNOSIS

Prostate cancer is often asymptomatic. Men with prostatism, chronic low backache, terminal hematuria, and/or nocturia should be evaluated for prostate cancer.

Digital rectal examination and measurement of the prostate-specific antigen (PSA) level can be combined to achieve a screening procedure with high sensitivity.[5] A hard, irregular, nodular prostate with an obliterated median sulcus on rectal examination combined with an increased PSA level is diagnostic of prostate cancer. A PSA level in excess of 10 ng/mL suggests prostate disease, and an increase in excess of 30 ng/mL rules out benign prostatic hypertrophy.[6] The PSA level increases with age. High normal PSA levels are 2.5 ng/mL for 49-year-olds, 3.5 ng/mL for 59-year-olds, 4.5 ng/mL for 69-year-olds, and up to 6.5 ng/mL for 79-year-olds. The serum acid phosphatase level is also elevated.

THERAPEUTIC STRATEGY

Carcinogenesis is a two-stage process involving initiation and promotion. Initiators irreversibly alter DNA, and promoters accelerate cell proliferation.

There is a long delay between initiation, the primary causative event, and overt disease.

Epidemiologic and laboratory evidence suggest that a diet low in fat, with good sources of soy proteins, vitamin E, and selenium, may have a protective effect against prostate cancer.[4] Epidemiologic evidence, in particular, suggests a positive relationship between prostate cancer and animal, but not vegetable, fat.[7] Furthermore, data from descriptive studies support the hypothesis that a dietary fat intake of around 40% of energy consumption promotes the progression of focal prostatic cancer to clinical disease.[8] The nuclear grade of prostatic carcinoma in situ appears proportional to the fat intake; higher fat intakes are associated with enhanced tumor aggression, and total fat consumption from meat, but not fish, is directly related to the risk of advanced prostate cancer.[9] Consistent with this finding is the observation, when erythrocyte phosphatidylcholine levels of eicosapentaenoic acid (EPA) and docosahexaenoic acid (DHA) are used as biomarkers, that a high dietary intake of fish oils may reduce the risk of prostate cancer.[10] In contrast to this finding, a case-control study showed that the risk of prostate cancer increased in proportion to intake of α-linolenic acid, the ω-3 precursor of EPA.[11] The apparent specificity of the effect of particular fatty acids on prostatic tissue may explain why, despite a high index of suspicion, correlation between a high animal fat diet and an increased risk of prostate cancer remains controversial.[12,13] Fat may initiate cancer by diverse mechanisms, which vary from increased free radical production resulting from consumption of an energy-dense diet to modification of the eicosanoid balance. It has even been surmised that a high-fat diet may enhance androgenic stimulation over time.[14]

Although total fat, animal fat, milk, and red meat are significant dietary risk factors for prostate cancer, the greatest risk correlation seems to be the nonfat portion of milk and its calcium content.[15] A significant increase in advanced prostate cancer and metastatic prostate cancer has been reported in subjects consuming more than 2000 mg of calcium per day, compared with individuals ingesting less than 500 mg of calcium per day.[16] A high calcium intake may suppress the conversion of 25-hydroxyvitamin D, the primary form of vitamin D in the circulation, to 1,25-dihydroxyvitamin D. The dihydroxy, fully active form of vitamin D has an antitumor effect on prostate cancer.

Strategies to prevent initiation of prostate cancer may differ from those to prevent spread. For metastasis to occur, cancerous cells must first clump together. Galectins located on the surface of cancer cells facilitate clumping and enable metastasis. Galactose-rich modified citrus pectin has a binding affinity for galectins on the surface of cancer cells, resulting in an inhibition, or blocking, of cancer cell aggregation, adhesion, and metastasis.[17] Results of animal studies indicated that oral modified citrus pectin did not affect primary tumor growth but significantly reduced metastases from injected prostate adenocarcinoma cell lines.[18] Experimental observation also suggests that a low-fat diet plus soy protein extract reduces progression of established tumors.[4]

Intervention strategies may target initiation, promotion, and/or progression of prostate cancer.

LIFESTYLE CHANGES

Although there is evidence that diet may play an important role in preventing prostate cancer, further research is necessary to define what role nutrition plays in preventing or promoting this disease.[19]

Good dietary advice may be to limit fat intake to around 25% of total energy. Olive oil is the preferred source of fat.[20] In a recent two-center cohort study, a consistent and significant inverse association was found between the premorbid intake of monounsaturated fat and the risk of death from prostate cancer.[21] In contrast, associations between animal products and prostate cancer have been detected in numerous observational studies. The Health Professionals Follow-Up Study showed that processed meats (beef, pork, or lamb) and dairy products each contributed to an elevated risk of metastatic prostate cancer.[22] Consumption of animal products, especially dairy products, should be limited.[23]

However, whether the high fat content of these foods or some other component accounts for the association is unclear. Calcium and fatty acids explain most of the observed association with dairy products.[22] Results from the Physicians' Health Study support the hypothesis that dairy products and calcium are associated with a greater risk of prostate cancer.[24] There are strategies to counteract the untoward effect of calcium. It has been suggested that 29 to 33 kcal of tomatoes may fully counter the effects of calcium contained in one cup of nonfat milk, which has 86 kcal and 300 mg of calcium.[15]

A diet rich in fruits and vegetables appears protective.[25] Cruciferous vegetables and tomatoes, especially cooked tomatoes, appear to be particularly beneficial.[8,12,14,25] Frequent tomato or lycopene intake was associated with a reduced risk of prostate cancer.[26] In a case-control study, significant inverse associations were found between prostate cancer and plasma concentrations of lycopene and zeaxanthin.[27] Tomatoes, with tomato sauce as the primary source of bioavailable lycopene, have been found, through epidemiologic studies, to correlate with high serum concentrations of lycopene and a reduced risk of prostate cancer.[28] Despite much support for the lycopene hypothesis and the contribution of red-colored fruits and vegetables to a lower risk of prostate cancer,[29] a recent study indicated that intake of tomatoes and fruit is unrelated to risk. This multicenter, case-control study showed that the intake of legumes and yellow-orange and cruciferous vegetables was inversely related to the risk of prostate cancer.[30] High fructose intake, achieved by eating five servings, rather than one serving, of fruit a day, has also been inversely related to the progression of prostate cancer.[31]

Like lycopene, soy phytonutrients are free radical quenchers. In addition, soy phytoestrogens have a hormonal influence. In a prospective study men who drank soy milk more than once a day were found to have a 70%

reduction in the risk of prostate cancer.[32] Although findings were not statistically significant, in one study, men who ate tofu five or more times a week had a lower risk of prostate cancer than those who ate it less than twice weekly.[33] Soy isoflavones have been found to inhibit the growth of prostate cancer cells in some animal studies.[34] Genistein is an isoflavone found in soy. It has an estrogenic effect and may inhibit metastasis of prostate cancer cells by decreasing tyrosine phosphorylase levels and modifying signal transduction, which inhibits growth of both androgen-dependent and androgen-independent prostate cells. Animal studies showed that genistein in the diet inhibited the development of invasive adenocarcinomas and reduced the incidence of poorly differentiated prostatic adenocarcinomas in a dose-dependent manner by regulating specific sex steroid receptors and growth factor signaling pathways.[35] Nonetheless, short-term exposure of elderly men with elevated serum PSA values to soy protein containing isoflavones did not alter serum PSA levels.[36] PSA is an enzymatic tumor marker, and its doubling time reflects the speed at which the cancer is growing. The effect of soy on the normal human prostate is unknown.

NUTRIENT THERAPY/DIETARY SUPPLEMENTS

Although results of a population-based, case-control study suggest that multivitamin use is not associated with prostate cancer risk, use of individual supplements of zinc, selenium, vitamins C, E, D, lycopene, or isoflavones may be protective.[37,38] In vitro studies suggest that zinc inhibits human prostatic cancer cell growth, possibly as a result of the induction of cell cycle arrest and apoptosis.[39] Daily supplementation with 30 mg of zinc may be helpful, as is daily supplementation with synthetic vitamin E.[40] Even small doses of vitamin E (50 mg, i.e., 55 IU *dl*-α-tocopherol) appear to offer significant protection against prostate cancer.[41] A nested case-control study demonstrated that the risk of prostate cancer declined, but not linearly, with increasing concentrations of α-tocopherol. Statistically significant protection with high levels of selenium and α-tocopherol is observed only when γ-tocopherol concentrations are high.[42] Alpha-Tocopherol is the major form of vitamin E in supplements, but γ-tocopherol is the major form of dietary vitamin E in the United States.

Despite a systematic analysis in which no association between smoking and prostate cancer was found,[43] 100 IU of vitamin E may reduce risk of metastases among smokers or recent quitters.[44] Because of these and other supportive epidemiologic and laboratory findings, a randomized, prospective, double-blind study designed to determine whether selenium and vitamin E decrease the risk of prostate cancer in healthy men is being undertaken.[45]

Converging evidence from epidemiologic, experimental animal, and molecular biology studies suggests that selenium has an antitumor effect.[46] Selenium, the catalytic center of a number of selenoenzymes including those with antioxidant and redox functions, may protect against cancer initiation. By serving as a source for selenium metabolites that affect carcinogenesis, selenium may also hinder cancer progression.

Modified citrus pectin (MCP) may reduce the risk of metastases. When administered orally at a dosage of 15 g/day in three divided doses, MCP lengthened the doubling time of PSA in four of seven patients tested.[47] Lengthening of the doubling time represents a decrease in the cancer growth rate. MCP, also known as *fractionated pectin*, is a complex polysaccharide obtained from the peel and pulp of citrus fruits. Shorter polysaccharide units give MCP its ability to access and bind tightly to galactose-binding lectins (galectins). MCP taken in divided doses to a daily total between 6 and 30 g is safe and produces a soft stool.

It may be advisable to avoid certain supplements. A prospective study of almost 50,000 men free of cancer in 1986 demonstrated that 8 years later, a higher consumption of calcium, 2000 versus 500 mg a day, was related to a higher risk of advanced and metastatic prostate cancer.[31] It may be wise for men with prostate cancer to avoid calcium supplementation.

HERBAL THERAPY

A Chinese herb combination that contains eight herbs (chrysanthemum, dyers woad, licorice, reishi, san-qi ginseng, rabdosia, saw palmetto, and baikal skullcap) benefited patients with prostate cancer and caused a decline in serum PSA levels, often to the undetectable range.[48]

Several herbal constituents are capable of interfering with carcinogenesis. Along with an estrogenic effect, herbs have a number of potential mechanisms through which they can influence prostate cancer. Albeit with different potency, bioflavonoids silymarin, genistein, and epigallocatechin 3-gallate all appear to inhibit mitogenic signaling pathways and alter cell cycle regulators, leading to growth inhibition and death of advanced and androgen-independent prostate carcinoma cells.[49] Experiments have shown that, in contrast to silymarin, higher doses of genistein showed cytotoxic effects causing 30% to 40% cell death. An even more profound cytotoxic effect was observed with epigallocatechin 3-gallate, which accounted for 50% cell death at lower doses. Higher doses resulted in a complete loss of cellular viability.

PRACTICE TIPS

- Sexual activity in early adulthood may be inversely associated with prostate cancer.[50]
- Experimental observations suggest that, rather than inhibiting etiologic factors, low-fat diets and soy protein extracts may influence the progression of established tumors.

- Nutritional prevention of prostate cancer remains unproven at the level of double-blind, placebo-controlled clinical trials.
- Daily use of nonsteroidal anti-inflammatory drugs (NSAIDs) may be associated with a lower incidence of prostate cancer in men aged 60 years or older; NSAIDs may prevent the progression of prostate cancer from latency to clinical disease.[51]
- Long-term supplementation with vitamin E (50 mg/day) and beta-carotene (20 mg/day) may reduce the risk of prostate cancer.
- Taking 160 mg phytoestrogens (e.g., red clover) for 1 week before prostatectomy may improve the prognosis for patients with prostate cancer.

REFERENCES

1. Yip I, Heber D, Aronson W: Nutrition and prostate cancer, *Urol Clin North Am* 26:403-11, 1999.
2. Meyer F, Bairati I, Fradet Y, et al: Dietary energy and nutrients in relation to preclinical prostate cancer, *Nutr Cancer* 29:120-6, 1997.
3. Kolonel LN, Nomura AM, Cooney RV: Dietary fat and prostate cancer: current status, *J Natl Cancer Inst* 91:414-28, 1999.
4. Fair WR, Fleshner NE, Heston W: Cancer of the prostate: a nutritional disease? *Urology* 50:840-8, 1997.
5. Pamies RJ, Crawford DR: Tumor markers. An update, *Med Clin North Am* 80:185-99, 1996.
6. Hostetler RM, Mandel IG, Marshburn J: Prostate cancer screening, *Med Clin North Am* 80:83-98, 1996.
7. Willett WC: Specific fatty acids and risks of breast and prostate cancer: dietary intake, *Am J Clin Nutr* 66(suppl 6):1557S-1563S, 1997.
8. Zhou J, Blackburn GL: Bridging animal and human studies: what are the missing segments in dietary fat and prostate cancer? *Am J Clin Nutr* 66(suppl 6):1572S-1580S, 1997.
9. Primack A: Complementary/alternative therapies in the prevention and treatment of cancer. In Spencer JW, Jacobs JJ, editors: *Complementary/alternative therapy: an evidence-based approach*, St Louis, 1998, Mosby.
10. Norrish AE, Skeaff CM, Arribas GL, et al: Prostate cancer risk and consumption of fish oils: a dietary biomarker-based case-control study, *Br J Cancer* 81:1238-42, 1999.
11. Ramon JM, Bou R, Romea S, et al: Dietary fat intake and prostate cancer risk: a case-control study in Spain, *Cancer Causes Control* 11:679-85, 2000.
12. Brawley OW, Knopf K, Thompson I: The epidemiology of prostate cancer part II: the risk factors, *Semin Urol Oncol* 16:193-201, 1998.
13. Veierod MB, Laake P, Thelle DS: Dietary fat intake and risk of prostate cancer: a prospective study of 25,708 Norwegian men, *Int J Cancer* 73:634-8, 1997.
14. Brawley OW, Parnes H: Prostate cancer prevention trials in the USA, *Eur J Cancer* 36:1312-5, 2000.
15. Grant WB: An ecologic study of dietary links to prostate cancer, *Altern Med Rev* 4:162-9, 1999.

16. Giovannucci E: Dietary influences of 1,25(OH)2 vitamin D in relation to prostate cancer: a hypothesis, *Cancer Causes Control* 9:567-82, 1998.
17. Raz A, Loton R: Endogenous galactoside-binding lectins: a new class of functional cell surface molecules related to metastasis, *Cancer Metastasis Rev* 6:433-52, 1987.
18. Pienta KJ, Naik H, Akhtar A, et al: Inhibition of spontaneous metastasis in a rat prostate cancer model by oral administration of modified citrus, *J Natl Cancer Inst* 87:348-53, 1995.
19. Blumenfeld AJ, Fleshner N, Casselman B, et al: Nutritional aspects of prostate cancer: a review, *Can J Urol* 7:927-35, 2000.
20. Tzonou A, Signorello LB, Lagiou P, et al: Diet and cancer of the prostate: a case-control study in Greece, *Int J Cancer* 80:704-8, 1999.
21. Kim DJ, Gallagher RP, Hislop TG, et al: Premorbid diet in relation to survival from prostate cancer (Canada), *Cancer Causes Control* 11:65-77, 2000.
22. Michaud DS, Augustsson K, Rimm EB, et al: A prospective study on intake of animal products and risk of prostate cancer, *Cancer Causes Control* 12:557-67, 2001.
23. Chan JM, Giovannucci E, Andersson SO, et al: Dairy products, calcium, phosphorous, vitamin D, and risk of prostate cancer, *Cancer Causes Control* 9:559-66, 1998.
24. Chan JM, Stampfer MJ, Ma J, et al: Dairy products, calcium, and prostate cancer risk in the Physicians' Health Study, *Am J Clin Nutr* 74:549-54, 2001.
25. Cohen JH, Kristal AR, Stanford JL: Fruit and vegetable intakes and prostate cancer risk, *J Natl Cancer Inst* 92:61-8, 2000.
26. Giovannucci E, Rimm EB, Liu Y, et al: A prospective study of tomato products, lycopene, and prostate cancer risk, *J Natl Cancer Inst* 94:391-8, 2002.
27. Lu QY, Hung JC, Heber D, et al: Inverse associations between plasma lycopene and other carotenoids and prostate cancer, *Cancer Epidemiol Biomarkers Prev* 10:749-56, 2001.
28. Gann PH, Ma J, Giovannucci E, et al: Lower prostate cancer risk in men with elevated plasma lycopene levels: results of a prospective analysis, *Cancer Res* 59:1225-30, 1999.
29. de la Taille A, Katz A, Vacherot F, Saint F, et al: Cancer of the prostate: influence of nutritional factors. Vitamins, antioxidants and trace elements, *Presse Med* 30:557-60, 2001.
30. Kolonel LN, Hankin JH, Whittemore AS, et al: Vegetables, fruits, legumes and prostate cancer: a multiethnic case-control study, *Cancer Epidemiol Biomarkers Prev* 9:795-804, 2000.
31. Giovannucci E, Rimm EB, Wolk A, et al: Calcium and fructose intake in relation to risk of prostate cancer, *Cancer Res* 58:442-7, 1998.
32. Jacobsen BK, Knutsen SF, Fraser GE: Does high soy milk intake reduce prostate cancer incidence? The Adventist Health Study (United States), *Cancer Causes Control* 9:553-7, 1998.
33. Messina MJ: Legumes and soybeans: overview of their nutritional profiles and health effects, *Am J Clin Nutr* 70(suppl 3):439S-450S, 1999.
34. Zhou JR, Gugger ET, Tanaka T, et al: Soybean phytochemicals inhibit the growth of transplantable human prostate carcinoma and tumor angiogenesis in mice, *J Nutr* 129:1628-35, 1999.

35. Lamartiniere CA, Cotroneo MS, Fritz WA, et al: Genistein chemoprevention: timing and mechanisms of action in murine mammary and prostate, *J Nutr* 132:552S-558S, 2002.

36. Urban D, Irwin W, Kirk M, et al: The effect of isolated soy protein on plasma biomarkers in elderly men with elevated serum prostate specific antigen, *J Urol* 165:294-300, 2001.

37. Kristal AR, Stanford JL, Cohen JH, et al: Vitamin and mineral supplement use is associated with reduced risk of prostate cancer, *Cancer Epidemiol Biomarkers Prev* 8:887-92, 1999.

38. Kumar NB, Besterman-Dahan K: Nutrients in the chemoprevention of prostate cancer: current and future prospects, *Cancer Control* 6:580-6, 1999.

39. Liang JY, Liu YY, Zou J, et al: Inhibitory effect of zinc on human prostatic carcinoma cell growth, *Prostate* 40:200-7, 1999.

40. Moyad MA, Brumfield SK, Pienta KJ: Vitamin E, alpha- and gamma-tocopherol, and prostate cancer, *Semin Urol Oncol* 17:85-90, 1999.

41. Heinonen OP, Albanes D, Virtamo J, et al: Prostate cancer and supplementation with alpha-tocopherol and beta-carotene: incidence and mortality in a controlled trial, *J Natl Cancer Inst* 90:440-6, 1998.

42. Helzlsouer KJ, Huang HY, Alberg AJ, et al: Association between alpha-tocopherol, gamma-tocopherol, selenium, and subsequent prostate cancer, *J Natl Cancer Inst* 92:2018-23, 2000.

43. Lumey LH: Prostate cancer and smoking: a review of case-control and cohort studies, *Prostate* 29:249-60, 1996.

44. Chan JM, Stampfer MJ, Ma J, et al: Supplemental vitamin E intake and prostate cancer risk in a large cohort of men in the United States, *Cancer Epidemiol Biomarkers Prev* 8:893-9, 1999.

45. Klein EA, Thompson IM, Lippman SM, et al: SELECT: the next prostate cancer prevention trial. Selenium and Vitamin E Cancer Prevention Trial, *J Urol* 166:1311-5, 2001.

46. Costello AJ: A randomized, controlled chemoprevention trial of selenium in familial prostate cancer: rationale, recruitment, and design issues, *Urology* 57 (4 suppl 1):182-4, 2001.

47. Strum S, Scholz M, McDermed J, et al: Modified citrus pectin slows PSA doubling time: a pilot clinical trial, Presentation: International Conference on Diet and Prevention of Cancer, Tampere, Finland, May 28-June 2, 1999.

48. Porterfield H: UsToo PC-SPES surveys: review of studies and update of previous survey results, *Mol Urol* 4:289-91, 2000.

49. Bhatia N, Agarwal R: Detrimental effect of cancer preventive phytochemicals silymarin, genistein and epigallocatechin 3-gallate on epigenetic events in human prostate carcinoma DU145 cells, *Prostate* 46:98-107, 2001.

50. Hsieh CC, Thanos A, Mitropoulos D, et al: Risk factors for prostate cancer: a case-control study in Greece, *Int J Cancer* 80:699-703, 1999.

51. Roberts RO, Jacobson DJ, Girman CJ, et al: A population-based study of daily nonsteroidal anti-inflammatory drug use and prostate cancer, *Mayo Clin Proc* 77:219-25, 2002.

■ CHAPTER 42 ■

PSORIASIS

Psoriasis is a common, chronic, recurrent inflammatory skin disorder associated with oxidative stress, abnormal plasma lipid metabolism, and an increased risk of cardiovascular events and arthritis. Although the cause is unknown, psoriasis occurs in families, suggesting genetic susceptibility.

The condition is characterized by increased mitosis and DNA synthesis, resulting in epidermal hyperproliferation with skin thickening and increased keratocytes and producing red, silver-scaled lesions. Attacks may be precipitated by trauma, physical illness, or emotional stress. Drugs and sunburn are other precipitating factors.

CLINICAL DIAGNOSIS

Psoriasis is a disorder with a history of exacerbations and remissions that affects the skin and, in some cases, the joints. The appearance of skin lesions depends on the anatomic site involved. Plaques—inflamed red patches with white flaking scales often found on the scalp, flexures, and extensor surfaces—are described as silvery scales on red plaques, which may itch. Pustular lesions are found on the palms and soles. The nails show pitting, transverse ridging, and yellowing destruction.

When present, psoriatic arthritis, although limited to a few joints, destroys mobility by an inflammatory resorptive process.

THERAPEUTIC STRATEGY

There is no cure for psoriasis. The cause is unproven, but chemical and food sensitivities are possible because it is a genetic imbalance of inflammatory mediators. Excessive stimulation of, or inadequate inhibition of, cyclic guanosine monophosphate and cyclooxygenase and lipoxygenase enzymes favors an inflammatory response. Enzyme and T-cell cytokine–mediated interactions induce cutaneous inflammation. Proinflammatory cytokines, including tumor necrosis factor, have been detected in skin lesions and joints of patients with psoriasis, and early results of treatment suggest that tumor necrosis factor–neutralizing agents may be helpful.[1] The aims of therapy are to reduce inflammation, promote growth of healthy skin, and provide symptomatic relief from severe attacks.

In addition to dampening inflammation for management of skin and joint lesions, some attention should also be given to a potential increased risk of cardiovascular disease. High-density lipoprotein cholesterol was found to be significantly reduced, and low-density lipoprotein cholesterol, significantly increased in a study of patients with psoriatic arthritis.[2] Results of another study confirmed that patients with mild and severe psoriasis have a lipid profile consistent with increased risk of ischemic heart disease, and the authors concluded that reductions in total antioxidant capacity and levels of vitamins A and E were present.[3] Worsening of psoriasis was paralleled by an increase in oxidative stress and changes in lipid risk factors.

LIFESTYLE CHANGES

Psoriasis can be improved by various physical measures, such as preventing dry skin and avoiding exposure to sunlight. Humidifiers are useful in winter, and aloe vera gel is a good moisturizer. Sunlight with both ultraviolet A and ultraviolet B radiation is effective in clearing psoriasis. Morning or late afternoon sun exposure for 15 to 30 minutes a day usually results in some improvement within 3 to 6 weeks.

Dietary changes can create a less proinflammatory environment. Fish has a beneficial effect. Patients should be advised to regularly eat oily fish (e.g., mackerel, sardines, salmon, pilchard, kipper, and herring). Eating four to six meals that include 170 g of oily fish each week contributes 1 to 2 g of ω-3 fatty acids and triples the recommended daily intake of vitamin D.[4] An increased intake of antioxidants can be achieved by eating fresh fruits and vegetables. Carrots and tomatoes appear to be particularly helpful.

NUTRIENT THERAPY/DIETARY SUPPLEMENTS

Clinical trials support the use of ω-3 fatty acids (5 g daily); topical application of 1% arachidonic acid, fumaric acid, or vitamin A; injections of vitamin B_{12} (1000 μg daily); and ingestion of bromine and nickel.[5] Uncontrolled studies have provided some support for the use of folic acid (20 mg four times daily) and vitamin C (500 mg twice daily), topical selenium sulfide (25 mg/mL), topical application of 10% zinc oxide, vitamin D supplementation, and correction of chromium deficiency.

One therapeutic option is fish oils (1000 mg three times daily). Psoriatic lesions are rich in leukotriene B_4, a major proinflammatory metabolite of arachidonic acid. Leukotriene B_4 is inhibited by metabolites generated by epidermal 15-lipoxygenase acting on eicosapentaenoic acid (EPA). EPA itself serves as a substrate for less proinflammatory eicosanoids. A randomized, open study showed that patients with chronic, stable psoriasis vulgaris responded better to low-dose etretinate when it was combined with EPA.[6] In a literature review, Chalmers et al[7] found only one trial in which an ω-3 fatty acid preparation was used to treat patients with guttate psoriasis and concluded that there appeared to be some benefit.[7] Another study indicated that within days of infusion of 4.2 g of both EPA and docosahexaenoic acid daily, the plasma-free EPA concentration and generation of neutrophil leukotriene B_5 and platelet thromboxane B_3 increased.[8] These eicosanoid changes did not occur in patients receiving ω-6 fatty acid supplements .However, a double-blind trial showed that combined supplementation with ω-3 and ω-6 fatty acids did appear to enhance efficacy,[9] although a double-blind parallel trial demonstrated that combined ω-3 and ω-6 fatty acid (EPA) supplementation did not significantly reduce the clinical severity of psoriasis or produce any meaningful change in transepidermal water loss in chronic stable plaque psoriasis.[10] Furthermore, in a 4-month, double-blind, multicenter trial, purified ethyl esters of ω-3 fatty acids containing 5 g of EPA and docosahexaenoic acid were found to be no more effective than corn oil supplementation in the treatment of psoriasis.[11] Scaling was reduced in both groups and, although the fish oil group had less cellular infiltration, the corn oil group had greater reduction in desquamation and redness. In the corn oil group, there was a significant correlation between clinical improvement and an increase in EPA and total ω-3 fatty acids.

Debate is not limited to oral supplementation. A multicenter, double-blind, placebo-controlled study of topical therapy for moderate plaque-type psoriasis with the use of ω-3 polyunsaturated fatty acids indicated that there was no significant benefit.[12] However, in another study, topical application of fish oil was found to be more effective than liquid paraffin.[13]

In addition to reducing the concentration of a proinflammatory substrate by limiting meat and egg consumption and increasing fish consumption, inflammation can be dampened by inhibiting lipoxygenase through supplementation with vitamin E, quercetin, garlic, curcumin, or chaparral and by avoiding cyclic guanosine monophosphate stimulants such as biotin, ginseng, calcium, and vitamin C in large amounts. Instead of targeting fatty acid metabolism to dampen inflammation, free radical quenching can be used to suppress the inflammatory response. Reduced concentrations of selenium in whole blood, plasma, and leukocytes have been observed in psoriasis. Selenium is required for activation of glutathione peroxidase, an inhibitor of the 5-lipoxygenase pathway. Topical application by means of selenium shampoo has been found to be beneficial.[14] However, a placebo-controlled trial showed that supplementation of 600 μg of selenium-enriched yeast, with and without 600 IU of vitamin E, failed to reduce the severity of psoriasis despite increased serum and platelet levels of these nutrients.[15]

Laboratory studies suggest treatment with vitamin D_3 might ameliorate psoriatic lesions by contributing to the completion of the apoptotic process.[16] Patients with psoriasis seem unable to produce a normal amount of fumaric acid on exposure to sunlight. Fumaric acid, the trans-isomer of malic acid and an intermediate in the tricarboxylic acid cycle, is formed in the skin on exposure to ultraviolet light. A combination of oral dimethylfumaric acid and topical fumaric acid has been effective in clinical trials.[17] Fumaric acid esters appear to have an immunosuppressive effect, with the lymphocyte count being linked to the clinical outcome.[18] A multicenter study of patients with psoriasis demonstrated that fumaric acid derivatives were effective and safe in the treatment of psoriasis.[19] Adverse events such as flushing and gastrointestinal disturbances were initially relatively frequent but decreased with time. A review of randomized, controlled trials of interventions for the treatment of moderate to severe chronic plaque psoriasis revealed that oral fumaric acid ester (fumarate) therapy was an effective systemic treatment, as were retinoids, especially with ultraviolet A radiation, and/or a combination treatment of phototherapy with a vitamin D_3 analogue such as calcipotriol.[20]

Although vitamin A, 25,000 IU per day for 30 days and 10,000 IU per day thereafter, and zinc, 30 mg/day, are popular treatments, vitamin A toxicity is a problem and the efficacy of zinc is questionable.

Other potentially useful interventions range from nickel dibromide[21] to grapeseed extract. The dose-dependent free radical scavenging ability of a grapeseed proanthocyanidin extract compared favorably with vitamins C, E, and beta-carotene in both in vitro and in vivo models.[22] Grapeseed proanthocyanidin extract containing 5000 ppm resveratrol facilitates oxidant-induced vascular endothelial growth factor expression in keratinocytes and may promote dermal healing.[23] Anecdotal evidence suggests that administration of grapeseed extract, 100 mg twice daily, without food is helpful. Alpha-lipoic acid, 150 mg, taken some time before eating each morning, is another possible intervention for quenching free radicals.

HERBAL THERAPY

Two herbs deserve mention for the treatment of psoriasis. Milk thistle (which contains the flavonoid silymarin), 150 mg twice daily, may be used to reduce inflammation and possibly slow proliferation of abnormal cells.[24] Silymarin exhibits several anti-inflammatory effects, including inhibition of leukotriene and prostaglandin synthesis, mast cell stabilization, and inhibition of neutrophil migration. However, its value in the treatment of psoriasis may be due to its ability to improve endotoxin removal by the liver, inhibit cyclic adenosine monophosphate phosphodiesterase, and inhibit leukotriene synthesis.[25] Abnormally high levels of cyclic adenosine monophosphate and leukotrienes have been observed in patients with psoriasis. Silymarin is nontoxic, although at doses exceeding 1500 mg daily, a laxative effect is possible. Mild allergic reactions have also been noted.

Topical aloe vera may be helpful. However, despite promising results, clinical effectiveness of topical aloe vera is not sufficiently defined at present.[26]

PRACTICE TIPS

- Eating at least a serving of tomatoes each day, a serving of carrots every second day, and/or two servings of fresh fruit daily may halve the risk of psoriasis.
- In some people, symptoms of psoriasis may be somewhat relieved by eating 6 ounces of oily fish every day.
- Patients with diabetes should limit fish oil to no more than 2000 mg/day to avoid disturbances in blood glucose regulation.
- Long-term zinc supplementation requires concurrent administration of 2 mg of copper daily to prevent mineral imbalance.
- Exercise is important.
- Supplementation with high-dose vitamins A and E may be helpful.
- Fish oil and evening primrose oil may be tried.
- Patients with psoriasis should get some sun exposure (ultraviolet B radiation).
- A rich intake of garlic may be beneficial.
- No more than 1g of vitamin C should be taken daily.
- Aspirin should not be taken.
- Exposure to food triggers (e.g., gluten) should be avoided by susceptible persons.
- No more than 50 µg of biotin should be taken daily.

REFERENCES

1. Mease PJ: Tumour necrosis factor (TNF) in psoriatic arthritis: pathophysiology and treatment with TNF inhibitors, *Ann Rheum Dis* 61:298-304, 2002.
2. Jones SM, Harris CP, Lloyd J, et al: Lipoproteins and their subfractions in psoriatic arthritis: identification of an atherogenic profile with active joint disease, *Ann Rheum Dis* 59:904-9, 2000.
3. Rocha-Pereira P, Santos-Silva A, Rebelo I, et al: Dislipidemia and oxidative stress in mild and in severe psoriasis as a risk for cardiovascular disease, *Clin Chim Acta* 303:33-9, 2001.
4. Collier PM, Ursell A, Zaremba K, et al: Effect of regular consumption of oily fish compared with white fish on chronic plaque psoriasis, *Eur J Clin Nutr* 47:251-4, 1993.
5. Werbach MR, Moss J: *Textbook of nutritional medicine*, Tarzana, CA, 1999, Third Line Press.
6. Danno K, Sugie N: Combination therapy with low-dose etretinate and eicosapentaenoic acid for psoriasis vulgaris, *J Dermatol* 25:703-5, 1998.
7. Chalmers RJ, O'Sullivan T, Owen CM, et al: Interventions for guttate psoriasis, *Cochrane Database Syst Rev* 2:CD001213, 2000.
8. Mayser P, Mrowietz U, Arenberger P, et al: Omega-3 fatty acid-based lipid infusion in patients with chronic plaque psoriasis: results of a double-blind, randomized, placebo-controlled, multicenter trial, *J Am Acad Dermatol* 38:539-47, 1998.

9. Grimminger F, Mayser P, Papavassilis C, et al: A double-blind, randomized, placebo-controlled trial of n-3 fatty acid based lipid infusion in acute, extended guttate psoriasis. Rapid improvement of clinical manifestations and changes in neutrophil leukotriene profile, *Clin Invest* 71:634-43, 1993.

10. Oliwiecki S, Burton JL: Evening primrose oil and marine oil in the treatment of psoriasis, *Clin Exp Dermatol* 19:127-9, 1994.

11. Soyland E, Funk J, Rajka G, et al: Effect of dietary supplementation with very-long-chain n-3 fatty acids in patients with psoriasis, *N Engl J Med* 328:1812-6, 1993.

12. Henneicke-von Zepelin HH, Mrowietz U, Farber L, et al: Highly purified omega-3-polyunsaturated fatty acids for topical treatment of psoriasis. Results of a double-blind, placebo-controlled multicentre study, *Br J Dermatol* 129:713-7, 1993.

13. Escobar SO, Achenbach R, Iannantuono R, et al: Topical fish oil in psoriasis—a controlled and blind study, *Clin Exp Dermatol* 17:159-62, 1992.

14. Borglund E, Enhamre A: Treatment of psoriasis with topical selenium sulphide, *Br J Dermatol* 117:665-6, 1987.

15. Fairris GM, Lloyd B, Hinks L, et al: The effect of supplementation with selenium and vitamin E in psoriasis, *Ann Clin Biochem* 26:83-8, 1989.

16. Fukuya Higaki M, HigakiY, Kawashima M: Effect of vitamin D(3) on the increased expression of Bcl-x(L) in psoriasis, *Arch Dermatol Res* 293:620-5, 2002.

17. Altmeyer PJ, Matthes U, Pawlak F, et al: Antipsoriatic effect of fumaric acid derivatives. Results of a multicenter double-blind study in 100 patients, *J Am Acad Dermatol* 30:977-81, 1994.

18. Hoxtermann S, Nuchel C, Altmeyer P: Fumaric acid esters suppress peripheral CD4- and CD8-positive lymphocytes in psoriasis, *Dermatology* 196:223-30, 1998.

19. Mrowietz U, Christophers E, Altmeyer P: Treatment of psoriasis with fumaric acid esters: results of a prospective multicentre study. German Multicentre Study, *Br J Dermatol* 138:456-60, 1998.

20. Griffiths CE, Clark CM, Chalmers RJ, et al: A systematic review of treatments for severe psoriasis, *Health Technol Assess* 4:1-125, 2000.

21. Smith SA, Young TR, Winsjansen E, et al: Improvement of psoriasis vulgaris with oral nickel dibromide, *Arch Dermatol* 133:661-3, 1997.

22. Bagchi D, Bagchi M, Stohs SJ, et al: Free radicals and grape seed proanthocyanidin extract: importance in human health and disease prevention, *Toxicology* 148:187-97, 2000.

23. Khanna S, Roy S, Bagchi D, et al: Upregulation of oxidant-induced VEGF expression in cultured keratinocytes by a grape seed proanthocyanidin extract, *Free Radic Biol Med* 31:38-42, 2001.

24. *Silybum marianum* (milk thistle), *Altern Med Rev* 4:272-4, 1999.

25. Vogler BK, Ernst E: Aloe vera: a systematic review of its clinical effectiveness, *Br J Gen Pract* 49:823-8, 1999.

26. Diefendorf D, Healey J, Kalyn W, editors: *The healing power of vitamins, minerals and herbs*, Surry Hills, Australia, 2000, Readers Digest.

■ CHAPTER 43 ■

RHEUMATOID ARTHRITIS

Rheumatoid arthritis is an autoimmune condition precipitated in genetically susceptible individuals on exposure to known and unknown triggers. It is an inflammatory disease characterized by dysregulation of the immune system. B lymphocytes become overactive and secrete antibodies that destroy synovial tissues of the joint.

Most conventional treatments include use of drugs designed to control pain and suppress the overall immune response rather than address the actual immune dysfunction. Nutritional management of this condition focuses both on suppressing inflammation and reducing exposure to immune response triggers. Because conventional therapy for rheumatoid arthritis is associated with significant side effects, there is considerable interest in the growing scientific justification for the use of dietary supplements as adjuncts.[1]

CLINICAL DIAGNOSIS

Patients complain of persistent joint pain and stiffness, especially in the morning. Joints are tender and swollen. Joint involvement is widespread and symmetrical, especially in the fingers and upper and lower limbs. Muscle wasting is common in the later stages of the disease.

THERAPEUTIC STRATEGY

Explanations for the significant objective improvement observed in placebo-controlled studies of dietary manipulation include reduced exposure to food allergens, normalization of gastrointestinal permeability, and favorable modification of eicosanoid fatty acid substrates.[2]

Intestinal integrity may be compromised by local intestinal inflammation or nonsteroidal anti-inflammatory drug (NSAID) therapy, which is routinely used to manage inflammatory conditions. Use of these drugs may exacerbate rheumatoid arthritis by increasing gut permeability and facilitating antigen absorption.[3] Increased intestinal permeability permits toxins and proteolytic enzymes, normally limited to the bowel lumen, to evade local mucosal defenses and effect systemic inflammatory responses. Absorption of microbial or dietary antigens, such as casein or gluten, may enable joint deposition of immune complexes or antigens.

In addition to food or microbial antigens forming immune complexes, cross-reactivity of foreign antigens with host endogenous antigens (molecular mimicry) may induce autoimmunity.[4,5] Lymphocytes may accumulate in the joint synovium of genetically susceptible persons exposed to these or other triggers. Rheumatoid factors that form immune complexes with complement are produced, and joint chemotaxis of inflammatory cells results.

Nitric oxide appears to play a pivotal role in the inflammatory response. Nitric oxide, produced within the synoviocytes and chondrocytes, produces highly toxic peroxynitrite radicals and may mediate some of the deleterious effects of cytokines on bone resorption. Several cytokines, including tumor necrosis factor α (TNF-α), are involved in the formation of free radicals, in part by increasing the activity of nitric oxide synthase. Aspirin, tetracyclines, steroids, and methotrexate—all drugs used in the treatment of rheumatoid arthritis—can suppress nitric oxide synthase. Eicosanoid products of arachidonic acid are also believed to be important mediators of inflammation in rheumatoid arthritis. Prostaglandin E_2 potentiates pain and inflammation through enhancing the action of bradykinin and histamine; enhances autoantibody production; stimulates osteoclasts, facilitating bone resorption; and damages cartilage by stimulating collagenase secretion by macrophages and inhibiting proteoglycan production by chondrocytes. In rheumatoid synovium, a cytokine network involving monocyte chemoattractant protein 1 and other proinflammatory cytokines (interleukin [IL]–1β, IL-6, IL-8, and TNF-α) has also been shown to contribute to the immunopathogenesis of rheumatoid arthritis.[6]

Nutritional measures to prevent or control rheumatoid arthritis focus on reducing exposure to antigens and dampening the inflammatory response. The former focuses on avoiding dietary allergens and enhancing intestinal integrity, and the latter, on reducing the proinflammatory nature of fatty acid metabolites and quenching free radicals.

LIFESTYLE CHANGES

Diet has long been believed to be an important trigger of the inflammatory response.[7] Avoidance of important dietary triggers for symptoms of arthritis and arthralgia such as wheat, dairy products, soy products, yeast, eggs, red meat, and food additives such as the benzoates, sulfite, nitrate, and glutamates may reduce the risk of exposure. Foods of the Solanaceae (nightshade) family such as potato, tomato, eggplant, and peppers are also known to promote inflammation, increase pain, and delay tissue repair.[7] Research supports the suggestion that avoidance of allergenic foods is beneficial for certain patients, especially younger females with less severe rheumatoid arthritis.[8]

In addition to avoiding specific allergens, use of the "living food' diet may reduce the signs and symptoms of rheumatoid arthritis.[9] The living food diet reduces proinflammatory fatty acids, avoids sources of common allergens (e.g., dairy products), and includes potentially anti-inflammatory compounds (e.g., enzymes) present in raw plant foods. The living food diet is an uncooked vegan diet rich in berries, fruits, vegetables, nuts, germinated seeds, and sprouts (i.e., rich sources of carotenoids, vitamins C and E, lactobacilli, and fiber). A small study that combined the notion of allergen elimination and "living food" showed that a vegan diet free of gluten may be of clinical benefit for certain patients with rheumatoid arthritis by reducing immunoreactivity to food antigens.[10] A significant, diet-induced change in fecal flora was observed in a group following an uncooked vegan diet.[11] Changes in fecal flora are associated with improvement in rheumatoid arthritis, even once the condition has been established. The use of prebiotics and probiotics can also improve the intestinal environment.

Although no significant improvement could be observed on a composite index, a controlled, double-blind study demonstrated that a diet high in unsaturated and low in saturated fats with hypoallergenic foods provided some clinical benefit.[12] A less profound dietary change, such as consumption of cooked vegetables and olive oil, is also inversely and independently associated with risk of rheumatoid arthritis.[13] A prospective cohort study suggested that decaffeinated coffee is independently and positively associated with the onset of rheumatoid arthritis, whereas tea consumption shows an inverse association with disease onset.[14]

Patients with rheumatoid arthritis may be prone to nutrient deficiencies. Patients with rheumatoid arthritis tend to have a lower mid-arm muscular circumference and lower serum albumin levels, suggesting impaired nutritional status despite the absence of an overtly deficient diet.[15] Another study demonstrated that, in spite of an equivalent dietary intake, patients with juvenile arthritis had significantly reduced serum concentrations of beta-carotene, retinol, and zinc compared with healthy control subjects.[16] These patients benefited from dietary supplements of nutrients when the dietary intake did not reach the recommended daily allowances. Given individual uniqueness, the optimal diet required may vary among patients.

NUTRIENT THERAPY/DIETARY SUPPLEMENTS

The risk of absorbing dietary triggers of the inflammatory response can be decreased by improving digestion and avoiding ingestion of high-risk allergens. Taking hydrochloric acid, pancreatic enzymes, and/or bromelain may aid digestion. Following a diet replete in zinc, folate, bioflavonoids, and vitamin C may enhance bowel integrity. Controlled clinical trials support management of rheumatoid arthritis by administration of one or a combination of polyunsaturated fatty acids, vitamin E, pantothenic acid, copper, selenium, and zinc.[17]

Dietary ω-3 fatty acids variably inhibit synthesis of platelet activating factor (PAF) and end products of cyclooxygenase and lipoxygenase. They can reduce production of substances that induce release of lysosomal enzymes, produce free radicals, and enhance aggregation of inflammatory cells. Studies of healthy volunteers and patients with rheumatoid arthritis have shown that up to 90% inhibition of proinflammatory cytokines (e.g., TNF-α and IL-1β) can be achieved after dietary supplementation with fish oils.[18] Use of flaxseed oil in domestic food preparation also reduced production of these cytokines. Flaxseed is rich in α-linoleic acid, the precursor of the fatty acids (eicosapentaenoic acid [EPA] and docosahexaenoic acid [DHA]) in fish oil. A placebo-controlled, double-blind, randomized study over 15 weeks demonstrated substantial cellular incorporation of ω-3 fatty acids and improved clinical status with fish oil supplementation at a daily dose of 40 mg ω-3 fatty acids per kilogram of body weight in persons on a diet in which the daily ω-6 fatty acid intake was less than 10 g.[19] A double-blind study indicated that ω-3 fatty acids, 130 mg/kg body weight daily, as ethyl esters of EPA and DHA significantly decreased the mean number of tender joints and duration of morning stiffness and improved patient activity.[20] Another study has shown that patients receiving MaxEPA were able to reduce their NSAID requirement without experiencing any deterioration in clinical or laboratory parameters of rheumatoid arthritis activity.[21] Benefit was experienced at 3 months and reached its peak at 12 months. There is good scientific evidence that patients with rheumatoid arthritis respond to ω-3 fatty acids.

Benefit may also be derived from ω-6 fatty acids. In a double-blind trial, patients who received a daily dose of 1.4 g of γ-linolenic acid (GLA), a ω-6 fatty acid from borage oil, reported less joint tenderness and swelling.[22] In a follow-up, double-blind study, 76% of patients showed meaningful improvement at 12 months when taking 2.8 g of GLA daily.[23] Concerns about the safety of borage oil because of its potentially toxic pyrrolozidine content can be eliminated by using the extracted oil, which is devoid of these alkaloids. GLA is the precursor of prostaglandin E_1, the eicosanoid that reduces the release of arachidonic acid from cell membranes, and various 15-hydroxyl derivatives that block transformation of arachidonic acid to leukotrienes.[24] In a review of herbal therapy, Little and Parsons[25] concluded that there appeared to be some potential benefit for the use of GLA in rheumatoid arthritis, although further studies are required to establish optimum dosage and duration of treatment.

Some other oils of marine origin (e.g., from the green-lipped mussel) and a range of vegetable oils (e.g., olive oil) also appear to have indirect anti-inflammatory actions.[26] This is consistent with the finding of abnormal fatty acid patterns for both ω-3 and ω-6 fatty acids in patients with rheumatoid arthritis.[5] Because both of these classes of fatty acids have been shown to have both immunosuppressive and anti-inflammatory effects[27] and to be associated with only occasional minor adverse reactions, such as bloating with ω-3 fatty acids and belching with ω-6 fatty acids, their use deserves serious consideration.

Although fatty acids may change the substrate in cell membranes, bioflavonoids can reduce the release of arachidonic acid from cell membranes. Quercetin, a bioflavonoid, has been shown to suppress TNF-α–induced expression of IL-8 and monocyte chemoattractant protein 1 in vitro.[27] TNF-α, present in synovial fluid of patients with rheumatoid arthritis, induces the expression of proinflammatory cytokines in synovial cells.

Clinical trials suggest that calcium with vitamin D and molybdenum can be used to prevent or treat complications.[17] Other minerals that have been used with varying success in the treatment of rheumatoid arthritis include zinc (50 mg three times daily), selenium (200 μg daily), and copper (4 mg/day).[28] Copper bracelets have traditionally been used for treatment of rheumatic conditions because copper is absorbed through the skin. Furthermore, copper salicylate is known to have analgesic and anti-inflammatory effects, and the efficacy of various copper-based anti-inflammatory drugs is under investigation.[29]

Clinical trials suggest that folic acid and vitamin E can reduce drug-related complications.[17] Both the well-documented efficacy and adverse effects of methotrexate in the treatment of rheumatoid arthritis are dose-dependent. Several of the adverse effects are related to folate deficiencies. Folic acid appears to reduce some side effects of methotrexate therapy without compromising its efficacy.[30] Numerous clinical investigations suggest that an individually adjusted supply of folic acid, rather than folinic acid, is helpful in patients for whom a properly balanced diet is insufficient to prevent folate deficiency.[31] Similarly, vitamin E reduces the adverse effects of aspirin. In a laboratory study, co-administration of vitamin E was found to render cyclooxygenase-2 more sensitive to inhibition by aspirin through an unknown mechanism.[32] Because the use of aspirin in rheumatoid arthritis is limited, since inhibition of the proinflammatory enzyme cyclooxygenase-2 occurs only at higher aspirin doses often associated with side effects such as gastric toxicity, such combination therapy may provide a safer anti-inflammatory therapy option with lower aspirin doses. Animal studies also showed that the beneficial effects of fish oil can be enhanced by the addition of 500 IU of vitamin E in the diet[33]; and 600 mg of vitamin E, administered twice daily, may exert a small but significant analgesic effect without suppressing inflammatory joint destruction.[34] A case-control study indicated that low α-tocopherol status may be a risk factor for rheumatoid arthritis, independently of rheumatoid factor status.[35] This study also suggested that low selenium status may be a risk factor for rheumatoid factor–negative rheumatoid arthritis.

HERBAL THERAPY

Phyto-anti-inflammatories appear to have considerable potential benefit in the symptomatic treatment of rheumatic disorders; however, further research is required to reach definitive conclusions.[36] Herbs that affect eicosanoid metabolism appear most promising.

Ginger is a traditional anti-inflammatory agent. Five constituents of ginger have been identified as inhibitors of prostaglandin synthesis.[37] Oral administration of ginger oil suppressed the induction of adjuvant-induced inflammation in rats.[38] A pilot study showed that patients with rheumatoid arthritis who consumed 5 g of fresh ginger or 0.5 to 1.0 g of powdered ginger daily reported less pain, better joint mobility, less swelling, and less morning stiffness within 3 months.[39]

Bromelain (20-40 mg three times daily), dried feverfew (70-86 mg/day), and curcumin (400 mg three times daily) have all been found to be beneficial in clinical studies.[40] *Urtica dioica* inhibits lipoxygenase, and clinical trials suggest that phytodolor may provide some symptomatic relief in certain patients.[40] There is a little evidence to suggest that boswellia offers clinical benefit without gastrointestinal side effects.

In addition to these traditional remedies, another avenue of natural intervention is emerging. Beta-sitosterol and its glycoside are sterol molecules synthesized by plants. In animals, these sterols exhibit anti-inflammatory, antineoplastic, antipyretic, and immune-modulating activity. A proprietary mixture of this phytosterol complex seems to target specific T-helper lymphocytes, the T_H1 and T_H2 cells, helping normalize their function and improve T-lymphocyte and natural killer cell activity.[41] By selectively activating or inhibiting certain aspects of the immune response, various combinations of these compounds may be able to effectively regulate and control the overactive immune response seen in rheumatoid arthritis and other autoimmune diseases.[42] Should this prove possible, specific therapy, rather than generalized immunosuppression, may be achieved.

PRACTICE TIPS

- *Spirulina*, the blue-green algae, has antioxidant and anti-inflammatory properties that may help patients with rheumatoid arthritis.
- Herbalists believe that, unlike synthetic salicylates, natural salicylates from willow bark, the poplar tree, black cohosh, and meadowsweet do not cause dyspepsia.
- Ginger and turmeric may be helpful.
- As of 2001, there is no scientifically documented evidence to support the use of green lipped mussels.
- NSAIDs may exacerbate arthritis by interfering with essential fatty acid metabolism and increasing gut permeability to microbial and food antigens.
- Copper complexes can reduce inflammation and heal NSAID-induced peptic ulcers.
- Nutritional intervention can be used to reduce the dose of NSAIDs required to control rheumatoid arthritis.
- Eating 224 g of herring supplies 3.2 g of ω-3 fatty acids; salmon provides 2.4 g, and tuna provides 1 g.

REFERENCES

1. Darlington LG, Stone TW: Antioxidants and fatty acids in the amelioration of rheumatoid arthritis and related disorders, *Br J Nutr* 85:251-69, 2001.
2. Darlington LG, Ramsey NW, Mansfield JR: Placebo-controlled, blind study of dietary manipulation therapy in rheumatoid arthritis, *Lancet* 1:236-8, 1986.
3. Sigthorsson G, Tibble J, Hayllar J, et al: Intestinal permeability and inflammation in patients on NSAIDs. *Gut* 43:506-11, 1998.
4. Inman RD: Arthritis and enteritis—an interface of protean manifestations, *J Rheumatol* 14:406-10, 1987.
5. Inman RD: Antigens, the gastrointestinal tract, and arthritis, *Rheum Dis Clin North Am* 17:309-21, 1991.
6. Harigai M, Hara M, Yoshimura T, et al: Monocyte chemoattractant protein-1 (MCP-1) in inflammatory joint diseases and its involvement in the cytokine network of rheumatoid synovium, *Clin Immunol Immunopathol* 69:83-91, 1993.
7. Henderson CJ, Panush RS: Diets, dietary supplements, and nutritional therapies in rheumatic diseases, *Rheum Dis Clin North Am* 25(4):937-68, 1999.
8. Gaby AR: Alternative treatments for rheumatoid arthritis, *Altern Med Rev* 4(6):392-402, 1999.
9. Hanninen P, Kaartinen K, Rauma AL, et al: Antioxidants in vegan diet and rheumatic disorders, *Toxicology* 155:45-53, 2000.
10. Hafstrom I, Ringertz B, Spangberg A, et al: A vegan diet free of gluten improves the signs and symptoms of rheumatoid arthritis: the effects on arthritis correlate with a reduction in antibodies to food antigens, *Rheumatology (Oxford)* 40:1175-9, 2001.
11. Peltonen R, Nenonen M, Helve T, et al: Faecal microbial flora and disease activity in rheumatoid arthritis during a vegan diet, *Br J Rheumatol* 36:64-8, 1997.
12. Sarzi-Puttini P, Comi D, Boccassini L, et al: Diet therapy for rheumatoid arthritis. A controlled double-blind study of two different dietary regimens, *Scand J Rheumatol* 29(5):302-7, 2000.
13. Linos A, Kaklamani VG, Kaklamani E, et al: Dietary factors in relation to rheumatoid arthritis: a role for olive oil and cooked vegetables? *Am J Clin Nutr* 70:1077-82, 1999.
14. Mikuls TR, Cerhan JR, Criswell LA, et al: Coffee, tea, and caffeine consumption and risk of rheumatoid arthritis: results from the Iowa Women's Health Study, *Arthritis Rheum* 46:83-91, 2002.
15. Gomez-Vaquero C, Nolla JM, Fiter J, et al: Nutritional status in patients with rheumatoid arthritis, *Joint Bone Spine* 68:403-9, 2001.
16. Helgeland M, Svendsen E, Forre O, et al: Dietary intake and serum concentrations of antioxidants in children with juvenile arthritis, *Clin Exp Rheumatol* 18:637-41, 2000.
17. Werbach MR: *Textbook of nutritional medicine*, Tarzana, CA, 1999, Third Line Press.
18. James MJ, Gibson RA, Cleland LG: Dietary polyunsaturated fatty acids and inflammatory mediator production, *Am J Clin Nutr* 71(suppl 1):343S-348S, 2000.
19. Volker D, Fitzgerald P, Major G, et al: Efficacy of fish oil concentrate in the treatment of rheumatoid arthritis, *J Rheumatol* 27:2343-6, 2000.

20. Kremer JM, Lawrence DA, Petrillo GF, et al: Effects of high-dose fish oil on rheumatoid arthritis after stopping nonsteroidal antiinflammatory drugs. Clinical and immune correlates, *Arthritis Rheum* 38:1107-14, 1995.

21. Lau CS, Morley KD, Belch JJ: Effects of fish oil supplementation on non-steroidal anti-inflammatory drug requirement in patients with mild rheumatoid arthritis—a double-blind placebo controlled study, *Br J Rheumatol* 32:982-9, 1993.

22. Leventhal LJ, Boyce EG, Zurier RB: Treatment of rheumatoid arthritis with gammalinolenic acid, *Ann Intern Med* 119:867-73, 1993.

23. Zurier RB, Rossetti RG, Jacobson EW, et al: Gamma-linolenic acid treatment of rheumatoid arthritis. A randomized, placebo-controlled trial, *Arthritis Rheum* 39:1808-17, 1996.

24. Belch JJ, Hill A: Evening primrose oil and borage oil in rheumatologic conditions, *Am J Clin Nutr* 71(suppl):352S-356S, 2000.

25. Little C, Parsons T: Herbal therapy for treating rheumatoid arthritis (Cochrane Review), *Cochrane Database Syst Rev* 1:CD002948, 2001.

26. Navarro E, Esteve M, Olive A, et al: Abnormal fatty acid pattern in rheumatoid arthritis. A rationale for treatment with marine and botanical lipids, *J Rheumatol* 27:298-303, 2000.

27. Calder PC: Sir David Cuthbertson Medal Lecture. Immunomodulatory and anti-inflammatory effects of n-3 polyunsaturated fatty acids, *Proc Nutr Soc* 55:737-74, 1996.

28. Sato M, Miyazaki T, Kambe F, et al: Quercetin, a bioflavonoid, inhibits the induction of interleukin 8 and monocyte chemoattractant protein-1 expression by tumor necrosis factor-alpha in cultured human synovial cells, *J Rheumatol* 24:1680-4, 1997.

29. Jackson GE, Mkhonta-Gama L, Voye A, et al: Design of copper-based anti-inflammatory drugs, *J Inorg Biochem* 79:147-52, 2000.

30. Griffith SM, Fisher J, Clarke S, et al: Do patients with rheumatoid arthritis established on methotrexate and folic acid 5 mg daily need to continue folic acid supplements long term? *Rheumatology (Oxford)* 39:1102-9, 2000.

31. Endresen GK, Husby G: Folate supplementation during methotrexate treatment of patients with rheumatoid arthritis. An update and proposals for guidelines, *Scand J Rheumatol* 30:129-34, 2001.

32. Abate A, Yang G, Dennery PA, et al: Synergistic inhibition of cyclooxygenase-2 expression by vitamin E and aspirin, *Free Radic Biol Med* 29:1135-42, 2000.

33. Venkatraman JT, Chu WC: Effects of dietary omega-3 and omega-6 lipids and vitamin E on serum cytokines, lipid mediators and anti-DNA antibodies in a mouse model for rheumatoid arthritis, *J Am Coll Nutr* 18:602-13, 1999.

34. Edmonds SE, Winyard PG, Guo R, et al: Putative analgesic activity of repeated oral doses of vitamin E in the treatment of rheumatoid arthritis. Results of a prospective placebo controlled double blind trial, *Ann Rheum Dis* 56:649-55, 1997.

35. Knekt P, Heliovaara M, Aho K, et al: Serum selenium, serum alpha-tocopherol, and the risk of rheumatoid arthritis, *Epidemiology* 11:402-5, 2000.

36. Ernst E, Chrubasik S: Phyto-anti-inflammatories. A systematic review of randomized, placebo-controlled, double-blind trials, *Rheum Dis Clin North Am* 26:13-27, vii, 2000.

37. Kiuchi F, Shibuya M, Sankawa U: Inhibitors of prostaglandin biosynthesis from ginger, *Chem Pharm Bull (Tokyo)* 30:754-7, 1982.

38. Sharma JN, Srivastava KC, Gan EK: Suppressive effects of eugenol and ginger oil on arthritic rats, *Pharmacology* 49:314-8, 1994.
39. Srivastava KC, Mustafa T: Ginger (*Zingiber officinale*) and rheumatic disorders, *Med Hypotheses* 29:25-8, 1989.
40. Pinn G: Herbal therapy in rheumatology, *Aust Fam Phys* 30:878-83, 2001.
41. Bouic PJD, Lamprecht JH: Plant sterols and sterolins: a review of their immune-modulating properties, *Altern Med Rev* 4:170-7, 1999.
42. Bouic PJD: Sterols/sterolins: the natural, nontoxic immuno-modulators and their role in the control of rheumatoid arthritis, *The Arthritis Trust* Summer:3-6, 1998.

■ CHAPTER 44 ■

STONES—CHOLELITHIASIS AND UROLITHIASIS

At least one in five persons has an asymptomatic stone or experiences stone-related colic during his or her lifetime. The gallbladder and urinary tract are the anatomic areas most prone to stone formation. Genetic predisposition, dietary choices, and infection all influence stone formation.

Most gallstones are composed of cholesterol; the remainder are composed of bile pigment. Cholesterol, derived mainly but not solely from the diet, is secreted in the bile. Cholesterol stones form when there is a relative excess of cholesterol compared with bile salts. As many as three in four gallstones are asymptomatic, and many persons with gallstone dyspepsia do not experience relief of symptoms after removal of their gallstones.

Urinary stones result from crystallization of urinary solutes. Predisposing factors are reduced urine flow, increased concentrations of urinary crystalloids (e.g., calcium salts, uric acid, and cystine), and changes in urinary pH. Common causes include infection, the presence of foreign bodies, dehydration, diet, and periods of immobility.[1]

Seven of 10 patients with urolithiasis will experience a recurrence within the next 5 years. Fortunately, spontaneous passage usually occurs when stones are less than 5 mm in diameter. In fact, more than 90% of stones pass without complication within 3 to 7 days of presentation.

CLINICAL DIAGNOSIS

Stones in the gallbladder or kidneys are asymptomatic; pain is precipitated once a stone moves into the bile duct or ureter. Pain occurs when a stone is impacted in or propelled along a narrow passage. Stones in the urinary or biliary system present as colic. The pain is severe and often associated with restlessness, nausea, vomiting, and sweating.

In the case of biliary colic, the patient experiences pain that lasts for hours, which may start in the back and later radiate between the shoulders. Typically, the pain occurs after eating or at night. Attacks recur as pain in the right hypochondrium. Murphy's sign is positive; that is, inspiration is arrested when the tender inflamed gallbladder is palpated during examination of the area under the right costal margin. The patient may become jaundiced. Biliary colic lacks the periodicity of renal colic.

Renal colic presents with the abrupt onset of pain. Depending on the site of impaction, renal colic may present as a relatively constant ache in the loin or as intense unilateral loin-to-groin pain that waxes and wanes. Pain radiates to the groin, testicles, labia, and/or suprapubic area. On physical examination, costovertebral angle tenderness is detected. Hematuria, dysuria, and urinary frequency are present. The abdomen may become distended as a result of an associated reflex ileus.

THERAPEUTIC STRATEGY

The aim of intervention is to prevent stasis and supersaturation of bile or urine. In the case of the former, this is largely achieved by causing contraction of the gallbladder; with respect to the latter, a high fluid intake ensures a good flow of dilute urine. A urine output in excess of 2 L/day is recommended.[1]

Aside from ensuring a good urine flow, the particular intervention required to prevent stone formation is determined by the particular predisposing factors in each patient. Dietary choices influence the consistency of bile and urine. Dietary changes are influenced by the particular composition of the stone involved. Low dietary potassium, magnesium, and oxalate intake, an increased body mass index, and a history of hypertension are associated with an increased risk of kidney stones; but supplemental calcium intake of more than 500 mg daily is inversely associated with stone occurrence.[2] Similarly, an adequate dietary phytate intake is required to maintain urinary levels that effectively inhibit crystallization of calcium salts and subsequent renal stone formation. Urinary phytate content is significantly lower in patients with a tendency for stone formation. A phytate-free diet decreases the urinary excretion of phytate by about 50% after 36 hours.[3]

LIFESTYLE CHANGES

Eating frequent small meals reduces the risk of gallstones by stimulating contraction and more frequent emptying of the gallbladder. Olive oil enhances gallbladder contraction and consequently reduces the risk of cholelithiasis.[4] However, lavish amounts of olive oil and lemon juice should be avoided in persons with large gallstones, because they may cause impaction. A low-energy diet of 860 calories or less a day increases the risk of gallstones, whereas a diet rich in wheat bran may reduce the cholesterol content of bile and the risk of gallstones. A high-fiber diet does not appear to directly reduce the risk of gallstones.[5]

The risk of urinary stones is reduced by drinking copiously; eight or more glasses of water daily is recommended. The importance of a good fluid intake should not be underestimated. Analysis of data from three Northern California Kaiser Permanente medical centers suggests that increased fluid intake alone is as effective as following a low–animal-protein, high-fiber, and high-fluid diet.[6] A cohort study demonstrated that magnesium intake and beer consumption were inversely associated, fiber intake was directly associated, and calcium intake was not associated with the risk of kidney stones.[7] Each bottle of beer consumed daily was estimated to reduce risk by 40%. At least part of this benefit is attributable to the fluid load.

Persons prone to calcium stones may benefit from a low-salt, moderately low-protein diet. Although a high-protein diet can elevate urinary calcium, uric acid, and sulfate levels and decrease urinary citrate levels, restriction of protein to less than the current recommended daily allowance for the management of stone disease is not currently recommended.[8] Persons prone to oxalate stones should follow a low-fat diet and avoid oxalate-rich foods (e.g., beetroot, dried figs, currants, rhubarb, parsley, spinach, grapefruit, and cranberry juice). Drinking herbal rather than black tea may help to reduce the risk of calcium oxalate stone formation.[9] Dietary oxalate restriction is particularly prudent for patients with a tendency for stone formation and hyperoxaluria.[10] Dietary factors and/or a molecular lesion may contribute to the pathophysiology of uric acid stone formation in persons with a very low urinary pH.[11] Persons prone to uric acid stones benefit from an alkaline urine and therefore should avoid dietary factors that tend to lower urinary pH (e.g., vitamin C). Animal protein, a good source of the sulfur-containing amino acids methionine and cystine, should be limited. Patients with uric acid stones should avoid liver, kidneys, sweetbreads, sardines, anchovies, fish roe, and yeast extracts (i.e., foods rich in purines), the precursors of uric acid. A high-carbohydrate diet enhances uric acid secretion; a low-fat diet retards uric acid secretion.

In general, there is compelling evidence that a diet high in sodium, animal protein, and sucrose increases the risk of stone formation, but undue reductions in calcium intake appear detrimental.[12]

NUTRIENT THERAPY/DIETARY SUPPLEMENTS

Cholesterol is an important component of gallstones. Ascorbic acid affects the catabolism of cholesterol to bile acids and the development of gallbladder disease in experimental animals. Serum ascorbic acid level is inversely related to the prevalence of clinical and asymptomatic gallbladder disease among women, but not men.[13] Women at risk of gallstones should, perhaps, avoid vitamin C supplementation. Fat seems less problematic. A diet rich in cholesterol and saturated fats was negatively associated with the risk of gallstone disease in a group of women.[14] A double-blind, placebo-controlled clinical trial demonstrated that fish oil probably results in the prevention of cholesterol gallstone formation in obese woman who are on rapid weight loss diets.[15] Omega-3 fatty acids decrease biliary cholesterol saturation in the bile of patients with gallstones. Results of clinical trials also support increasing the intake of essential fatty acids to reduce the risk of urinary stone formation.[16]

Urinary oxalate, an important determinant of calcium oxalate kidney stone formation, is amenable to modification by dietary supplements. Cranberry concentrates increase the risk of oxalate stones. In a study of healthy volunteers, cranberry tablets taken to avoid urinary tract infections were found to increase urinary oxalate content.[17] Patients at risk for nephrolithiasis should be cautioned against ingestion of these supplements. On the other hand, high doses of vitamin B_6 may decrease oxalate production. Results of a prospective cohort study indicated that a high intake of vitamin B_6 was inversely associated with the risk of stone formation. In this study, the relative risk of incident stone formation for women in the highest intake group taking at least 40 mg of vitamin B_6 daily was 0.66, compared with the lowest intake group.[18]

Magnesium appears to reduce urinary saturation of calcium oxalate by forming a more soluble magnesium oxalate complex when it is administered with a meal. Magnesium (200 mg twice daily) taken alone[16] or magnesium oxide (300 mg/day), combined with pyridoxine hydrochloride (10 mg/day), causes a gradual and significant decline in oxalate excretion during the therapy.[19] The risk of formation of calcium oxalate stones was decreased within 120 days.

In a case study of persons at risk for recurrent urinary stones, Williams et al[20] concluded that regular calcium supplementation (500 mg daily) does not raise the product of calcium and oxalate in urine and the proportion of oxalate to calcium is reduced. Furthermore, two powerful, prospective, observational studies suggested that increased dietary calcium reduced the risk of the first kidney stone.[21] A dietary calcium intake of at least 1000 mg daily should be encouraged.

Vitamin C has long been debated as a risk factor for urinary stones. Ascorbate breakdown reportedly accounts for 30% to 55% of urinary oxalate excreted. Although vitamin C can be metabolized to oxalate, routine restriction of vitamin C to prevent stone formation appears unwarranted.[18] Despite concerns that megadose vitamin C supplementation may precipitate urinary oxalate stones, a study of the pathophysiologic role of ascorbic acid in renal calcium stone formation failed to demonstrate that vitamin C facilitated stone formation or directly modulated calcium oxalate crystallization.[22] Daily vitamin C supplementation of 1500 mg does not appear to be associated with risk. However, it should be noted that vitamin C may increase the risk of stone formation in a subgroup of persons with a urinary tract infection caused by a particular organism. Urinary ascorbate, if present at a high concentration in association with *Proteus mirabilis* infection, appears to be locally degraded to oxalate, potentially leading to calcium oxalate deposition on infection stones.[23]

HERBAL THERAPY

Choleretics stimulate bile production by hepatocytes; cholagogues stimulate release of bile from the biliary system. Herbs that have choleretic and cholagogic effects include barberry, Oregon grape, dandelion, and wild yam. They should be avoided by persons with large or impacted gallstones. On the other hand, chamomile, a spasmolytic, may theoretically ease gallbladder pain. A terpene mixture reminiscent of peppermint oil is reputed to dissolve gallstones.

Results of animal studies suggest that beneficial effects caused by herb infusions on urolithiasis can be attributed to some disinfectant action, and tentatively, to the presence of saponins. Herbs believed to prevent and treat kidney stone formation are *Verbena officinalis*, *Lithospermum officinale*, *Taraxacum officinale*, *Equisetum arvense*, *Arctostaphylos uva-ursi*, *Arctium lappa*, and *Silene saxifraga*.[24]

PRACTICE TIPS

- Herbal diuretics such as parsley, celery, and nettle, by increasing urinary flow, may reduce the risk of stone formation.
- Calcium supplementation with calcium citrate is preferred because citrate is a major anion used to inhibit calcium oxalate crystal formation in the kidneys.
- Magnesium supplements should be taken with meals to maximize their efficacy.

REFERENCES

1. Steggall MJ: Urinary tract stones: cause, complications and treatment, *Br J Nurs* 10:1452-6, 2002.
2. Hall WD, Pettinger M, Oberman A, et al: Risk factors for kidney stones in older women in the southern United States, *Am J Med Sci* 322:12-8, 2001.
3. Grases F, March JG, Prieto RM, et al: Urinary phytate in calcium oxalate stone formers and healthy people—dietary effects on phytate excretion, *Scand J Urol Nephrol* 34:162-4, 2000.
4. Alarcon de la Lastra C, Barranco MD, Motilva V, Herrerias JM: Mediterranean diet and health: biological importance of olive oil, *Curr Pharm Des* 7:933-50, 2001.
5. Bennett WG, Cerda JJ: Benefits of dietary fiber. Myth or medicine? *Postgrad Med* 99:153-6, 166-8, 171-2, 1996.
6. Hiatt RA, Ettinger B, Caan B, et al: Randomized controlled trial of a low animal protein, high fiber diet in the prevention of recurrent calcium oxalate kidney stones, *Am J Epidemiol* 144:25-33, 1996.
7. Hirvonen T, Pietinen P, Virtanen M, et al: Nutrient intake and use of beverages and the risk of kidney stones among male smokers, *Am J Epidemiol* 150:187-94, 1999.
8. Martini LA, Wood RJ: Should dietary calcium and protein be restricted in patients with nephrolithiasis? *Nutr Rev* 58:111-7, 2000.
9. Mills S, Bone K: *Principles and practice of phytotherapy*, Edinburgh, 2000, Churchill Livingstone.

10. Assimos DG, Holmes RP: Role of diet in the therapy of urolithiasis, *Urol Clin North Am* 27:255-68, 2000.
11. Kamel KS, Cheema-Dhadli S, Halperin ML: Studies on the pathophysiology of the low urine pH in patients with uric acid stones, *Kidney Int* 61:988-94, 2002.
12. Colussi G, De Ferrari ME, Brunati C, et al: Medical prevention and treatment of urinary stones, *J Nephrol* 13(suppl 3):S65-S70, 2000.
13. Simon JA, Hudes ES: Serum ascorbic acid and gallbladder disease prevalence among US adults: the Third National Health and Nutrition Examination Survey (NHANES III), *Arch Intern Med* 160:931-6, 2000.
14. Devesa F, Ferrando J, Caldentey M, et al: Cholelithiasic disease and associated factors in a Spanish population, *Dig Dis Sci* 46:1424-36, 2001.
15. Mendez-Sanchez N, Gonzalez V, Aguayo P, et al: Fish oil (n-3) polyunsaturated fatty acids beneficially affect biliary cholesterol nucleation time in obese women losing weight, *J Nutr* 131:2300-3, 2001.
16. Werbach MR: *Textbook of nutritional medicine*, Tarzana, CA, 1999, Third Line Press.
17. Terris MK, Issa MM, Tacker JR: Dietary supplementation with cranberry concentrate tablets may increase the risk of nephrolithiasis, *Urology* 57:26-9, 2001.
18. Curhan GC, Willett WC, Speizer FE, et al: Intake of vitamins B_6 and C and the risk of kidney stones in women, *J Am Soc Nephrol* 10:840-5, 1999.
19. Rattan V, Sidhu H, Vaidyanathan S, et al: Effect of combined supplementation of magnesium oxide and pyridoxine in calcium-oxalate stone formers, *Urol Res* 22:161-5, 1994.
20. Williams CP, Child DF, Hudson PR, et al: Why oral calcium supplements may reduce renal stone disease: report of a clinical pilot study, *J Clin Pathol* 54:54-62, 2001.
21. Heller HJ: The role of calcium in the prevention of kidney stones, *J Am Coll Nutr* 18(suppl 5):373S-378S, 1999.
22. Schwille PO, Schmiedl A, Herrmann U, et al: Ascorbic acid in idiopathic recurrent calcium urolithiasis in humans—does it have an abettor role in oxalate, and calcium oxalate crystallization? *Urol Res* 28:167-77, 2000.
23. Hokama S, Toma C, Jahana M, et al: Ascorbate conversion to oxalate in alkaline milieu and *Proteus mirabilis* culture, *Mol Urol* 4:321-8, 2000.
24. Grases F, Melero G, Costa-Bauza A, et al: Urolithiasis and phytotherapy, *Int Urol Nephrol* 26:507-11, 1994.

■ CHAPTER 45 ■

RECURRENT URINARY TRACT INFECTIONS

> Because they have short urethras, women are at particular risk for urinary tract infections.

CLINICAL DIAGNOSIS

Urinary symptoms such as frequency, burning, or urgency suggest infection. Diagnosis is confirmed by urinalysis. Indications for urine culture are relapsing or recurrent infection, suspected pyelonephritis, complicated infections, or an uncertain history coupled with a dipstick positive for nitrites and/or leukocytes.

THERAPEUTIC STRATEGY

Strategies for preventing recurrent urinary tract infections include use of antibiotics or antiseptics, probiotics, functional foods, or natural peptides; avoidance of spermicides; and maintenance of good hygiene.[1] Natural measures focus on preventing bacteriuria.

LIFESTYLE CHANGES

Good urinary hygiene aims to reduce urinary stasis and includes emptying the bladder completely before going to sleep and drinking at least 2.5 L of water a day. A popular natural approach to treating urinary tract infection is consumption of 800 mg (400 mg twice daily) of cranberries or 500 mL of undiluted cranberry juice mixed with apple or pear juice to taste. Half this amount is taken to prevent recurrences. Cranberry juice appears to significantly reduce adhesion of bacteria to cells.[2] This may be due to proanthocyanidin trimers, which have been shown to prevent adherence of P-fimbriated *Escherichia coli* to the surfaces of uroepithelial cells.[3] Despite popular belief and support from some clinical trials, a recent review indicated that no trials of scientifically acceptable quality were available to assess the efficacy of cranberry juice for the treatment of urinary tract infections.[4] Nonetheless, a randomized, double-blind, placebo-controlled trial showed that consumption of 300 mL of a commercially available standard cranberry beverage per day did reduce the frequency of bacteriuria with pyuria in older women.[5] Urine samples obtained after cranberry or ascorbic acid supplementation had reduced initial deposition rates and reduced numbers of adherent *E. coli* and *Enterococcus faecalis* but not *Pseudomonas aeruginosa, Staphylococcus epidermidis,* or *Candida albicans.*[6] Cranberry may be selectively protective.

In addition to attempts to prevent adherence of bacteria to the bladder wall, a possible prophylactic approach is colonization of the vulvovaginal area with commensals. A crossover trial demonstrated that daily ingestion of 150 mL of yogurt enriched with live *Lactobacillus acidophilus* organisms increased colonization of the rectum and vagina by these bacteria and may have reduced episodes of bacterial vaginosis.[7] Competitive exclusion of pathogens and production of inhibitory substances, including bacteriocins, by these commensals may explain any protective effect. Intravaginal *L. acidophilus* therapy reduces the recurrence rate of uncomplicated lower urinary tract infections in women.[8] Weekly vaginal insertion of lactobacilli may be helpful.[9] Use of *Lactobacillus* strains resistant to nonoxynol 9, a spermicide that kills members of the protective normal vaginal flora, may also be useful in women with recurrent cystitis who use this contraceptive agent.

An integrated approach may be required. However, an open, randomized, controlled trial (over 1 year) of consumption of 50 mL of cranberry-lingonberry juice concentrate daily for 6 months or regular consumption of 100 mL of lactobacilli 5 days a week showed that cranberry juice, but not lactobacilli, seemed to reduce the recurrence of urinary tract infections.[10]

NUTRIENT THERAPY/DIETARY SUPPLEMENTS

Urinary acidification with vitamin C is used to treat and prevent urinary tract infections. Nitric oxide, a bacteriostatic gas, is formed when nitrite is acidified. Infected urine may contain considerable amounts of nitrite as a result of bacterial nitrate reductase activity. In fact, detection of nitrite in urine is routinely used in the diagnosis of bacterial cystitis. Results of a laboratory study confirmed that nitrite-producing bacteria, such as *E. coli,* induce their own death in acidic urine by supplying substrate for generation of bacteriostatic compounds such as nitric oxide.[11] Results of another laboratory study confirmed that mildly acidified nitrite-containing urine generated large amounts of nitric oxide and this production was greatly potentiated by ascorbic acid.[12] The growth of *E. coli, Pseudomonas aeruginosa,* and *Staphylococcus saprophyticus* were all markedly reduced by the addition of nitrite to acidified urine. However, the clinical relevance of urinary acidification with ascorbic acid is doubtful, because 1.8 g of ascorbic acid daily failed to cause a statistically significant reduction in urinary pH,[13] and 1 g, administered four times daily, only caused a statistically and clinically insignificant mean decrease in urinary pH of 0.58.[14]

HERBAL THERAPY

Cranberry and bilberry, berries of the heather family, appear to impair adhesion of bacteria. Cranberry tablets are available, but results of a small trial suggest that they may increase the risk of urinary stones.[15] Furthermore, cranberry reduces the efficacy of other herbs and therefore should not be used in conjunction with bearberry (*Arctostaphylos uva-ursi*).

Other herbs that may be useful include goldenseal, a urinary antiseptic, and dandelion, an herbal diuretic.[16] Other herbal diuretics are nettle (*Urtica dioica*), parsley, and celery. Drinking one cup of hot nettle tea made from a teaspoon of the dried herb may be helpful.[17]

PRACTICE TIPS

- Women troubled by recurrent urinary tract infections may benefit from drinking 10 ounces of cranberry or blueberry juice daily.
- Eating a cup of cranberries daily reduces the risk of recurrent urinary tract infections.
- Cranberry deodorizes urine and my be useful for persons with an incontinence problem.
- A high fluid intake including cranberry juice and/or barley water (30 g of barley in 1 L of water reduced by boiling to 500 mL) is helpful.
- Sodium citrate neutralizes acidic urine, which reduces burning, but does not eliminate and may encourage multiplication of bacteria.

REFERENCES

1. Reid G: Potential preventive strategies and therapies in urinary tract infection, *World J Urol* 17:359-63, 1999.
2. Reid G, Hsiehl J, Potter P, et al: Cranberry juice consumption may reduce biofilms on uroepithelial cells: pilot study in spinal cord injured patients, *Spinal Cord* 39:26-30, 2001.
3. Foo LY, Lu Y, Howell AB, et al: A-type proanthocyanidin trimers from cranberry that inhibit adherence of uropathogenic P-fimbriated *Escherichia coli, J Nat Prod* 63:1225-8, 2000.
4. Jepson RG, Mihaljevic L, Craig J: Cranberries for treating urinary tract infections, *Cochrane Database Syst Rev* 2:CD001322, 2000.
5. Avorn J, Monane M, Gurwitz JH, et al: Reduction of bacteriuria and pyuria after ingestion of cranberry juice, *JAMA* 271:751-4, 1994.
6. Habash MB, Van der Mei HC, Busscher HJ, et al: The effect of water, ascorbic acid, and cranberry derived supplementation on human urine and uropathogen adhesion to silicone rubber, *Can J Microbiol* 45:691-4, 1999.

7. Shalev E, Battino S, Weiner E, et al: Ingestion of yogurt containing *Lactobacillus acidophilus* compared with pasteurized yogurt as prophylaxis for recurrent candidal vaginitis and bacterial vaginosis, *Arch Fam Med* 5:593-6, 1996.

8. Reid G, Bruce AW, McGroarty JA, et al: Is there a role for lactobacilli in prevention of urogenital and intestinal infection? *Clin Microbiol Rev* 3:335-44, 1990.

9. Bruce AW, Reid G, McGroanty JA: Preliminary study on the prevention of recurrent urinary tract infection in adult women using intravaginal lactobacilli, *Int Urogynecol J Pelvic Floor Dysfunct* 103:22-5, 2000.

10. Kontiokari T, Sundqvist K, Nuutinen M, et al: Randomised trial of cranberry-lingonberry juice and Lactobacillus GG drink for the prevention of urinary tract infections in women, *BMJ* 322:1571, 2001.

11. Lundberg JO, Carlsson S, Engstrand L, et al: Urinary nitrite: more than a marker of infection, *Urology* 50:189-91, 1997.

12. Carlsson S, Wiklund NP, Engstrand L, et al: Effects of pH, nitrite, and ascorbic acid on nonenzymatic nitric oxide generation and bacterial growth in urine, *Nitric Oxide* 5:580-6, 2001.

13. Wall I, Tiselius HG: Long-term acidification of urine in patients treated for infected renal stones, *Urol Int* 45:336-41, 1990.

14. Hetey SK, Kleinberg ML, Parker WD, et al: Effect of ascorbic acid on urine pH in patients with injured spinal cords, *Am J Hosp Pharm* 37:235-7, 1980.

15. Terris MK, Issa MM, Tacker JR: Dietary supplementation with cranberry concentrate tablets may increase the risk of nephrolithiasis, *Urology* 57:26-9, 2001.

16. Mills S, Bone K: *Principles and practice of phytotherapy*, Edinburgh, 2000, Churchill Livingstone.

17. Diefendorf D, Healey J, Kalyn W, editors: *The healing power of vitamins, minerals and herbs*, Surry Hills, Australia, 2000, Readers Digest.

■ CHAPTER 46 ■

VENOUS DISORDERS

More than one in 10 men and one in five women have varicose veins. Three in four persons have hemorrhoids at some point in their lives. A loss of vascular integrity is associated with the pathogenesis of both hemorrhoids and varicose veins. Less prevalent, but potentially more serious, is chronic venous insufficiency. Any prolonged obstruction to venous draining is accompanied by varying degrees of venous insufficiency.

CLINICAL DIAGNOSIS

The clinical presentation of hemorrhoids, varicose veins, and chronic venous insufficiency is determined by the pathophysiologic changes of the vessel involved. Hemorrhoids, varices of the superior hemorrhoidal vein that drains the anorectal area, present as bleeding on defecation. Blood may splatter the bedpan or be streaked on the toilet paper or the stool's surface. Depending on the magnitude of the hemorrhoid, bleeding may be associated with varying degrees of protrusion of the anal mucosa. The larger and more persistent the prolapse, the greater is the likelihood of a mucoid discharge and anal pruritus.

Varicose veins are varices of the superficial leg veins. They are abnormally dilated, tortuous veins. Although often asymptomatic, varicose veins may present as a dull, aching heaviness exacerbated by standing and improved by walking or elevating the leg. Because superficial veins are poorly supported, they tend to become tortuous if exposed to high venous back pressure, as may occur with valvular incompetence or deep vein thrombosis.

Deep vein thrombosis is an important cause of impaired drainage that results in venous insufficiency. Chronic venous insufficiency is most commonly encountered in the lower limbs as a result of thrombosis of the deep veins of the lower limbs. The mildest form of venous insufficiency is minimal edema after prolonged standing. More clinically relevant is chronic venous insufficiency, which presents as progressive leg edema, pruritic atrophic skin, a cyanotic limb, and chronic recurrent ulceration.

THERAPEUTIC STRATEGY

When possible, the goal of intervention is to modify factors that predispose to venous insufficiency or varicosity. Excess pressure on a normal or weakened vessel wall predisposes the vessel to tortuosity. The likelihood of venous tortuosity is increased by pressure such as that which occurs with venous valvular incompetence or straining on defecation as in constipation. The aim of intervention is to prevent undue pressure on the vessel wall.

Impaired blood flow may result from partial or complete occlusion of the vessel lumen, most often caused by thrombosis. Preventing deep vein thrombosis reduces the risk of both varicose veins and venous insufficiency. The risk of thrombosis is increased by stasis, damage to the intima of the vessel wall, or increased blood coagulability. The aims of intervention are to prevent external occlusive pressure on the vessel wall, to improve venous tone, and to prevent blood coagulation.

LIFESTYLE CHANGES

Exercise and hydration reduce the risk of both hemorrhoids and venous thrombosis. Good bowel habits are fundamental to decreasing the risk of hemorrhoids, constipation, and straining on defecation. Strategies include not suppressing the urge to defecate, a high fluid intake, and a fiber-rich diet. Fiber shortens and fat tends to prolong bowel transit time.[1] Insoluble fiber draws fluid into the bowel, increasing the bulk and softness of the stool. Good sources of dietary fiber include nuts, whole-grain products, fruits, and vegetables. Particularly good sources of insoluble fiber are figs, raspberries, dried fruit, and whole-grain cereals. Stone fruits, pineapple, and citrus fruits have good fiber content, as do cabbage, peas, beans, cauliflower, and brussels sprouts. An adequate total dietary fiber intake appears to be one that yields a stool of 200 to 250 g in one or two passes a day. Prunes and kiwi fruit, in addition to their fiber content, have other chemicals conducive to the regular passage of a soft stool.

The risk of venous thrombosis may be reduced by a number of dietary choices. Alcohol and phenolics in wine have demonstrated platelet inhibition in vitro.[2] Persons at risk of thrombosis may benefit from regular consumption of red wine or even grape juice. Omega-3 fatty acids are believed to be responsible for the prolonged bleeding tendency observed among Eskimos. A diet rich in fish oil, which favors decreased production of thromboxane A_2 and increased production of thromboxane A_3 and prostaglandin I_3, inhibits platelet aggregation.[3] A diet rich in deep sea cold water fish is protective.

NUTRIENT THERAPY/DIETARY SUPPLEMENTS

Initial intervention for constipation routinely includes dietary measures and fiber supplements.[4] Fiber supplements such as wheat bran increase the frequency of defecation, lead to softer stools, and are safe for use during pregnancy.[5] Vitamin C supplementation beyond bowel tolerance is another strategy for preventing constipation. Megadoses of vitamin C cause osmotic diarrhea, as does magnesium hydroxide. Iatrogenic constipation may result from use of calcium and iron supplements. Supplements may be taken to reduce the risk of thrombosis. Daily doses of vitamin E in excess of 400 IU may impair platelet function and 1200 IU per day may impair the effects of vitamin K, prolonging clotting time.[6] MaxEPA, although it has a more potent antithrombotic effect in arteries, does reduce the risk of venous thrombosis.[7] Dietary supplementation for 1 month of 2.28 g of ω-3 fatty acids twice daily impaired platelet aggregation; the antiplatelet effect persisted for 8 weeks after the supplement was discontinued.[8]

HERBAL THERAPY

Several botanical extracts have been shown to improve microcirculation, capillary flow, and vascular tone and to strengthen the connective tissue of the perivascular amorphous substrate.[9] Active constituents include oligomeric proanthocyanidin complexes and flavonoids, especially hesperidin.[9] Bioflavonoids exhibit phlebotonic activity and vasculoprotective effects and antagonize biochemical mediators of inflammation. Animal studies have shown that flavonoids reduce neutrophil activation, mediate inflammation, and decrease soluble endothelial adhesion molecules.[10] Results of trials in humans have confirmed the ability of flavonoids to improve venous tone and vein elasticity as assessed by plethysmography.[11] Oligomeric proanthocyanidin complexes effectively decrease vascular permeability and enhance capillary strength and peripheral circulation. Symptoms of venous insufficiency have been reduced in patients receiving 300 mg of oligomeric proanthocyanidin complexes from grapeseed daily, and venous tone and low capillary resistance improved in patients receiving 150 mg.[9]

Oral supplementation with *Aesculus hippocastanum*, *Ruscus aculeatus*, *Centella asiatica*, *Hamamelis virginiana*, and bioflavonoids may prevent time-consuming, painful, and expensive complications of varicose veins and hemorrhoids.[9] Topical or oral horse chestnut (*Aesculus hippocastanum*) is a key herb for improving circulation by increasing venous tone.[12] Clinical trials support the use of horse chestnut in treating chronic venous insufficiency, varicose veins, and pedal edema. Pittler and Ernst[13] concluded, from a systematic review, that horse chestnut seed extract decreased the lower-leg volume, reduced leg circumference at the calf and ankle, and lessened symptoms such as leg pain, pruritus, and feelings of fatigue and tenseness. The active constituents appear to be saponins (escin) and flavonoids, lipids, and sterols. Escin reduces the edema of inflammation by reducing capillary permeability and increasing capillary strength as determined by the petechiae test. It has been used with some success in patients with chronic venous insufficiency. Horse chestnut should only be applied to intact skin, and enteric-coated preparations are recommended to avoid gastric irritation.

R. aculeatus has vasoconstrictive and venotonic properties, making it ideally suited to treat peripheral blood pooling caused by lack of venous tone and neurally mediated vasoconstriction.[14] *R. aculeatus* contains ruscogenins and flavonoids; it is an α-adrenergic agonist that causes venous constriction by directly activating postjunctional α1- and α2-receptors. It reduces venous capacity and pooling of blood in the legs. Its flavonoid content strengthens blood vessels, reduces capillary fragility, and helps maintain healthy circulation. It is an extremely safe, inexpensive, over-the-counter botanical medicine.

Clinical trials support the topical use of arnica flowers (*Arnica montana L*) in chronic venous insufficiency to relieve muscle aches[12] and bruising. Arnica flowers contain, among other substances, sesquiterpene lactones, flavonoids, and phenolic acids. They have anti-inflammatory, antimicrobial, and antitumor activity.

Other herbal options are sweet clover (meliotus), which improves venous return and reduces edema, and ginkgo, which is also useful for circulatory problems.[12]

An herbal regimen for treatment of hemorrhoids includes[12] mucilage-containing herbs such as slippery elm and psyllium to maintain a soft stool, horse chestnut or flavonoid-containing herbs (e.g., hawthorn) to improve venous and connective tissue tone, and topical witch hazel or horse chestnut to act as an astringent and enhance healing.

PRACTICE TIPS

- Horse chestnut should not be taken by persons receiving anticoagulants or aspirin.

REFERENCES

1. Ron Y, Wainstein J, Leibovitz A, et al: The effect of acarbose on the colonic transit time of elderly long-term care patients with type 2 diabetes mellitus, *J Gerontol A Biol Sci Med Sci* 57:M111-M114, 2002.
2. Ruf JC: Wine and polyphenols related to platelet aggregation and atherothrombosis, *Drugs Exp Clin Res* 25:125-31, 1999.
3. Simopoulos AP: Omega-3 fatty acids in health and disease and in growth and development, *Am J Clin Nutr* 54:438-63, 1991.
4. Borum ML: Constipation: evaluation and management, *Prim Care* 28:577-90, 2001.
5. Jewell DJ, Young G: Interventions for treating constipation in pregnancy, *Cochrane Database Syst Rev* 2:CD001142, 2001.
6. Kim JM, White RH: Effect of vitamin E on the anticoagulant response of warfarin, *Am J Cardiol* 77:545-6, 1996.
7. Andriamampandry MD, Leray C, Freund M, et al: Antithrombotic effects of (n–3) polyunsaturated fatty acids in rat models of arterial and venous thrombosis, *Thromb Res* 93:9-16, 1999.

8. Cerbone AM, Cirillo F, Coppola A, et al: Persistent impairment of platelet aggregation following cessation of a short-course dietary supplementation of moderate amounts of N-3 fatty acid ethyl esters, *Thromb Haemost* 82:128-33, 1999.

9. MacKay D: Hemorrhoids and varicose veins: a review of treatment options, *Altern Med Rev* 6:126-40, 2001.

10. Smith PD: Neutrophil activation and mediators of inflammation in chronic venous insufficiency, *J Vasc Res* 36(suppl 1):24-36, 1999.

11. Struckmann JR: Clinical efficacy of micronized purified flavonoid fraction: an overview, *J Vasc Res* 36(suppl 1):37-41, 1999.

12. Mills S, Bone K: *Principles and practice of phytotherapy*, Edinburgh, 2000, Churchill Livingstone.

13. Pittler MH, Ernst E: Horse-chestnut seed extract for chronic venous insufficiency. A criteria-based systematic review, *Arch Dermatol* 134:1356-60, 1998.

14. Redman DA: *Ruscus aculeatus* (butcher's broom) as a potential treatment for orthostatic hypotension, with a case report, *J Altern Complement Med* 6:539-49, 2000.

PART THREE

DIETARY SUPPLEMENTS

■ CHAPTER 47 ■

ASTRAGALUS MEMBRANACEUS

> Astragalus is an immunostimulant, but overdosing may cause immunosuppression.

Astragalus membranaceus is a Chinese herb often used as a "Qi tonifier." The root of the plant is used for medicinal purposes. Despite having been used to increase vitality and as an immunostimulant for many years, conclusive data from clinical trials are lacking. Nonetheless, astragalus has demonstrated a wide range of immunopotentiating effects and has proven efficacious as an adjunct cancer therapy.[1]

MECHANISM OF ACTION

Astragalus is rich in high–molecular-weight polysaccharides (astragalans), triterpenoid glycosides (saponins or astragalosides I-X), and flavonoids (quercetin and phytosterols). The root of the plant contains some unique flavones, including kumatakenin and 3',7 -dihydroxy-4' methoxyisoflavone, and their glucosides.

Astragalus' immunostimulatory properties lie, in part, in the saponins and polysaccharides present in the root. Astragalus enhances the cytotoxicity of natural and lymphokine-activated killer cells. Studies have shown that injected Astragalus membranaceus extracts enhance the antibody response to a T-cell–dependent antigen in normal, immunosuppressed, and elderly mice.[2] Astragalus extract was also found to exert an anticarcinogenic effect in carcinogen-treated mice through activation of cytotoxic activity and the production of cytokines.[3] Astragali Radix, the root of *A. membranaceus* Bunge, was shown to have inhibitory effects on lipid peroxidation and protein oxidative modification by copper.[4] Its proven antioxidant activity is one mechanism used to explain clinical efficacy.[5] Astragalus lowers mitochondrial oxygen consumption and enhances longevity in tissue cultures. This may explain its beneficial effects in angina and early heart failure and its energizing effects in mice.

DOSE

Traditionally, 10 to 30 g of dried root or 4 to 8 mL of 1:2 liquid extract are taken per day. Doses of 20 mg every 6 hours may be taken for bronchitis, and

200 mg twice a day for 3 weeks may be taken to boost the immune system. It is often alternated with echinacea and pau d'arco.

CLINICAL USES

Clinical trials provide some support for the use of astragalus in viral infections (e.g., coryza and herpes cervicitis) and in situations of impaired immunity (e.g., cancer or leukopenia).[1,6] Astragalus may be helpful if taken at the first sign of an upper respiratory tract infection.

It may also benefit persons with ischemic heart disease, myocardial infarction, heart failure, or anginal pain by enhancing perfusion and reducing free radical damage to the myocardium.

TOXICITY/DRUG INTERACTIONS

Astragalus is considered safe in recommended doses, but adverse reactions have been reported. Overdosing may cause immunosuppression.

The Chinese herb used for medicinal purposes should not be confused with locoweed, an American variant that is toxic to cattle.

CLINICAL CAUTION

Astralagus is contraindicated in acute infections. It should be avoided or used only under supervision during pregnancy.

PRACTICE TIPS

- Astragalus can be used safely with conventional medicine.
- It may act as a diuretic, lowering blood pressure and leading to dizziness and fatigue.
- It should not be prescribed during acute episodes of infection.
- Astragalus is available as a dietary supplement in the United States.

REFERENCES

1. Sinclair S: Chinese herbs: a clinical review of Astragalus, Ligusticum, and Schizandrae, *Altern Med Rev* 3:338-44, 1998.
2. Zhao KS, Mancini C, Doria G: Enhancement of the immune response in mice by Astragalus membranaceus extracts, *Immunopharmacology* 20:225-33, 1990.
3. Kurashige S, Akuzawa Y, Endo F: Effects of astragali radix extract on carcinogenesis, cytokine production, and cytotoxicity in mice treated with a carcinogen, N-butyl-N'-butanolnitrosoamine, *Cancer Invest* 17:30-5, 1999.

4. Toda S, Yase Y, Shirataki Y: Inhibitory effects of astragali radix, crude drug in Oriental medicines on lipid peroxidation and protein oxidative modification of mouse brain homogenate by copper, *Phytother Res* 14:294-6, 2000.
5. Miller AL: Botanical influences on cardiovascular disease, *Altern Med Rev* 3: 422-31, 1998.
6. Mills S, Bone K: *Principles and practice of phytotherapy*, Edinburgh, 2000, Churchill Livingstone.

■ CHAPTER 48 ■

BILBERRY FRUIT (*VACCINIUM MYRTILLUS*)

> Different blueberry sources have their own patterns of anthocyanin distribution and amounts in the extracts. Could this account for discrepancies detected between anecdotal and scientific reports of the efficacy of bilberry?

Vaccinium species include lowbush blueberry, bilberry, and cranberry. A rich source of various flavonoids, bilberry is a particularly good source of anthocyanins. These flavonoids are believed to improve perfusion, reduce capillary permeability, and enhance ocular health.

MECHANISM OF ACTION

Bilberry is rich in various flavonoids, which in combination have an antioxidant effect, inhibit platelet aggregation, stabilize collagen, and enhance wound healing.

Bilberry is a particularly rich source of anthocyanins. These flavonoids have antiplatelet activity and prolong bleeding time. Anthocyanins normalize capillary permeability and are more effective than bioflavonoids in decreasing edema after microvascular trauma. Anthocyanins also enhance regeneration of rhodopsin and may improve night vision. Although anthocyanins have great biologic importance, it has been suggested that they have little pharmacologic significance.

Fresh bilberries are also a source of flavonols. The flavonol content of fresh bilberries is around 41 mg/kg.[1] These flavonoids lose substantial antioxidant activity when subject to processing. Cooking bilberries in water and sugar results in a 40% loss of quercetin, as does storing bilberries at 20° C for 9 months. Myricetin and kaempferol are even more susceptible than quercetin to depletion during storage.

DOSE

Traditionally, the daily dose is 3 to 6 mL of 1:1 liquid extract or one tablet containing 50 to 120 mg of anthocyanins. This equates to around 20 to 50 g of fresh fruit.

CLINICAL USES

There is clinical support for use of bilberry in conditions involving dysfunction of small blood vessels, particularly capillaries. Bilberry has been used to enhance microcirculation, counteract venous insufficiency, and hasten vascular repair.[2] Anecdotal reports suggest that administration of 57 to 115 mg of anthocyanins reduces venous congestion and can be used to relieve hemorrhoids. A dose of 173 mg of anthocyanins per day over 30 to 60 days has been reported to inhibit platelet aggregation, prolonging bleeding time without affecting blood coagulation. Research is required.

Unconfirmed reports do suggest that 50 to 115 mg of anthocyanins per day may be beneficial in treating visual disorders. However, two double-blind, placebo-controlled trials of anthocyanins in healthy volunteers failed to show improved night visual acuity or night contrast sensitivity.[3,4] High doses were used—160 mg of bilberry extract (25% anthocyanosides) three times daily.

TOXICITY/DRUG INTERACTIONS

Fresh fruit is regarded as safe, although eating the whole fruit does cause intestinal irritation in sensitive individuals. Mild gastrointestinal, dermatologic, and neurologic side effects have been reported.

High doses interact with and may enhance the effects of warfarin and antiplatelet drugs. Patients taking warfarin should be under medical supervision if they are taking anthocyanins in doses greater than 170 mg/day.[5]

CLINICAL CAUTION

Bilberry should be avoided or used with caution by patients with hemorrhagic disorders.

PRACTICE TIPS

- Bilberry tea or gargle may be used to ease mucosal inflammation, whether this presents as nonspecific mild diarrhea or a sore throat.
- Bilberry may be helpful for people who bruise easily.
- Bilberry is available as a dietary supplement in the United States.

REFERENCES

1. Hakkinen SH, Karenlampi SO, Mykkanen HM, et al: Influence of domestic processing and storage on flavonol contents in berries, *J Agric Food Chem* 48: 2960-5, 2000.

2. Mills S, Bone K: *Principles and practice of phytotherapy*, Edinburgh, 2000,Churchill Livingstone.
3. Muth ER, Laurent JM, Jasper P: The effect of bilberry nutritional supplementation on night visual acuity and contrast sensitivity, *Altern Med Rev* 5:164-73, 2000.
4. Zadok D, Levy Y, Glovinsky Y: The effect of anthocyanosides in a multiple oral dose on night vision, *Eye* 13:734-6, 1999.
5. Braun L: Herb-drug interaction guide, *Aust Fam Phys* 30:259-60, 2001.

CHAPTER 49

BIOTIN

Eating raw egg white over prolonged periods can lead to biotin deficiency; thus, natural may not always be best.

Biotin is a member of the B group of vitamins. This water-soluble vitamin has previously been known as *vitamin H* or *coenzyme R*. Its name is derived from the Greek word *bios*, meaning life. Biotin is involved in glucose utilization and therefore in energy metabolism. It is also necessary for formation of fatty acids and is important for the metabolism of amino acids.

MECHANISM OF ACTION

Many enzymes containing biotin catalyze carboxylation reactions. Important reactions in which biotin participates include the following: gluconeogenesis, by adding carbon dioxide to pyruvate to form oxaloacetate; fatty acid synthesis, by elongating the fatty acid chain; and energy production, by facilitating entry of both fatty acids and certain amino acids into the citric acid cycle. Biotin also participates in DNA synthesis.

FOOD SOURCES

Biotin tends to be protein-bound and is found in meat (especially liver), whole-grain cereals, soy products, nuts, and yeast. Intestinal bacteria synthesize biotin, but this is not believed to contribute much to the absorption of biotin.

Cooking and preserving reduce the biotin content of food. Raw egg white contains avidin, a protein that binds biotin and prevents its absorption in eggnog. Egg yolk is a source of biotin.

DOSE

The adequate intake for adults is 30 µg/day and is increased to 35 µg/day during lactation.

The recommended daily allowance from birth to 3 years of age is 10 to 20 µg, increasing to 30 µg by the age of 7 years. The upper limit has not been set. The therapeutic dose range is 300 to 3000 µg/day.[1]

CLINICAL USES

Supplements are necessary for persons with biotinase deficiency, a rare genetic condition. Deficiency may manifest as dry flaking skin, depression, drowsiness, anorexia, myalgia, and anemia. There is speculation that biotin may facilitate blood sugar control in diabetes and reduce the risk of diabetic neuropathy. It has been suggested that 1000 to 1200 µg of biotin promotes the growth and health of hair and nails.[2]

TOXICITY/DRUG INTERACTIONS

No side effects have been reported for biotin in amounts up to 10 mg a day. Long-term use of antibiotics or anticonvulsants may increase the requirement for biotin.

CLINICAL CAUTION

A deficiency of biotin is rare. However, if it occurs, it may lead to skin rash, loss of hair, high blood levels of cholesterol, and heart problems.

Avidin, a protein found in high concentrations in egg white, binds biotin and prevents its absorption. A diet rich in raw egg white may cause biotin deficiency, which manifests as a red, scaly, facial skin rash, hair thinning, loss of hair color, and neurologic symptoms (e.g., depression, lethargy, and paresthesia).

PRACTICE TIPS

• Dietary supplements provide 100 to 300 µg of biotin daily.

REFERENCES

1. Brighthope I: Nutritional medicine tables, *J Aust Coll Nutr Env Med* 17:20-5, 1998.
2. Diefendorf D, Healey J, Kalyn W, editors: *The healing power of vitamins, minerals and herbs*, Surrey Hills, Australia, 2000, Readers Digest.

BLACK COHOSH (*CIMICIFUGA RACEMOSA*)

Clinical reports suggest that black cohosh alleviates menopausal symptoms such as flushing, depression, and anxiety; yet in vitro assays suggest that it has no estrogenic activity.

Black cohosh is tall plant with a gnarled, dark root. It is used to relieve menopausal symptoms, premenstrual tension, and dysmenorrhea.

MECHANISM OF ACTION

Black cohosh is rich in phytoestrogens. It mimics estrogen by providing a negative feedback to the pituitary and reducing luteinizing hormone (LH) but not follicle-stimulating hormone. Black cohosh is believed to relieve hot flashes by reducing circulating LH levels. Although flushing is related to a decline in estrogen, rather than any fluctuation in estrogen levels, it appears that an increase in the LH level triggers a flush.

Triterpenes are the active components in black cohosh.

DOSE

Traditional doses were 0.5 to 1 g of dried root or rhizome three to four times a day. Currently, the dosage is 40 to 200 mg of dried rhizome or root per day. The standard dose is 40 mg of black cohosh taken twice daily for menopausal symptoms, taken for 10 days before menses for premenstrual tension, and taken as required up to three times daily for dysmenorrhea. An extract that contains 2.5% triterpenes should be selected.

CLINICAL USES

Black cohosh is used to treat symptoms arising from ovarian failure. Remifemin, a standardized extract of black cohosh, is commonly prescribed as an alternative to hormone replacement therapy for menopause.[1] In a review of eight human studies on the effectiveness of an extract of *Cimicifuga racemosa* in alleviating menopausal symptoms, Lieberman[2] concluded that it is a safe, effective alternative to estrogen replacement therapy for those patients who refuse estrogen replacement therapy or for whom it is contraindicated. However, a randomized clinical trial of patients with breast cancer receiving tamoxifen showed that black cohosh was not significantly more efficacious than placebo; however, menopausal symptoms, including the number and intensity of hot flashes, were reduced in both groups.[3] Nonetheless, another review of current literature suggested that for relief of menopausal symptoms, although black cohosh root extract and dong quai have good safety profiles, only black cohosh had demonstrated efficacy.[4] In addition, of eight botanical preparations that are commonly used for the treatment of menopausal symptoms, only black cohosh showed no activity in any of the in vitro assays for estrogenic activity.[5] In this study, dong quai showed weak affinity for estrogen receptors. Contradictions abound.

TOXICITY/DRUG INTERACTIONS

At recommended doses, black cohosh has a positive safety profile with low toxicity, few and mild side effects, and good tolerability.[1] It may be used during labor but not pregnancy. Nonetheless, it is potentially dangerous if taken in excess. High doses cause a dull or bursting frontal headache. Overdose produces vertigo, visual and neural disturbances, nausea, and vomiting.

Black cohosh may interfere with administration of female sex hormones. In vitro black cohosh augments the antiproliferative action of tamoxifen; however, it is contraindicated for women with estrogen-dependent breast cancer.

It may augment the action of antihypertensive drugs, resulting in an untoward drop in blood pressure.

CLINICAL CAUTION

Black cohosh should not be used during pregnancy or lactation.

PRACTICE TIPS

- It may take 8 weeks before benefits of black cohosh are detected, and it is probably wise to discontinue regular use after 6 months.
- A popular but scientifically unproven use is to relieve smooth and striated muscle pain.
- Aching muscles and joints may be relieved by warm compresses soaked in water boiled with dried black cohosh root for 30 minutes.
- Patients receiving antihypertensive agents who start taking black cohosh may need to have their doses adjusted.

REFERENCES

1. McKenna DJ, Jones K, Humphrey S, et al: Black cohosh: efficacy, safety, and use in clinical and preclinical applications, *Altern Ther Health Med* 7:93-100, 2001.
2. Lieberman S: A review of the effectiveness of *Cimicifuga racemosa* (black cohosh) for the symptoms of menopause, *J Womens Health* 7:525-9, 1998.
3. Jacobson JS, Troxel AB, Evans J, et al: Randomized trial of black cohosh for the treatment of hot flashes among women with a history of breast cancer, *J Clin Oncol* 19:2739-45, 2001.
4. Hardy ML: Herbs of special interest to women, *J Am Pharm Assoc (Wash)* 40: 234-42, 2000.
5. Liu J, Burdette JE, Xu H, et al: Evaluation of estrogenic activity of plant extracts for the potential treatment of menopausal symptoms, *J Agric Food Chem* 49: 2472-9, 2001.

■ CHAPTER 51 ■

BORON

Although no discrete deficiency disease has been identified and no defined biochemical function described, the total health effects of boron suggest that patients should be advised to include it in their diets; chromium and fluoride enjoy similar status.

Recent thinking suggests that boron is an essential ultratrace mineral in humans. A diet rich in boron is believed to be beneficial for macromineral, energy, nitrogen, and reactive oxygen metabolism.[1] Epidemiologic evidence and results of animal and human experiments demonstrate that boron is essential for healthy bones and joints.[2]

MECHANISM OF ACTION

Boron is important in calcium metabolism and may influence metabolism of copper, magnesium, potassium, and vitamin D. It may influence certain enzymes. Boron is thought to contribute to bone health by preventing calcium loss and enhancing bone maintenance by activating estrogen. Boron increases the ability of 17β-estradiol, but not parathyroid hormone, to improve trabecular bone quality in ovariectomized rats.[3]

FOOD SOURCES

Plant-based foods are good sources of boron, especially prunes, almonds, raisins (2.7 mg/100 g food), wine (0.8 mg/100 mL), parsley, hazelnuts, peanuts, apples, and peaches.

DOSE

No recommended daily allowance (RDA) has been established, but an acceptable range of boron for adults could well be 1 to 13 mg daily. Individuals consuming 0.25 mg/day respond positively to boron supplementation of 1 mg/day. A daily intake of 2 to 3 mg boron can be obtained from a 100-g serving of dried prunes.[4]

CLINICAL USES

Calcium appears to be more readily stripped from bones in persons with low boron intake. Boron may be particularly effective in protecting bone mass in persons with vitamin D, magnesium, and potassium deficiencies.[5]

The concentration of boron in the femoral heads and synovial fluid of people with arthritis is low, and the bones of patients using boron supplements are much harder to cut.[2] In areas where boron intakes are 1.0 mg or less per day, the estimated incidence of arthritis ranges from 20% to 70%, whereas in areas of the world where boron intakes are usually 3 to 10 mg, the estimated incidence of arthritis ranges from 0% to 10%.[2] Low boron intakes may also worsen rheumatoid arthritis and osteoarthritis and decrease the ability to engage in physical exercise that requires a high energy output.

Anecdotal suggestions that boron supplementation may reduce postmenopausal night sweats and hot flashes lack clinical support[6]; nonetheless, animal studies do suggest that the beneficial effects of hormone replacement therapy would be reduced in individuals with boron deficiency. In addition to potentially enhancing the response to estrogen therapy, a boron-rich diet is believed to improve psychomotor skills and cognitive processes.[1] Studies indicate that boron deprivation impairs cognitive and psychomotor function in humans, resulting in decreased mental alertness and poorer performance of tasks requiring motor speed and dexterity, attention, and/or short-term memory.[6]

TOXICITY/DRUG INTERACTIONS

Boron is safe in doses of up to 10 mg/day. Gastrointestinal upsets, dermatitis, and lethargy are likely to result from ingestion of boron in doses in excess of 100 mg daily.

CLINICAL CAUTION

Although no deficiency state has been described, recent findings indicate that a significant number of people do not consistently consume more than 1 mg of boron daily. This suggests that boron deficiency could be of clinical concern.[1]

PRACTICE TIPS

- A boron deficiency may upset calcium metabolism.
- Deficiencies of calcium and magnesium may increase requirements for boron.

REFERENCES

1. Nielsen FH: The justification for providing dietary guidance for the nutritional intake of boron, *Biol Trace Elem Res* 66:319-30, 1998.
2. Newnham RE: Essentiality of boron for healthy bones and joints, *Environ Health Perspect* 102(suppl 7):83-5, 1994.
3. Sheng MH, Taper LJ, Veit H, et al: Dietary boron supplementation enhanced the action of estrogen, but not that of parathyroid hormone, to improve trabecular bone quality in ovariectomized rats, *Biol Trace Elem Res* 82:109-23, 2001.
4. Stacewicz-Sapuntzakis M, Bowen PE, Hussain EA, et al: Chemical composition and potential health effects of prunes: a functional food? *Crit Rev Food Sci Nutr* 41:251-86, 2001.
5. Schaafsma A, de Vries PJ, Saris WH: Delay of natural bone loss by higher intakes of specific minerals and vitamins, *Crit Rev Food Sci Nutr* 41:225-49, 2001.
6. Penland JG: The importance of boron nutrition for brain and psychological function, *Biol Trace Elem Res* 66:299-317, 1998.

■ CHAPTER 52 ■

BROMELAIN (*ANANAS COMOSUS*)

It is a myth that bromelain, a protein extracted from the stem of pineapples, cannot be effective when it is administered orally.

The stem and, to a lesser extent, the fruit of the pineapple contain a number of sulfhydryl-containing proteolytic enzymes collectively known as *bromelain*. Some 40% of ingested bromelain is absorbed unchanged from the intestine.[1] Bromelain is glycosylated, which may protect it from gastrointestinal breakdown.

Bromelain has anti-inflammatory, anticoagulant, and antineoplastic effects and may enhance absorption of drugs, particularly antibiotics.[2] It also has the potential to facilitate skin debridement and accelerate wound healing.

MECHANISM OF ACTION

Bromelain contains cysteine proteases, protease inhibitors, mannosidases, and glucosaminidase. Although its proteolytic fraction is important, many of the beneficial effects of bromelain are due to other factors.

Bromelain's anti-inflammatory action results from blocking bradykinin and its modulation of prostaglandin synthesis.[3] It achieves an anticoagulant effect through both reduced platelet aggregation, by increasing relative concentrations of prostacyclin and prostaglandin E_2 over the concentration of thromboxane A_2, and fibrinolyis by activation of plasmin. Plasmin further suppresses inflammation by blocking the mobilization of endogenous arachidonic acid by phospholipases.

Bromelain's antineoplastic effects result from its ability to affect T-cell activation, induce cytokine production in circulating monocytes, and enhance production of tumor necrosis factor and interleukins.[4] However, its immunomodulating activity is complex. Data indicate that bromelain can simultaneously enhance and inhibit T-cell responses in vitro and in vivo by means of a stimulatory action on accessory cells and a direct inhibitory action on T cells.[5] Bromelain's immunostimulatory properties are also mediated by enhanced phagocytosis.[6] As an adjunct in cancer therapy, bromelain may act as an immunomodulator by raising the impaired immunocytotoxicity of monocytes against tumor cells and by inducing the production of distinct cytokines such as tumor necrosis factor-α, interleukin (IL)–1β, IL-6, and IL-8.[7]

DOSE

Rorer units (ru), gelatin dissolving units (gdu), and milk clotting units (mcu) are the most commonly used measures of activity. One gram of bromelain standardized to 2000 mcu would be approximately equal to 1 g with 1200 gdu of activity or 8 g with 100,000 ru of activity.[3] Bromelain, with activity in the range of 1200 to 1800 mcu, is usually given as a dose of 250 to 500 mg three times a day. Doses of up to 1000 mg/day correspond to 15 mg/kg weight.

Clinical results of bromelain therapy are dose-dependent. Bromelain has demonstrated therapeutic benefits in doses as small as 160 mg/day; however, it is thought that for most conditions, best results occur at doses of 750 to 1000 mg/day.[3]

Bromelain should be taken on an empty stomach.

CLINICAL USES

Claims have been made suggesting that bromelain may provide a clinical benefit in angina pectoris, bronchitis, sinusitis, surgical traumas, thrombophlebitis, pyelonephritis, and cancer care.[7]

Bromelain's most common use is in the treatment of inflammation and soft tissue injuries. It reduces swelling, pain, and tenderness.[8] It is useful for debriding wounds when it is applied topically as a cream (35% bromelain in a lipid base). It may be used before surgery and in the treatment of acute thrombophlebitis, and bromelain in doses of 120 to 400 mg/day has been used to treat patients with myocardial infarction.

Bromelain also appears to enhance the effect of cancer chemotherapy (in doses of 1000 mg/day) and antibiotics.[3] It may aid digestion and enhance absorption of drugs.[2] Bromelain is emerging as a promising antidiarrheal agent.[9]

TOXICITY/DRUG INTERACTIONS

Bromelain is considered to have very low toxicity. However, because of its use as a meat tenderizer and a beer clarifier, bromelain is a potential ingestive allergen. It may induce allergic reactions, especially immunoglobulin E–mediated respiratory problems, in sensitive individuals.

Bromelain interacts with anticoagulants (e.g., warfarin) and antiplatelet drugs (e.g., aspirin) to inhibit platelet aggregation and increase prothrombin time.

CLINICAL CAUTION

Bromelain is contraindicated in persons who are allergic to pineapple or have a peptic ulcer.

PRACTICE TIPS

- For best results, 750 to 1000 mg of bromelain should be taken in four divided doses daily on an empty stomach.
- Bromelain should be used with caution by persons with hypertension.

REFERENCES

1. Lotz-Winter H: On the pharmacology of bromelain: an update with special regard to animal studies on dose-dependent effects, *Planta Med* 56:249-53, 1990.
2. Taussig SJ, Batkin S: Bromelain, the enzyme complex of pineapple (*Ananas comosus*) and its clinical application. An update, *J Ethnopharmacol* 22:191-203, 1988.
3. Bromelain, *Altern Med Rev* 3:302-5, 1998.
4. Hinck G: The role of herbal products in the prevention of cancer, *Topics Clin Chiro* 6:54-62, 1999.
5. Engwerda CR, Andrew D, Ladhams A, et al: Bromelain modulates T cell and B cell immune responses in vitro and in vivo, *Cell Immunol* 210:66-75, 2001.
6. Brakebusch M, Wintergerst U, Petropoulou T, et al: Bromelain is an accelerator of phagocytosis, respiratory burst and killing of *Candida albicans* by human granulocytes and monocytes, *Eur J Med Res* 6:193-200, 2001.
7. Maurer HR: Bromelain: biochemistry, pharmacology and medical use, *Cell Mol Life Sci* 58:1234-45, 2001.
8. Masson M: Bromelain in blunt injuries of the locomotor system. A study of observed applications in general practice, *Fortschr Med* 113:303-6, 1995.
9. Thomson AB, Keelan M, Thiesen A, et al: Small bowel review: normal physiology part 1, *Dig Dis Sci* 46:2567-87, 2001.

■ CHAPTER 53 ■

CALCIUM

The efficacy of nutrient supplementation may be influenced by the stage of the host's life cycle at which supplementation is prescribed; calcium alone increases bone density before and around puberty. Calcium and vitamin D reduce the decline of bone density in the elderly, but calcium probably does not attenuate menopausal bone loss.

Calcium, the most abundant mineral in the body, is largely stored in bones where it provides structural strength. When blood levels of calcium decline, calcium is drawn from bones. A lifelong dietary deficiency of calcium manifests in later life as osteoporosis, a major health problem in developed countries.

Calcium intake is an important determinant of peak bone mass, and the risk of osteoporotic fractures is strongly influenced by bone mass. Low calcium intake has also been implicated in the development of several chronic conditions including hypertension, colon cancer, nephrolithiasis, and even premenstrual syndrome[1]; calcium supplementation has been used in the prevention of these diseases. Calcium is an essential component of antiresorptive agent therapy for osteoporosis.[2]

MECHANISM OF ACTION

Calcium is a divalent metal essential for maintenance of the neuromusculoskeletal system. It influences cell membrane and capillary permeability and is important for bone strength, blood coagulation, and electrical conduction in nerves and the heart. Hormones, or first messengers, interact with cell membrane receptors and produce signals that generate second messengers inside cells. Calcium and the calcium-calmodulin complex, like cyclic adenosine monophosphate, can act as second messengers. When calcium combines with calmodulin, this small regulatory protein undergoes a conformational change that allows it to interact with several enzymes, resulting in an increase in the catalytic activity of various protein kinases, including those that regulate membrane permeability to calcium and control the intracellular contractile proteins actin and myosin. About 99% of calcium is stored in bones as hydroxyapatite.

FOOD SOURCES

Good sources of calcium are milk, cheese, dolomite, bone meal, sesame seeds, dark green vegetables, dried legumes, sardines, tuna, and salmon. The concentration of calcium in foods varies. One cup of reconstituted non-fat dry milk contains 375 mg of calcium, a cup of low-fat, skim or whole milk has 290 to 300 mg, a cup of yogurt has 275 to 400 mg, low-fat cottage cheese has 154 mg, and part-skim ricotta cheese has 680 mg. One ounce of Swiss cheese contains 272 mg, and one ounce of cheddar has 204 mg. Among nondairy sources, 3 ounces of sardines with bones contains 370 mg, and an equivalent amount of canned salmon with bones contains 285 mg calcium. The best vegetable source is tofu: 4 ounces contains 154 mg.

Absorption of calcium from dairy products is most efficient. However, it is unclear whether dairy foods promote bone health in all populations and whether all dairy foods are equally beneficial.[3] A review of 57 outcomes of the effects of dairy foods on bone health indicated that 53% were not significant, 42% were favorable, and 5% were unfavorable. In 21 stronger-evidence studies, 57% of outcomes were not significant, 29% were favorable, and 14% were unfavorable. The authors concluded that foods such as milk and yogurt are likely to be beneficial; others, such as cottage cheese, may adversely affect bone health. The amount of dietary fat consumed relative to dietary fiber appears to have an important role in determining differences in calcium absorption.[4] Fractional calcium absorption is positively associated with dietary fat intake, body mass index and serum 1,25 dihydroxyvitamin D and parathyroid hormone concentrations. It is inversely associated with total calcium intake, dietary fiber intake, alcohol consumption, and, to a lesser extent, with physical activity and symptoms of constipation. Dietary fat, fiber, and alcohol are independent predictors of calcium absorption. Calcium absorption varies from 17% to 58% among individuals.[4]

DOSE

The recommended daily allowance (RDA) for calcium is 800 to 1400 mg. Recommended intakes escalate on a sliding scale from 400 to 800 mg per day for infants and children up to the age of 3 years, through 800 mg/day for children aged 4 to 10 years, and 800 to 1200 mg/day for children older than 10 years and adults. An intake of 1200 mg/day has been proposed for pregnant and lactating woman. The supplementary range for calcium is 1000 to 2000 mg. The RDA for calcium has been revised upward, and this trend may continue.

One factor determining the RDA of calcium is urinary excretion of this mineral. Calcium excretion below the dietary threshold for calcium correlates negatively with peak bone mass. The dietary threshold for calcium in the average teenager is about 1500 mg daily. Overall, calciuria plateaus when calcium intake is between 500 and 2000 mg. Urinary losses of calcium can be minimized by administration of calcium supplements in doses in excess of 500 mg and by avoiding foods and beverages with high sodium, protein, sugar, and/or caffeine content. An additional 6 mg of calcium is lost when caffeine intake reaches 175 mg/day, and 1 mg is lost for every gram of protein consumed.[5] Calciuria appears to correlate with the concentration of sulfur-containing amino acids.

Another factor influencing the RDA for calcium is calcium absorption. Calcium supplements should not be taken with fiber-rich meals. Phytates and oxalates found in bran, whole-grain cereals, and breads impede absorption. On the other hand, lactose enhances absorption, and dairy products are particularly good sources. Absorption of calcium is increased when supplements are taken in divided doses. Calcium supplements are best taken 60 to 90 minutes after meals, unless the patient has achlorhydria, in which case supplements are best taken with meals. Calcium is better absorbed from lactate, citrate, or gluconate than carbonate; this is particularly important in elderly people and those with hypochlorhydria. Although inexpensive, calcium carbonate is of limited value as either a calcium supplement or an antacid. Any benefit derived from calcium carbonate reducing gastric irritation by neutralizing gastric acid is compromised by calcium's stimulation of gastrin production.

CLINICAL USES

Calcium intake levels greater than 2500 mg/day are not recommended.[2] For osteoporosis prevention, at least 1200 mg of calcium per day is required. A daily intake of 400 to 600 IU of vitamin D is also recommended—achieved through sun exposure, diet, and/or supplementation—to ensure adequate calcium absorption.[2] Higher intakes of calcium are associated with increased bone density and a reduced risk of gastrointestinal tract cancers.

Calcium absorption and bone deposition vary at different stages of the life cycle, peaking in early puberty and decreasing gradually after menarche.[6] A study of twins showed that calcium supplementation (1000 mg daily) increased the rate of increase in bone mineral density in children even when their mean dietary intake approximated the RDA, provided that they had not reached puberty.[7] A bone mineralization study showed that size-adjusted bone mineral content in school-aged children was positively associated with average calcium intake; however, size-adjusted accretion in bone mineral content was only positively associated with changes in the dietary calcium intake in boys.[8] Although there is no convincing evidence that young girls need more than 900 mg of calcium daily to achieve peak bone mass, it is the dose, not the requirement for calcium, that is unclear.[9] Studies have also shown that dietary calcium slows osteoporotic bone loss, and the preventive effect of calcium supplements is most evident in women more than 10 years after menopause.[10] In Europe, low calcium intake and suboptimal vitamin D status are common in the elderly, and evidence indicates that routine daily supplementation is beneficial for people at risk for osteoporosis with 700 to 800 mg of calcium and 400 to 800 IU of vitamin D.[11]

Calcium has a protective effect on bowel epithelium; it may precipitate toxic bile acids in the colonic lumen, thus reducing the rate of proliferation of colonic epithelium. Calcium has been found to protect against colon carcinogenesis in animal models, and a human intervention trial demonstrated that supplementation with 1200 mg of calcium carbonate per day led to a significant reduction in the risk of recurrent colonic adenomas.[12] Both men and women with high dietary intakes of calcium have been found to have a lower risk for colon cancer.[13] Calcium supplementation (1.5 g daily) over 12 months in patients with adenoma was found to significantly suppress rectal epithelial proliferation.[14] However, a randomized intervention trial indicated that calcium supplementation (2.0 g) was associated with a modest but nonsignificant reduction in the risk of adenoma recurrence.[15] Long-term dietary habits influence the outcome of these studies. Supplementation with fiber, such as ispaghula husk (3.5 g), may have adverse effects on colorectal adenoma recurrence, especially in patients with high dietary calcium intakes.

Calcium is also postulated to affect the risk of cancer at other sites. High calcium concentrations in drinking water correlate with a significantly reduced risk of breast cancer,[16] and analysis of data from the Alpha-Tocopherol Beta-Carotene Cancer Prevention Study suggests a possible association between the interaction of calcium and phosphorus with the risk of prostate cancer.[17]

Hypercalcemia is associated with hypertension, although calcium supplementation to RDA levels may lower blood pressure. Persons with a calcium intake of less than 700 mg daily tend to have higher blood pressure. Results of epidemiologic studies consistently show an inverse relationship between dietary calcium intake and blood pressure, but results of clinical trials with calcium supplements have been less consistent. Nonetheless, recommendations from the Sixth Report of the Joint National Committee on Prevention, Detection, Evaluation, and Treatment of High Blood Pressure include increasing calcium, potassium, and magnesium intake; reducing sodium intake; controlling obesity; and avoiding heavy alcohol intake, along with aggressive blood pressure control.[18]

Calcium is important for blood pressure control during pregnancy. A randomized trial of pregnant women at high risk of developing preeclampsia showed that 2 g of calcium daily was helpful in preventing preeclampsia.[19] This is consistent with a review of 10 studies, all of good quality, which suggested a modest reduction in high blood pressure and the risk of preeclampsia with calcium supplementation.[20] The reviewers concluded that calcium supplementation appeared to be beneficial for women at high risk of gestational hypertension and in communities with low dietary calcium intake.

Human studies have also shown that calcium depletion appears to be an important consequence of potassium depletion in subjects with hypertension and a higher salt sensitivity index.[21] Therefore treatment of salt-sensitive patients with hypertension may best be undertaken with sodium restriction, plus potassium and calcium supplementation. Although the mechanism by which calcium reduces blood pressure requires elucidation, animal studies have shown that calcium supplementation reduces blood pressure during chronic nitric oxide synthase inhibition and abrogates the associated impairments in endothelium-dependent and endothelium-independent arterial relaxation.[22] It has also been postulated that increased calcium intake may improve calmodulin activity, which has the potential to interfere with various cellular processes linked to vascular tone.[23] Increased calcium intake is also associated with the following:

- A reduced risk of nephrolithiasis. Calcium possibly prevents kidney stones by reducing urinary oxalate content.[24]

Reduced symptoms of premenstrual tension. Premenstrual syndrome may represent the clinical manifestation of a calcium deficiency state that is unmasked after the increase in ovarian steroid hormone concentrations during the menstrual cycle.[25] A prospective, randomized, double-blind, placebo-controlled, parallel-group, multicenter clinical trial demonstrated that supplementation with 1200 mg of elemental calcium daily resulted in a major reduction in overall luteal phase symptoms of premenstrual tension.[26]

An improved serum lipid profile. Calcium may increase excretion of saturated fats and reduce serum low-density lipoprotein cholesterol and apolipoprotein B levels.[27]

TOXICITY/DRUG INTERACTIONS

Constipation is commonly associated with calcium supplementation. Calcium supplements are poorly absorbed when taken without vitamin D_3. In fact, serum calcium levels need only be monitored when calcium is used in combination with vitamin D_3. Vitamin D_3 (cholecalciferol) increases calcium absorption, but vitamin D_2 (ergocalciferol) does not. Excessive cholecalciferol and calcium supplementation may cause hypercalcemia. Hypercalcemia presents clinically with the following signs symptoms: weakness, dehydration, metastatic calcification, impaired concentration, increased sleep, altered state of consciousness, polydipsia, anorexia, nausea, vomiting, constipation, pancreatitis, peptic ulceration, polyuria, nephrolithiasis, nephrocalcinosis, and hypertension.

In the absence of vitamin D supplementation, hypercalcemia is unlikely. Oral calcium supplements may interfere with other medications if they are taken within 2 hours of each other. Supplementation with 1800 mg of calcium gluconate decreases net zinc absorption from a balanced diet that supplies 216 mg of calcium and 13.1 mg of zinc. When calcium is consumed in the form of calcium carbonate (in an antacid), it may impair absorption of other minerals such as iron and zinc, acetaminophen, phenytoin, and thyroid hormones. Although calcium carbonate is less expensive, the bioavailability of marketed calcium carbonate is equivalent to that of calcium citrate.[28]

CLINICAL CAUTION

Mild calcium deficiency may present as anxiety, irritability, and insomnia. More severe deficiency presents as muscle cramps and palpitations in the short term and as stunted growth, osteoporosis, and rickets in the long term.

Persons at risk are those with lactose intolerance and those avoiding dairy products.

PRACTICE TIPS

- Children, adolescents, and pregnant, lactating, perimenopausal, or post-menopausal women may need more calcium than they normally obtain from eating calcium-rich foods.
- Bone meal and dolomite should not be used as sources of calcium, because these products may contain lead.
- The elemental calcium content of a supplement should always be ascertained because the proportion of calcium varies among compounds.
- When long-term calcium supplementation is prescribed, the patient's magnesium status should be checked.
- Water softeners remove calcium from water.
- Calcium can temporarily control cardiac arrhythmia associated with hypokalemia.
- Nocturnal cramps may be relieved by administration of 4.8 g of calcium gluconate at bedtime.
- Persons whose urine turns pinkish after eating 250 g of beetroot may have hypochlorhydria and impaired calcium absorption.
- Hypercalcemia should be suspected in patients receiving calcium and vitamin D supplementation who complain of a dry mouth, persistent headache, irritability, anorexia, and depression.

REFERENCES

1. Power ML, Heaney RP, Kalkwarf HJ, et al: The role of calcium in health and disease, *Am J Obstet Gynecol* 181:1560-9, 1999.
2. The role of calcium in peri-and postmenopausal women: consensus opinion of The North American Menopause Society, *Menopause* 8:84-95, 2001.
3. Weinsier RL, Krumdieck CL: Dairy foods and bone health: examination of the evidence, *Am J Clin Nutr* 72:681-9, 2000.
4. Wolf RL, Cauley JA, Baker CE, et al: Factors associated with calcium absorption efficiency in pre- and perimenopausal women, *Am J Clin Nutr* 72:466-71, 2000.
5. Kerstetter JE, Allen LH: Dietary protein increases urine calcium, *J Nutr* 120:134-6, 1989.
6. Abrams SA: Calcium turnover and nutrition through the life cycle, *Proc Nutr Soc* 60:283-9, 2001.

7. Johnston CC Jr, Miller JZ, Slemenda CW, et al: Calcium supplementation and increases in bone mineral density in children, *N Engl J Med* 327:119-20, 1992.

8. Molgaard C, Thomsen BL, Michaelsen KF: The influence of calcium intake and physical activity on bone mineral content and bone size in healthy children and adolescents, *Osteoporos Int* 12:887-94, 2001.

9. Lloyd T, Taylor DS: Calcium intake and peak bone mass, *J Am Med Womens Assoc* 56:49-52, 2001.

10. Murray TM: Prevention and management of osteoporosis: consensus statements from the Scientific Advisory Board of the Osteoporosis Society of Canada. 4. Calcium nutrition and osteoporosis, *CMAJ* 155:935-9, 1996.

11. Gennari C: Calcium and vitamin D nutrition and bone disease of the elderly, *Public Health Nutr* 4:547-59, 2001.

12. Baron JA, Beach M, Mandel JS, et al: Calcium supplements for the prevention of colorectal adenomas. Calcium Polyp Prevention Study Group, *N Engl J Med* 340:101-7, 1999.

13. Kampman E, Slattery ML, Caan B, et al: Calcium, vitamin D, sunshine exposure, dairy products and colon cancer risk, *Cancer Causes Control* 11:459-66, 2000.

14. Rozen P, Lubin F, Papo N, et al: Calcium supplements interact significantly with long-term diet while suppressing rectal epithelial proliferation of adenoma patients, *Cancer* 91:833-40, 2001.

15. Bonithon-Kopp C, Kronborg O, Giacosa A, et al: Calcium and fibre supplementation in prevention of colorectal adenoma recurrence: a randomised intervention trial. European Cancer Prevention Organisation Study Group, *Lancet* 356:1300-6, 2000.

16. Yang CY, Chiu HF, Cheng MF, et al: Calcium and magnesium in drinking water and risk of death from breast cancer, *J Toxicol Environ Health* 60:231-41, 2000.

17. Chan JM, Pietinen P, Virtanen M, et al: Diet and prostate cancer risk in a cohort of smokers, with a specific focus on calcium and phosphorus (Finland), *Cancer Causes Control* 11:859-67, 2000.

18. Davis MM, Jones DW: The role of lifestyle management in the overall treatment plan for prevention and management of hypertension, *Semin Nephrol* 22:35-43, 2002.

19. Niromanesh S, Laghaii S, Mosavi-Jarrahi A: Supplementary calcium in prevention of pre-eclampsia, *Int J Gynaecol Obstet* 74:17-21, 2001.

20. Atallah AN, Hofmeyr GJ, Duley L: Calcium supplementation during pregnancy for preventing hypertensive disorders and related problems, *Cochrane Database Syst Rev* 3:CD001059, 2000.

21. Coruzzi P, Brambilla L, Brambilla V, et al: Potassium depletion and salt sensitivity in essential hypertension, *J Clin Endocrinol Metab* 86:2857-62, 2001.

22. Jolma P, Kalliovalkama J, Tolvanen JP, et al: High-calcium diet enhances vasorelaxation in nitric oxide-deficient hypertension, *Am J Physiol Heart Circ Physiol* 279:H1036-H1043, 2000.

23. McCarron DA, Hatton D, Roullet JB, et al: Dietary calcium, defective cellular Ca^+ handling, and arterial pressure control, *Can J Physiol Pharmacol* 72:937-44, 1994.

24. Curhan GC, Willett WC, Rimm EB, et al: A prospective study of dietary calcium and other nutrients and the risk of symptomatic kidney stones, *N Engl J Med* 328:833-8, 1993

25. Thys-Jacobs S: Micronutrients and the premenstrual syndrome: the case for calcium, *J Am Coll Nutr* 19:220-7, 2000.
26. Thys-Jacobs S, Starkey P, Bernstein D, et al: Calcium carbonate and the premenstrual syndrome: effects on premenstrual and menstrual symptoms. Premenstrual Syndrome Study Group, *Am J Obstet Gynecol* 179:444-52, 1998.
27. Denke MA, Fox MM, Schulte MC: Short-term dietary calcium fortification increases fecal saturated content and reduces serum lipids in men, *J Nutr* 123:1047-53, 1993.
28. Heaney RP, Dowell SD, Bierman J, et al: Absorbability and cost effectiveness in calcium supplementation, *J Am Coll Nutr* 20:239-46, 2001.

■ CHAPTER 54 ■

CAROTENOIDS

Carotenes cannot cause vitamin A toxic effects; the extent to which the body converts beta-carotene to vitamin A is determined and controlled by vitamin A levels.

Carotenoids are a family of conjugated polyene molecules that give fruits and vegetables their pink, orange, and yellow colors. More than 600 carotenoids have been isolated in nature, around 50 have been found in the human diet, and 20 have been identified in plasma and tissues.

The best known of the carotenes is beta-carotene, the nontoxic water-soluble precursor of vitamin A. As beta-carotene is being absorbed, it can be split into two molecules of retinol. One retinol equivalent (RE), the vitamin A activity in food, is equivalent to 6 µg of all-trans beta-carotene.

Carotenoids may reduce the risk of chronic diseases, particularly those attributable to free radical pathology.[1]

MECHANISM OF ACTION

A number of carotenoids, such as cryptoxanthin, alpha-carotene, and beta-carotene, are converted to fat-soluble vitamin A. In addition, carotenoids have an antioxidant effect. Carotenoids are important dietary free radical scavengers. Lutein, followed by beta-carotene, alpha-carotene, and lycopene are the most effective quenchers of singlet oxygen in this nutrient group.[2] In addition to quenching singlet oxygen and reducing peroxyl radicals at a low partial oxygen pressure, beta-carotene has been shown to modulate immunity.[3] However, its health impact is modified by its concentration and stereochemistry. Although the natural cis form of beta-carotene is an antioxidant, the synthetic trans form may be a prooxidant.[4]

FOOD SOURCES

Vegetables and fruits are the major dietary sources of carotenoids. The clinically important carotenes are beta-carotene, alpha-carotene, lycopene, lutein, and the xanthins. Beta-carotene is present in leafy green vegetables such as spinach and in yellow vegetables such as carrots and sweet potatoes;

alpha-carotene is plentiful in yellow-orange vegetables such as carrots and pumpkin; lycopene is found in red fruits such as tomatoes and guavas; lutein is found in dark green vegetables such as spinach; and the xanthins are found in orange fruits such as mangoes and mandarins.

Processing adversely affects the carotene concentration in food. As much as one third of bioavailable beta-carotene can be lost on heating. Sun-drying depletes almost all of the beta-carotene in food; frying for 15 minutes causes a 70% loss; boiling for 60 minutes causes a 40% loss; and freezing, canning, and controlled drying cause a 20% loss of this nutrient.

In the United States, the average daily consumption of beta-carotene is approximately 1.5 mg; the U.S. National Cancer Institute has suggested that the daily dietary intake of beta-carotene be increased to 5.6 to 6.0 mg. At least five servings of fruits or vegetables are required each day to obtain the 6 mg of beta-carotene recommended by the U.S. National Cancer Institute. A diet of 25 to 35 g of whole grains, 100 g of fruit, and 500 g of vegetables per day increases blood levels of lutein, lycopene, beta-carotene, and vitamin C. Dietary carotenes are better absorbed if eaten with foods that contain some fat.

DOSE

Adults and teenagers require a daily intake of 6 to 15 mg of beta-carotene, the equivalent of 10,000 to 25,000 IU of vitamin A activity. Children require 3 to 6 mg of beta-carotene daily, the equivalent of 5000 to 10,000 IU of vitamin A activity. Intakes of carotenoids up to 5 mg/kg body weight are considered acceptable.

The following conversions should be considered:

- Retinal equivalent (RE) = retinal intake + carotene/6
- 1 RE = 3.33 IU retinol = 10 IU beta-carotene
- 1 RE = 1 µg retinol = 6 µg or 10 IU beta-carotene = 12 µg carotenoids
- 1 mg all-*trans* beta-carotene = 1667 IU of vitamin A activity
- 1 µg dietary beta-carotene = 0.167 µg retinol

CLINICAL USES

Beta-carotene intake of no more than 10 mg/day from diet and supplements is suggested for populations with serum concentrations of less than 0.15 µmol/L or intakes of less than 700 µg/day.[5] In addition to use of other antioxidants, an intake of 9 to 12 mg of beta-carotene per day with a plasma concentration of 0.4 µmol/L is recommended for reducing the risk of degenerative diseases.[6] However, despite strong evidence that vitamin C and beta-carotene have a protective effect against stroke[7] and positive reports that beta-carotene reduces the risk of heart disease in current smokers by 70%, former smokers by 40%, and lifetime nonsmokers by 0%,[6] there is skepticism about the usefulness of beta-carotene supplementation, particularly in healthy persons.

A review of patient-oriented evidence on the effectiveness of supplementation indicated that although available evidence may be insufficient to recommend the routine use of vitamin E, vitamin C, or folate supplements for the prevention of myocardial infarction or stroke, the evidence does suggest that beta-carotene supplementation not be used for this purpose.[8] In fact, "clinical trials with beta-carotene supplements have been disappointing and their use as a preventive intervention for cancer and coronary heart disease should be discouraged."[9] Such conclusions are consistent with the finding that apparently healthy women, taking a 50-mg beta-carotene supplement on alternate days for just over 2 years, neither benefited nor experienced harm and showed no change in their anticipated incidence of cancer and/or cardiovascular disease.[10] Such conclusions are also supported by the following three beta-carotene intervention trials: the Beta-Carotene and Retinol Efficacy Trial, the Alpha-Tocopherol, Beta-Carotene Cancer Prevention Study, and the Physicians' Health Study. All conclusions pointed to failure of synthetic beta-carotene to decrease the risk of cardiovascular disease or cancer in well-nourished populations.[11] In the Physicians' Health Study I—a randomized, double-blind, placebo-controlled trial—22,071 healthy U.S. male physicians took 50 mg of beta-carotene on alternate days.[12] The final results of this study indicated that beta-carotene supplementation had no significant effect on cardiovascular disease, but benefits of beta-carotene supplementation on subsequent vascular events were detected among a small subgroup of 333 men with prior angina or revascularization. This may be related to beta-carotene reducing the oxidation of low-density lipoprotein cholesterol at doses of 6 to 20 mg/day.[13]

The Physicians' Health Study I also showed no overall effect on either incidence of total cancer or incidence of prostate, colon, and lung cancers, the three most common site-specific cancers.[12] However, final results after more than 12 years did indicate a possible reduced incidence of total cancer and prostate cancer in those with low baseline carotenoid levels who were assigned to receive beta-carotene.[14] Despite disappointing clinical results, epidemiologic evidence continues to strongly associate beta-carotene intake with a reduced risk of many different types of cancer.[15] In vitro and animal studies have demonstrated that beta-carotene can inhibit carcinogenesis through its antioxidant activity, vitamin A precursor status, enhancement of gap junction communication, immunologic effect, and induction of hepatic detoxification of carcinogens.[16] One explanation for the discrepancy between epidemiologic and animal study data and human experimental data is that in human studies synthetic beta-carotene was used and may not have provided the right nutrient mixture for chemoprevention. Mixed carotenes have a better chemopreventive action than synthetic beta-carotene.

Controversy surrounding the efficacy of carotene supplementation in trials may be a consequence of synthetic carotenes lacking an effective concentration of cis beta-carotene and/or the absence of other carotenes (lycopene, lutein, cryptoxanthine, or zeaxanthin) found in dietary sources. In addition to failing to provide a protective dose, synthetic beta-carotene, with its ability to behave as a prooxidant in vivo,[17] is potentially carcinogenic, given particular circumstances.

Failure of beta-carotene to meet initial expectations does not obviate the potential value of the carotenoid group. The American Institute of Cancer Research reported that consumption of 400 to 600 g of fruits and vegetables each day is associated with a reduced risk of lung cancer.[18] Over a 12-year follow-up period, it was concluded that the lung cancer risk was significantly lower in subjects who consumed a diet high in a variety of carotenoids.[19] Increased alpha-carotene intake is inversely associated with the risk of lung cancer in nonsmokers.[18] Other carotenes are also associated with a reduced risk, but this is not statistically significant. However, smoking attenuates this risk relationship for all carotenes except lycopene. Although controversial, there are those who advocate, for primary prevention of both cancer and cardiovascular disease, that nonsmokers may only need to take 2.5 to 4 mg (0.005-0.007 mmol) and smokers need 9 mg (0.017 mmol) of beta-carotene.[20] Furthermore, beta-carotene (6-25 mg/day), in combination with vitamins C (100-1500 mg) and E (50-1500 mg), is still considered to have possible cardioprotective and cancer-protective effects.[21]

A study of 3000 Americans showed that consumption of one carrot a day reduced the chances of macular degeneration in elderly patients by 40%.[22] Although beta-carotene may protect against cataracts, lutein found in high concentrations in the eye filters out blue light and may protect against macular degeneration. The free radical scavenging of lycopene may also be helpful. A therapeutic dose of 30 to 300 mg of beta-carotene daily for adults and teenagers, and 30 to 150 mg for children, is used to protect patients with photosensitive erythropoietic protoporphyria.

TOXICITY/DRUG INTERACTIONS

Plasma carotene levels reflect intake of precursors. No toxicity for carotene has been recorded for doses of up to 150,000 IU.

Hypercarotenemia occurs in people taking about 30 mg of beta-carotene per day over several weeks. It is completely reversible. Occasionally, individuals complain of bloating, which is dose-related and reversible. Excessive intake of carotenoids results in yellowing of the palms, hands, soles of the feet, and to a lesser extent, the face. In rare cases, patients complain of diarrhea, dizziness, joint pain, unusual bleeding, or bruising.

Several clinical trials have failed to demonstrate any serious interaction between vitamin E and beta-carotene that would compromise availability of α-tocopherol in individuals taking beta-carotene supplements.

CLINICAL CAUTION

Although intake of large amounts of beta-carotene must be viewed with caution, there is no evidence at present that consuming small amounts of supplemental beta-carotene (i.e., the amount in foods or in a multivitamin tablet) is unwise for any population. However, current findings do suggest that smokers and those with a history of asbestos exposure should avoid taking large amounts of beta-carotene supplements (20-30 mg/day) for prolonged periods (i.e., several years). Despite data from two cohort studies (male and female) that suggest that several carotenoids may reduce the risk of lung cancer,[19] the results of three large-scale clinical trials have cast doubt on the desirability of beta-carotene supplementation.[23] The populations involved were Finnish male heavy smokers (the Alpha Tocopherol Beta Carotene trial), male asbestos workers and male and female heavy smokers (Beta-Carotene and Retinol Efficacy Trial), and U.S. male physicians, 11% of whom were current smokers (Physician's Health Study). All three trials demonstrated that beta-carotene provided no protection against lung cancer, and in two trials a higher risk for lung cancer was found among subjects given beta-carotene.

Any protective action of carotenoids may be largely attributed to their singlet oxygen quenching and antioxidant activity. Any cancer-enhancing actions in lung tissue may be ascribed to the prooxidant action of carotenoid free radicals in damaged cells. On the other hand, beta-carotene's effect in vivo may be unrelated to its antioxidant properties and may be due to its effect on any number of biochemical systems.

PRACTICE TIPS

- Megadose dietary consumption of beta-carotene does not result in vitamin A toxicity.
- Use of a mixed carotenoid supplement (15 mg/day), rather than beta-carotene as a single supplement, is recommended.
- Blood concentrations of carotenoids have been proposed as integrated biochemical markers of vegetable, fruit, and synthetic supplements consumed.[24]

REFERENCES

1. Lamson DW, Brignall MS: Natural agents in the prevention of cancer, part two: preclinical data and chemoprevention for common cancers, *Altern Med Rev* 6: 167-87, 2001.
2. Arab L, Steck S: Lycopene and cardiovascular disease, *Am J Clin Nutr* 71(suppl 6):1691S-1695S, 2000.
3. Patrick L: Beta-carotene: the controversy continues, *Altern Med Rev* 5:530-45, 2000.

4. Levin G, Yeshurun M, Mockady S: In vitro antiperoxidative effect of 9-cis beta-carotene compared with that of the all trans isomer, *J Nutr Cancer* 27:293-7, 1997.

5. Burri BJ: Beta-carotene and human health: a review of current research, *Nutr Res* 17:547-80, 1997.

6. Charleux J: Beta-carotene, vitamin C, and vitamin E: the protective micronutrients, *Nutr Rev* 54:S109-S114, 1996.

7. Ascherio A: Antioxidants and stroke, *Am J Clin Nutr* 72:337-8, 2000.

8. Pearce KA, Boosalis MG, Yeager B: Update on vitamin supplements for the prevention of coronary disease and stroke, *Am Fam Physician* 62:1359-66, 2000.

9. Marchioli R: Antioxidant vitamins and prevention of cardiovascular disease: laboratory, epidemiological and clinical trial data, *Pharmacol Res* 40:227-38, 1999.

10. Lee IM, Cook NR, Manson JE, et al: Beta-carotene supplementation and incidence of cancer and cardiovascular disease: the Women's Health Study, *J Natl Cancer Inst* 91:2102-6, 1999.

11. Patrick L: Beta-carotene: the controversy continues, *Altern Med Rev* 5:530-45, 2000.

12. Cook NR, Le IM, Manson JE, et al: Effects of beta-carotene supplementation on cancer incidence by baseline characteristics in the Physicians' Health Study (United States), *Cancer Causes Control* 11:617-26, 2000.

13. Dixon ZR, Burri BJ, Clifford A, et al: Effects of carotene-deficient diet on measures of oxidative susceptibility and superoxide dismutase activity in adult women, *Free Radic Biol Med* 17:537-44, 1994.

14. Christen WG, Gaziano JM, Hennekens CH: Design of Physicians' Health Study II—a randomized trial of beta-carotene, vitamins E and C, and multivitamins, in prevention of cancer, cardiovascular disease, and eye disease, and review of results of completed trials, *Ann Epidemiol* 10:125-34, 2000.

15. Cooper DA, Eldridge AL, Peters JC: Dietary carotenoids and certain cancers, heart disease, and age-related macular degeneration: a review of recent research, *Nutr Rev* 57:201-14, 1999.

16. Wang XD, Russell RM: Procarcinogenic and anticarcinogenic effects of beta-carotene, *Nutr Rev* 57:263-72, 1999.

17. Omaye ST, Krinsky NI, Kagan VE, et al: Beta-carotene: friend or foe? *Fundam Appl Toxicol* 40:163-74, 1997.

18. Heber D: Colorful cancer prevention: alpha-carotene, lycopene, and lung cancer, *Am J Clin Nutr* 72:901-2, 2000.

19. Michaud DS, Feskanich D, Rimm EB, et al: Intake of specific carotenoids and risk of lung cancer in 2 prospective US cohorts, *Am J Clin Nutr* 72:990-7, 2000.

20. Gey KF: Vitamins E plus C and interacting conutrients required for optimal health. A critical and constructive review of epidemiology and supplementation data regarding cardiovascular disease and cancer, *Biofactors* 7:113-74, 1998.

21. Brighthope I: Nutritional medicine-its presence and power, *J Aust Coll Nutr Environ Med* 17:5-18, 1998.

22. Lachance P: Dietary intake of carotenes and the carotene gap, *Clin Nutr* 7: 118-22, 1988.

23. Pryor WA, Stahl W, Rock CL: Beta-carotene: from biochemistry to clinical trials, *Nutr Rev* 58:39-53, 2000.

24. Toniolo P, Van Kappel AL, Akhmedkhanov A, et al: Serum carotenoids and breast cancer, *Am J Epidemiol* 153:1142-7, 2001.

■ CHAPTER 55 ■

CHAMOMILE (*MATRICARIA RECUTITA*)

> The potential cost-benefit ratio of scientifically unproven interventions with chamomile approximates infinity.
> Although allergic responses in atopic individuals devaluate the potential benefit of proven mediations, they make use of unproven interventions intolerably hazardous.

The healing properties of chamomile are largely linked to its volatile oils. It is reputed to have soothing qualities, including calming, anti-inflammatory, and antispasmodic effects.

MECHANISM OF ACTION

The active substances in chamomile belong to chemically different structural types. The largest group of medically important compounds is found among the essential oils. Flavonoids, coumarins, mucilages, monosaccharides, and oligosaccharides all have beneficial effects.

DOSE

Traditional doses are 2 to 3 g of dried flower heads per day and 3 to 6 mL of 1:2 liquid extract or 7 to 14 mL of 1:5 tincture per day. Infusion of chamomile (3%-10% wt/wt flowers) is for external use. Only creams that contain at least 3% chamomile should be used.

CLINICAL USES

Chamomile tea is used as a mild sedative. Chamomile creams are used to soothe inflamed, irritated skin. They are useful for providing symptomatic relief of sunburn and eczema. In a partially double-blind, randomized study Kamillosan, a cream that contains chamomile extract rich in active principles without any chamomile-related allergen potential, was found to be slightly superior to 0.5% hydrocortisone in topical treatment of atopic eczema.[1] There is clinical evidence to support the topical use of chamomile for wound healing and for the treatment of varicose eczema.[2]

Chamomile has also traditionally been used to treat flatulence, nervous dyspepsia, and nervous diarrhea.

TOXICITY/DRUG INTERACTIONS

Chamomile is safe when used as recommended. Anaphylaxis has been reported and contact dermatitis may rarely occur.

In one study, chamomile was one of the aromatherapy oils used to treat children with eczema.[3] Children who were treated with essential oil massage experienced initial improvement but later showed a deterioration in their eczematous condition.[3]

CLINICAL CAUTION

The herb is contraindicated in persons with hay fever.

PRACTICE TIPS

• Chamomile may be used with other medications.
• Chamomile should not be used for prolonged periods.

REFERENCES

1. Patzelt-Wenczler R, Ponce-Poschl E: Proof of efficacy of Kamillosan® cream in atopic eczema, *Eur J Med Res* 5:171-5, 2000.
2. Mills S, Bone K: *Principles and practice of phytotherapy*, Edinburgh, 2000, Churchill Livingstone.
3. Anderson C, Lis-Balchin M, Kirk-Smith M: Evaluation of massage with essential oils on childhood atopic eczema, *Phytother Res* 14:452-6, 2000.

■ CHAPTER 56 ■

CHASTE TREE (*VITEX AGNUS-CASTUS*)

A clinical response to herbal and other natural interventions may be gradual; it may take at least 6 weeks of treatment before any clinical changes are detectable.

Despite its name and the traditional belief that the berries of the chaste tree encourage chastity, there is little evidence to suggest it decreases libido in therapeutic doses. Today the herb is used largely for women's complaints including hot flashes, premenstrual tension, amenorrhea, and infertility.

MECHANISM OF ACTION

Chasteberry acts on the anterior pituitary to normalize menstruation and encourage ovulation. It reduces prolactin production and increases progesterone production by reducing secretion of follicle-stimulating hormone and increasing production of luteinizing hormone. Its active principle appears to bind to dopamine receptors in the pituitary.

Chasteberry contains essential oils, flavonoids, and iridoid glycosides.

DOSE

A daily dose of 1 to 5 mL of a 1:5 tincture, 1 to 4 mL of a 1:2 extract, or 500 mg of chaste tree tablets is often used. The 225 mg of powdered extract containing 0.5% agnoside is a standard dose used once or twice daily for a number of symptoms.

Chaste tree is most effective when taken on an empty stomach. If this causes gastric irritation, the herb may be prescribed in divided doses or in capsule form.

CLINICAL USES

Chasteberry, useful for menstrual disorders, is particularly effective in women who have a short luteal phase and inadequate luteal progesterone production. It is most effective in women with mild or moderately low progesterone levels. Clinical trials have demonstrated that chasteberry is effective for managing menstrual disorders, including correction of disturbances in the length, frequency, and volume of menses.[1] It has also been shown to be beneficial in the treatment of premenstrual symptoms, infertility attributable to low progesterone levels, and acne. Results of a multicenter, open study confirmed that an extract of the fruit of the chaste tree reduced or eliminated the premenstrual syndrome symptoms of depression, anxiety, food craving, and hyperhydration.[2] Irritability, bloating, and depression are most likely to be relieved in women who produce insufficient progesterone in the 2 weeks before menstruation. Mastodynia is less severe after therapy. Less prolactin production may reduce premenstrual breast tenderness.

It has been suggested that 225 mg of chaste tree tea twice daily enhances milk production in breast-feeding mothers.[3]

TOXICITY/DRUG INTERACTIONS

Chasteberry appears to be a safe herb but should be avoided or used with caution during pregnancy and lactation. Occasionally, abdominal pain or a skin rash is reported.

Chasteberry contains progesterones and should not be taken in conjunction with progesterone, the contraceptive pill, or hormone replacement therapy. It intensifies effects of dopamine antagonists and should not be used in patients receiving phenothiazides.

CLINICAL CAUTION

Chaste tree may exacerbate certain types of spasmodic dysmenorrhea.

PRACTICE TIPS

- Although 6 weeks of therapy reduces symptoms of premenstrual syndrome, it may take 6 or more months before amenorrhea or infertility is corrected.
- Use of the herb should be discontinued if the menstrual cycle is markedly altered.

REFERENCES

1. Mills S, Bone K: *Principles and practice of phytotherapy*, Edinburgh, 2000, Churchill Livingstone.

2. Loch EG, Selle H, Boblitz N: Treatment of premenstrual syndrome with a phytopharmaceutical formulation containing *Vitex agnus castus*, *J Womens Health Gend Based Med* 9:315-20, 2000.

3. Diefendorf D, Healey J, Kalyn W, editors: *The healing power of vitamins, minerals and herbs*, Surry Hills, Australia, 2000, Readers Digest.

■ CHAPTER 57 ■

CHOLINE

Dietary supplements for which no known clinical application is proven can be readily purchased.

Choline is a vitamin-like compound synthesized from methionine by the body. It is a precursor for acetylcholine, phospholipid (lecithin), sphingomyelin, platelet-activating factor, and the methyl donor betaine.

MECHANISM OF ACTION

Choline is a source of methyl groups for transmethylation reactions. It is also a component of various other molecules including the following:

• Acetylcholine, a neurotransmitter important for transmembrane signaling and cholinergic neurotransmission
• Phosphatidylcholine (lecithin) and sphingomyelin, phospholipids important for maintaining the structural integrity of cell membranes and for signal transduction
• Platelet-activating factor, which is important for clot formation

Choline plays a role in the transport and metabolism of lipids (including cholesterol)

FOOD SOURCES

Choline can be absorbed from the diet or synthesized de novo. It is widely distributed, and milk and cell membranes (e.g., liver, eggs, peanuts) are particularly good sources of choline.

Lecithins added during food processing may increase the average intake of phosphatidylcholine by 1.5 mg/kg body weight or the intake of choline by 0.225 mg/kg body weight.

DOSE

The adequate intake of choline is 550 mg/day for men and 425 mg/day for women. The AI for pregnant women is 450 mg/day and increases to 550 mg/day during lactation. The upper limit of choline for adults is 3.5 g/day.

CLINICAL USES

Despite various claims, there are no scientifically proven benefits of choline supplementation.[1]

TOXICITY/DRUG INTERACTIONS

Toxic effects of choline include hypotension. At a dose of 10 g/day, cholinergic side effects include diarrhea, dizziness, sweating, and electrocardiographic changes.

CLINICAL CAUTION

Deficiency may result in liver damage.

PRACTICE TIPS

• Persons with a fishy body odor may have choline toxicosis.

REFERENCE

1. Mason P: *Dietary supplements*, ed 2, London, 2001, Pharmaceutical Press.

■ CHAPTER 58 ■

CHROMIUM

> Suboptimal chromium intake increases susceptibility to diabetes, which in turn predisposes to chromium deficiency.

Chromium is a trace mineral. In its trivalent state, chromium is an essential trace element required for carbohydrate, lipid, and nucleic acid metabolism. Its primary function is to enhance the effects of insulin.

Contrary to popular belief, chromium has not been shown to increase muscle mass or decrease body fat.

MECHANISM OF ACTION

Chromium has an important influence on carbohydrate, fat, and protein metabolism and appears to have an impact on nucleic acid synthesis and gene expression.

Chromium increases insulin binding to cells and insulin receptor numbers and activates insulin receptor kinase, leading to increased insulin sensitivity.[1] As a component of glucose tolerance factor, chromium is believed to mediate insulin's effects and aid glucose transport across cell membranes. Glucose tolerance factor is composed of trivalent chromium, two nicotinic acid molecules, and a small oligopeptide. The chromium-binding oligopeptide chromodulin is thought to play a unique role in the auto-amplification of insulin signaling.[2]

FOOD SOURCES

Chromium is found in various foods, including brewers' yeast, calf liver, American cheese, wheat germ, molasses, sugar beets, seafood, eggs, meat, and whole grains. Barley is a good source of chromium and should be included in the diet of patients with diabetes. Absorption is around 10%.

DOSE

The estimated safe and adequate daily dietary intake of chromium is 50 to 200 µg for adults. The therapeutic dose range is 200 to 2000 µg/day.[3]

CLINICAL USES

Chromium has been shown to improve glucose metabolism in subjects with glucose intolerance and type 1, type 2, gestational, and steroid-induced diabetes.[1] A clinical trial demonstrated that 1000 µg of chromium daily, in the form of chromium picolinate, had significant beneficial effects on hemoglobin A_{1c}, glucose, insulin, and cholesterol levels in subjects with type 2 diabetes.[4] However, the beneficial effects of chromium in diabetes may only be detected at levels around fivefold higher than the upper limit of the estimated safe and adequate daily dietary intake.[5]

The requirement for chromium is related to the degree of glucose intolerance. Although higher intakes are more effective, 200 µg of supplemental chromium daily is adequate to improve glucose levels in individuals with mild glucose intolerance. In gestational diabetes, chromium in doses of 8 µg/kg body weight is more effective than 4 µg/kg,[6] and steroid-induced diabetes can be reversed by chromium supplementation in doses of 600 µg daily.[7] Corticosteroid treatment increases chromium losses. Results of a recent double-blind, crossover trial confirmed that chromium supplementation improved control of glucose and lipid levels while decreasing drug dosage in patients with type 2 diabetes.[8] Brewers' yeast (23.3 µg of chromium per day) and chromium chloride ($CrCl_{13}$) (200 µg of chromium per day) were used. Brewers' yeast was marginally more effective.

Other indications for chromium supplementation are less well documented. Preliminary observations suggest that chromium, 200 µg once or twice daily, may enhance antidepressant therapy for dysthymic disorder, with symptomatic improvement occurring within 3 days of treatment.[9]

Athletes who restrict calories to maintain low body weights could compromise their chromium status. Although chromium has been touted as an agent for increasing lean body mass and decreasing body fat,[10] chromium supplementation does not appear to promote muscle accretion or fat loss or to enhance strength in young men and women.[11] Acute, intense activity results in short-term increases in both urine and sweat losses of minerals, including chromium. Losses apparently diminish during recovery in the days after exercise.

TOXICITY/DRUG INTERACTIONS

There is little information available on the long-term use of chromium supplements, but at present, supplements within the estimated safe and adequate daily dietary allowance level do not appear to be harmful.[12] Trivalent chromium has a very large safety range, and there have been no documented signs of chromium toxic effects at doses up to 1 mg/day in any of the nutritional studies.[4] Long-term intake of chromium in excess of 100 mg/day may lead to growth retardation, cardiomyopathy, and hepatic and renal damage.

Chromium and iron compete for binding on transferrin. Supplementation with chromium picolinate, but not chromium chloride, decreases transferrin saturation. The bioavailability of chromium is better in oral chromium picolinate or nicotinate salt supplements.

Chromium supplementation is likely to alter the amount of insulin required by patients with diabetes and a chromium deficiency. Chromium may reduce insulin requirements and enhance the effects of oral hypoglycemic agents. Patients taking hypoglycemic agents may require dose adjustments.[11]

CLINICAL CAUTION

The dietary intake of chromium in humans is often suboptimal, and assessment is problematic because of the absence of a reliable indicator of chromium status. Furthermore, suboptimal dietary intake of chromium appears to be associated with risk factors for diabetes and cardiovascular diseases, such as impaired glucose tolerance, increased circulating insulin levels, glucosuria, and hyperlipidemia. Studies also suggest that even the lowest normal chromium intake (25%) has a detrimental effect on glucose tolerance and insulin and glucagon levels in subjects with mildly impaired glucose tolerance.[13] Chromium (200 μg/day) increased by 50% the number of insulin receptors in subjects with hyperglycemia. Diabetes itself may exacerbate chromium deficiency. Patients with type 2 diabetes lose more chromium in their urine than individuals without diabetes, and diets low in chromium may have adverse effects on patients with borderline diabetes.[14]

Peripheral neuropathy, encephalopathy, and impaired protein and fat metabolism have been reported in persons with an inadequate chromium status.

PRACTICE TIPS

- The use of chromium supplements in excessive doses or for prolonged periods is not advisable, because the long-term effects of chromium accumulation in humans are unknown.
- Adults who consume a diet of refined foods over prolonged periods are at risk for chromium deficiency.

REFERENCES

1. Anderson RA: Chromium in the prevention and control of diabetes, *Diabetes Metab* 26:22-7, 2000.
2. Vincent JB: Elucidating a biological role for chromium at a molecular level, *Acc Chem Res* 33:503-10, 2000.

3. Brighthope I: Nutritional medicine tables, *J Aust Coll Nutr Environ Med* 17:20-5, 1998.
4. Anderson RA, Cheng N, Bryden NA, et al: Elevated intakes of supplemental chromium improve glucose and insulin variables in individuals with type 2 diabetes, *Diabetes* 46:1786-91, 1997.
5. Preuss HG, Anderson RA: Chromium update: examining recent literature 1997-1998, *Curr Opin Clin Nutr Metab Care* 1:509-12, 1998.
6. Anderson RA: Chromium, glucose intolerance and diabetes, *J Am Coll Nutr* 17:548-55, 1998.
7. Ravina A, Slezak L, Mirsky N, et al: Reversal of corticosteroid-induced diabetes mellitus with supplemental chromium, *Diabet Med* 16:164-7, 1999.
8. Bahijiri SM, Mira SA, Mufti AM, et al: The effects of inorganic chromium and brewer's yeast supplementation on glucose tolerance, serum lipids and drug dosage in individuals with type 2 diabetes, *Saudi Med J* 21:831-7, 2000.
9. McLeod MN, Gaynes BN, Golden RN: Chromium potentiation of antidepressant pharmacotherapy for dysthymic disorder in 5 patients, *J Clin Psychiatry* 60:237-40, 1999.
10. Kobla HV, Volpe SL: Chromium, exercise, and body composition, *Crit Rev Food Sci Nutr* 40:291-308, 2000.
11. Lukaski HC: Magnesium, zinc, and chromium nutriture and physical activity, *Am J Clin Nutr* 72(suppl 2):585S-593S, 2000.
12. Clarkson PM: Effects of exercise on chromium levels. Is supplementation required? *Sports Med* 23:341-9, 1997.
13. Anderson RA, Polansky MM, Bryden NA, et al: Supplemental-chromium effects on glucose, insulin, glucagon, and urinary chromium losses in subjects consuming controlled low-chromium diets, *Am J Clin Nutr* 54:909-16, 1991.
14. Morelli V, Zoorob RJ: Alternative therapies: part I. Depression, diabetes, obesity, *Am Fam Physician* 62:1051-60, 2000.

■ CHAPTER 59 ■

COENZYME Q10 (UBIQUINONE)

> Health gains achieved by correcting a nutrient deficiency are not necessarily augmented by using nutrients for medicinal purposes.

Coenzyme Q10 is a vital cell membrane antioxidant and facilitates cellular respiration. Coenzyme Q10 is often included in anti-aging potions in view of its role in energy generation and the finding that cellular levels decrease with age.

MECHANISM OF ACTION

The primary biochemical action of coenyzme Q10 is as a cofactor in the electron transport chain, a series of oxidation-reduction reactions involved in cellular respiration and the synthesis of energy (adenosine triphosphate). As an electron and proton carrier, it is essential for production of adenosine triphosphate in the electron transport chain. In addition to its role in energy production, coenzyme Q10 is thought to have membrane-stabilizing properties. It also acts as a free radical scavenger and antioxidant.

FOOD SOURCES

Coenzyme Q10 is produced in the body. Rich dietary sources are fatty fish such as sardines and beans, nuts, whole grains, and meat.

DOSE

A typical dose for treatment of most conditions is 30 to 60 mg twice daily; however, certain conditions require higher doses. Some studies on breast cancer treatment report use of 400 mg daily.[1] No adverse effects have been reported at doses of 200 mg daily for 1 year,[2] and no important adverse effects have been reported from experiments in which daily supplements of up to 200 mg of coenzyme Q10 were used for 6 to 12 months and daily supplements of 100 mg were used for up to 6 years. Some patients do lose their appetite and have skin eruptions during supplementation with coenzyme Q10.

A synthetic analogue of coenzyme Q10, idebenone [2,3-dimethoxy-5-methyl-6-(10-hydroxydecyl)-1,4-benzoquinone], is available.[3]

493

CLINICAL USES

In view of its central role in energy metabolism, it is not surprising that coenzyme Q10 is postulated to have a plethora of clinical effects. It may improve immune function, preventing metastasis and enhancing remission in certain cancers; reduce the risk of obesity; enhance myocardial contractility; reduce male infertility; protect gastric mucosa as a result of its antioxidant effects; and improve blood sugar control in patients with diabetes.[1]

Of all its possible functions, most clinical interest has focused on its potential impact on cardiovascular health. However, clinical trials in which coenzyme Q10 (100-200 mg daily) was used for the management of congestive heart failure have had conflicting results.[4] One year-long, double-blind trial showed that, compared with a placebo group, patients with chronic congestive heart failure given coenzyme Q10, 2 mg/kg per day, required less hospitalization for worsening heart failure and had fewer episodes of pulmonary edema.[5] Another randomized, double-blind, controlled trial of coenzyme Q10 (200 mg/day) showed no change in ejection fraction, peak oxygen consumption, or exercise duration in patients with congestive heart failure receiving standard medical therapy.[6] Before this study, randomized trials had indicated that administration of coenzyme Q10, 100 mg twice daily, in conjunction with standard medical therapy augmented myocardial kinetics, increased cardiac output, elevated the ischemic threshold, and enhanced functional capacity in patients with congestive heart failure.[7, 8] It is premature to discount the possibility that coenzyme Q10 may enhance cardiac output both by exerting a positive inotropic effect on the myocardium and by causing mild vasodilatation.

Coenzyme Q10 is also of interest with respect to energy production in patients with chronic fatigue syndrome. Patients with chronic fatigue syndrome are often deficient in coenzyme Q10, and in one study, supplementation with 100 mg daily over 3 months improved exercise tolerance and reduced clinical symptoms.[9]

Another possible use for coenzyme Q10 is as an anti-aging agent. Two potential dietary means of delaying the effects of free radicals on cellular aging are enrichment of mitochondrial membranes with monounsaturated fatty acids and supplementation with antioxidants. A preliminary study of elderly male rats suggests that dietary supplementation with coenzyme Q10 and enrichment of cell membranes with monounsaturated fatty acids protect mitochondrial membranes from free radical insult.[10]

TOXICITY/DRUG INTERACTIONS

Drugs such as lovastatin and pravastatin, used to reduce blood cholesterol levels by inhibiting the enzyme 3-hydroxy-3-methyl glutaryl–coenzyme A reductase, also impair synthesis of coenzyme Q10. Antihypertensive agents—such as the β-blockers propranolol and metoprolol, phenothiazines, and tricyclic antidepressants—inhibit coenzyme Q10–dependent enzymes.[11]

CLINICAL CAUTION

The ability to synthesize coenzyme Q10 decreases with age.

PRACTICE TIPS

- Absorption of coenzyme Q10 is greatest from supplements in an oil base.
- It may take 8 weeks before any clinical changes are detected.
- Concurrent supplementation of coenzyme Q10 with vitamin B_6 is recommended; the endogenous biosynthesis of the quinone nucleus of coenzyme Q10 is dependent on adequate vitamin B_6 levels.

REFERENCES

1. Coenzyme Q10, *Altern Med Rev* 3:58-61, 1998.
2. Overvad K, Diamant B, Holm L, et al: Coenzyme Q10 in health and disease, *Eur J Clin Nutr* 53:764-70, 1999.
3. Idebenone—monograph, *Altern Med Rev*;6:83-6, 2001.
4. Morelli V, Zoorob RJ: Alternative therapies: part II. Congestive heart failure and hypercholesterolemia, *Am Fam Physician* 62:1325-30, 2000.
5. Morisco C, Trimarco B, Condorelli M: Effect of coenzyme Q10 therapy in patients with congestive heart failure: a long-term multicenter randomized study, *Clin Investig* 71(suppl 8):S134-S136, 1993.
6. Khatta M, Alexander BS, Krichten CM, et al: The effect of coenzyme Q10 in patients with congestive heart failure, *Ann Intern Med* 132:636-40, 2000.
7. Munkholm H, Hansen HH, Rasmussen K: Coenzyme Q10 treatment in serious heart failure, *Biofactors* 9:285-9, 1999.
8. Sacher HL, Sacher ML, Landau SW, et al: The clinical and hemodynamic effects of coenzyme Q10 in congestive cardiomyopathy, *Am J Ther* 4:66-72, 1999.
9. Werbach MR: Nutritional strategies for treating chronic fatigue syndrome, *Altern Med Rev* 5:93-108, 2000.
10. Huertas JR, Martinez-Velasco E, Ibanez S, et al: Virgin olive oil and coenzyme Q10 protect heart mitochondria from peroxidative damage during aging, *Biofactors* 9:337-43, 1999.
11. Willis R, Anthony M, Sun L, et al: Clinical implications of the correlation between coenzyme Q10 and vitamin B_6 status, *Biofactors* 9:359-63, 1999.

■ CHAPTER 60 ■

COPPER

Copper can have an antioxidant effect in vivo, but a prooxidant effect in vitro.

Copper is an essential trace element. The total body content of copper is primarily regulated by means of excretion rather than absorption. Regulation is by bile excretion. Copper is excreted attached to taurochenodeoxycholic acid, a sulfur-containing bile acid that is stored in the liver. When mobilized, copper is found in the plasma firmly attached to protein as ceruloplasmin.

Copper (Cu) plays a role in hemoglobin synthesis, neural function, glucose utilization, and skeletal and cardiovascular health. It is required for iron utilization. Copper salicylate is known to have analgesic and anti-inflammatory effects, and the efficacy of various copper-based anti-inflammatory drugs is under investigation.[1]

MECHANISM OF ACTION

Copper acts as an activating ion in a number of enzymatic reactions. Its efficacy is often mediated by oxidation-reduction reactions in which Cu^+ is converted to Cu^{2+}. Copper is involved in the following:

- Control of free radicals. Copper is an essential component of superoxide dismutase, an enzyme that protects cell membranes by contributing to the breakdown of toxic free radicals, and cytochrome C oxidase, an enzyme of the electron transport chain involved in oxidative energy production
- Iron metabolism. Copper plays an important role in the oxidation-reduction, mobilization, and transport of iron (Fe), which is stored as Fe^{3+}, mobilized as Fe^{2+}, and deoxidized as Fe^{3+} for transport as transferrin.
- Activation of enzymes important for tissue formation and repair. Lysyl oxidase, a copper requiring enzyme, cross-links lysine in collagen and elastin.
- Skin pigmentation. Tyrosinase, a copper-activated enzyme, contributes to the synthesis of melanin.
- Metabolism of glucose, cholesterol, and myelin.

FOOD SOURCES

Copper is found in various foods including organ meats (especially liver), seafood, mushrooms, beans, nuts, whole grains, and chocolate. Additional copper can be obtained by drinking water that flows through copper pipes, by using copper cookware, and by eating farm products sprayed with copper-containing chemicals. The copper content of acidic foods decreases when they are stored in tin cans for long periods. The absorption of copper is regulated by the thioneines, sulfur-rich binding proteins found in the intestinal lining and other body cells. The thioneines are responsible for binding copper, zinc, and various other divalent metals. The efficiency of copper absorption is reduced by sulfides, ascorbic acid, zinc, and molybdenum.

DOSE

There is no estimated average requirement or reference nutrient intake for copper. However, normally recommended intakes are 1 to 3 mg/day. A safe and adequate dietary intake is 2 to 3 mg/day. The therapeutic dose range is 2 to 4 mg/day.[2]

CLINICAL USES

Results of animal studies suggest that diets low in copper increase the risk of skeletal and cardiovascular disease, as well as copper deficiency anemia. Both men and women fed diets close to 1 mg of copper per day experienced reversible, potentially harmful changes in blood pressure control, in cardiac electrical conduction as shown on electrocardiograms, cholesterol levels, and glucose metabolism.[3] These changes are similar to those in copper-deficient animals. Animal studies also suggest that copper deficiency below a threshold level can induce atherosclerotic lesions.[4]

Osteoporosis, like ischemic heart disease, is a likely consequence of diets low in copper. A longitudinal study of young men demonstrated that although most indices of copper status were unchanged, biomarkers of bone resorption were significantly increased on switching from medium (1.6 mg) to low (0.7 mg) daily copper intakes.[5] However, a double-blind, placebo-controlled, randomized, crossover trial of copper supplementation consisting of 3 and 6 mg of elemental copper daily indicated that, despite an apparently improved copper status, there was no change in biochemical markers of either bone formation or bone resorption over the 4-week periods.[6] Nonetheless, women supplemented with trace elements, including copper, experience beneficial effects on bone density.[3] The interaction of trace elements, rather than the presence of any one trace element, may hold the key to prevention.

TOXICITY/DRUG INTERACTIONS

Ingestion of copper in excess of 10 mg/day reduces absorption of zinc and iron. Nausea, abdominal and muscle pain, irritability, and depression may indicate copper toxicosis.

CLINICAL CAUTION

Intestinal absorption of copper is inhibited by zinc. When zinc to copper ratios exceed 10:1, copper absorption is impaired. Daily zinc supplementation of 150 mg over 2 years will precipitate copper deficiency. Similarly, simultaneous use of oral zinc supplements with copper supplements may decrease copper absorption. Copper and zinc supplements should be taken at least 2 hours apart to obtain the maximum benefit from each. Persons receiving penicillamine or trientine should delay taking their medication until at least 2 hours have elapsed after administration of a copper supplement.[7]

Copper deficiency is rare but is associated with hypochromic microcytic anemia in which iron stores are normal. However, the anemia is an iron deficiency anemia because iron stores lack the copper necessary for iron mobilization. Patients do not respond to iron supplements. Copper deficiency also presents with depigmented, grayish hair that has lost its regular wave. Weakened collagen and elastin predispose patients with copper deficiency to skeletal and vascular disorders.

A useful indicator of copper status is the copper-zinc–superoxide dismutase level in erythrocytes, which is depressed in copper deficiency.

PRACTICE TIPS

- A 2-mg copper supplement should be taken daily during zinc supplementation over periods exceeding 4 weeks.
- A low-copper diet has an adverse effect on the cholesterol ratio, increasing low-density lipoprotein cholesterol levels and decreasing high-density lipoprotein cholesterol levels.
- Administration of a 3-mg copper supplement daily may help to prevent osteoporosis (unproven).
- Persons with Wilson's disease, a hereditary disorder, should avoid copper.

REFERENCES

1. Jackson GE, Mkhonta-Gama L, Voye A, et al: Design of copper-based anti-inflammatory drugs, *J Inorg Biochem* 79:147-52, 2000.
2. Brighthope I: Nutritional medicine tables, *J Aust Coll Nutr Environ Med* 17:20-5, 1998.

3. Klevay LM: Lack of a recommended dietary allowance for copper may be hazardous to your health, *J Am Coll Nutr* 17:322-6, 1998.
4. Hamilton IM, Gilmore WS, Strain JJ: Marginal copper deficiency and atherosclerosis, *Biol Trace Elem Res* 78:179-89, 2000.
5. Baker A, Harvey L, Majask-Newman G, et al: Effect of dietary copper intakes on biochemical markers of bone metabolism in healthy adult males, *Eur J Clin Nutr* 53:408-12, 1999.
6. Cashman KD, Baker A, Ginty F, et al: No effect of copper supplementation on biochemical markers of bone metabolism in healthy young adult females despite apparently improved copper status, *Eur J Clin Nutr* 55:525-31, 2001.
7. Sandstead HH: Requirements and toxicity of essential trace elements, illustrated by zinc and copper, *Am J Clin Nutr* 61(suppl 3):621S-624S, 1995.

■ CHAPTER 61 ■

ECHINACEA

Short-term use of echinacea is thought to counteract the effect of immunosuppressants; however, long-term use of the herb my enhance immunosuppression.

Three species of *Echinacea* (purple cornflower) are used therapeutically. *E. purpurea* is the most easily cultivated, and the whole plant can be used. Only the root and rhizome of *E. pallida* and *E. angustifolia* are used medicinally. *E. purpurea* and *E. pallida* have been approved by European health authorities as supportive therapy for colds and flu-like symptoms. Topical preparations of *E. purpurea* have also been approved to assist poor wound healing and chronic ulceration. More work is needed to clearly distinguish between the efficacy of various species and the different plant parts (roots versus upper plant parts) and to ascertain the bioavailability, relative potency, and synergistic effects of the active compounds.

MECHANISM OF ACTION

Studies show that echinacea affects the nonspecific immune system but has little or no effect on the specific or acquired immune system. In vitro studies suggest that echinacea enhances the immune response and has an antiviral and weak antibacterial effect. Although echinacea has no direct bactericidal or bacteriostatic properties, in vitro studies have shown that it enhances phagocytosis, triggers proliferation of T lymphocytes, and increases macrophage release of tumor necrosis factor, interleukin 1, and β-interferon.

DOSE

Parenteral, oral, and topical extracts from the roots and aerial portions of the plant are available. Active constituents include caffeic acid derivatives, flavonoids, essential oils, polyacetylenes, alkylamides, and polysaccharides. However, the purity of some commercial products is doubtful; many have been found to be adulterated with various plant extracts. Furthermore, because active constituents vary slightly according to species and because echinacea's immune-stimulating effect probably results from interaction between various constituents, standardization of an extract is problematic. Discrepancies in the source and dose of echinacea are, in fact, one explanation for the variable results found in reviews of placebo-controlled, randomized studies investigating the immunomodulatory activity of echinacea preparations in healthy volunteers.[1]

Typical dosages for dried root are 0.5 to 1.0 g three times daily; for tincture (1:5), a half to one teaspoon three times daily; for dry, powdered extract standardized to 3.5% echinacoside, 300 mg three times daily; for liquid extract (1:1), a quarter to one half a teaspoon three times daily. Freeze-dried echinacea can be taken as one to two capsules or tablets three times daily. In general, fresh-pressed juice with 2.4% β-1, 2-fructo-furanosides or pills with 3.5% echinacosides should be selected.[2]

Because the purity and potency of preparations vary, no standard dose recommendations are possible. However, to prevent illness or to treat chronic conditions, any one of the following may be useful: 1 to 3 g/day dried root of *E. pallida* and/or *E. angustifolia*, 2.5 to 4.5 g/day *E. purpurea* dried root or 2.5 to 6.5 g/day dried aerial parts, 3 to 5.5 mL/day of 1:1 fresh plant tincture of roots and flowering tops of *E. purpurea* or 1:1 of whole dried plant, 3 to 9 mL/day of 1:2 liquid extract of *E. purpurea* dried root or 7.5 to 22.5 mL/day of 1:5 tincture of *E. purpurea* dried root. Considerably higher doses, up to 10 times, may be used for acute conditions. Scrutiny and selection of individual products by the user is recommended.

CLINICAL USES

Echinacea is used to enhance immunity and may be particularly beneficial for persons with upper respiratory tract or urinary tract infections. Recent evidence suggests that echinacea is likely to be more effective when used therapeutically rather than for prophylaxis. Symptomatic relief is reported when therapy is initiated at the first sign of infection, but there is insufficient evidence to support prevention of respiratory tract infections by long-term prophylactic use of echinacea.[3] Although echinacea appears to reduce the duration and severity of symptoms, it should be noted that this effect is achieved only with certain preparations of echinacea.[4]

Product discrepancies make it difficult to determine the true efficacy of this herb. A review of 12 clinical studies suggested that methodological problems such as small populations and use of noncommercially available, non-standardized dosage forms make it difficult to determine whether echinacea provides effective therapy for upper respiratory tract infections.[5] Yet many people do use *E. purpurea* at the first sign of colds and *E. pallida* as supportive treatment for flu-like symptoms. Such popularity among patients would seem to demand that professionals at least cautiously explore echinacea as an option offering immune support for persons with upper respiratory tract infections. A randomized, double-blind, placebo-controlled study demonstrated that echinacea concentrate and Echinaforce provided a low-risk and effective alternative to the standard symptomatic medicines in the acute treatment of the common cold.[6] However, another randomized, controlled trial showed that a fluid extract of *E. purpurea* did not significantly decrease the incidence, duration, or severity of colds and respiratory tract infections compared with placebo.[7] A recent review of the literature concurred, concluding that, although the majority of available studies report positive results, there is not enough evidence to recommend a specific echinacea product, or echinacea preparations for the treatment or prevention of the common cold.[8] Other reviewers concluded that despite somewhat dubious methodology, evidence from published trials does suggest that echinacea may be beneficial for the early treatment of acute upper respiratory tract infections.[9] Although uncertainty prevails regarding use of echinacea in treatment, there is stronger consensus that very little evidence supports prolonged use of echinacea for the prevention of upper respiratory tract infections.[3,9,10]

Echinacea may also be helpful if cautiously used in persons with impaired immunity (e.g., candidiasis) receiving chemotherapy. Topical use of echinacea may be considered for skin problems (e.g., for temporary relief of pain and as an antiseptic for cold sores). *E. purpurea*, applied every 6 to 8 hours, is used for poorly healing wounds and chronic ulcers.

TOXICITY/DRUG INTERACTIONS

Although evidence for echinacea's efficacy is inconclusive, it does appear to be safe at recommended doses. It even appears safe during the first trimester of pregnancy.[11]

Side effects primarily involve gastrointestinal upset, with patients complaining of dyspepsia, nausea, and vomiting. Numbness and tingling of the tongue and alterations to taste have been reported. Allergic reactions are rare, but anaphylaxis and contact dermatitis have been reported.

Atopic subjects appear to be at increased risk. The possibility that cross-reactivity between echinacea and other environmental allergens may trigger allergic reactions in "echinacea-naive" subjects is supported by Australian data.[12] Topical echinacea should not be applied to eyes or over large areas.

Echinacea may exacerbate symptoms of autoimmune disorders such as lupus or rheumatoid arthritis and multiple sclerosis. It is considered prudent to avoid prescribing echinacea for patients having treatment with immunosupressives including corticosteroids, cytotoxic drugs, and antiretroviral drugs. A review of the literature to determine the possible interactions between seven top-selling herbal medicines found no reported interactions between echinacea (*E, angustifolia, E purpurea, E. pallida*) and the prescribed drugs reviewed.[13]

CLINICAL CAUTION

The duration and circumstances in which echinacea should be used are disputed.[14,15] Some authorities suggest that avoiding use of echinacea in immune-modulated conditions is unnecessary[11]; others believe that echinacea is contraindicated in persons with immunologic dysfunction. Some authorities advise against taking echinacea for longer than 8 weeks; others believe that long-term ingestion is acceptable. Because prolonged use of echinacea may diminish its immune-boosting effects over time, another approach is to rotate echinacea with cat's claw, goldenseal, astragalus, pau d'arco, or reishi and maitake mushrooms. Another potentially useful treatment protocol for patients with poor immunity is the following[16]:

A daily maintenance dose of 5 mL of a 1:2 preparation (2.5 g) of the root of *E. angustifolia* or *E. purpurea*. This dose may be doubled in patients with markedly impaired immunity.

Double or triple the daily maintenance dose at the earliest suspicion of infection and only return to the maintenance dose once the threat has passed.

If the infection progresses, maintain the higher dose until fully recovered, then return to the maintenance dose.

Patients with renal or hepatic impairment should limit or avoid use of echinacea. Because parental administration alters blood sugar levels, patients with diabetes should take care when using any form of echinacea.

PRACTICE TIPS

- Use of echinacea should be started at the first signs of cold or flu and continued for 14 days or until symptoms remit, whichever is shorter.
- High-quality liquid echinacea causes tingling of the tongue.

REFERENCES

1. Melchart D, Linde K, Worku F, et al: Results of five randomized studies on the immunomodulatory activity of preparations of Echinacea, *J Altern Complement Med* 1:145-60, 1995.
2. Diefendorf D, Healey J, Kalyn W, editors: *The healing power of vitamins, minerals and herbs*, Surry Hills, Australia, 2000, Readers Digest.
3. Hoheisel O, Sandberg M, Bertram S: Echinacea shortens the course of the common cold: a double-blind placebo controlled clinical trial, *Eur J Clin Res* 9:261-9, 1997.
4. Percival SS: Use of echinacea in medicine, *Biochem Pharmacol* 60:155-8, 2000.
5. Giles JT, Palat CT, Chien SH, et al: Evaluation of echinacea for treatment of the common cold, *Pharmacotherapy* 20:690-7, 2000.

6. Brinkeborn RM, Shah DV, Degenring FH: Echinaforce and other Echinacea fresh plant preparations in the treatment of the common cold. A randomized, placebo controlled, double-blind clinical trial, *Phytomedicine* 6:1-6, 1999.

7. Grimm W, Muller HH: A randomized controlled trial of the effect of fluid extract of *Echinacea purpurea* on the incidence and severity of colds and respiratory infections, *Am J Med* 106:138-43, 1999.

8. Melchart D, Linde K, Fischer P, et al: Echinacea for preventing and treating the common cold, *Cochrane Database Syst Rev* 2:CD000530, 2000.

9. Barrett B, Vohmann M, Calabrese C: Echinacea for upper respiratory infection, *J Fam Pract* 48:628-35, 1999.

10. Melchart D, Walther E, Linde K, et al: Echinacea root extracts for the prevention of upper respiratory tract infections: a double-blind, placebo-controlled randomized trial, *Arch Fam Med* 7:541-5, 1998.

11. Gallo M, Koren G: Can herbal products be used safely during pregnancy? Focus on echinacea, *Can Fam Physician* 47:1727-8, 2001.

12. Mullins RJ, Heddle R: Adverse reactions associated with echinacea: the Australian experience, *Ann Allergy Asthma Immunol* 88:42-51, 2002.

13. Izzo AA, Ernst E: Interactions between herbal medicines and prescribed drugs: a systematic review, *Drugs* 61:2163-75, 2001.

14. Echinacea, *Altern Med Rev* 6:411-4, 2001.

15. Bone K: Echinacea: when should it be used? *Altern Med Rev* 2:451-8, 1997.

16. Mills S, Bone K: *Principles and practice of phytotherapy*, Edinburgh, 2000, Churchill Livingstone.

▪ CHAPTER 62 ▪

EVENING PRIMROSE OIL

Different brands of evening primrose oil (EPO) contain different quantities of γ-linolenic acid (GLA), the active principle and, when possible, doses of dietary supplements are based on the concentration of the active principle.

EPO is rich in GLA, an 18-carbon polyunsaturated fatty acid of the ω-6 series. Other sources of GLA are the oils from starflower, borage, and blackcurrant seeds. GLA can modify cellular lipid composition and eicosanoid biosynthesis. It and other fatty acids maintain cell structure and are key determinants of membrane functions such as activation of receptor sites and enzyme binding.

EPO has anti-inflammatory, antiallergic, and hypotensive effects. It has been postulated to have a prophylactic role in treating various chronic disease states.

MECHANISM OF ACTION

EPO is a rich source of the ω-6 essential fatty acid, linoleic acid, and GLA. Essential fatty acids are incorporated into cell membranes where they play a vital role in the structure of cell membranes, influencing membrane flexibility, fluidity, and the behavior of membrane-bound proteins. Essential fatty acids serve as a source of eicosanoids. Consumption of GLA (18:3 ω-6) favors an increase in the dihomogammalinolenic acid (DGLA) content of cell membranes without a corresponding increase the arachidonic acid concentration.[1] Ingestion of EPO elevates concentrations of DGLA (20:3 ω-6), enhancing production of eicosanoids of the prostaglandin 1 series (PG1). In addition, DGLA, which itself cannot be converted to leukotrienes, can form a 15-hydroxyl derivative that blocks the transformation of arachidonic acid to leukotrienes. Increased DGLA may act as a competitive inhibitor of the proinflammatory eicosanoids, prostaglandin 2 and leukotriene 4 series produced from arachidonic acid (20:4 ω-6) (see Figure 62-1). Membranes rich in DGLA favor formation of the prostaglandin 1 series of eicosanoids and reduce leukotriene synthesis. Membranes rich in DGLA favor a less inflammatory state.

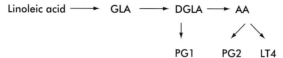

FIG. 62-1 Omega-6 eicosanoids.

On stimulation, DGLA can be converted by inflammatory cells into compounds that possess both anti-inflammatory and antiproliferative properties. Chronic inflammation is reduced by suppression of T lymphocytes. EPO may be beneficial in the treatment of diabetic neuropathy, mastalgia, premenstrual syndrome, atopic dermatitis, and rheumatoid arthritis. EPO is also used to correct an ω-6 fatty acid deficiency.

DOSE

The recommended dose of EPO varies depending on the condition. Low to medium doses of 2.6 to 5.2 g/day (250-600 mg/day GLA) are recommended for mastalgia and atopic dermatitis. Medium to high doses, 4.2 to 21 g/day(400-2000 mg/day GLA), are suggested for diabetes, inflammatory disorders, and cardiovascular problems (e.g., hypertension, hyperlipidemia). Persons with diabetic neuropathy may require 480 mg of GLA per day, whereas those with rheumatoid arthritis may receive an initial dose of 500 mg daily but only experience significant benefit when doses of 2.8 g daily are reached.

CLINICAL USES

Although treatment with EPO tends to normalize the fatty acid profile, clinical benefit should not be assumed. Direct evidence of a clinical response is required. This is available from at least one clinical trial with respect to diabetic neuropathy, mastalgia, rheumatoid arthritis, and migraine. Animal studies have shown that GLA increases nerve conduction velocity in diabetic rats.[2] A randomized, double-blind, placebo-controlled, parallel study in humans showed that GLA (480 mg/day) had beneficial effects on the course of mild diabetic neuropathy over a 12-month period.[3]

GLA supplementation is often used to relieve pain or discomfort. Results from a clinical trial suggest that EPO should be recommended as a first-line specific treatment for women with distressing cyclic mastalgia.[4] Patients with active rheumatoid arthritis benefited from GLA (2.8 g/day) over 6 months.[5] Several well-controlled, randomized clinical studies suggest that essential fatty acids are promising options in the treatment of rheumatoid arthritis and related conditions.[6] Combination therapy involving GLA and fish oil (ω-3 fatty acids) provided greater benefit.

Combination therapy may also be helpful for migraine prophylaxis. Polyunsaturated fatty acids—administered for 6 months in an open-label, uncontrolled study—reduced the severity, frequency, and duration of migraine attacks in 86% of participants.[7] Self-medication changed to simple analgesics in the majority of patients.

Animal studies suggest that the cardiovascular system may benefit from EPO. These studies suggest that GLA may retard atherosclerosis,[8] inhibit the development of hypertension,[9] reduce tissue lipid peroxidation, and increase the antithrombotic capacity of the endothelium in animals on a high-fat diet.[10,11]

The use of EPO remains controversial. Although some authors suggest that according to the available evidence, EPO may be a reasonable treatment alternative for some patients with premenstrual syndrome,[12] others disagree.[13] GLA has been shown to correct deficiencies in skin lipids associated with reduced δ-6-desaturase activity, which should result in improved regulation of inflammation and immunity in atopic eczema. However, clinical studies with EPO containing 10% GLA have yielded contradictory results. These contradictory findings may be due to discrepancies in patient groups and the delivery system. The stabilizing effect of EPO on the stratum corneum barrier is only apparent with the water-in-oil emulsion, not the amphiphilic emulsion.[14] Although most studies have indicated that GLA relieves skin roughness and reduces the elevated blood catecholamine concentrations of patients with atopic eczema,[15] there is insufficient evidence to recommend EPO for the treatment of these patients.[16] Although pragmatic trials of at least 4 months' duration are required to determine the dose and effect of EPO, there is evidence to suggest that EPO causes more effective dampening of inflammation than other sources of ω-6 fatty acids. For patients undergoing hemodialysis, oral supplementation with GLA-rich EPO (2 g/day) seems to be more favorable than supplementation with α-linolenic acid in terms of shifting eicosanoid metabolism toward a less inflammatory status.[17]

An interesting new proposal is that GLA may have selective antitumor properties with negligible systemic toxicity. In a study of 38 elderly patients with breast cancer who were treated with GLA and tamoxifen, GLA was well-tolerated with no major side effects and achieved a significantly faster clinical response than tamoxifen alone in controlling an endocrine-sensitive cancer.[18] Proposed mechanisms of action include modulation of steroid hormone receptors.

TOXICITY/DRUG INTERACTIONS

When used in recommended doses, EPO is considered safe. However, EPO should be avoided by patients taking phenothiazides, because it lowers the seizure threshold level and increases the risk of temporal lobe epilepsy.

Bloating and gastrointestinal complaints occur in a small percentage of patients.

CLINICAL CAUTION

Long-term use may carry a risk of arachidonic acid buildup. Theoretically, this may lead to enhanced inflammatory and thrombotic responses.

PRACTICE TIPS

- EPO should be used in conjunction with ω-3 fatty acids to favor creation of a less proinflammatory cellular environment.
- Long-term use appears safe; however, caution should be exercised in the treatment of rheumatoid arthritis.

REFERENCES

1. Fan YY, Chapkin RS: Importance of dietary gamma-linolenic acid in human health and nutrition, *J Nutr* 128:1411-4, 1998
2. Head RJ, McLennan PL, Raederstorff D, et al: Prevention of nerve conduction deficit in diabetic rats by polyunsaturated fatty acids, *Am J Clin Nutr* 71(suppl 1):386S-392S, 2000.
3. Keen H, Payan J, Allawi J, et al: Treatment of diabetic neuropathy with gamma-linolenic acid. The gamma-Linolenic Acid Multicenter Trial Group, *Diabetes Care* 16:8-15, 1993.
4. Cheung KL: Management of cyclical mastalgia in oriental women: pioneer experience of using gamolenic acid (Efamast) in Asia, *Aust N Z J Surg* 69:492-4, 1999.
5. Zurier RB, Rossetti RG, Jacobson EW, et al: Gamma-linolenic acid treatment of rheumatoid arthritis. A randomized, placebo-controlled trial, *Arthritis Rheum* 39:1808-17, 1996.
6. Belch JJ, Hill A: Evening primrose oil and borage oil in rheumatologic conditions, *Am J Clin Nutr* 71(Suppl 1):352S-356S, 2000.
7. Wagner W, Nootbaar-Wagner U: Prophylactic treatment of migraine with gamma-linolenic and alpha-linolenic acids, *Cephalalgia* 17:127-30, 1997.
8. Fan YY, Ramos KS, Chapkin RS: Modulation of atherogenesis by dietary gamma-linolenic acid, *Adv Exp Med Biol* 469:485-91, 1999.
9. Engler M: Comparative study of diets enriched with evening primrose, black currant, borage or fungal oils on blood pressure and pressor responses in spontaneously hypertensive rats, *Prostaglandins Leukot Essent Fatty Acids* 49:809-14, 1993.
10. De La Cruz JP, Quintero L, Galvez J, et al: Antioxidant potential of evening primrose oil administration in hyperlipemic rabbits, *Life Sci* 65:543-55, 1999.
11. Villalobos MA, De La Cruz JP, Martin-Romero M, et al: Effect of dietary supplementation with evening primrose oil on vascular thrombogenesis in hyperlipemic rabbits, *Thromb Haemost* 80:696-701, 1998.
12. Hardy ML: Herbs of special interest to women, *J Am Pharm Assoc (Wash)* 40:234-42, 2000.

13. Budeiri D, Li Wan Po A, Dornan JC: Is evening primrose oil of value in the treatment of premenstrual syndrome? *Control Clin Trials* 17:60-8, 1996.

14. Gehring W, Bopp R, Rippke F, et al: Effect of topically applied evening primrose oil on epidermal barrier function in atopic dermatitis as a function of vehicle, *Arzneimittelforschung* 49:635-42, 1999.

15. Horrobin DF: Essential fatty acid metabolism and its modification in atopic eczema, *Am J Clin Nutr* 71(suppl 1):367S-372S, 2000.

16. Hoare C, Li Wan Po A, Williams H: Systematic review of treatments for atopic eczema, *Health Technol Assess* 4:1-191, 2000.

17. Yoshimoto-Furuie K, Yoshimoto K, Tanaka T, et al: Effects of oral supplementation with evening primrose oil for six weeks on plasma essential fatty acids and uremic skin symptoms in hemodialysis patients, *Nephron* 81: 151-9, 1999.

18. Kenny FS, Pinder SE, Ellis IO, et al: Gamma linolenic acid with tamoxifen as primary therapy in breast cancer, *Int J Cancer* 85:643-8, 2000.

■ CHAPTER 63 ■

FEVERFEW (*TANACETUM PARTHENIUM*)

> Despite a persuasively plausible mode of action, the clinical efficacy of feverfew is questionable; just as there is many a slip betwixt cup and lip, there is many an oversight between biologic plausibility and clinical efficacy.

Tanacetum parthenium (feverfew) has a long history of medicinal use for the treatment of fever, arthritis, migraine, and tension headaches. The leaves, without the stem, are picked when the plant is in flower and used medicinally. The odor of feverfew is offensive to insects and can act as a natural repellent.

MECHANISM OF ACTION

Feverfew exerts its anti-inflammatory effect by both irreversibly inhibiting eicosanoid generation and inhibiting release of granules from platelets and polymorphonuclear leukocytes, possibly through interaction with the protein kinase C pathway. Degranulation of platelets results in serotonin-enhancing platelet aggregation, and release of lysosomal enzymes from polymorphonuclear leukocytes enhances inflammation. Crude extracts of fresh feverfew leaves (rich in sesquiterpene lactones) and of commercially available powdered leaves (lactone-free) produce dose-dependent inhibition of leukocyte-generated thromboxane B_2 and leukotriene B_4.[1] Parthenolide is the important biologically active sesquiterpene lactone.

Parthenolide is believed to achieve its antimigraine effect by inhibiting release of serotonin and histamine from platelets, by its dose-dependent inhibition of inflammatory leukotrienes and thromboxane B_2, and by decreasing the smooth muscle response to endogenous vasoactive substances, including norepinephrine, acetylcholine, prostaglandins, bradykinin, histamine, and serotonin.[1]

DOSE

Traditionally, daily treatment has involved 0.7 to 2 mL of 1:1 fresh plant tincture or 1 to 2 mL of 1:5 dried plant tincture. Dose recommendations range from one or two 150-mg tablets, standardized to contain at least 0.6%

parthenolide daily, to 0.25 mg of parthenolide for treating migraine. In addition to tablets, a sublingual spray is available.

Commercial preparations of feverfew leaves are known to vary widely in parthenolide content. Plants from commercial sources and dark-leafed varieties have lower mean parthenolide levels than plants from wild-collected seeds and light green– or yellow–leafed varieties.[2]

Products that contain less than 2% parthenolide should be avoided.

CLINICAL USES

Scientific validation of feverfew in the management of arthritis is lacking and is questionable with respect to controlling headaches. Although reviews of randomized, placebo-controlled, double-blind trials suggest that feverfew prevents migraine more effectively than placebo,[3,4] a large, methodologically rigorous trial failed to demonstrate a significant difference between the clinical efficacy of feverfew and placebo.[4]

In vitro experiments suggest that feverfew may have some future application in cancer management. However, the dose and circumstances of parthenolide use are likely to be critical.[5] Feverfew may be useful in increasing the sensitivity of cancers with constitutively active NF-kappaB to chemotherapeutic drugs.[6] Parthenolide may inhibit NF-kappaB binding to genes. NF-kappaB regulates genes important for tumor invasion, metastasis, and chemoresistance.

TOXICITY/DRUG INTERACTIONS

Although it is believed to be a serotonin antagonist, feverfew is regarded as a potentially safe herb.[7] Side effects are mild and include abdominal pain, diarrhea, and tingling. Allergic contact dermatitis, mouth ulcers, and a swollen, tender tongue or lips may result from chewing fresh leaves.

CLINICAL CAUTION

Feverfew has an additive anticoagulant, antiplatelet effect when used in patients receiving aspirin, warfarin, or dipyridamole. Feverfew—like fish oils, garlic, *Gingko biloba*, and willow bark—increases the potential for bleeding in patients who are taking aspirin.

PRACTICE TIPS

- Product potency varies.
- Feverfew leaves may be chewed, but this is not recommended because oral ulceration has been reported.

- Treatment may be required for more than 4 months before clinical benefits are achieved.
- When therapy is being terminated, the dose should be gradually tapered to reduce the risk of headaches recurring in patients with migraine.
- Nonsteroidal anti-inflammatory drugs may negate the usefulness of feverfew in the treatment of migraine headaches.

REFERENCES

1. Sumner H, Salan U, Knight DW, et al: Inhibition of 5-lipoxygenase and cyclo-oxygenase in leukocytes by feverfew. Involvement of sesquiterpene lactones and other components, *Biochem Pharmacol* 43:2313-20, 1992.
2. Cutlan AR, Bonilla LE, Simon JE, et al: Intra-specific variability of feverfew: correlations between parthenolide, morphological traits and seed origin, *Planta Med* 66:612-7, 2000.
3. Vogler BK, Pittler MH, Ernst E: Feverfew as a preventive treatment for migraine: a systematic review, *Cephalalgia* 18:704-8, 1998.
4. Pittler MH, Vogler BK, Ernst E: Feverfew for preventing migraine, *Cochrane Database Syst Rev* 3:CD002286, 2000.
5. Ross JJ, Arnason JT, Birnboim HC: Low concentrations of the feverfew component parthenolide inhibit in vitro growth of tumor lines in a cytostatic fashion, *Planta Med* 65:126-9, 1999.
6. Patel NM, Nozaki S, Shortle NH, et al: Paclitaxel sensitivity of breast cancer cells with constitutively active NF-kappaB is enhanced by IkappaBalpha super-repressor and parthenolide, *Oncogene* 19:4159-69, 2000.
7. Klepser TB, Klepser ME: Unsafe and potentially safe herbal therapies, *Am J Health Syst Pharm* 56:125-38, 1999.

■ CHAPTER 64 ■

FISH OILS

Fish oils do not have identical health effects; oil derived from the flesh of fish does not carry a risk of vitamin A or D toxicosis, as do halibut, shark, and to a lesser extent, cod liver oil.

Fish is the major dietary source of long-chain omega-3 (ω-3) polyunsaturated fatty acids. The essential acid precursor of the 20-carbon ω-3 fatty acid eicosapentaenoic acid (EPA) and the 22-carbon ω-3 fatty acid docosahexaenoic acid (DHA) found in fish oil is linolenic acid, an 18-carbon ω-3 polyunsaturated fatty acid. Linolenic acid and linoleic acid, an 18 carbon ω-6 polyunsaturated fatty acid, are both essential fatty acids. Linoleic acid is found in vegetable oils and is the precursor of arachidonic acid (AA). Linolenic acid is found in flaxseed.

The typical American diet has a high ratio of ω-6 to ω-3 fatty acids (10:1).[1] The relatively low intake of ω-3 fatty acids has health implications. The long-chain ω-3 polyunsaturated fatty acids dampen inflammation and modulate immunity. Patients with immune disorders are often found have deficiencies of ω-3 fatty acids.[2]

MECHANISM OF ACTION

The longer-chain ω-3 fatty acids found in fish oil are rapidly incorporated into phospholipids in the cell membrane, where they influence cellular metabolism. Animal studies have shown that fish oil has an anti-inflammatory and immunomodulatory effect.[3] Mechanisms by which these changes are achieved include the following:

• Alteration in the fluidity of membranes. This can cause subtle changes in receptor function, alterations in cell signaling mechanisms, and membrane-bound enzyme activity.
• Regulation of gene expression. Through their ability to modulate the activity of protein kinase C and T-cell and B-cell responses, lymphokine secretion, cell proliferation, free radical generation, and lipid peroxidation, these polyunsaturated fatty acids have antimutagenic and antimicrobial (including antiviral) properties.[4]
• Regulation of eicosanoid synthesis (see Figure 64-1). EPA and DHA can replace AA in the cell membrane and compete with AA for the enzymes

cyclooxygenase and 5-lipoxygenase. In the presence of EPA, instead of 5-lipoxygenase in leukocytes and macrophages converting AA into the powerful proinflammatory leukotriene 4 series (e.g., leukotriene B$_4$), EPA is converted into leukotriene B$_5$, a weak inducer of inflammation, chemotaxis, and adherence. Omega-3 fatty acids also inhibit synthesis and release of proinflammatory cytokines such as tumor necrosis factor α, interleukin 1 (IL-1), and IL-2.[5] Along with the anti-inflammatory effects, the antithrombotic effects of fish oils appear, to date, to have provided the greatest benefit to human health. In the presence of EPA, instead of cyclooxygenase in platelets converting AA into thromboxane A$_2$, a potent platelet aggregator and vasoconstrictor, EPA is converted into thromboxane A$_3$ and prostacyclin. Thromboxane A$_3$ is a weak platelet aggregator and vasoconstrictor, and prostacyclin is a vasodilator and inhibitor of platelet aggregation.[6] This eicosanoid modification, in combination with an unchanged concentration of prostacyclin, results in an overall decrease in platelet aggregation and adhesion.

- Modification of blood lipids. Fish oil affects lipid metabolism by decreasing both very low density lipoproteins and triglycerides as a result of inhibition of hepatic triglyceride synthesis. Daily supplementation with 4 g of ω-3 fatty acids has been shown to reduce triglyceride and total cholesterol concentrations and to increase high-density lipoprotein (HDL) cholesterol concentrations.[7] However, a review did not support this finding, suggesting that total cholesterol was not materially affected by ω-3 fatty acid consumption because both low-density lipoprotein (LDL) and HDL cholesterol concentrations tended to rise by 5% to 10% and 1% to 3%, respectively.[8] This review also indicated that unless very large amounts of flaxseed oil were consumed, the effect of α-linolenic acid (18:3 ω-3) would be equivalent to that of ω-6-rich oils rather than EPA as compared with lipid and lipoprotein effects.

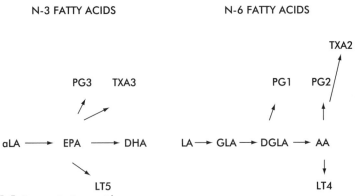

FIG. 64-1 Omega-3 eicosanoids.

FOOD SOURCES

Fish is the major dietary source of ω-3 fatty acids. Fish rich in EPA and DHA include kippers, mackerel, pilchards, Atlantic salmon, trout, blue grenadier, herring, sardines, tuna, yellowtail, and perch. Flaxseed oil, spinach, and walnuts are good sources of α-linolenic acid (18:3 ω-3), which can be converted, after ingestion, to EPA (20:5 ω-3). Flaxseed, also called *linseed*, is a potent source α-linolenic acid and contains ω-6 fatty acids and lignans. The oil has a nutty flavor, and one teaspoon contains around 2.5 g of ω-3 fatty acids.

DOSE

The U.S. Department of Agriculture has not established a recommended daily intake for ω-3 fatty acids, but Canada recommends that 0.5% of energy be derived from this source.[9] Recommendations in the United Kingdom and Europe range from a low daily intake of 200 mg through 300 and 650 mg, to 1250 mg, and even 1500 mg.[10] The therapeutic dosage ranges from 1 to 10 g daily; a number of clinical trials have used 4 g/day.

Fish is the best source of long-chain ω-3 fatty acids, and at least one meal that includes fish per week is recommended. Fish oil capsules can be purchased. Around 1 g of ω-3 fatty acids provides 860 mg of EPA and DHA in a ratio of 2:1, which corresponds to a dietary intake of 100 g of fatty fish.

People who do not eat fish should consider obtaining at least 200 mg of very-long-chain ω-3 fatty acids daily from other sources.[11] One option is "functional food" eggs. Feeding flaxseed to hens increases linolenic acid in the egg yolk about 30-fold, and the longer-chain DHA increases nearly four-fold.[9] Persons obtaining their ω-3 fatty acids from α-linolenic acid probably require an intake of 2 g per day or 1% of energy.[11]

CLINICAL USES

The cardiovascular health benefits of fish oils include improved lipoprotein metabolism, a reduced tendency to coagulation through both platelet and vessel wall interactions, an antiarrhythmic effect, and inhibition of smooth muscle cell proliferation in the arterial wall.[12] Atherogenesis may be reduced by means of inhibition of vascular smooth muscle cell proliferation at the gene expression level, reduced expression of inflammatory mediators, and altered lipid metabolism. The risk of vascular occlusion is reduced by changes in the eicosanoid profile and nitric oxide, which decrease the risk of vasospasm and thrombosis. Omega-3 fatty acids may protect the myocardium from ventricular arrhythmias. Vagal stimulation by ω-3 fatty acids is thought to increase parasympathetic tone, leading directly to modulation of heart rate and indirectly, through acetylcholine transmission, to attenuation of the release of tumor necrosis factor, IL-1β, IL-6, and IL-18.[4]

This latter effect is of particular interest, because fish appears to more effectively reduce the risk of death from myocardial infarction than to protect against heart disease.[13] Animal studies have shown that supplementing diets with tuna oil significantly reduces the incidence and severity of arrhythmia, preventing ventricular fibrillation during both coronary artery occlusion and reperfusion.[14] Prospective studies and secondary prevention trials have also provided strong evidence that an increased intake of ω-3 fatty acids substantially lowers the risk of cardiovascular mortality.[15] Moreover, supplementation with 875-mg fish oil capsules, containing 850 to 882 mg EPA and DHA, reduced mortality but did not reduce the incidence of nonfatal heart attacks.[16] After 3.5 years, those taking the ω-3 fatty acids had experienced a 20% reduction in overall mortality and a 45% decrease in the risk for sudden cardiac death. Research suggests that relatively small intakes of ω-3 fatty acids are cardioprotective and may operate by stabilizing the myocardium itself.[17] However, consumption of fatty, rather than lean, fish is associated with this reduction in cardiovascular mortality.[18] Furthermore, although long-chain ω-3 polyunsaturated fatty acids (EPA) have an antiarrhythmic effect, α-linolenic acid, its plant-derived precursor, appears devoid of any such aptitude.[19]

Patients with diabetes may benefit from a diet rich in fish. Animal studies suggest that fish oil enhances insulin secretion from beta cells.[20] However, a review of 18 trials in which doses of fish oil ranging from 3 to 18 g/day were used indicated that fish oil supplementation in type 2 diabetes lowers triglyceride levels and raises LDL cholesterol levels but has no statistically significant effect on glycemic control.[21] Regardless of the efficacy of fish oil in enhancing insulin secretion, improved lipid control can benefit patients with diabetes. Fish oil significantly lowers serum triglyceride levels in patients with hyperlipidemia but is only marginally effective in individuals with normal lipid levels.[22] The smallest amount of ω-3 fatty acid needed to significantly lower serum triglyceride levels appears to be approximately 1 g daily, as provided by a fish diet.[22] In addition to patients with diabetes, postmenopausal women have demonstrated marked reductions in serum triglyceride concentrations and the ratio of triglycerides to HDL cholesterol with fish oil supplementation, regardless of whether they are receiving hormone replacement therapy.[23]

Fish oil has long been recognized as a viable option for patients with rheumatoid arthritis who wish to reduce the dosage of their anti-inflammatory drug without precipitating an exacerbation of symptoms. Several double-blind, placebo-controlled trials of γ-linolenic acid and fish oil have demonstrated significant improvements in various clinical parameters; it has been suggested that these polyunsaturated fatty acids should be included as part of the normal therapeutic approach to rheumatoid arthritis.[24] Because the overall clinical improvement with fish oil supplementation is only moderate, it has been suggested that simultaneous vitamin E supplementation might have an additional positive effect by further decreasing the production of proinflammatory cytokines and eicosanoids.[25]

Although fish oils may be useful for certain immunologic disorders, they do not seem to benefit others. Analysis of randomized, controlled trials, in which marine ω-3 fatty acid supplementation was compared with placebo in patients with asthma, showed no consistent effect on forced expiratory volume in 1 second, peak flow rate, asthma symptoms, asthma medication use, or bronchial hyperreactivity after 4 or more weeks.[26]

Mood disorders have been associated with abnormalities in ω-3 fatty acid levels. Geographic areas where consumption of DHA is high are associated with decreased rates of depression. DHA deficiency states, such as alcoholism and the postpartum period, are positively linked with depression, and individuals with major depression show marked depletion of ω-3 fatty acids in their erythrocyte cell membranes.[27] Further investigation is needed into the potentially beneficial effects of ω-3 fatty acids in major depression, bipolar disorders, schizophrenia, and dementia.[28] Several studies have shown that patients with schizophrenia often have low levels of essential fatty acids; one review indicated that although data are preliminary, results look encouraging for use of fish oil supplements in the treatment of schizophrenia.[29] Symptoms of schizophrenia may result from altered neuronal membrane structure and metabolism.

DHA is found in unusually high concentrations in the brain and retina and is selectively accumulated during fetal and infant brain growth. Recent studies have suggested that DHA is involved in dopamine and serotonin metabolism, but clinical studies on the potential benefits of dietary DHA for neural development have yielded conflicting results.[30] Significantly lower amounts of DHA in breast milk have been directly correlated to the decreased amount of fish eaten,[31] and studies suggest that preterm and possibly term infants may benefit from feedings that contain ω-3 and ω-6 long-chain polyunsaturated fatty acids.[32]

There is epidemiologic and experimental evidence that the long-chain ω-3 fatty acids exert protective effects against some common cancers, notably breast and colon cancer and, perhaps, prostate cancer.[33,34] Inhibition of eicosanoid production from ω-6 fatty acid precursors appears to underlie much of the chemopreventive activity of ω-3 fatty acids, regardless of whether it is caused by suppression of neoplastic transformation, cell growth inhibition, enhanced apoptosis, or antiangiogenicity.[33] Epidemiologic, experimental, and mechanistic data suggest that long-chain ω-3 fatty acids, but not ω-6 fatty acids, impair carcinogenesis.[35,36] Animal studies suggest that the antitumor effect of EPA is largely related to suppression of cell proliferation, whereas DHA's efficacy appears related to its ability to induce apoptosis.[37] The dietary ω-3/ω-6 fatty acid ratio, rather than the quantity administered, may emerge as the principal factor in the antitumor effect of ω-3 fatty acids. Animal experiments suggest an effective ratio in the range of 1.8 to 1.9.[37]

Other potential clinical applications of fish oil are for increasing bone density,[38] as combination therapy with etretinate for chronic psoriasis,[39] and in the management of various renal problems. Daily treatment with ω-3 fatty acids may reduce hypercalciuria in patients who have kidney stones and may benefit those receiving maintenance hemodialysis by helping to control immunoglobulin A nephropathy.[40] Immunoglobulin A nephropathy, the most common form of primary glomerulonephritis, may lead to progressive renal failure.

TOXICITY/DRUG INTERACTIONS

In one study, the maximum tolerated daily dose of fish oil capsules was found to be 0.3 g per kilogram of body weight.[41] Fish oil supplementation is generally safe and well-tolerated with few side effects. Gastrointestinal complaints, mainly diarrhea, have been reported.

CLINICAL CAUTION

Increasing the intake of polyunsaturated fatty acids may increase oxidative stress. A trial showed that daily supplements of fish oil, providing 2.5 g of EPA and 1.8 g of DHA, did cause a small, but statistically significant, increase in oxidative stress.[42] Administration of α-tocopherol acetate up to 400 mg as a daily supplement had no effect. The common practice of vitamin E supplementation after consumption of EPA and DHA may need to be reviewed.

PRACTICE TIPS

- Consumption of 30 to 35 g of fish per day reduces the risk of death from ischemic heart disease.
- The American Heart Association recommends at least two meals of fatty fish weekly.

REFERENCES

1. Kris-Etherton PM, Taylor DS, Yu-Poth S, et al: Polyunsaturated fatty acids in the food chain in the United States, *Am J Clin Nutr* 71(suppl 1):179S-188S, 2000.
2. Holman RT: The slow discovery of the importance of omega-3 essential fatty acids in human health, *J Nutr* 128(suppl 2):427S-433S, 1998.
3. Calder PC: Polyunsaturated fatty acids, inflammation, and immunity, *Lipids* 36:1007-24, 2001.
4. Das UN: Essential fatty acids in health and disease, *J Assoc Physicians India* 47:906-11, 1999.
5. Das UN: Beneficial effect(s) of n-3 fatty acids in cardiovascular diseases: but, why and how? *Prostaglandins Leukot Essent Fatty Acids* 63:351-62, 2000.

6. Fish oil, *Altern Med Rev* 5:576-80, 2000.

7. Nilsen DW, Albrektsen G, Landmark K, et al: Effects of a high-dose concentrate of n-3 fatty acids or corn oil introduced early after an acute myocardial infarction on serum triacylglycerol and HDL cholesterol, *Am J Clin Nutr* 74:50-6, 2001.

8. Harris WS: N-3 fatty acids and serum lipoproteins: human studies, *Am J Clin Nutr* 65(suppl 5):1645S-1654S, 1997.

9. Lewis NM, Seburg S, Flanagan NL: Enriched eggs as a source of n-3 polyunsaturated fatty acids for humans, *Poult Sci* 79:971-4, 2000

10. Mason P: *Dietary supplements*, ed 2, London, 2001, Pharmaceutical Press.

11. de Deckere EA, Korver O, Verschuren PM, et al: Health aspects of fish and n-3 polyunsaturated fatty acids from plant and marine origin, *Eur J Clin Nutr* 52:749-53, 1998.

12. Abeywardena MY, Head RJ: Longchain n-3 polyunsaturated fatty acids and blood vessel function, *Cardiovasc Res* 52:361-71, 2001.

13. Brown AA, Hu FB: Dietary modulation of endothelial function: implications for cardiovascular disease, *Am J Clin Nutr* 73:673-86, 2001.

14. McLennan PL, Abeywardena MY, Charnock JS: Dietary fish oil prevents ventricular fibrillation following coronary artery occlusion and reperfusion, *Am Heart J* 116:709-17, 1988.

15. Hu FB, Manson JE, Willett WC: Types of dietary fat and risk of coronary heart disease: a critical review, *J Am Coll Nutr* 20:5-19, 2001.

16. Stone NJ: The Gruppo Italiano per lo Studio della Sopravvivenza nell'Infarto Miocardio (GISSI)-Prevenzione Trial on fish oil and vitamin E supplementation in myocardial infarction survivors, *Curr Cardiol Rep* 2:445-51, 2000.

17. Harris WS, Isley WL: Clinical trial evidence for the cardioprotective effects of omega-3 fatty acids, *Curr Atheroscler Rep* 3:174-9, 2001.

18. Oomen CM, Feskens EJ, Rasanen L, et al: Fish consumption and coronary heart disease mortality in Finland, Italy, and The Netherlands, *Am J Epidemiol* 151:999-1006, 2000.

19. Christensen JH, Christensen MS, Toft E, et al: Alpha-linolenic acid and heart rate variability, *Nutr Metab Cardiovasc Dis* 10:57-61, 2000.

20. Ajiro K, Sawamura M, Ikeda K, et al: Beneficial effects of fish oil on glucose metabolism in spontaneously hypertensive rats, *Clin Exp Pharmacol Physiol* 27:412-5, 2000.

21. Montori VM, Farmer A, Wollan PC, et al: Fish oil supplementation in type 2 diabetes: a quantitative systematic review, *Diabetes Care* 23:1407-15, 2000.

22. Weber P, Raederstorff D: Triglyceride-lowering effect of omega-3 LC-polyunsaturated fatty acids—a review, *Nutr Metab Cardiovasc Dis* 10:28-37, 2000.

23. Stark KD, Park EJ, Maines VA, et al: Effect of a fish-oil concentrate on serum lipids in postmenopausal women receiving and not receiving hormone replacement therapy in a placebo-controlled, double-blind trial, *Am J Clin Nutr* 72:389-94, 2000.

24. Calder PC, Zurier RB: Polyunsaturated fatty acids and rheumatoid arthritis, *Curr Opin Clin Nutr Metab Care* 4:115-21, 2001.

25. Tidow-Kebritchi S, Mobarhan S: Effects of diets containing fish oil and vitamin E on rheumatoid arthritis, *Nutr Rev* 59:335-8, 2001.

26. Woods RK, Thien FC, Abramson MJ: Dietary marine fatty acids (fish oil) for asthma, *Cochrane Database Syst Rev* 2:CD001283, 2000.

27. Mischoulon D, Fava M: Docosahexanoic acid and omega-3 fatty acids in depression, *Psychiatr Clin North Am* 23:785-94, 2000.

28. Freeman MP: Omega-3 fatty acids in psychiatry: a review, *Ann Clin Psychiatry* 12:159-65, 2000.

29. Joy CB, Mumby-Croft R, Joy LA: Polyunsaturated fatty acid (fish or evening primrose oil) for schizophrenia, *Cochrane Database Syst Rev* 2:CD001257, 2000.

30. Innis SM: The role of dietary n-6 and n-3 fatty acids in the developing brain, *Dev Neurosci* 22:474-80, 2000.

31. Smit EN, Oelen EA, Seerat E, et al: Breast milk docosahexaenoic acid (DHA) correlates with DHA status of malnourished infants, *Arch Dis Child* 82:493-4, 2000.

32. Forsyth JS, Carlson SE: Long-chain polyunsaturated fatty acids in infant nutrition: effects on infant development, *Curr Opin Clin Nutr Metab Care* 4:123-6, 2001.

33. Rose DP, Connolly JM: Omega-3 fatty acids as cancer chemopreventive agents, *Pharmacol Ther* 83:217-44, 1999.

34. Kontogiannea M, Gupta A, Ntanios F, et al: Omega-3 fatty acids decrease endothelial adhesion of human colorectal carcinoma cells, *J Surg Res* 92:201-5, 2000.

35. Bougnoux P: N-3 polyunsaturated fatty acids and cancer, *Curr Opin Clin Nutr Metab Care* 2:121-6, 1999.

36. de Deckere EA: Possible beneficial effect of fish and fish n-3 polyunsaturated fatty acids in breast and colorectal cancer, *Eur J Cancer Prev* 8:213-21, 1999.

37. Calviello G, Palozza P, Piccioni E, et al: Dietary supplementation with eicosapentaenoic and docosahexaenoic acid inhibits growth of Morris hepatocarcinoma 3924A in rats: effects on proliferation and apoptosis, *Int J Cancer* 75:699-705, 1998.

38. Kruger MC, Coetzer H, de Winter R, et al: Calcium, gamma-linolenic acid and eicosapentaenoic acid supplementation in senile osteoporosis, *Aging (Milano)* 10:385-94, 1998

39. Danno K, Sugie N: Combination therapy with low-dose etretinate and eicosapentaenoic acid for psoriasis vulgaris, *J Dermatol* 25:703-5, 1998.

40. Donadio JV: N-3 Fatty acids and their role in nephrologic practice, *Curr Opin Nephrol Hypertens* 10:639-42, 2001.

41. Burns CP, Halabi S, Clamon GH, et al: Phase I clinical study of fish oil fatty acid capsules for patients with cancer cachexia: cancer and leukemia group B study 9473, *Clin Cancer Res* 5:3942-7, 1995.

42. Wander RC, Du SH: Oxidation of plasma proteins is not increased after supplementation with eicosapentaenoic and docosahexaenoic acids, *Am J Clin Nutr* 72:731-7, 2000.

■ CHAPTER 65 ■

FLAVONOIDS

High dietary intakes of flavonoids have been linked with a reduced risk of disease, but authoritative evidence that dietary supplements are beneficial is largely lacking.

Polyphenols are a large and diverse class of compounds, many of which occur naturally in a wide range of plant foods. The flavonoids are the largest and best studied of the polyphenols. There are several thousand individual compounds known. The more clinically important flavonoids are categorized as flavonols, flavones, catechins, flavanones, anthocyanidins, and isoflavonoids. Many plant polyphenols are either being actively developed or currently sold as dietary supplements and/or herbal remedies. Flavonoids and carotenes are largely responsible for the color in fruit and vegetables. In plants, flavonoids act as antioxidants, antimicrobials, photoreceptors, and visual attractors; they also repel feeding insects. Animal and human studies suggest that flavonoids have potential as antiallergenic, antiviral, anti-inflammatory, vasodilating, and antioxidant agents.[1,2] Moreover, through several different mechanisms of action, particular flavonoids may exert significant anticarcinogenic activity and even promote cellular differentiation.[3]

In addition to this brief overview, more important clinical information can be found in the sections on quercetin (flavonol), soy (isoflavones), and bilberry (anthocyanidins). For a broader overview, refer to the section on phytonutrients. The flavonoids have also been reviewed recently.[4,5]

MECHANISM OF ACTION

Flavonoids are low molecular weight polyphenolic compounds composed of a three-ring structure similar to vitamin E. An oxy group at position 4, a double bond between carbon atoms 2 and 3, or a hydroxyl group in position 3 of the C (middle) ring enhances potency, especially antioxidant and antiproliferative activity.[6]

In in vitro studies, the inhibitory effect of flavonoids on low-density lipoprotein (LDL) cholesterol oxidation was observed to be, in order of efficacy:

luteolin > epicatechin gallate > epicatechin > quercetin > catechin > epigallocatechin gallate > epigallocatechin > myricetin > kaempferol > apigenin.[7] Radical trapping effects of flavonoids differ according to their structure, and flavonoids act as hydrogen donors to α-tocopherol radicals, further augmenting their potential to delay the oxidation of LDL cholesterol. In addition to acting as antioxidants and protecting LDL cholesterol from oxidation, flavonoids enhance the activity of vitamin C and inhibit platelet aggregation.[8]

Plant flavonoids attenuate inflammation and the immune response both by modulation of regulatory enzymes involved in the biosynthesis of prostaglandins and cytokines and by inhibition of kinases through competitive binding of flavonoids with adenosine triphosphate at enzyme catalytic sites.[9] Flavonoids have an inhibitory effect on several enzyme systems intimately connected to cell activation processes such as protein kinase C, protein tyrosine kinases, phospholipase A_2, cyclooxygenase, and lipoxygenase.[3] Evidence suggests that only activated cells (i.e., cells that are responding to a stimulus) are susceptible to the modulating effects of flavonoids. Such cells include mast cells, basophils, neutrophils, eosinophils, T and B lymphocytes, macrophages, platelets, smooth muscle cells, and hepatocytes.[3]

FOOD SOURCES

Flavonoids commonly cited in clinical circles are quercitin, rutin and hesperidin, proanthocyanidins, anthocyanosides, epigallocatechin gallate, and genistein. Although flavonoids are widely distributed, certain fruits and vegetables are better sources of particular flavonoids.[2] Onions and apples are a rich source of quercetin, and citrus fruits have rutin and hesperidin. Bilberry is the preferred source of anthocyanosides, soy products are a good source of genistein, and epigallocatechin gallate is found in green tea. Of the flavanols, proanthocyanidins are widely available naturally occurring plant metabolites found in wine, cranberries, and the leaves of bilberry, birch, ginkgo, and hawthorn. The preferred source of oligomeric proanthocyanidin complexes (OPCs) is grapeseed extract. Among the medicinal botanicals rich in flavonoids are *Ginkgo biloba*, *Hypericum perforatum* (St. John's wort), and *Sambucus canadensis* (elderberries).

The flavonoid content of foods varies widely. Eating the white pulp of citrus fruits and the peel of apples can enhance dietary intake. Grape juice, particularly rich purple varieties, has a protective effect. However, processing ensures that small volumes of wine provide a more potent concentration of flavonoids. Although flavonoids are present in both black and green tea, green tea appears to be a stronger antioxidant than black tea. The maximum effect of flavonoids in green tea peaks earlier, around 30 minutes after consumption.[10]

DOSE

There is no recommended daily allowance for flavonoids. In fact, despite a considerable amount of in vitro data, some animal and epidemiologic studies, plus a few well-controlled human trials, it is premature to recommend specific polyphenolic supplements at specific doses in the human population.[11] The therapeutic dose range is 50 to 5000 mg/day.[12]

The sugar moiety of flavonoids is an important determinant of their absorption and bioavailability. Flavonoids present in foods used to be considered nonabsorbable because they are bound to sugars as β-glycosides. More recently, however, it was found that human absorption of the quercetin glycosides from onions (52% absorption) is better than that from the pure aglycone (24%). It now appears that glycosylation increases the water solubility of flavonoids.

CLINICAL USES

Despite overlapping functions, individual flavonoids promise to have particular clinical strengths.[2] The flavonols, notably OPCs, inhibit lipid peroxidation, platelet aggregation, and capillary permeability and fragility; flavonols also affect enzymes including phospholipase A_2, cyclooxygenase, and lipoxygenase. They have demonstrated preferential binding to areas characterized by a high content of glycosaminoglycans, such as epidermis, capillary wall, and mucosa. Their antioxidant, antibacterial, antiviral, anticarcinogenic, anti-inflammatory, antiallergic, and vasodilatory actions make them clinically versatile. They are regarded as particularly useful for enhancing perfusion and increasing vascular integrity.[13]

Despite documentation that flavonoids are powerful antioxidants in vitro, their overall function as an antioxidant, anti-inflammatory, enzyme inhibitor; enzyme inducer; and/or inhibitor of cell division has yet to be clarified in vivo.[14] Dietary investigations are further complicated by the plethora of bioflavonoids present in foods and the difficulty in appropriately attributing efficacy. Experimental studies suggest that flavonols and flavones are effective free radical scavengers, metal chelators, and antithrombotic agents. Some epidemiologic studies suggest an inverse association between intake of flavonols and flavones and the risk of cardiovascular disease. In a randomized, double-blind, placebo-controlled trial, in which subjects had daily supplementation of α-tocopherol (50 mg/day) and/or beta-carotene (20 mg/day), dietary analysis showed that, compared with men consuming 4 mg/day, those ingesting 18 mg of flavonols and flavones per day had a decreased risk of nonfatal myocardial infarction.[15] Flavonols and flavones are found in tea, vegetables, fruits, and wine.

Flavonoids may promote cardiovascular health by reducing LDL cholesterol peroxidation, by scavenging reactive oxygen/nitrogen species in macrophages and other cells in the arterial wall, by chelating transition metal ions, and by sparing LDL cholesterol–associated antioxidants either through inhibiting cellular oxygenases or activating cellular antioxidants (e.g., the glutathione system).[16]

Flavonoids may also reduce the risk of cancer.[2] Possible mechanisms of action whereby isoflavones and flavones may prevent cancer include estrogenic/antiestrogenic activity, antiproliferation, induction of cell-cycle arrest and apoptosis, prevention of oxidation, induction of detoxification enzymes, regulation of the host's immune system, and changes in cellular signaling.[17] Various flavonoids have different effects on the cell cycle of cancer cells.[18]

TOXICITY/DRUG INTERACTIONS

Toxicity is related to dose and the flavonoid involved. The citrus flavonoids show little effect on normal, healthy cells and thus typically exhibit remarkably few toxic effects in animals.[19] The citrus flavonoids extend their influence in vivo through their induction of hepatic phase I and phase II enzymes, their interactions with key regulatory enzymes involved in cell activation and receptor binding, and the biologic actions of their metabolites. On the other hand, at higher doses, certain flavonoids may act as mutagens, prooxidants that generate free radicals, and as inhibitors of key enzymes involved in hormone metabolism.[20]

Caution should be exercised when flavonoids are ingested at levels above that which would be obtained from a typical vegetarian diet.

CLINICAL CAUTION

Even though polyphenol extracts or high-polyphenol diets may lead to transitory changes in the antioxidative capacity of plasma in humans, not all polyphenols and not all actions of individual polyphenols are necessarily beneficial.[11]

An unborn fetus may be especially at risk, since flavonoids readily cross the placenta.

PRACTICE TIPS

- Flavonoids are often taken with vitamin C to enhance the protective effect of both supplements.
- Adding milk to tea destroys the antioxidant effect of flavonoids.
- Flavonoids may prevent clotting and vascular occlusion more effectively than aspirin, because their efficacy appears to be unchanged by stress-induced increases in adrenaline.

- In addition to a high-fiber diet and drinking lots of fluids, consumption of berries, which are rich in proanthocyanidins, may prevent bleeding hemorrhoids.
- Flavonoids can protect vitamins C and E from oxidative degradation in the growing plant, during food storage and cooking, and during digestion and absorption in the human body.[21]

REFERENCES

1. Pietta PG: Flavonoids as antioxidants, *J Nat Prod* 63:1035-42, 2000.
2. Diefendorf D, Healey J, Kalyn W, editors: *The healing power of vitamins, minerals and herbs*, Surry Hills, Australia, 2000, Readers Digest.
3. Middleton E Jr: Effect of plant flavonoids on immune and inflammatory cell function, *Adv Exp Med Biol* 439:175-82, 1998.
4. Nijveldt RJ, van Nood E, van Hoorn DE, et al: Flavonoids: a review of probable mechanisms of action and potential applications, *Am J Clin Nutr* 74:418-25, 2001.
5. Wang HK: The therapeutic potential of flavonoids, *Expert Opin Investig Drugs* 9:2103-19, 2000.
6. Middleton E Jr, Kandaswami C, Theoharides TC: The effects of plant flavonoids on mammalian cells: implications for inflammation, heart disease, and cancer, *Pharmacol Rev* 52:673-751, 2000.
7. Hirano R, Sasamoto W, Matsumoto A, et al: Antioxidant ability of various flavonoids against DPPH radicals and LDL oxidation, *J Nutr Sci Vitaminol (Tokyo)* 47:357-62, 2001.
8. Craig WJ: Health-promoting properties of common herbs, *Am J Clin Nutr* 70(suppl 3):491S-499S, 1999.
9. Manthey JA: Biological properties of flavonoids pertaining to inflammation, *Microcirculation* 7:S29-S34, 2000.
10. Mills S, Bone K: *Principles and practice of phytotherapy*, Edinburgh, 2000, Churchill Livingstone.
11. Ferguson LR: Role of plant polyphenols in genomic stability, *Mutat Res* 475: 89-111, 2001.
12. Brighthope I: Nutritional medicine tables, *J Aust Coll Nutr Env Med* 17:20-5, 1998.
13. Fine AM: Oligomeric proanthocyanidin complexes: history, structure, and phytopharmaceutical applications, *Altern Med Rev* 5:144-51, 2000.
14. Rice-Evans C: Flavonoid antioxidants, *Curr Med Chem* 8:797-807, 2001.
15. Hirvonen T, Pietinen P, Virtanen M, et al: Intake of flavonols and flavones and risk of coronary heart disease in male smokers, *Epidemiology* 12:62-7, 2001.
16. Fuhrman B, Aviram M: Flavonoids protect LDL from oxidation and attenuate atherosclerosis, *Curr Opin Lipidol* 12:41-8, 2001.
17. Birt DF, Hendrich S, Wang W: Dietary agents in cancer prevention: flavonoids and isoflavonoids, *Pharmacol Ther* 90:157-77, 2001.
18. Kobayashi T, Nakata T, Kuzumaki T: Effect of flavonoids on cell cycle progression in prostate cancer cells, *Cancer Lett* 176:17-23, 2002.
19. Manthey JA, Grohmann K, Guthrie N: Biological properties of citrus flavonoids pertaining to cancer and inflammation, *Curr Med Chem* 8:135-53, 2001.

20. Skibola CF, Smith MT: Potential health impacts of excessive flavonoid intake, *Free Radic Biol Med* 29: 375-83, 2000.
21. Miller NJ, Ruiz-Larrea M: Flavonoids and other plant phenols in the diet: their significance as antioxidants, *J Nutr Env Med* 12:39-51, 2002.

■ CHAPTER 66 ■

FLUORIDE

> The increase in bone density after fluoride supplementation does not necessarily translate into increased bone strength; appearances can be deceptive.

Fluoride is of potential value in the prevention of dental caries and the treatment of postmenopausal osteoporosis.

MECHANISM OF ACTION

Fluoride is an anion absorbed from the intestine by diffusion. More than 90% of retained fluoride is deposited in the skeleton; the remainder is excreted in the urine. Fluoride can replace the hydroxy ion in bone. The basic structure of bone mineral is hydroxyapatite $(Ca_3(PO_4)_2)_3.Ca(OH)_2$. Substitution of fluoride in the hydroxyapatite crystal is a reversible process.

The plasma fluoride level is well regulated to 0.7 to 0.9 mmol/L on a diet in which the fluoride concentration varies between 1 and 8 ppm (parts per million). The margin of safety for fluoride is about 100:1 between the dosage effective for reversal of osteoporotic lesions in the elderly and a toxic level for adults not forming teeth.

FOOD SOURCES

Fluoride is present naturally in drinking water; however, in some areas the fluoride content is very low. Artificially fluoridated water contains 0.7 to 1.2 mg of fluoride per liter. Dietary sources of fluoride are tea and seafood; fluoride-enriched toothpaste is also readily available.

DOSE

An adequate daily intake of fluoride is 3 mg for women and 4 mg for men. Fluoride has a narrow therapeutic window. Supplementation in the form of sodium fluoride at levels around 60 mg should always be accompanied by an adequate calcium intake. Potentially toxic adult levels are reached when 10 mg is taken for a prolonged period.

CLINICAL USES

Fluoride protects against dental caries. In fact, optimal (1 ppm) water fluoridation is seen as the most socially equitable way to prevent dental caries. Studies strongly suggest that fluoride at concentrations of up to 1 ppm has no adverse effect on bone strength, bone mineral density, or fracture incidence.[1] Another approach, which offers the individual more personal control, is use of fluoride toothpaste. A study comparing one toothpaste with 0.243% sodium fluoride in a silica base with another containing 0.76% sodium monofluorophosphate in a dicalcium phosphate dihydrate base showed that both effectively reduced dental caries.[2] Topical application, as a fluoride varnish by dentists and by means of everyday brushing with fluoride-enriched toothpaste, is accepted as a routine measure to prevent dental caries.[3] Although there is insufficient evidence of the efficacy of fluoride varnish for prevention of caries in primary teeth, a review of the methods available to prevent dental caries indicated that there is good evidence for the effectiveness of fluoride gel and varnish to prevent caries in permanent teeth of children and adolescents.[4]

Fluoride exerts a biphasic action at the level of osteoblasts. Its effect on bone mineral content has consequences for bone structure and function and for the treatment of osteoporosis.[5] At low circulating concentrations, skeletal uptake of fluoride is limited, and the effects are beneficial. At higher concentrations with greater skeletal uptake, fluoride may cause the formation of abnormally mineralized bone of impaired quality. Concern has been expressed that fluoride may increase bone density without increasing bone strength. A meta-analysis to determine the efficacy of fluoride therapy in preventing bone loss and vertebral and nonvertebral fractures in postmenopausal women indicated that although fluoride has the ability to increase bone mineral density at the lumbar spine, it does not result in a reduction in vertebral fractures.[6] Furthermore, increasing the dose of fluoride increases the risk of nonvertebral fractures and gastrointestinal side effects without any effect on the vertebral fracture rate. On the other hand, a combination of sustained-release sodium fluoride, calcium citrate, and cholecalciferol significantly decreased the risk for vertebral fractures and increased spinal bone mass without reducing bone mass at either the femoral neck or total hip.[7] Selecting the correct regimen is important.[8] Fluoride may be particularly beneficial for women with postmenopausal osteoporosis who have low bone turnover. Given with calcium, it can stimulate bone formation and preserve bone mass.

TOXICITY/DRUG INTERACTIONS

Excess fluoride retention can result in skeletal fluorosis, a condition of hyperossification. The early stages of skeletal fluorosis are asymptomatic. The first radiologic signs are those of increased bone density. Osteosclerosis is most marked in the vertebrae and pelvis. It must be emphasized that a bone with increased radiologic density caused by fluoride incorporation is not necessarily stronger or harder.

With fluoride accumulation from a diet with a fluoride concentration of greater than 5000 ppm, bone changes include the following:

- Patchy osteoporosis
- Patchy osteosclerosis/hypermineralization
- Bands of uncalcified osteoid tissue, as seen in osteomalacia
- Severe chronic osteofluorosis (On microscopic examination, this manifests as a mixture of normal bone and dense, rarefied, disorganized bone. The sclerotic, porotic bone resembles that found in osteomalacia.)
- Exostoses and osteophytes are detectable on x-ray films. Calcification of ligaments and tendons can present clinically as a poker spine or hunch back.
- For the purpose of perspective, it should be noted that radiologic evidence of fluorosis is found in the form of osteosclerosis in 10% to 15% people who consume fluoride at a concentration of 8 ppm for prolonged periods. After 3 years of fluoride treatment, patients with osteoporosis supplemented with calcium and 30 to 60 mg fluoride each day had a reduced fracture rate compared with those not receiving fluoride. The fluoride serum levels of these patients were 0.5 to 1.0 mmol/L. Fluoride, although not without risk, is worthy of consideration in osteoporosis treatment.

CLINICAL CAUTION

White, brown, or black spots on the teeth may indicate excess fluoride consumption. Acute severe fluoride overdose may cause melena, hemoptysis, and abdominal pain. Early signs of possible chronic fluoride overdose are bone pain, skin rashes, and tooth discoloration.

PRACTICE TIPS

- It is inadvisable to prescribe fluoride in areas where its concentration in water exceeds 70 µg/L.
- Swallowing of fluoride toothpaste should be avoided.
- Fluoride supplements are best taken at bedtime, after the teeth have been thoroughly brushed.

REFERENCES

1. Demos LL, Kazda H, Cicuttini FM, et al: Water fluoridation, osteoporosis, fractures—recent developments, *Aust Dent J* 46:80-7, 2001.

2. Saporito RA, Boneta AR, Feldman CA, et al: Comparative anticaries efficacy of sodium fluoride and sodium monofluorophosphate dentifrices. A two-year caries clinical trial on children in New Jersey and Puerto Rico, *Am J Dent* 13: 221-6, 2000.
3. Newbrun E: Topical fluorides in caries prevention and management: a North American perspective, *J Dent Educ* 65:1078-83, 2001.
4. Rozier RG: Effectiveness of methods used by dental professionals for the primary prevention of dental caries, *J Dent Educ* 65:1063-72, 2001.
5. Pak CY, Zerwekh JE, Antich P: Anabolic effects of fluoride on bone, *Trends Endocrinol Metab* 6:229-34, 1995.
6. Haguenauer D, Welch V, Shea B, et al: Fluoride for the treatment of postmenopausal osteoporotic fractures: a meta-analysis, *Osteoporos Int* 11:727-38, 2000.
7. Rubin CD, Pak CY, Adams-Huet B, et al: Sustained-release sodium fluoride in the treatment of the elderly with established osteoporosis, *Arch Intern Med* 161:2325-33, 2001.
8. Reginster JY, Rovati LC, Setnikar I: Correct regimen of fluoride and calcium reduces the risk of vertebral fractures in postmenopausal osteoporosis, *Osteoporos Int* 12:800, 2001.

■ CHAPTER 67 ■

FOLATE

Routine supplementation of folic acid in doses up to 400 μg daily deserves consideration, particularly in women of childbearing age.

Folates are water-soluble vitamins of the B group. Folate coenzymes are involved in the synthesis of nucleic acids, interconversion of amino acids, and single-carbon metabolism (e.g., formate generation and transmethylation). Folate is involved in the formation of glutamic acid, norepinephrine, and serotonin. It is critical to the formation of nucleic acid and has an important role in cell maturation. Folate deficiency has a particularly adverse effect on the neural tube, erythrocytes, and epithelial cells of the gastrointestinal tract.

Folate deficiency is a common nutritional problem. The low cost and safety profile of folic acid favor its empiric supplementation in recommended doses.[1]

MECHANISM OF ACTION

Folate functions as a single-carbon donor in the synthesis of nucleotides from purine precursors and, indirectly, in the synthesis of transfer RNA.[2] It is essential for the synthesis, methylation, and repair of DNA. Folate deficiency leads to impaired cell division, a problem that becomes apparent first in rapidly regenerating tissue (e.g., bowel mucosa and erythrocytes).

Folate is involved in amino acid metabolism, including the synthesis of serine from glycine and the methylation of homocysteine to methionine. Methionine is activated by adenosine triphosphate to produce S-adenosylmethionine, the primary intracellular methyl donor.

FOOD SOURCES

Folate is synthesized by intestinal bacteria and found in a variety of foods, especially green leafy vegetables, yeast, organ meats, potatoes, fruits, and sprouts. As few as 10 asparagus spears supply half the recommended daily allowance (RDA) of folate. It is best to eat fresh fruits and vegetables whenever possible, since they contain the most vitamins. Food processing (e.g., heat) destroys some of the vitamin. Dietary folates are a complex and variable mixture of compounds that are readily destroyed.

Folates in food occur naturally as pteroylpolyglutamates. Folic acid, pteroylmonoglutamic acid, is the inactive precursor of tetrahydrofolic acid and methyltetrahydrofolate. It is the most oxidized and stable form of folate and is the form used in vitamin supplements and food fortification. Fortified foods include cereals, flour, and bread. However, the other supplemental form, folinic acid, does appear to be more metabolically active. Folinic acid is capable of boosting levels of the coenzyme forms of the vitamin in circumstances in which folic acid has little or no effect. Synthesis of the active forms of folic acid is a complex process requiring several enzymes, as well as adequate supplies of riboflavin (B_2), niacin (B_3), pyridoxine (B_6), zinc, and serine.

DOSE

The RDA for folic acid is 200 µg/1000 kcal or 400 µg/day with a world range of 100 to 400 µg. The estimated average requirement is 320 µg/day for adults. This is increased to 500 to 520 µg/day in pregnant women and women contemplating pregnancy and drops to 450 µg/day during lactation. Children require 120 to 250 µg/day, and the requirement increases with age. An upper limit for folate has been set as 1 mg/day or 1000 µg/day from fortified foods or supplements. The upper limit of folate applies to folic acid and not to the folate occurring naturally in food. Dietary equivalence is as follows:

- 1 µg of food folate = 0.7 µg of folate added to food (food fortification) or 0.5 µg of folate taken as a supplement on an empty stomach
- 1 µg of folic acid supplementation = 2 µg of dietary folate
- 1 µg of folate consumed as fortified food = 1.7 µg of dietary folate in unfortified food

The therapeutic dose range is 400 to 5000 µg/day.[3]

CLINICAL USES

Folic acid deficiency causes anemia. A maintenance dose of folic acid, 0.6 to 0.8 mg/day, is therefore recommended during pregnancy and lactation, and a therapeutic dose of 1 mg of folic acid daily is used to treat megaloblastic anemia. This is later reduced to a maintenance dose of 0.4 mg/day.

Administration of folic acid during the periconceptional period reduces the risk of neural tube defects.[4] All women should have a minimum of 0.4 to 0.5 mg/day during childbearing years; those at high risk for folate deficiency may increase their intake to 5 mg/day during pregnancy. Women who have had a neural tube defect detected in a previous pregnancy should take 4 mg/day for 1 month before and 3 months after becoming pregnant. Dietary supplementation with a folic acid–containing multivitamin (0.8 mg of folate) may be more effective than high doses of folic acid (6 mg) taken alone during the periconceptual period.[5]

A prospective study of almost 5000 persons demonstrated that the plasma total homocysteine level was significant for all causes of cardiovascular and cancer deaths in patients aged 65 to 72 years.[6] Epidemiologic studies have shown that higher blood homocysteine levels are inversely related to blood levels of folate, vitamin B_{12}, and vitamin B_6. Oral folate therapy (2.5 mg) reduces homocysteinemia.[7] Results of the 1998 Nurses' Health Study showed cardiovascular disease risk was lowest among those women with the highest intakes of folate and B_6.[8] A combination of folic acid (500 µg) and pyridoxine (100 mg) reduced fasting plasma homocysteine concentrations by 32% in 49 patients with hyperhomocysteinemia.[9] However, meta-analysis of 12 randomized trials suggested that daily supplementation with both 0.5 to 5 mg folic acid and about 0.5 mg of vitamin B_{12} without vitamin B_6 would be expected to reduce homocysteine levels by one quarter to one third to about 8 to 9 µmol/L.[10] Laboratory evidence suggests that folic acid and vitamin B_{12} supplementation improves vascular endothelial function in patients with coronary artery disease, and this effect is likely to be mediated through reduced concentrations of free plasma homocysteine concentrations.[11] However, pharmacologic doses of folic acid increased plasma total homocysteine in one in five subjects in another study.[12] In addition to and independent of its effect on homocysteine, folic acid supplementation may benefit the cardiovascular system through its antioxidant properties, direct scavenging effects, and improved nitric oxide production by enhancing nitric oxide synthetase.[13]

Folate deficiency has been linked with fatigue[14] and depression, and less convincingly, with other neuropsychiatric disorders such as dementia, insomnia, irritability, forgetfulness, peripheral neuropathy, myelopathy, and restless legs syndrome. An oral dose of 5 to 10 mg of folic acid for 6 to 12 months often eliminates or controls these symptoms. Folate, 400 µg daily taken as part of a B complex, may help relieve depression by combating high levels of homocysteine and by increasing the efficacy of antidepressants.

Poor folate status is believed to create an environment that facilitates expression of a predisposition to cancer, particularly colorectal cancer.[15] Epidemiologic evidence supports the notion that a high folate intake is protective against colon cancer.[16] Folate depletion appears to enhance carcinogenesis, whereas folate supplementation above that presently considered to be the basal requirement appears to be protective.[17] Persons with a high folate intake have a lower risk for adenomas. A high alcohol intake is associated with low folate levels. Adenomas and a high alcohol intake correlate with an increased risk of colorectal cancer.[18] Folate supplementation appears to reduce the risk of neoplasia in patients with ulcerative colitis. The effect is dose-dependent, with a dose of 1 mg of folate per day reducing the relative risk of cancer in patients with ulcerative colitis to 0.54.[19]

Folate deficiency may cause immunodepression. DNA hypomethylation is thought to be the link between the observed relationship between inadequate folate status and cancer.[20] Gene expression is controlled in part by DNA methylation, and epidemiologic studies have shown low folate status to correlate with increased risk of cancers of the colon, cervix, lung, esophagus, brain, pancreas, and breast.[17] Although folate deficiency might play a role in the initiation of cervical dysplasia, folic acid supplements do not appear to be very effective in altering the course of established disease. Nonetheless, for many individuals, a daily multivitamin that contains folic acid may be part of a reasonable overall cancer prevention strategy.[21]

TOXICITY/DRUG INTERACTIONS

Folate is a safe nutrient. Excess folate intake results in restlessness, and megadoses may alter sleep patterns and cause insomnia. Its toxicity is linked to its metabolic interaction with vitamin B_{12}.

The metabolic relationship between vitamin B_{12} and folate ensures that a deficiency of one affects the function of the other. Masking of vitamin B_{12} deficiency with folate supplementation results in improvement of the hematologic picture while neurologic damage progresses. Therefore it has been suggested that the safe upper limit of routine folate supplementation in food or tablets is 1 mg/day. In fact, erring on the side of caution, doses of folic acid in excess of 400 µg daily should be avoided until pernicious anemia has been ruled out. In vitamin B_{12} deficiency, the erythrocyte folate level is low because vitamin B_{12} is required for folate entry into cells. If both serum folate and serum vitamin B_{12} levels are low, a combined deficiency should be suspected. The serum folate level reflects intake, and the erythrocyte folate level reflects cellular stores.

Sulfasalazine, cimetidine, and antacids appear to reduce folate absorption. Several drugs such as aminopterin, methotrexate, pyrimethamine, trimethoprim, and triamterene act as folate antagonists.[21] Oral contraceptives may cause depletion of folic acid, as may high therapeutic doses of nonsteroidal anti-inflammatory drugs. This is not a problem at the low doses routinely used.

Persons taking anticonvulsants have an increased requirement for folate, but folate supplements may precipitate convulsions in patients with epilepsy. Folic acid in doses approximating 6 mg daily impairs the activity of anticonvulsants, and dose adjustment may be necessary. Careful patient monitoring is required.

Folate deficiency associated with alcoholism is due to an inadequate diet rather than a drug interaction.

CLINICAL CAUTION

A serum folate level of 7 mmol/L (3 ng/mL) indicates a negative folate balance. The sequence of deficiency after inadequate intake is sequentially a decrease in serum folate concentration, a decrease in erythrocyte folate concentration, increased homocysteine levels, megaloblastic changes in bone marrow, and finally impaired production of cells with a rapid turnover (e.g., erythrocytes, leukocytes, and intestinal epithelium cells). Clinical findings include megaloblastic anemia, insomnia, irritability, malaise, apathy, and irritability. Other signs of deficiency are poor memory, cheilosis (cracks is corners of mouth), and glossitis. Mucosal defects result in impaired absorption, further exacerbating folate deficiency. Peripheral neuropathy, tendon hyperreflexia, diarrhea, weight loss, and cerebral disturbances may develop.[7]

Erythrocyte folate levels provide an indicator of long-term folate status and should be around 305 nmol/L (140 ng/mL).

PRACTICE TIPS

- Smaller-than-average babies, those who are breast fed, and those receiving unfortified formulas (e.g., evaporated milk or goat's milk) may need folic acid supplementation.
- A mouthwash containing 5 mg of folate per 5 mL of mouthwash used twice daily for 4 weeks, with a rinsing time of 1 minute, improves gingival health.
- Doses in excess of 1 mg per day may mask a vitamin B_{12} deficiency and possibly interfere with zinc absorption; 0.5 mg seems to be a safe daily dose.
- Folic acid, 1 mg/day 5 times a week (5 mg/week), may be used as prophylaxis for toxic effects of methotrexate in patients treated for rheumatoid arthritis.
- A deficiency of folate and/or vitamin B_{12} depresses both cellular and humoral immunity.

REFERENCES

1. Pearce KA, Boosalis MG, Yeager B: Update on vitamin supplements for the prevention of coronary disease and stroke, *Am Fam Physician* 62:1359-66, 2000.
2. Fowler B: The folate cycle and disease in humans, *Kidney Int* 59(suppl 78): S221-S229, 2001.
3. Brighthope I: Nutritional medicine tables, *J Aust Coll Nutr Env Med* 17:20-5,1998.
4. Thompson S, Torres M, Stevenson R, et al: Periconceptional vitamin use, dietary folate and occurrent neural tube defected pregnancies in a high risk population, *Ann Epidemiol* 10:476, 2000.

5. Czeizel AE: Primary prevention of neural-tube defects and some other major congenital abnormalities: recommendations for the appropriate use of folic acid during pregnancy, *Paediatr Drugs* 2:437-49, 2000.

6. Vollset SE, Refsum H, Tverdal A, et al: Plasma total homocysteine and cardiovascular and noncardiovascular mortality: the Hordaland Homocysteine Study, *Am J Clin Nutr* 74:130-6, 2001.

7. Kelly GS: Folates: supplemental forms and therapeutic applications, *Altern Med Rev* 3:208-20, 1998.

8. Rimm EB, Willett WC, Hu FB, et al: Folate and vitamin B$_6$ from diet and supplements in relation to risk of coronary heart disease among women, *JAMA* 279:359-64, 1998.

9. Van der Griend R, Haas FJ, Biesma DH, et al: Combination of low-dose folic acid and pyridoxine for treatment of hyperhomocysteinaemia in patients with premature arterial disease and their relatives, *Atherosclerosis* 143:177-83, 1999.

10. Clarke R, Armitage J: Vitamin supplements and cardiovascular risk: review of the randomized trials of homocysteine-lowering vitamin supplements, *Semin Thromb Hemost* 26:341-8, 2000.

11. Chambers JC, Ueland PM, Obeid OA, et al: Improved vascular endothelial function after oral B vitamins: an effect mediated through reduced concentrations of free plasma homocysteine, *Circulation* 102:2479-83, 2000.

12. Malinow MR: Plasma concentrations of total homocysteine predict mortality risk, *Am J Clin Nutr* 74:3, 2001.

13. Brown AA, Hu FB: Dietary modulation of endothelial function: implications for cardiovascular disease, *Am J Clin Nutr* 73:673-86, 2001.

14. Werbach MR: Nutritional strategies for treating chronic fatigue syndrome, *Altern Med Rev* 5:93-108, 2000.

15. Mason JB, Levesque T: Folate: effects on carcinogenesis and the potential for cancer chemoprovention, *Oncology* 10:1727-36, 1996.

16. Prinz-Langenohl R, Fohr I, Pietrzik K: Beneficial role for folate in the prevention of colorectal and breast cancer, *Eur J Nutr* 40:98-105, 2001.

17. Choi SW, Mason JB: Folate and carcinogenesis: an integrated scheme, *J Nutr* 130:129-32, 2000.

18. Lamson DW, Brignall MS: Natural agents in the prevention of cancer, part two: preclinical data and chemoprevention for common cancers, *Altern Med Rev* 6:167-87, 2001.

19. Lashner BA, Provencher KS, Seidner DL, et al: The effect of folic acid supplementation on the risk for cancer or dysplasia in ulcerative colitis, *Gastroenterology* 112:29-32, 1997.

20. Selhub J: Folate, vitamin B$_{12}$ and vitamin B$_6$ and one carbon metabolism, *J Nutr Health Aging* 6:39-42, 2002.

21. Willett WC: Goals for nutrition in the year 2000, *CA Cancer J Clin* 49:331-52, 1999.

■ CHAPTER 68 ■

GARLIC (*ALLIUM SATIVUM*)

> Garlic should be discontinued for 2 to 3 weeks before surgical procedures; this includes stopping routine consumption of one to two cloves for culinary purposes or as self-mediation.

Garlic has been used as a culinary herb and medicinal agent for thousands of years. Garlic cloves can be eaten raw or roasted. When garlic is roasted, the bulb is cut to expose just the tips of the cloves, then the bulb is rubbed in olive oil, wrapped in silver foil, and baked at 350°C for 45 minutes. Garlic is frequently used as a flavoring agent in sauces and pasta dishes.

Most of garlic's medicinal properties are found in the sulfur compounds concentrated in the bulb. Mincing, crushing, or pressing garlic increases the surface area and maximizes production and release of health-promoting compounds; the same applies to onions. In fact, both garlic and onion have been shown to have antimicrobial, antithrombotic, antitumor, hypolipidemic, antiarthritic, and hypoglycemic properties.[1] Recent interest in garlic has primarily focused on its potential in the fields of cardiovascular and cancer research.

MECHANISM OF ACTION

Garlic is rich in natural sulfur products including alliin, a sulfur-containing amino acid. When garlic is crushed or chewed, alliin is exposed to the enzyme alliinase and converted into the active compound allicin. It is unstable and, on exposure to heat and/or acid, forms various diallyl and dimethyl sulfides, as well as E-ajoene and Z-ajoene. Allicin is responsible for the characteristic odor of garlic. The biologic activity of garlic lies in its ability to produce allicin.

Garlic reduces the risk of arterial occlusion by lowering serum lipids, retarding inflammatory processes that favor atherosclerosis, and reducing thrombosis. The antihyperlipidemic effect is believed to be due to the formation of sulfide bridges between the disulfides in garlic and the 3-hydroxy-3-methylglutaryl–coenzyme A reductase enzyme involved in cholesterol synthesis. Prevention of atherosclerosis may also be mediated through other pathways including reduced lipid oxidation and increased nitric oxide synthetase activity. Nitric oxide facilitates relaxation of endothelium-dependent smooth muscle, and increased blood levels of catalase and glutathione peroxidase reduce the risk of free radical damage.

Explaining garlic's antithrombotic effect is more problematic.[2] Methyallyltrisulfide and the ajoenes are believed to be responsible for garlic's antithrombotic actions, but although ajoene is being developed as a drug for treatment of thromboembolic disorders, it is not naturally present in garlic, garlic powders, or other commercial garlic preparations and is only found in small amounts in garlic oil macerates. Furthermore, although allicin and adenosine are the most potent antiplatelet constituents of garlic in vitro, both are rapidly metabolized in blood and other tissues and consequently may not contribute to garlic's antithrombotic actions in the body. Garlic may inhibit platelet activity through inhibition of thromboxane synthesis. It has been suggested that the potent enzyme-inhibiting activities of adenosine deaminase and cyclic adenosine monophosphate phosphodiesterase in garlic extracts may play a significant role in the antithrombotic, vasodilatory, and anticancer actions of garlic.

Animal and in vitro studies have provided evidence of garlic's anticarcinogenic effect. Both water- and lipid-soluble allyl sulfur compounds are effective in blocking a myriad of chemically induced tumors. Garlic seems to prevent carcinogenesis by detoxifying chemical carcinogens and directly inhibiting the growth of cancer cells. It is reported to enhance immunity both through stimulating the activity of immunocompetent cells such as macrophages, natural killer cells, and killer cells and through increasing the production of interleukin 2, tumor necrosis factor, and interferon-γ.[3] In addition to modifying immunocompetence, garlic's other mechanisms of action include blocking nitrosamine formation and metabolism, blocking initiation and promotion phases of the carcinogenicity of various compounds (e.g., polycyclic hydrocarbons), altering several phase I and phase II reactions, inducing apoptosis, and effecting DNA repair.[4] The anticarcinogenic potential of garlic may be influenced by several dietary components including specific fatty acids, selenium, and vitamin A.

Garlic achieves a hypoglycemic effect through increased serum insulin levels and enhanced glycogen storage. Garlic achieves an antimicrobial effect through reacting with the sulfhydryl group on enzymes used by microorganisms for nutrition (e.g., alcohol dehydrogenase) and tissue invasion (e.g., cysteine proteinase).

DOSE

The potency of garlic preparations varies depending on the manufacturer. An extract standardized to 1.3% alliin is recommended. Fresh garlic yields around 0.4% allicin, whereas garlic powder contains 1.3% allicin. Dried garlic contains alliin and allinase. However, the reaction required to activate alliin in dried garlic cannot occur in the acid environment of the stomach. Dried garlic must be enteric-coated and activated in the intestines if it is to be effective.

A frequently used dose is 400 to 1000 mg of dried garlic or 2 to 5 g of fresh garlic. One clove of fresh garlic contains around 4000 μg of allicin activity. As a rough guide, 800 mg of garlic powder is roughly equivalent to 2.7 g or one largish clove of fresh garlic. For maximum effect, garlic should be used over a prolonged period.

CLINICAL USES

The clinical efficacy of garlic is controversial. An analysis of eight reviews indicated that although garlic has a modest short-term lipid-lowering effect, its clinical relevance is uncertain.[5] Despite promising results with respect to fibrinolysis and platelet aggregation, there is insufficient information from which to draw any definitive conclusions.[6,7] Furthermore, garlic does not appear to achieve any consistent reduction in blood pressure; to have any effect on glucose or insulin sensitivity; or to decrease the risk of breast, lung, gastric, colon, or rectal cancer.[7] However, a report by the Agency for Healthcare Research and Quality[7] does emphasize that short follow-up periods, unclear randomization processes, the absence of intention-to-treat analyses, missing data, and variability in techniques used to assess outcomes make it impossible to draw firm conclusions. Consequently, potential benefits from garlic ingestion cannot yet be definitely excluded.

It remains possible, albeit improbable, that regular daily ingestion of 4 g or 2 average-sized cloves of fresh garlic may help prevent atherosclerosis and hypertension. Consuming 300 to 900 mg of standardized garlic powder over 2 or more years may protect against age-related changes in aortic elasticity.[6] An earlier review of randomized, controlled trials in which garlic preparations were consumed for 4 or more weeks also suggested that Kwai garlic powder preparation may be of some clinical use in subjects with mild hypertension.[8] Garlic intake may have a protective effect on the elastic properties of the aorta in aging humans.

Despite inconsistency in dosage, standardization of garlic preparations, and period of treatment, most findings suggest that garlic decreases cholesterol and triglyceride levels in patients with increased levels of these lipids.[2] Meta-analysis of the controlled trials of garlic to reduce hypercholesterolemia reveals a significant reduction in total cholesterol levels.[9] Thirty-seven randomized trials, all but one in adults, consistently demonstrated that, compared with placebo, various garlic preparations led to small, statistically significant reductions in total cholesterol levels at 1 month and 3 months. When analyses of eight placebo-controlled trials were pooled, total cholesterol outcomes at 6 months showed no significant reductions in total cholesterol with garlic as compared with placebo. The reasons for statistically significant positive short-term effects, but negative longer-term effects, are unclear.[7] The best available evidence at that time suggested that garlic, in an amount approximating one half to one clove per day, decreased total serum cholesterol levels by about 9% in the groups of patients studied.

More recently, the hypolipdemic effect of garlic has been disputed. A randomized, double-blind, placebo-controlled, parallel treatment study showed that administration of garlic powder for 12 weeks (900 mg/d, 300 mg taken with meals three times daily) was ineffective in lowering cholesterol levels in patients with hypercholesterolemia.[10] Another double-blind, randomized, placebo-controlled trial demonstrated that after 3 months of therapy at a similar dose, levels of major plasma lipoproteins, high-density lipoprotein cholesterol, lipoprotein(a), apolipoprotein B subfractions, and postprandial triglycerides were all unchanged in subjects with moderate hypercholesterolemia.[11] Commercial garlic oil has similarly failed to influence serum lipoproteins, cholesterol absorption, or cholesterol synthesis.[12] A recent meta-analysis indicated that although garlic is superior to placebo in reducing total cholesterol levels, the size of the effect is so modest that its usefulness as a hypocholesterolemic agent is questionable.[13]

Although 10 small, randomized trials showed promising effects of various garlic preparations on platelet aggregation and mixed effects on plasma viscosity and fibrinolytic activity, there are insufficient data to confirm or refute effects of garlic on clinical outcomes such as myocardial infarction and intermittent claudication.[7] Nonetheless, in two double-blind studies of patients with atherosclerotic lower-extremity disease, garlic was found to increase pain-free walking distance at 12 to16 weeks compared with placebo. Despite several positive results, a review of trials suggests that the benefit of garlic to the cardiovascular system is limited; garlic has possible small short-term beneficial effects on some lipid and antiplatelet factors, insignificant effects on blood pressure, and no effect on glucose levels.[14,15]

Garlic is also of interest with respect to other conditions. Meta-analyses of the epidemiologic literature suggests that a high intake of garlic (28 g/day) may be associated with a protective effect against stomach and colorectal cancers.[16] Although evidence for a protective effect against cancer at other sites, including the breast, is still insufficient, diets rich in garlic and other allium vegetables, such as onions, leeks, and chives, have been reported to protect against stomach and colorectal cancers.[7,17] Ajoene, extracted from garlic, is helpful in treating fungal infection such as tinea pedis.[18] Daily consumption of garlic capsules with a concentration of 2 to 5 mg of allicin is recommended. Topical use of sliced cloves or garlic oil three times daily for 1 to 2 weeks may also be useful for managing superficial infections. An extensive current review of the medicinal activities of garlic is available.[19]

TOXICITY/DRUG INTERACTIONS

Liberal consumption by humans over millennia and experimental and clinical data suggest that garlic is very safe for therapeutic use.[20] An adverse effect of oral ingestion of garlic is "smelly" breath and body odor. Chewing parsley or taking enteric-coated garlic may prevent garlic breath.

Other, more common adverse reactions reported are gastrointestinal complaints such as dyspepsia, flatulence, and heartburn. Headache has been reported by children. Some persons have experienced contact dermatitis.

Garlic should be used with caution or avoided by patients taking drugs or herbs that increase the risk of bleeding. This includes aspirin, nonsteroidal anti-inflammatory drugs, anticoagulants, platelet inhibitors, ginger, ginseng, *Ginko biloba*, feverfew, and willow bark.[21] Garlic changes the pharmacokinetic variables of acetaminophen (paracetamol) and produces hypoglycemia when taken with chlorpropamide.[22]

CLINICAL CAUTION

Garlic taken in quantities in excess of 4 g should be used with caution. Patients taking aspirin or warfarin should avoid taking garlic in doses of 4 g or more and should only take garlic in these quantities if under medical supervision.[23]

PRACTICE TIPS

- Despite controversy, current thinking suggests that deodorized garlic preparations do remain clinically effective.
- Blood sugar monitoring should be increased in patients with diabetes who intend to consume therapeutic doses of garlic.
- Enteric-coated garlic tablets with at least 9.6 mg of allicin-releasing potential may be of value for patients with mild to moderate hypercholesterolemia in combination with a low-fat diet.[24]

REFERENCES

1. Ali M, Thomson M, Afzal M: Garlic and onions: their effect on eicosanoid metabolism and its clinical relevance, *Prostaglandins Leukot Essent Fatty Acids* 62:55-73, 2000.
2. Agarwal KC: Therapeutic actions of garlic constituents, *Med Res Rev* 16:111-24, 1996.
3. Lamm DL, Riggs DR: The potential application of *Allium sativum* (garlic) for the treatment of bladder cancer, *Urol Clin North Am* 27:157-62, xi, 2000.
4. Milner JA: A historical perspective on garlic and cancer, *J Nutr* 131(3s):1027S-31S, 2001.
5. Linde K, ter Riet G, Hondras M, et al: Systematic reviews of complementary therapies—an annotated bibliography. Part 2: herbal medicine, *BMC Complement Altern Med* 1:5, 2001.
6. Breithaupt-Grogler K, Ling M, Boudoulas H, et al: Protective effect of chronic garlic intake on elastic properties of aorta in the elderly, *Circulation* 96:2649-55, 1997.

7. Garlic: effects on cardiovascular risks and disease, protective effects against cancer, and clinical adverse effects. *Summary, Evidence Report/Technology Assessment*, No. 20. AHRQ Publication No. 01-E022, Rockville, MD, October 2000, Agency for Healthcare Research and Quality. http://www.ahrq.gov/clinic/epcsums/garlicsum.htm.

8. Silagy CA, Neil HA: A meta-analysis of the effect of garlic on blood pressure, *J Hypertens* 12:463-8, 1994.

9. Warshafsky S, Kamer RS, Sivak SL: Effect of garlic on total serum cholesterol. A meta-analysis, *Ann Intern Med* 119:599-605, 1993.

10. Isaacsohn JL, Moser M, Stein EA, et al: Garlic powder and plasma lipids and lipoproteins: a multicenter, randomized, placebo-controlled trial, *Arch Intern Med* 158:1189-94, 1998.

11. Superko HR, Krauss RM: Garlic powder, effect on plasma lipids, postprandial lipemia, low-density lipoprotein particle size, high-density lipoprotein subclass distribution and lipoprotein(a), *J Am Coll Cardiol* 35:321-6, 2000.

12. Berthold HK, Sudhop T, von Bergmann K: Effect of a garlic oil preparation on serum lipoproteins and cholesterol metabolism: a randomized controlled trial, *JAMA* 279:1900-2, 1998.

13. Stevinson C, Pittler MH, Ernst E: Garlic for treating hypercholesterolemia. A meta-analysis of randomized clinical trials, *Ann Intern Med* 133:420-9, 2000.

14. Ackermann RT, Mulrow CD, Ramirez G, et al: Garlic shows promise for improving some cardiovascular risk factors, *Arch Intern Med* 161:813-24, 2001.

15. Spigelski D, Jones PJ: Efficacy of garlic supplementation in lowering serum cholesterol levels, *Nutr Rev* 59:236-41, 2001.

16. Fleischauer AT, Poole C, Arab L: Garlic consumption and cancer prevention: meta-analyses of colorectal and stomach cancers, *Am J Clin Nutr* 72:1047-52, 2000.

17. Bianchini F, Vainio H: Allium vegetables and organosulfur compounds: do they help prevent cancer? *Environ Health Perspect* 109:893-902, 2001.

18. Ledezma E, Marcano K, Jorquera A, et al: Efficacy of ajoene in the treatment of tinea pedis: a double-blind and comparative study with terbinafine. *J Am Acad Dermatol* 43(5 Pt 1):829-832, 2000.

19. Kaul PN, Joshi BS: Alternative medicine: herbal drugs and their critical appraisal—part II, *Prog Drug Res* 57:1-75, 2001

20. Klepser TB, Klepser ME: Unsafe and potentially safe herbal therapies, *Am J Health Syst Pharm* 56:125-38, 1999.

21. Evans V: Herbs and the brain: friend or foe? The effects of ginkgo and garlic on warfarin use, *J Neurosci Nurs* 32:229-32, 2000.

22. Izzo AA, Ernst E: Interactions between herbal medicines and prescribed drugs: a systematic review, *Drugs* 61:2163-75, 2001.

23. Braun L: Herb-drug interaction guide, *Aust Fam Physician* 30:259-60, 2001.

24. Kannar D, Wattanapenpaiboon N, Savige GS, et al: Hypocholesterolemic effect of an enteric-coated garlic supplement, *J Am Coll Nutr* 20:225-31, 2001.

CHAPTER 69

GINGER (*ZINGIBER OFFICINALE*)

> Ginger demonstrates that old wives' tales may acquire scientific respectability.

The rhizome of *Zingiber officinale* (ginger) is used both as a spice and a medicinal. It is closely related to turmeric. Ginger has been used for centuries as a carminative and intestinal spasmolytic. In fact, there is scientific approval for using this ancient medicine to stimulate digestion in persons with gastrointestinal problems. Its ability to increase gastrointestinal activity has resulted in its use as an appetite stimulant for anorexia and for relief of dyspepsia, nausea, and flatulence. It has also been used to stimulate circulation and treat migraine.

MECHANISM OF ACTION

Various essential oils (e.g., zingiberene) and pungent principles (e.g., gingerols) are present in fresh ginger and decompose on drying and storage. The active ingredients, gingerols and shogaols, affect eicosanoid metabolism. Gingerols are potent inhibitors of prostaglandin synthesis and are also effective inhibitors of leukotriene biosynthesis. By modifying thromboxane and prostacyclin synthesis, ginger reduces arachidonate-induced platelet aggregation.[1] Ginger affects blood coagulation by inhibiting arachidonic acid activity. Gingerol has a structure similar to that of aspirin.

DOSE

For cooking or eating, the tough outer peel should be removed; and fresh ginger should be thinly sliced, grated, or crushed for maximum flavor. Fresh, unpeeled ginger, if tightly wrapped in plastic, will last for up to 14 days in the refrigerator or for up to 2 months in the freezer. African and Indian varieties are the most potent.

Recommended therapeutic doses are 500 to 1000 mg of fresh root three times daily or 500 mg of dried root two to four times a day. Other suggested doses are one 500-mg ginger tablet two to four times a day, 0.7 to 2 mL of 1:2 liquid extract per day, and 1.7 to 5 mL of 1:5 tincture per day.

CLINICAL USES

It has been suggested that administration of 2 to 5 g of ginger per day eases dyspepsia. The efficacy of ginger rhizome for the prevention of nausea, dizziness, and vomiting in motion sickness has been well documented and proved beyond doubt in numerous high-quality clinical studies.[2] Oral ginger, taken twice daily as a 10-mg rhizome extract, improved gastroduodenal motility both in the fasting state and after a standard test meal.[3] Furthermore, evidence from six randomized, controlled trials favored ginger over placebo in the treatment of nausea and vomiting.[4] In a double-blind study of pregnant women, administration of 1 g of ginger daily was found to be effective for relief of morning sickness.[5] No side effects were detected.

However, although ginger may be of benefit, pyridoxine (vitamin B_6) appears to be more effective in reducing the severity of nausea in pregnancy.[6] On the other hand, medicinal ginger is a well-recognized option for preventing the symptoms of travel sickness.[2] A dose of 1 g orally, taken immediately then every 4 hours as required to a maximum of 4 g in 24 hours, is recommended to prevent motion sickness. The first dose of ginger should be taken at least 3 hours before departure.

The ability of ginger to inhibit prostaglandin and leukotriene biosynthesis from arachidonic acid favors a less inflammatory state and may explain the symptomatic relief reported by some patients with arthritis and fibromyalgia. An effective dose may be achieved by taking 100 to 1000 mg of ginger in tablet form per day or by consuming 50 g of lightly cooked ginger or 5 g of raw ginger per day.[7] Some patients with arthritis seem to experience some pain relief from taking up to 6 teaspoons of ginger daily. Although eugenol (33 mg/kg) and ginger oil (33 mg/kg), given orally to rats for 26 days, caused a significant suppression of both paw and joint swelling,[8] a controlled, double-blind, double-dummy, crossover study in which ginger extract was compared with placebo in patients with osteoarthritis failed to show significant benefit.[9]

In addition to affecting pain and inflammation, inhibition of cyclooxygenase activity by ginger also affects platelet activity. Ginger has an antithrombotic effect. A randomized, placebo-controlled, crossover study, in which healthy volunteers consumed 15 g of raw ginger root or 40 g of cooked stem ginger or placebo over 2 weeks, demonstrated that thromboxane production decreased 9% for ginger root and 8% for stem ginger compared with placebo.[10] The effect of ginger on thromboxane synthetase activity is dose-dependent. Four grams of powdered ginger per day had no effect, but a single dose of 10 g produced a significant reduction in platelet aggregation.[11] Results of a randomized, double-blind study confirmed that 2 g or less of dried ginger is unlikely to cause platelet dysfunction.[12]

Inadequately proven uses for ginger are attenuation of atherosclerosis (possibly through its antioxidant and anti-inflammatory effects[13]) and prophylaxis for migraine headache without side effects.[14] One third of a teaspoon of fresh or powdered ginger may abort a migraine attack in certain people.

TOXICITY/DRUG INTERACTIONS

Liberal consumption by humans over millennia and experimental and clinical data suggest that ginger is very safe for therapeutic use.[15] Although safe at prescribed doses, ginger may enhance the effects of other drugs (e.g., antiplatelet agents, including aspirin and nonsteroidal anti-inflammatory drugs) and affect antiarrhythmics (inotropic agents and vasopressors). In doses of less than 4 g/day, ginger may be used with caution in patients receiving antacids or warfarin. Patients being treated with warfarin require medical supervision if they are taking ginger in doses of 4 or more grams daily.[1]

CLINICAL CAUTION

High doses of ginger may cause heartburn as a result of increased gastric secretion. The dose of ginger should not exceed 2 g/day during pregnancy. Ingestion of 6 g of fresh ginger causes exfoliation of gastric epithelium cells; therefore, ginger should be avoided or used cautiously by patients with peptic ulceration.

Ginger has the potential to cause cardiac arrhythmia, bleeding, and central nervous system depression. Ginger may have a glycemic effect and should be used with caution by patients with diabetes. Further information on the pharmacology and ethnomedical use of ginger is available.[16]

PRACTICE TIPS

- Ginger, like turmeric, fenugreek, cloves, and red chili peppers, reduces platelet clumping.
- Ginger stimulates the gall bladder and is contraindicated for patients with gallstones, unless patients are under medical supervision.
- Spicing beans with one teaspoon of ground ginger will reduce the risk of flatulence (soaking beans and pouring off the fluid before cooking also reduces gas-producing compounds).
- A cup of ginger tea, prepared by adding four thin slices of ginger to a cup of boiling water, may settle an upset stomach.
- Spices exhibit synergistic antioxidant activity: any mixture of ginger, onion, and/or garlic shows cumulative inhibition of lipid peroxidation.[17]
- The antioxidant activity of spice extracts is retained even after boiling for 30 minutes at 100°C.

REFERENCES

1. Braun L: Herb-drug interaction guide, *Aust Fam Physician* 30:259-60, 2001.

2. Langner E, Greifenberg S, Gruenwald J: Ginger: history and use, *Adv Ther* 15:25-44, 1998.

3. Micklefield GH, Redeker Y, Meister V, et al: Effects of ginger on gastroduodenal motility, *Int J Clin Pharmacol Ther* 37:341-6, 1999.

4. Ernst E, Pittler MH: Efficacy of ginger for nausea and vomiting: a systematic review of randomized clinical trials, *Br J Anaesth* 84:367-71, 2000.

5. Vutyavanich T, Kraisarin T, Ruangsri R: Ginger for nausea and vomiting in pregnancy: randomized, double-masked, placebo-controlled trial, *Obstet Gynecol* 97:577-82, 2001.

6. Jewell D, Young G: Interventions for nausea and vomiting in early pregnancy, *Cochrane Database Syst Rev* 2:CD000145, 2000.

7. Srivastava KC, Mustafa T: Ginger (*Zingiber officinale*) in rheumatism and musculoskeletal disorders, *Med Hypotheses* 39:342-8, 1992.

8. Sharma JN, Srivastava KC, Gan EK: Suppressive effects of eugenol and ginger oil on arthritic rats, *Pharmacology* 49:314-8, 1994.

9. Bliddal H, Rosetzky A, Schlichting P, et al: A randomized, placebo-controlled, cross-over study of ginger extracts and ibuprofen in osteoarthritis, *Osteoarthritis Cartilage* 8:9-12, 2000.

10. Janssen PL, Meyboom S, van Staveren WA, et al: Consumption of ginger (*Zingiber officinale roscoe*) does not affect ex vivo platelet thromboxane production in humans, *Eur J Clin Nutr* 50:772-4, 1996.

11. Bordia A, Verma SK, Srivastava KC: Effect of ginger (*Zingiber officinale Rosc.*) and fenugreek (*Trigonella foenumgraecum L.*) on blood lipids, blood sugar and platelet aggregation in patients with coronary artery disease, *Prostaglandins Leukot Essent Fatty Acids* 56:379-84, 1997.

12. Lumb AB: Effect of dried ginger on human platelet function, *Thromb Haemost* 71:110-1, 1994.

13. Fuhrman B, Rosenblat M, Hayek T, et al: Ginger extract consumption reduces plasma cholesterol, inhibits LDL oxidation and attenuates development of atherosclerosis in atherosclerotic, apolipoprotein E-deficient mice, *J Nutr* 130:1124-31, 2000.

14. Mustafa T, Srivastava KC: Ginger (*Zingiber officinale*) in migraine headache, *J Ethnopharmacol* 29:267-73, 1990.

15. Kaul PN, Joshi BS: Alternative medicine: herbal drugs and their critical appraisal—part II, *Prog Drug Res* 57:1-75, 2001.

16. Afzal M, Al-Hadidi D, Menon M, et al: Ginger: an ethnomedical, chemical and pharmacological review, *Drug Metabol Drug Interact* 18:159-90, 2001.

17. Shobana S, Naidu KA: Antioxidant activity of selected Indian spices, *Prostaglandins Leukot Essent Fatty Acids* 62:107-10, 2000.

■ CHAPTER 70 ■

GINKGO BILOBA (GINKGO)

Ginkgo may benefit older persons, but because it may interfere with drug metabolism, with patients who are receiving other medications, medical supervision is required.

Ginkgo enhances perfusion, inhibiting vasospasm and thrombus formation. Its potential to improve cerebral ischemia has resulted in its use for symptomatic treatment of dementia, vertigo, and tinnitus of vascular origin. Similarly, ginkgo has been used to increase peripheral perfusion. Current publications suggest that although ginkgo is of questionable use for memory loss and tinnitus, there is more convincing evidence that it has some effect on dementia and intermittent claudication.[1] Results of clinical studies also suggest that ginkgo extracts exhibit therapeutic potential for management of poor ocular blood flow and congestive symptoms of premenstrual syndrome and for the prevention of altitude sickness.[2]

MECHANISM OF ACTION

Ginkgo extracts contain approximately 24% flavone glycosides and 6% terpene lactones (ginkgolides A, B, and C and bilobalide).[3] The former act as antioxidants and anticoagulants; the latter enhance perfusion. Ginkgo is recognized as a specific platelet-activating factor antagonist. Other constituents include proanthocyanidins, glucose, rhamnose, and organic acids.

Ginkgo enhances perfusion. It achieves vascular relaxation via a nitrous oxide pathway. It reduces inflammation and thrombosis by its antioxidant activity and potent platelet-activating factor inhibition. Platelet-activating factor is a phospholipid released by platelets, macrophages, and monocytes, which aggregates platelets and enhances inflammation. Ginkgo lowers fibrinogen levels and decreases plasma viscosity. It may influence the metabolism of neurotransmitters, possibly by stimulation of prostaglandin synthesis.

The anti-stress and neuroprotective effects of *Ginkgo biloba* extract may be related to suppression of glucocorticoid biosynthesis.

DOSE

The usual dose is 120 mg per day of 50:1 ginkgo standardized extract, equivalent to 27 to 30 mg of ginkgo flavone glycosides and 10 mg terpenoids per day (4-8 g of leaf). This is usually available in the form of 40-mg tablets or in liquid form at a concentration of 40 mg/mL. The dose is three tablets per day or 3 mL of liquid. Extracts require standardization for the major active constituents.

CLINICAL USES

There is considerable clinical evidence supporting the use of ginkgo in the management of conditions that benefit from increased perfusion. Clinical trials support the use of ginkgo in the treatment of patients with mental deterioration associated with aging such as problems with memory, concentration, and alertness; dizziness; and tinnitus.[4] Ginkgo extracts appear to be capable of stabilizing and, in some cases, improving cognitive performance and the social functioning of patients with dementia. Most, although not all, clinical trials support the use of ginkgo extracts in the treatment of dementia.[5] Administration of ginkgo results in clinically significant improvements in memory and concentration and reduces symptoms of fatigue, anxiety, and depressed mood in these patients. A double-blind, placebo-controlled, parallel-group, multicenter study demonstrated that patients with uncomplicated Alzheimer's disease or multi-infarct dementia showed significantly less decline in cognitive function when they received a 120-mg dose (40 mg three times daily) of *Ginkgo biloba* extract over a 26-week period.[6] Placebo-controlled efficacy studies indicated that second-generation cholinesterase inhibitors (donepezil, rivastigmine, and metrifonate) and ginkgo special extract EGb 761 were equally effective in delaying symptom progression or achieving a response rate in the treatment of mild to moderate Alzheimer's disease.[7] *G. biloba* extract (EGb 761) is a well-defined plant extract containing two major groups of constituents (i.e., flavonoids and terpenoids).

A study in which hippocampal primary cultured cells were used demonstrated that *G. biloba* extract protected hippocampal neurons, possibly in part through its antioxidant properties.[8] Substantial evidence suggests that the accumulation of β-amyloid, and to a lesser extent, free radicals may contribute to the etiology and/or progression of Alzheimer's disease. Animal studies have shown that chemical induction of a permanent deficit in cerebral energy metabolism can be reversed and ongoing deterioration in learning, memory, and cognition partially compensated by using *G. biloba* extract.[9] The recommended dosage for Alzheimer's disease is at the higher end of the dose range, around 240 mg daily.[3] A review of trials indicated that ginkgo extracts were effective in managing minor cognitive impairment, although more evidence was needed to ascertain its efficacy in more severe forms of dementia.[10]

In addition to improving cerebral perfusion, gingko is of value in treating peripheral vascular disease. Even though some reviewers have deemed the clinical relevance of the improvement moderate, gingko has also been found to increase walking distance.[10] Meta-analysis of randomized, placebo-controlled, double-blind trials confirmed that *G. biloba* extract is superior to placebo in the symptomatic treatment of intermittent claudication.[11]

In a German study of eight controlled trials, the authors reported that *G. biloba* special extract EGb 761 was well tolerated and benefited patients with tinnitus caused by cerebrovascular insufficiency or labyrinthine disorders.[12] Therapeutic success in these and open trials was not directly correlated with either the genesis or the duration of tinnitus, but short-standing disorders did appear to have a better prognosis. Early intervention was recommended. Although gingko deserves consideration for the treatment of tinnitus,[13] its use in the management of age-related macular degeneration has yet to be clarified.[14] Nonetheless, ginkgo does significantly increase blood flow to the ophthalmic artery.[15]

Animal studies showed that a combination of *G. biloba* and *Zingiber officinale* (ginger) had anxiolytic effects comparable to those of diazepam, but at high doses, anxiogenic properties were also noted.[16]

TOXICITY/DRUG INTERACTIONS

Ginkgo is regarded as a potentially safe herb at recommended doses.[17] The median lethal dose of *G. biloba* extract is 15.3 g per kilogram body weight.[3] No side effects have been reported in healthy volunteers given 120-mg doses of a ginkgolide mixture. Nonetheless, *G. biloba* extract has been reported to cause spontaneous bleeding, and it may interact with anticoagulants and antiplatelet agents.[18] Interaction of ginkgo with warfarin, aspirin, and other anticoagulant or antiplatelet drugs may potentiate bleeding. Other potential repercussions of interactions are increased blood pressure when gingko is combined with a thiazide diuretic and coma when it is combined with trazodone.[19] There is also a risk of allergy in susceptible individuals.

Side effects are uncommon; however, gastrointestinal disturbances, headaches, dizziness, tinnitus, peripheral visual shimmering, and hypersensitivity reactions (e.g., skin rash) have been reported.

CLINICAL CAUTION

Medical supervision is required to adjust doses of aspirin and warfarin when patients receiving these medications take gingko.[20]

PRACTICE TIPS

- Because it may take 6 to 8 weeks for ginkgo to reach maximal efficacy, patients require at least 6 weeks of therapy before clinical benefit is assessed.
- Gingko should not be used by patients who are sensitive to the plant.
- Adverse effects (e.g., headache, gastrointestinal upsets, or rashes) are usually only observed with doses in excess of 180 mg/day.

REFERENCES

1. Ernst E: The risk-benefit profile of commonly used herbal therapies: ginkgo, St. John's wort, ginseng, echinacea, saw palmetto, and kava, *Ann Intern Med* 136:42-53, 2002.
2. McKenna DJ, Jones K, Hughes K: Efficacy, safety, and use of ginkgo biloba in clinical and preclinical applications, *Altern Ther Health Med* 7:70-86, 88-90, 2001.
3. Ginkgo biloba, *Altern Med Rev* 3:54-7, 1998.
4. Mills S, Bone K: *Principles and practice of phytotherapy*, Edinburgh, 2000, Churchill Livingstone.
5. Beaubrun G, Gray GE: A review of herbal medicines for psychiatric disorders, *Psychiatr Serv* 51:1130-4, 2000.
6. Le Bars PL, Kieser M, Itil KZ: A 26-week analysis of a double-blind, placebo-controlled trial of the ginkgo biloba extract Egb 761 in dementia, *Dement Geriatr Cogn Disord* 11:230-7, 2000.
7. Wettstein A: Cholinesterase inhibitors and Gingko extracts—are they comparable in the treatment of dementia? Comparison of published placebo-controlled efficacy studies of at least six months' duration, *Phytomedicine* 6: 393-401, 2000.
8. Bastianetto S, Ramassamy C, Dore S, et al: The *Ginkgo biloba* extract (Egb 761) protects hippocampal neurons against cell death induced by beta-amyloid, *Eur J Neurosci* 12:1882-90, 2000.
9. Hoyer S, Lannert H, Noldner M, et al: Damaged neuronal energy metabolism and behavior are improved by *Ginkgo biloba* extract (Egb 761), *J Neural Transm* 106:1171-88, 1999.
10. Linde K, ter Riet G, Hondras M, et al: Systematic reviews of complementary therapies—an annotated bibliography. Part 2: herbal medicine, *BMC Complement Altern Med* 1:5, 2001.
11. Pittler MH, Ernst E: *Ginkgo biloba* extract for the treatment of intermittent claudication: a meta-analysis of randomized trials, *Am J Med* 108:276-81, 2000.
12. Holstein N: Ginkgo special extract Egb 761 in tinnitus therapy. An overview of results of completed clinical trials, *Fortschr Med* 118:157-64, 2001 (abstract).
13. Ernst E, Stevinson C: *Ginkgo biloba* for tinnitus: a review, *Clin Otolaryngol* 24: 164-7, 1999.
14. Evans JR: *Ginkgo biloba* extract for age-related macular degeneration, *Cochrane Database Syst Rev* 2:CD001775, 2000.
15. Chung HS, Harris A, Kristinsson JK, et al: *Ginkgo biloba* extract increases ocular blood flow velocity, *J Ocul Pharmacol Ther* 15:233-40, 1999.

16. Hasenohrl RU, Nichau CH, Frisch CH, et al: Anxiolytic-like effect of combined extracts of *Zingiber officinale* and *Ginkgo biloba* in the elevated plus-maze, *Pharmacol Biochem Behav* 53:271-5, 1996.
17. Klepser TB, Klepser ME: Unsafe and potentially safe herbal therapies, *Am J Health Syst Pharm* 56:125-38, 1999.
18. Cupp MJ: Herbal remedies: adverse effects and drug interactions, *Am Fam Physician* 59:1239-45, 1999.
19. Izzo AA, Ernst E: Interactions between herbal medicines and prescribed drugs: a systematic review, *Drugs* 61:2163-75, 2001.
20. Braun L: Herb-drug interaction guide, *Aust Fam Physician* 30:259-60, 2001.

CHAPTER 71

GINSENG (*ELEUTHEROCOCCUS SENTICOSUS* AND *PANAX GINSENG*)

Despite its popularity and use over many centuries, scientific evidence supporting the clinical use of ginseng is weak.

The name *Panax* is derived from the term *panacea*, and ginseng is regarded as a cure-all. Ginseng is known as an adaptogen, capable of normalizing physiologic disturbances. It has traditionally been used as a tonic to adapt to stress and restore vitality. Ginseng is reputed to enhance vitality, boost the immune response, and promote cellular metabolism and longevity. It is available as tea, capsules, extracts, and chewing gum.

The efficacy of ginseng is influenced by its source. Several plants from the genus *Panax* are grown in China, Korea, Japan, and Russia. *Panax ginseng* (Korean or Asian ginseng), *P. quinquefolius* (American ginseng), and *P. vietnamensis* (Vietnamese ginseng) are considered to be more potent than Siberian ginseng (*Eleutherococcus senticosus*). Analysis of commercial ginseng preparations from the genera *Panax* and *Eleutherococcus* made in the United States revealed that the products were correctly labeled as to plant genus; however, marked variability was observed in the concentrations of constituents.[1] The concentration of ginsenosides varied by 15-fold in capsules and 36-fold in liquids, and the concentration of eleutherosides varied by 43-fold in capsules and 200-fold in liquids.[1] This may explain the mixed clinical results attributed to this herb.[2] Despite its popular uses, which range from treating impotence and male infertility to boosting energy and combating physical stress, well-conducted clinical trials do not support the efficacy of ginseng to treat any condition.[3] However, laboratory studies do suggest that Siberian ginseng has immunity-enhancing and anti-fatigue, anti-stress, and antidepressant effects.[4]

MECHANISM OF ACTION

Constituents of most ginseng species include ginsenosides, polysaccharides, peptides, polyacetylenic alcohols, and fatty acids. The activity of ginseng is largely related to the combination and relative concentration of the ginsenosides found in the main and lateral roots of the plant. The ginsenoside content of different species of ginseng varies widely, as does the ginsenoside content within a single species cultivated in two different locations.[5] The Asian root contains some 13 ginsenosides, the active principles of which are triterpenoid saponin glycosides. Although elements of ginseng (e.g., the diols) tend to sedate, the overall balance favors stimulation and ginseng is regarded as a tonic herb.

Ginseng appears to enhance stress adaptation through modulation of adrenal activity via the hypothalamo-pituitary-adrenocorticol pathway. By targeting the hypothalamus, ginseng appears to create an environment in which both the response to stressors and feedback from the stress response are rapid and effective. The ability of ginsenosides to independently target multireceptor systems at the plasma membrane, as well as to activate intracellular steroid receptors, may explain some of the other pharmacologic effects.[6] Ginseng saponins have been reported to demonstrate antimutagenic, anticancer, anti-inflammatory, antidiabetic, and neurovascular effects.[7] Ginseng enhances immune function, increasing natural killer cell activity and interferon production.

Platelet aggregation may be prevented by a nonsaponin fraction in the root that inhibits thromboxane A_2.[8]

DOSE

Enormous variation in the potency of products has been reported. A standard daily dose of 4 to 6 g of high-quality ginseng root or 200 mg of root extract containing 5% ginsenosides one to three times a day is recommended.

Extracts are often standardized so that 200 mg corresponds to about 1 g of root. At levels of 1 g of crude root, ginseng is well tolerated. Higher doses may cause side effects. Use of standardized ginseng preparations is required to achieve consistent results and reduce the risk of toxic effects. *Panax ginseng*, with the steroidal nature of its active constituents, is a more powerful herb than *Eleutherococcus senticosus* (Siberian ginseng) (see Table 71-1).

Because of its possible hormone-like or hormone-inducing effects, ginseng is usually used for up to 3 months, but continuous use may be appropriate for elderly people. Cyclic use of ginseng for 2 to 3 weeks, followed by an herb-free period of 2 weeks, is recommended for long-term administration.

TABLE 71-1 ■ A Comparison of Ginseng from Different Sources

	SIBERIAN GINSENG	AMERICAN GINSENG
Potency	Less potent	More potent
Safety	Safer	Less safe
Cost	Cheaper	More expensive

CLINICAL USES

Despite popular use, evidence of the efficacy of ginseng from both animal and human studies is equivocal.[3,9-11] A review of 16 double-blind, randomized, placebo-controlled trials of ginseng root extract revealed no compelling evidence for use of ginseng to enhance physical and psychomotor performance, cognitive function, or immunomodulation or to control diabetes mellitus and herpes simplex type II infections.[11] On the other hand, in a comparative, randomized, double-blind study, multivitamins plus ginseng were found to be more effective than the multivitamins alone in improving the quality of life in a population subjected to high physical and mental stress.[12] A prospective, double-blind, placebo-controlled, randomized, clinical trial demonstrated that neither 200 mg nor 400 mg of ginseng taken over 60 days had any effect on mood or affect in healthy young adults.[13] On the other hand, a double-blind study showed that administration of 350 mg of ginseng daily for 6 weeks improved psychomotor performance by shortening reaction time, although it did not alter exercise capacity.[14] Results of another study confirmed that long-term supplementation of up to 2 g of *P. ginseng* root (400 mg of ginseng) failed to improve maximal aerobic exercise performance.[15] Improvements in learning, memory, and physical capability may be influenced by the dose administered. Furthermore, discrepancies in clinical outcome may also be explained by the low bioavailability of ginsenosides until they are acted on by digestive enzymes and colonic bacteria.

The incidence of human cancer appears to decrease with the duration of ginseng use. Case-control studies suggest that *P. ginseng* C.A. Meyer is a nonorgan-specific cancer preventive agent.[16] The effect is dose-dependent, and only ginseng extract or powder appears to be effective. Although both animal and epidemiologic studies suggest that ginseng may have a cancer-preventive effect, particularly at the initiation phase of carcinogenesis,[17,18] this protective effect remains unproven in humans. Its antioxidant properties, as demonstrated by attenuation of lipid peroxidation in rat brain homogenates with extracts of red ginseng,[19] and its immune-boosting effect, demonstrated by use of a standardized extract of ginseng root in vaccination against influenza,[20] may contribute to its potential to reduce the risk of cancer. In a study of breast cancer cell growth, investigators found that American ginseng, in contrast to estradiol, caused a dose-dependent decrease in cell proliferation.[21] Estradiol significantly increased the proliferative phase and decreased the resting phase. In vitro testing of various breast cancer therapeutic agents with American ginseng resulted in a significant suppression of cell growth for most drugs evaluated.[21]

In nondiabetic individuals, 3, 6, or 9 g of American ginseng taken 40, 80, or 120 minutes before a glucose challenge improved glucose tolerance.[22] American ginseng, which appears to have postabsorptive effects and may enhance insulin secretion, is postulated to improve diabetes control, ameliorate insulin resistance, and reduce associated risk factors such as hyperlipidemia and hypertension.[23] Its potential appears most likely to be realized when used in conjunction with konjac-mannan.

Ginsenosides are thought to have an effect at different levels of the hypo-thalamo-pituitary-testis axis and may influence reproduction. A clinical study indicated that *P. ginseng* extract increased the number of spermatozoa, progressive oscillating motility, and testosterone levels.[24] Ginsenosides may also influence diurnal rhythms. Ginseng may help to maintain a normal sleep and wakefulness cycle.[25] A double-blind study, in which the influence of ginseng on the quality of life of urban dwellers was investigated, showed that a daily dose of 40 mg of ginseng extract for 12 weeks significantly improved quality of life, including sleep.[26] One mechanism for the central nervous system–depressant action of ginseng extract and ginsenosides is through regulation of GABAergic neurotransmission. Ginsenosides have been reported to compete with agonists for binding to (-aminobutyric acid A and B receptors.

TOXICITY/DRUG INTERACTIONS

Ginseng is regarded as a potentially safe herb.[27] It is well tolerated at thera-peutic doses, and a recent study demonstrated no advantage to increasing the dose of American ginseng above 3 g to reduce postprandial glycemia in patients with type 2 diabetes.[28]

Ginseng may alter the antiplatelet or anticoagulant effect of drugs or herbs. It interacts with warfarin, phenelzine, monoamine oxidase inhibitors, amphetamines, and caffeine.[29] It may reverse the effects of tranquilizers. Ginseng (*Panax* species) induces mania if used concomitantly with antide-pressants such as phenelzine, a monoamine oxidase inhibitor.[30] In fact, the most commonly reported side effects are arousal and anxiety, but these diminish with continued use or dosage reduction. Although the root con-tains both stimulatory and sedative agents, the net impact is considered to be stimulatory.

Ginseng may impair digoxin action or monitoring, and it should not be used with estrogens or corticosteroids because of possible additive effects.[31]

CLINICAL CAUTION

High doses may cause hypertension, euphoria, insomnia, and anxiety. Contraindications are pregnancy, hypertension, and a coagulation defect. Persons with malignant hypertension or cardiac arrhythmia should avoid ginseng, as should those with acute asthma or a tendency to bleed. In view of its possible estrogenic activity, ginseng should be avoided in estrogen-dependent conditions (e.g., uterine leiomyomas, endometriosis, breast can-cer, and fibrocystic breast disease).

A ginseng abuse syndrome—presenting with hypertension, nervous euphoria, insomnia, skin lesions, and morning diarrhea—has been described.[32]

PRACTICE TIPS

- *Panax ginseng* may decrease the effectiveness of antihypertensive agents and potentiate the anticoagulant effects of warfarin.
- For prevention of unintended hypoglycemia in nondiabetic subjects, American ginseng should probably be taken with a meal.[22]
- Ginseng should not be prescribed when a patient has an acute infection or breast cancer.
- Health care practitioners should caution patients against mixing herbs and prescription drugs.
- Women taking ginseng may experience breast tenderness.

REFERENCES

1. Harkey MR, Henderson GL, Gershwin ME, et al: Variability in commercial ginseng products: an analysis of 25 preparations, *Am J Clin Nutr* 73:1101-6, 2001.
2. Bucci LR: Selected herbals and human exercise performance, *Am J Clin Nutr* 72(suppl 2):624S-636S, 2000.
3. Ernst E: The risk-benefit profile of commonly used herbal therapies: ginkgo, St. John's wort, ginseng, echinacea, saw palmetto, and kava, *Ann Intern Med* 136: 42-53, 2002.
4. Deyama T, Nishibe S, Nakazawa Y: Constituents and pharmacological effects of Eucommia and Siberian ginseng, *Acta Pharmacol Sin* 22:1057-70, 2001.
5. Yuan CS, Wu JA, Lowell T, et al: Gut and brain effects of American ginseng root on brainstem neuronal activities in rats, *Am J Chin Med* 26:47-55, 1998.
6. Attele AS, Wu JA, Yuan CS: Ginseng pharmacology: multiple constituents and multiple actions, *Biochem Pharmacol* 58:1685-93, 1999.
7. Ong YC, Yong EL: Panax (ginseng)—panacea or placebo? Molecular and cellular basis of its pharmacological activity, *Ann Acad Med Singapore* 29:42-6, 2000.
8. Craig WJ: Health-promoting properties of common herbs, *Am J Clin Nutr* 70(suppl 3):491S-499S, 1999.
9. Bahrke MS, Morgan WR: Evaluation of the ergogenic properties of ginseng: an update, *Sports Med* 29:113-33, 2000.
10. Kitts D, Hu C: Efficacy and safety of ginseng, *Public Health Nutr* 3:473-8, 2000.
11. Vogler BK, Pittler MH, Ernst E: The efficacy of ginseng. A systematic review of randomised clinical trials, *Eur J Clin Pharmacol* 55:567-75, 1999.
12. Caso Marasco A, Vargas Ruiz R, Salas Villagomez A, et al: Double-blind study of a multivitamin complex supplemented with ginseng extract, *Drugs Exp Clin Res* 22:323-9, 1996.
13. Cardinal BJ, Engels HJ: Ginseng does not enhance psychological well-being in healthy, young adults: results of a double-blind, placebo-controlled, randomized clinical trial, *J Am Diet Assoc* 101:655-60, 2001.

14. Ziemba AW, Chmura J, Kaciuba-Uscilko H, et al: Ginseng treatment improves psychomotor performance at rest and during graded exercise in young athletes, *Int J Sport Nutr* 9:371-7, 1999.

15. Engels HJ, Wirth JC: No ergogenic effects of ginseng (Panax ginseng C.A. Meyer) during graded maximal aerobic exercise, *J Am Diet Assoc* 97:1110-5, 1997.

16. Yun TK, Choi SY, Yun HY: Epidemiological study on cancer prevention by ginseng: are all kinds of cancers preventable by ginseng? *J Korean Med Sci* 16(suppl):S19-S27, 2001.

17. Hinck G: The role of herbal products in the prevention of cancer, *Topics Clin Chiro* 6:54-62, 1999.

18. Shin HR, Kim JY, Yun TK, et al: The cancer-preventive potential of *Panax ginseng*: a review of human and experimental evidence, *Cancer Causes Control* 11:565-76, 2000.

19. Keum YS, Park KK, Lee JM, et al: Antioxidant and anti-tumor promoting activities of the methanol extract of heat-processed ginseng, *Cancer Lett* 150:41-8, 2000.

20. Scaglione F, Cattaneo G, Alessandria M, et al: Efficacy and safety of the standardised Ginseng extract G115 for potentiating vaccination against the influenza syndrome and protection against the common cold, *Drugs Exp Clin Res* 22:65-72, 1996.

21. Duda RB, Zhong Y, Navas V, et al: American ginseng and breast cancer therapeutic agents synergistically inhibit MCF-7 breast cancer cell growth, *J Surg Oncol* 72:230-9, 1999.

22. Vuksan V, Stavro MP, Sievenpiper JL, et al: American ginseng improves glycemia in individuals with normal glucose tolerance: effect of dose and time escalation, *J Am Coll Nutr* 19:738-44, 2000.

23. Vuksan V, Sievenpiper JL, Xu Z, et al: Konjac-Mannan and American ginseng: emerging alternative therapies for type 2 diabetes mellitus, *J Am Coll Nutr* 20(suppl 5):370S-380S, 2001.

24. Salvati G, Genovesi G, Marcellini L, et al: Effects of Panax Ginseng C.A. Meyer saponins on male fertility, *Panminerva Med* 38:249-54, 1996.

25. Attele AS, Xie JT, Yuan CS: Treatment of insomnia: an alternative approach, *Altern Med Rev* 5:249-59, 2000.

26. Marasco AC, Ruiz RV, Villagomex AS, et al: Double-blind study of a multivitamin complex supplemented with ginseng extract, *Drugs Exp Clin Res* 22:323-9, 1996.

27. Klepser TB, Klepser ME: Unsafe and potentially safe herbal therapies, *Am J Health Syst Pharm* 56:125-38, 1999.

28. Vuksan V, Stavro MP, Sievenpiper JL, et al: Similar postprandial glycemic reductions with escalation of dose and administration time of American ginseng in type 2 diabetes, *Diabetes Care* 23:1221-6, 2000.

29. Cupp MJ: Herbal remedies: adverse effects and drug interactions, *Am Fam Physician* 59:1239-45, 1999.

30. Izzo AA, Ernst E: Interactions between herbal medicines and prescribed drugs: a systematic review, *Drugs* 61:2163-75, 2001.

31. Miller LG: Herbal medicinals: selected clinical considerations focusing on known or potential drug-herb interactions, *Arch Intern Med* 158:2200-11, 1998.

32. Mills S, Bone K: *Principles and practice of phytotherapy*, Edinburgh, 2000, Churchill Livingstone.

■ CHAPTER 72 ■

GOLDENSEAL (*HYDRASTIS CANADENSIS*)

> *Berberis* species are freely available as dietary supplements, yet authoritative opinion suggests that although there is no evidence for the efficacy of these herbs, there are risks associated with plant parts containing berberine.

Hydrastis canadensis (goldenseal) is one of a number of plants that contain the alkaloid berberine. Berberine extracts and decoctions have demonstrated significant antimicrobial activity against a variety of organisms. Berberine is used clinically to treat bacterial diarrhea, intestinal parasite infections, and ocular trachoma infections. Goldenseal is also used topically to treat aphthous ulcers.

MECHANISM OF ACTION

Berberine contains alkaloids that have an anti-inflammatory effect, resulting in dose-dependent inhibition of arachidonic acid release from cell membranes. It also appears to have immunostimulant and antimicrobial effects. It may prevent cellular adherence of bacteria and appears toxic to a number of parasites.

DOSE

The therapeutic dosage of berberine for most clinical situations is 200 mg orally two to four times daily.[1]

CLINICAL USES

Results of animal studies have confirmed that berberine is effective in the treatment of gastrointestinal infections caused by endotoxin-producing bacteria (e.g., cholera, enteropathogenic *Escherichia coli*) and parasites such as *Giardia lamblia* and *Entamoeba histolytica*.[2] Berberine may also inhibit intestinal fluid accumulation and ion secretion. Goldenseal may be used in rotation with, in combination with, or as an alternative to echinacea in the early treatment of upper respiratory tract infections (125 mg five times a day) or herpes infections (125 mg four times a day).[3] Results of clinical studies have also confirmed the superiority of berberine chloride in treating trachoma.[2]

In addition to its antimicrobial action, berberine has an anti-inflammatory effect. In vitro studies with human cell lines have demonstrated that berberine inhibits activator protein 1, a key transcription factor in inflammation and carcinogenesis.[4] Inhibition of COX-2 transcription and N-acetyltransferase activity in colon cancer cell lines supports the notion that berberine may possess antitumor properties.[5]

Berberine may have a role in the treatment of ischemia-induced ventricular tachyarrhythmia,[2] chronic fatigue syndrome (125 mg twice daily),[3] and, in combination with hamamelis, varicose veins. It may influence smooth muscle contraction, ventricular tachyarrhythmia, and platelet aggregation.

TOXICITY/DRUG INTERACTIONS

Goldenseal is considered safe in recommended doses. Side effects, such as dry mouth and, rarely, dyspepsia, lethargy, and photosensitivity, are possible if more than 0.5 g of berberine is ingested. High doses of berberine cause gastrointestinal discomfort, dyspnea, low blood pressure, flu-like symptoms, and cardiac damage.

Because berberine induces several isoenzymes of the hepatic cytochrome P-450 enzyme system, it may influence the metabolism of numerous drugs. The efficacy of warfarin may be decreased, as may the efficacy of oral contraceptives and estrogen.

CLINICAL CAUTION

Berberine displaces bilirubin and can precipitate jaundice in susceptible neonates. Because of its potential for causing uterine contractions and miscarriage, it should also be avoided during pregnancy.

In vitro experiments in which keratinocytes were irradiated with ultraviolet A in the presence of 50 μmol/L berberine resulted in an 80% decrease in cell viability and a threefold increase in DNA damage.[6] These findings suggest that exposure to sunlight or artificial light sources emitting ultraviolet A radiation should be avoided when topical preparations derived from goldenseal or products containing berberine are used.

PRACTICE TIPS

- Berberine may be effective in treating warts.
- Goldenseal in doses of 2 or more grams daily requires medical monitoring, because it decreases effectiveness of antihypertension therapy (e.g., β-blockers).

- Berberine increases the toxic effects of alcohol, and berberine and alcohol should not be used concurrently.

REFERENCES

1. Birdsall TC, Kelly GS: Berberine: therapeutic potential of an alkaloid found in several medicinal plants, *Altern Med Rev* 2:94-103, 1997.
2. Berberine, *Altern Med Rev* 5:175-7, 2000.
3. Diefendorf D, Healey J, Kalyn W, editors: *The healing power of vitamins, minerals and herbs*, Surry Hills, Australia, 2000, Readers Digest.
4. Fukuda K, Hibiya Y, Mutoh M, et al: Inhibition of activator protein 1 activity by berberine in human hepatoma cells, *Planta Med* 65:381-3, 1999.
5. Fukuda K, Hibiya Y, Mutoh M, et al: Inhibition by berberine of cyclooxygenase-2 transcriptional activity in human colon cancer cells, *J Ethnopharmacol* 66:227-33, 1999.
6. Inbaraj JJ, Kukielczak BM, Bilski P, et al: Photochemistry and photocytotoxicity of alkaloids from goldenseal (*Hydrastis canadensis* L.) 1. Berberine, *Chem Res Toxicol* 14:1529-34, 2001.

■ CHAPTER 73 ■

New Zealand Green-Lipped Mussel (*Perna canaliculus*)

> Despite lay enthusiasm, evidence to show that green-lipped mussel is
> clinically effective is equivocal.

The New Zealand green-lipped mussel (*Perna canaliculus*) is attracting interest for the treatment of arthritis. It, like other ω-3 fatty acids, has potential anti-inflammatory activity.

MECHANISM OF ACTION

Analysis of an extract of green-lipped mussel, Lyprinol, revealed that the main lipid classes are sterol esters (predominantly desmosterol and brassicasterol), triglycerides, free fatty acids (predominantly eicosapentaenoic acid and docosahexaenoic acid), sterols (predominantly cholesterol), and phospholipids.[1] This contrasts with other major sources of ω-3 fatty acids, such as tuna and flaxseed. In tuna, triglycerides are the main lipids, the dominant ω-3 fatty acid is docosahexaenoic acid, and the major sterol is β-sitosterol. In flaxseed oil, triglycerides are the main lipids, aminolevulinic acid is the main ω-3 fatty acid, and β-sitosterol is the main sterol.

Like fish oil supplements, green-lipped mussel may potentially benefit rheumatoid arthritis by ω-3 fatty acid suppression of the immune system and its cytokine repertoire.[2] Green-lipped mussel extract contains a weak prostaglandin inhibitor. Lyprinol subfractions have been shown to inhibit leukotriene B_4 biosynthesis by polymorphonuclear leukocytes in vitro and prostaglandin E_2 production by activated macrophages.[3] Much of this anti-inflammatory activity is associated with ω-3 fatty acids and natural antioxidants such as carotenoids.

DOSE

No dosage consensus has been achieved. Dietary supplements provide approximately 1000 mg daily.

CLINICAL USES

A placebo-controlled trial of patients with rheumatoid arthritis demonstrated, after 6 months of therapy, that green-lipped mussel extract did not significantly improve any laboratory or clinical indices of disease activity.[4] Some years later, Lyprinol, a lipid-rich freeze-dried extract of green-lipped mussel, was shown to have significant anti-inflammatory activity in humans and animals.[3] The doses of Lyprinol required to achieve a demonstrable benefit were lower than those of nonsteroidal anti-inflammatory drugs and 200-fold lower than doses of other seed or fish oils.

TOXICITY/DRUG INTERACTIONS

Anorexia, nausea, and vomiting are possible side effects. However, animal studies suggest that Lyprinol, in contrast to nonsteroidal anti-inflammatory drugs, is not gastrotoxic and does not affect platelet aggregation.[3]

CLINICAL CAUTION

A hypersensitivity reaction may occur.

PRACTICE TIPS

• The heavy metal content of mussels grown in potentially polluted water may create a health hazard.

REFERENCES

1. Sinclair AJ, Murphy KJ, Li D: Marine lipids: overview "news insights and lipid composition of Lyprinol," *Allerg Immunol (Paris)* 32:261-71, 2000.
2. Darlington LG, Stone TW: Antioxidants and fatty acids in the amelioration of rheumatoid arthritis and related disorders, *Br J Nutr* 85:251-69, 2001.
3. Halpern GM: Anti-inflammatory effects of a stabilized lipid extract of Perna canaliculus (Lyprinol), *Allerg Immunol (Paris)* 32:272-8, 2000.
4. Larkin JG, Capell HA, Sturrock RD: Seatone in rheumatoid arthritis: a six-month placebo-controlled study, *Ann Rheum Dis* 44:199-201, 1985.

■ CHAPTER 74 ■

HAWTHORN (*CRATAEGUS OXYACANTHA*)

> Hawthorn contains diverse constituents, some that have similar and others that have opposing physiologic effects. When given in isolation, particular compounds extracted from hawthorn may have a very different clinical effect from that of the whole fruit extract.

Hawthorn has cardiotonic, hypotensive, antiarrhythmic, and antioxidant activity. Hawthorn's cardiovascular effects appear to be primarily due to its inotropic and chronotropic effects on the myocardium, its effects on coronary blood flow and oxygen utilization, and its ability to enhance the integrity of blood vessels.

Its current uses include treatment for angina, hypertension, arrhythmias, and congestive heart failure. It is the herbal practitioner's digitalis.

MECHANISM OF ACTION

The main constituents of hawthorn are flavonoids, triterpene saponins, and a few cardioactive amines. Leaves are good sources of oligomeric procyanidins and flowers are also good sources of flavonoids. The flavonoids, especially the oligomeric procyanidins, are believed to be primarily responsible for the cardiovascular protective activity of hawthorn. Hawthorn exerts its cardioprotective actions through the following[1-5]:

- Increasing coronary flow and the strength (positive ionotropic effect) and rate (positive chronotropic effect) of cardiac contraction. Although certain flavonoids have antagonistic actions, in vivo the dominant flavonoid effects are cardiotropic and vasodilatory. By prolonging the refractory period, hawthorn also achieves an antiarrhythmic effect. Hawthorn is an effective treatment option for cardiac conditions for which digitalis is not yet indicated.
- Enhancing the integrity of the blood vessels. Flavonoids have significant antioxidant activity and collagen-stabilizing effects. They work synergistically with vitamin C, enhancing its activity and promoting capillary stability. Both radical scavenging and inhibition of human neutrophil elastase by the oligomeric procyanidin fragment of the leaves and flowers may enhance cardioprotection.

- Beneficially influencing the lipid profile. In addition to directly protecting low-density lipoprotein (LDL) from oxidation, hawthorn may indirectly protect LDL from oxidation by maintaining the concentration of α-tocopherol.[6] Blood cholesterol levels are reduced by suppression of endogenous cholesterol production and exogenous cholesterol absorption. Cholesterol biosynthesis is reduced by upregulating hepatic LDL receptors, resulting in greater influx of plasma LDL cholesterol into the liver. Cholesterol degradation to bile acids is enhanced, and animal studies suggest that cholesterol absorption is reduced by downregulation of intestinal acyl coenzyme A/cholesterol acyltransferase activity.[7]
- Reducing blood pressure. By interfering with angiotensin-converting enzyme, a vasoconstrictor, hawthorn may normalize blood pressure in mild hypertension.

Different flavonoid constituents have differing effects on the heart. Some flavonoids increase coronary flow, left ventricular pressure, and heart rate; some have no effect; and others may even decrease these parameters.[4] This type of balanced effect is seen in many plant species.

DOSE

Traditionally, a daily dose has consisted of one of the following: 1.5 to 3.5 g of dried flower, leaf, or berry as infusion or decoction; two or three tablets with 1 g of leaves and flowers standardized to contain 15 to 20 mg of oligomeric procyanidins and 6 to 7 mg of flavonoids; 3 to 6 mL of 1:2 liquid extract of hawthorn berry; or 7.5 to 17.5 mL of 1:5 tincture of hawthorn berry.

A typical therapeutic dose of an extract, standardized to contain 1.8% vitexin-4 rhamnoside, is 100 to 250 mg three times daily.[1] A standardized extract containing 18% procyanidolic oligomers is dosed in the range of 250 to 500 mg daily.[1]

CLINICAL USES

Hawthorn fruit extract has been shown to have many health benefits including cardiovascular protective, hypotensive, and hypocholesterolemic effects.

In Europe, hawthorn is used as frequently as digoxin for treatment of heart failure and arrhythmia.[8] Doses of 5 g or 160 to 900 mg extract of hawthorn for 6 or more weeks seems to increase coronary perfusion and decrease peripheral resistance in patients with cardiac failure. Animal studies have shown that hawthorn extract prolongs the refractory phase, potentially reducing the risk of arrhythmias.[9] This gives it an advantage over other cardioprotective drugs (e.g., digoxin) that shorten the refractory period of the myocardium.

The antioxidant and anti-inflammatory effects, the peripheral and coronary vasodilation, the protection afforded against ischemia-induced ventricular arrhythmias and the cyclic adenosine monophosphate–independent positive inotropic effect detected in vitro, and experimental animal studies have resulted in an international study. A randomized, placebo-controlled, double-blind study is underway to investigate whether *Crataegus* Special Extract WS 1442 (hawthorn leaves with flowers) alters the mortality rate of patients with congestive heart failure.[4] There is growing clinical support for use of this herb in the treatment of congestive cardiac failure caused by ischemia or hypertension.[8,10] Results of a pilot study suggest that 500 mg of hawthorn extract may reduce resting diastolic blood pressure by week 10 of supplementation.[11] A tendency toward less anxiety was also observed.

TOXICITY/DRUG INTERACTIONS

Theoretically, hawthorn may act synergistically with digitalis, glycosides, β-blockers, and antihypertensive agents. The additive vasodilatory effect of hawthorn and antihypertensive agents may result in hypotension.

CLINICAL CAUTION

Acute oral toxic effects are encountered in animals at doses of 6 mg/kg body weight. Hawthorn is regarded as safe in humans in recommended doses.

PRACTICE TIPS

- It is safe to combine hawthorn with conventional drugs in the treatment of cardiac ischemia.
- Doses of digitalis and antihypertensive drugs may need modification if patients take hawthorn.
- Hawthorn should be used for more than 2 months in the treatment of cardiac conditions.
- Hawthorn appears to have a calming effect and may relieve insomnia in patients with heart disease.

REFERENCES

1. *Crataegus oxycantha*: hawthorne, *Altern Med Rev* 3:138-9, 1998.
2. Miller AL: Botanical influences on cardiovascular disease, *Altern Med Rev* 3:422-31, 1998.
3. Morelli V, Zoorob RJ: Alternative therapies: part II. Congestive heart failure and hypercholesterolemia, *Am Fam Physician* 62:1325-30, 2000.

4. Hertog MG, Kromhout D, Aravanis C, et al: Flavonoid intake and long-term risk of coronary heart disease and cancer in the seven countries study, *Arch Intern Med* 155:381-6, 1995.

5. Diefendorf D, Healey J, Kalyn W, editors: *The healing power of vitamins, minerals and herbs*, Surry Hills, Australia, 2000, Readers Digest.

6. Zhang Z, Chang Q, Zhu M, et al: Characterization of antioxidants present in hawthorn fruits, *J Nutr Biochem* 12:144-52, 2001.

7. Zhang Z, Ho WK, Huang Y, et al: Hawthorn fruit is hypolipidemic in rabbits fed a high cholesterol diet, *J Nutr* 132:5-10, 2002.

8. Pinn G: Herbs and cardiovascular disease, *Aust Fam Physician* 29:1149-53, 2000.

9. Holubarsch CJ, Colucci WS, Meinertz T, et al: Survival and prognosis: investigation of *Crataegus* extract WS 1442 in congestive heart failure (SPICE)— rationale, study design and study protocol, *Eur J Heart Fail* 2:431-7, 2000.

10. Mills S, Bone K: *Principles and practice of phytotherapy*, Edinburgh, 2000, Churchill Livingstone.

11. Walker AF, Marakis G, Morris AP, et al: Promising hypotensive effect of hawthorn extract: a randomized double-blind pilot study of mild, essential hypertension, *Phytother Res* 16:48-54, 2002.

■ CHAPTER 75 ■

IODINE

> Iodine deficiency is considered the single greatest cause of preventable brain damage and mental retardation.

Iodine is required for the synthesis of thyroid hormones. The thyroid gland may enlarge as a result of either iodine deficiency or iodine excess.

MECHANISM OF ACTION

Iodine is incorporated into an amino acid tyrosine, two molecules of which are then linked to form thyroid hormones. Thyroxine is more plentiful, but triiodothyronine is the more biologically potent hormone. Thyroid hormones increase the basal metabolic rate, speeding up metabolism. They control the rate of oxygen utilization and release energy from energy-producing nutrients.

When the dietary intake of iodine is inadequate, plasma levels of thyroid hormones fall, and more thyroid-stimulating hormone is released from the pituitary. If iodine deficiency persists, the thyroid gland enlarges in a vain attempt to trap more iodine and produce more thyroid hormones. Depending on the amount of iodine present, the glandular response, and the stage of the disease, the concentration of thyroid hormones may be increased or decreased. Epidemiologic studies suggest that the major consequence of mild to moderate iodine deficiency is hyperthyroidism, potentially complicated by cardiac arrhythmia, osteoporosis, and muscle wasting in the elderly.[1]

FOOD SOURCES

Good sources of iodine are kelp, seafood, dairy products, and iodized salt. Appreciable amounts of iodine are lost in cooking, possibly as much as 70%.[2] Iodized salt should be added to food after, rather than before, cooking. In addition to iodine, kelp contains carotenoids, fatty acids, and various other minerals.

DOSE

The recommended daily allowance for iodine is 0.14 mg (120-200 µg) or 75 µg/1000 kcal. Supplementary doses range from 1000 to 10,000 µg. In adults, prolonged intake of 1000 µg may result in toxicosis. Absorption is 100%.

In areas of Poland classified as being mildly to moderately iodine-deficient, iodine prophylaxis based only on iodized household salt (30 mg potassium iodide/kg salt) is highly effective.[3] Iodized salt in the United States contains around 76 µg of iodine per gram; however, depending on the region, inconsistency in the iodine content of iodized salt may result in iodine concentrations that exceed or fail to meet specific standards.[4]

CLINICAL USES

Iodine supplementation is used in the treatment of hypothyroidism in areas where soil is deficient in iodine. Hypothyroidism presents clinically as changes in menstruation, altered bowel function, a tendency to gain weight, increased sensitivity to heat or cold, and mood changes.

Although pregnant women and small children are not immediately endangered, an adequate iodine supply in utero and shortly after birth is crucial for physical and mental development. Iodine deficiency during pregnancy may lead to enlargement of the thyroid (goiter) in both mother and child and may cause neuropsychologic and intellectual impairment in the child. In adults, iodine deficiency may lead to mental slowness; however, the consequence of severe iodine deficiency in utero and in infancy is cretinism, a form of mental retardation. Although elevated hearing thresholds have been demonstrated in populations with endemic cretinism caused by severe iodine deficiency, a randomized, placebo-controlled trial has demonstrated that even children with mild iodine deficiencies have significantly higher hearing thresholds in the higher frequency range ($\geq$2000 Hz).[5] Adequate iodine supplementation, 200 µg/day, given early during pregnancy results in almost complete prevention of maternal and neonatal goitrogenesis.[6] Another double-blind study of children demonstrated that improvement in iodine status, rather than iodine status itself, determined mental performance in an initially iodine-deficient population. The authors suggest that iodine supplementation of schoolchildren with iodine deficiency may have a "catch-up" effect in terms of mental performance.[1]

TOXICITY/DRUG INTERACTIONS

Iodine excess inhibits thyroid hormone synthesis and can result in a goiter. A grossly enlarged thyroid gland may obstruct the airway in infants. There is also evidence that a high iodine intake may be associated with autoimmune hypothyroidism and that Graves' disease may manifest at a younger age and be more difficult to treat.[7] Goitrogens found in foods such as cabbage or turnips impair utilization of iodine and increase the dietary requirement for this mineral.

CLINICAL CAUTION

In iodine-deficient areas, nodules are frequently associated with Graves' disease, and the incidence of carcinoma is high in palpable cold nodules.

PRACTICE TIPS

- Urinary iodine content reflects intake; plasma-bound iodine or thyroxine reflects function.
- Inadequate iodine consumption leads to inadequate thyroid hormone production, and excess consumption can depress thyroid activity.

REFERENCES

1. Laurberg P, Nohr SB, Pedersen KM, et al: Thyroid disorders in mild iodine deficiency, *Thyroid* 10:951-63, 2000.
2. Verma M, Raghuvanshi RS: Dietary iodine intake and prevalence of iodine deficiency disorders in adults, *J Nutr Environ Med* 11:175-80, 2001.
3. Szybinski Z, Delange F, Lewinski A, et al: A programme of iodine supplementation using only iodised household salt is efficient—the case of Poland, *Eur J Endocrinol* 144:331-7, 2001.
4. Kumarasiri JP, Fernandopulle BM, Lankathillake MA: Iodine content of commercially available iodised salt in the Sri Lankan market, *Ceylon Med J* 43:84-7, 1998.
5. van den Briel T, West CE, Hautvast JG, et al: Mild iodine deficiency is associated with elevated hearing thresholds in children in Benin, *Eur J Clin Nutr* 55:763-8, 2001.
6. Glinoer D: Pregnancy and iodine, *Thyroid* 11:471-81, 2001.
7. van den Briel T, West CE, Bleichrodt N, et al: Improved iodine status is associated with improved mental performance of schoolchildren in Benin, *Am J Clin Nutr* 72:1179-85, 2000.
8. Mishra A, Mishra SK: Thyroid nodules in Graves' disease: implications in an endemically iodine deficient area, *J Postgrad Med* 47:244-7, 2001.

■ CHAPTER 76 ■

IRON

> Free iron is toxic to cells, yet heme-bound iron (hemoglobin) is essential for cellular viability.

Iron is a constituent of hemoglobin and of enzymes involved in energy metabolism. Functional iron makes up 75% of total body iron and equals 4.0 g in adults. Approximately 2.5 g of iron is found in hemoglobin. The rest is found in myoglobin and enzymes, such as ribonucleotide reductase, a key enzyme in DNA synthesis. Adult males store around 1.0 g of iron, but iron stores are lower in adult females. The time required to deplete reserves of iron is 750 days in men but only 125 days in women.

In Australia, about 4% of all women and 8% of women aged 30 to 49 years have iron deficiency. One in 10 female blood donors, pregnant women, teenage girls, and infants have depleted iron stores. Twenty-seven percent of vegetarians have iron deficiency. About 20 mg of iron is lost per menstrual cycle. Blood donation of 1 L results in a loss of 0.5 mg of iron. During pregnancy 2.5 mg of maternal iron is utilized per day, and breast-feeding depletes up to 1 mg of iron per day.[1]

Iron deficiency causes anemia, has been linked to learning problems in children and adults, and increases susceptibility to infection.

MECHANISM OF ACTION

Iron is essential for a number of oxidation-reduction reactions. Electrons are readily transferred between ferrous (Fe^{2+}) and ferric (Fe^{3+}) iron, a property that makes iron physiologically invaluable. As a component of heme, iron is involved through hemoglobin in the transport of oxygen in the blood. The iron in myoglobin facilitates movement of oxygen into muscle cells. As a component of cytochromes, iron contributes to energy production through the electron transport chain. Iron is also a cofactor for antioxidant enzymes.

Iron deficiency anemia increases nitric oxide production. Endothelium-derived nitric oxide favors vasodilation and increased perfusion provides an interim compensatory mechanism. Iron supplementation restores circulating haemoglobin levels and the elevated nitric oxide concentrations detected in iron deficiency anemia return to normal.[2]

Iron is transported as transferrin and stored as ferritin and hemosiderin. Iron status is regulated by balancing absorption, transport, storage, and loss. Except in patients with a high mean cellular volume or erythrocyte disorders such as thalassemia, a low reticulocyte hemoglobin content is a sensitive and specific predictor of inadequate bone marrow iron stores.[3]

FOOD SOURCES

Iron is found in the diet in two forms—heme iron, which is more readily absorbed (25%), and nonheme (inorganic) iron, which is poorly absorbed (<7%). Important sources of dietary iron include the following:

- Lean red meat, fish, and poultry, which contain heme iron.
- Fruits and vegetables, which contain variable amounts of nonheme iron and possess various enhancers and inhibitors of absorption. High levels of available iron are found in citrus fruit, tomatoes, papaya, broccoli, pumpkin, and cabbage. Chickpeas are also a good source.
- Cereal-based foods with low levels of inorganic iron.

Acidity promotes conversion of ferric to ferrous iron, the form most easily absorbed. Foods rich in vitamin C (e.g., citrus fruits and fresh vegetables), eaten with small amounts of heme iron–containing foods, such as meat, may increase the amount of inorganic iron absorbed from cereals, beans, and other vegetables. Otherwise, maximal iron absorption from a meal that includes inorganic iron can be achieved by simultaneous ingestion of 50 to 100 mg of vitamin C. As little as 50 mg of vitamin C can double the absorption of iron from other components in a meal. Other foods decrease the amount of inorganic iron absorbed from foods. Phytates (found in most grains, cereals, and spinach), polyphenols (found in tea, coffee, sorghum, and legumes), tannins (found in St. John's wort and saw palmetto), and calcium (found in dairy products) can inhibit iron absorption.

DOSE

The recommended daily allowance for iron is 10 to 20 mg or 8 mg/1000 kcal. Menstruating woman require more iron than men, as do pregnant (30 mg/day) and breast-feeding (15 mg/day) women. The therapeutic dose range is 10 to 50 mg/day.[4] In adults, prolonged intake of 100 mg of iron per day may result in toxicosis.

Iron is best absorbed when taken on an empty stomach with water or fruit juice. Iron salts used for supplementation differ little in their absorption capacity and likelihood of inducing side effects. Absorption and side effects are related to the concentration of iron present and to dose.

CLINICAL USES

Iron supplements are prescribed to treat iron deficiency anemia. At the clinical level, hypochromic microcytic anemia presents as pale conjunctivae, edematous atrophic papillae on the tongue, dysphagia, koilonychia, brittle nails, parasthesia, reduced resistance to infection, pica, and behavioral changes (e.g., irritability). Poor learning may persist after the anemia is corrected. Iron deficiency induces ventricular hypertrophy; and cardiac function demonstrates an increased inotropic, but not chronotropic response, to norepinephrine, the sympathetic neurotransmitter.[5] Immune function is depressed in both iron deficiency and excess.

Although iron deficiency may follow a hemorrhage, it is more frequently the result of a chronic problem. Iron deficiency may result from an inadequate diet, a physiologically determined increased demand for iron, or blood loss. A diagnosis of iron deficiency anemia is incomplete until a cause has been identified.

Iron deficiency attributable to chronic blood leakage from an underlying neoplasm or ulcer may be detected by means of an occult blood test. The heme-porphyrin (HemoQuant) test detects occult upper gastrointestinal tract blood loss significantly more frequently than the guaiac (Hemoccult II) or immunochemical (HemeSelect) test.[6] The kidneys are another potential source of microscopic blood loss. Women with menorrhagia have an increased requirement for iron.

During periods of increased demand, oral iron supplementation can prevent a deficiency state. Oral iron supplements are routinely given during pregnancy to meet the increased iron demand of around 1.23 g. In late pregnancy, the lowest acceptable hemoglobin level is 10.5 g; and 200 mg ferrous sulfate or equivalent, administered three times daily, is frequently recommended early in pregnancy to ensure that this level is met or exceeded.

Suspected dietary inadequacy can be detected early because sequential biochemical changes result from iron undernutrition. The progressive steps toward iron deficiency anemia are as follows:

- Reduced iron stores. Depletion of bone marrow stores presents clinically as reduced serum ferritin levels. Although a low serum ferritin level is diagnostic, an increased serum ferritin level does not preclude iron deficiency, because this level is also increased in infection.
- Reduced functional iron. This presents with decreased transferrin receptors, and as the residual binding capacity of iron increases (increased total iron binding capacity), transferrin saturation and protoporphyrin saturation are decreased.
- Reduced hemoglobin levels and decreased hematocrit.
- Decrease in erythrocyte mean corpuscular volume, mean corpuscular hemoglobin, and mean corpuscular hemoglobin concentration.

TOXICITY/DRUG INTERACTIONS

Long-term excess iron supplementation may cause constipation or diarrhea, leg cramps, nausea, and vomiting. Iron excess can result in hemosiderosis. Long-term ingestion in excess of 500 mg/day causes liver and heart damage.

Symptoms of acute iron overdose may not occur for up to 60 minutes or more after the overdose was taken. Early symptoms of iron overdose are diarrhea, fever, nausea, abdominal colic, and vomiting. Late symptoms of iron overdose are peripheral cyanosis, convulsions, drowsiness, and shock.

Hereditary hemochromatosis, a common inborn error of iron metabolism, is characterized by excess dietary iron absorption and iron deposition. In this condition, dysregulated iron homeostasis may cause hepatic failure, hepatocellular carcinoma, diabetes, cardiac failure, impotence, and arthritis.[7] Excess iron catalyzes formation of free radicals and increases the requirement for vitamins E and C and other antioxidants. Iron supplements and dimercaprol may combine in the body to form a harmful chemical.

CLINICAL CAUTION

Persons complaining of persistent fatigue, shortness of breath, and a decrease in physical performance should be checked for iron deficiency anemia.

PRACTICE TIPS

- Iron supplements and antacids or tetracyclines should not be taken within at least 1 hour, and preferably 2 hours, of each other.
- About half the iron in breast milk is absorbed, compared with only 10% in cow's milk.
- Staining of teeth caused by liquid forms of iron supplements can be reduced by mixing each dose in fruit or tomato juice and using a straw or dropper to prevent the solution from making contact with teeth.
- Iron stains on teeth can usually be removed by brushing with baking soda (sodium bicarbonate) or medicinal peroxide (hydrogen peroxide 3%).
- Cooking acidic food or fermenting beer in iron pots can increase the iron content to hazardous levels.

REFERENCES

1. Presgrave P, Biggs JC: The diagnosis and management of iron deficiency, *Mod Med Aust* 37:76-86, 1994.
2. Choi W, Pai H, Kim K, et al: Iron deficiency anemia increases nitric oxide production in healthy adolescents, *Ann Hematol* 81:1-6, 2002.

3. Mast AE, Blinder MA, Lu Q, et al: Clinical utility of the reticulocyte hemoglobin content in the diagnosis of iron deficiency, *Blood* 99:1489-91, 2002.
4. Brighthope I: Nutritional medicine tables, *J Aust Coll Nutr Env Med* 17:20-5, 1998.
5. Turner LR, Premo DA, Gibbs BJ, et al: Adaptations to iron deficiency: cardiac functional responsiveness to norepinephrine, arterial remodeling, and the effect of beta-blockade on cardiac hypertrophy, *BMC Physiol* 2:1, 2002.
6. Harewood GC, McConnell JP, Harrington JJ, et al: Detection of occult upper gastrointestinal tract bleeding: performance differences in fecal occult blood tests, *Mayo Clin Proc* 77:23-8, 2002.
7. Fleming RE, Sly WS: Mechanisms of iron accumulation in hereditary hemochromatosis, *Annu Rev Physiol* 64:663-80, 2002.

CHAPTER 77

KAVA KAVA (*PIPER METHYSTICUM*)

A herb that is contraindicated in pregnancy and breast-feeding and that should not be given to neonates, infants, and children is used as a traditional beverage in Fiji.

Kava kava is a bitter herb from the lateral roots of the *Piper methysticum* plant, a member of the black pepper family. It is believed to have sedative, anticonvulsive, antispasmodic, and central muscular relaxant effects. Kava is regarded as a natural relaxant and is used to treat anxiety, stress, and nervous restlessness without causing mental sluggishness. It has been used for relief of mild exogenous depression and menopausal symptoms. Its euphoretic and mild hallucinogenic properties have made it a popular choice for certain religious rites.

MECHANISM OF ACTION

Kavapyrones extracted from *P. methysticum* are pharmacologically active compounds with anticonvulsive, analgesic, and central muscle-relaxing properties.[1] Kava kava is thought to achieve its effect on the central nervous system through a number of mechanisms. Four lactones from kava (kavain, dihydrokavain, methysticin, and dihydromethysticin) have been found to have significant analgesic effects in animal studies. The analgesia appears to occur via nonopiate pathways. Gamma-aminobutyric acid binding is probably one mechanism for some of kava's sedative effects.[2] It is thought that the limbic system is the preferred site of action, with kavalactones possibly acting on γ-aminobutyric acid receptors to produce a mild sedative and anxiolytic effect.[3] In vitro studies have demonstrated that although kavalactones were not found to efficiently block uptake of serotonin, inhibition of norepinephrine uptake was demonstrated by three lactones.[4] Kava, which has been shown to inhibit experimentally induced convulsions in animals, is thought to achieve its anticonvulsive effect through affecting sodium and calcium ion channels.[5] Animal studies suggest that kavain is an effective in modulating excitatory signals in the hippocampus.[6] Kava kava also contains flavonoids.

DOSE

The recommended dosage for kava depends on the concentration of kavalactones. The therapeutic dosage is in the range of 50 to 70 mg of kavalactones three times daily. This may be taken as 1.5 to 3 g of dried root per day, 3 to 6 mL of 1:2 liquid extract per day, or one kava tablet (1.2-1.8 g standardized to contain 60 mg of kavalactones) two to four times daily. A total dosage of kavalactones in excess of 300 mg/day is regarded as undesirable.

CLINICAL USES

Kava kava is used to treat anxiety. Although several double-blind, placebo-controlled trials have demonstrated the anxiolytic effects of kava, these studies had ill-defined patient populations, small sample sizes, and short treatment duration.[7] Nonetheless, a review and meta-analysis of the efficacy of kava extract as a symptomatic treatment for anxiety indicated that kava extract was superior to placebo in all seven reviewed trials.[8] Kava is an efficacious short-term treatment for anxiety.[9] Clinical trials have demonstrated its superiority to placebo and have shown it to be roughly equivalent to oxazepam, 15 mg/day, or bromazepam, 9 mg/day.[10] Another study indicated that a kava extract is an acceptable alternative to tricyclic antidepressants and benzodiazepines in the treatment of anxiety disorders, with proven long-term efficacy and none of the tolerance problems associated with tricyclic antidepressants and benzodiazepines.[11] In fact, in a 5-week randomized, placebo-controlled, double-blind study of nonpsychotic nervous anxiety, tension, and restlessness, investigators found that not only was kava extract a well-tolerated, effective anxiolytic, it also achieved further symptom reduction after a change-over from benzodiazepine treatment.[12] A dose of 40 to 70 mg of kavalactone, administered orally two or three times daily, or 1.5 to 3.0 g of dried root, administered in divided doses throughout the day, has been found to be effective in reducing anxiety in a number of double-blind, placebo-controlled studies.[1] Kava improves concentration without altering reaction time. The effective dose of kava extract (standardized to contain 70% kavalactones) is 100 mg three times daily. This dose is similar to that used to treat mild insomnia.

Taking 150 mg of kavalactones or 2 g of dried root 30 to 60 minutes before going to bed aids sleep. Studies in animals have shown that kava extracts and kavalactones induce sleep and muscle relaxation. Several relatively short-term clinical studies provide favorable evidence that kava kava is effective in the treatment of insomnia.[13]

Kavain appears to be an effective surface anesthesia, comparable to cocaine in strength and duration of action. Subcutaneous injections have been known to provide anesthesia for several hours to several days. A 120 mg/kg dose of either dihydromethysticin or dihydrokavain was equivalent to 2.5 mg/kg morphine.[1]

Other observations of potential clinical relevance include the possible antimicrobial, antithrombotic, and antineoplastic effects. Kava may inhibit cyclooxygenase, leading to inhibition of thromboxane A_2.[1] Kavain reduces platelet aggregation and may predispose to easy bruising. Data from a recent epidemiologic study suggest that there is a close inverse relationship between cancer incidence and kava consumption.[14]

TOXICITY/DRUG INTERACTIONS

Kava has a number of adverse effects.[15] Persons taking more than 300 g of kava root per week are most likely to have poor health and experience temporary paresis, progressive ataxia, and muscle weakness. Kava ichthyosis, characterized by a dry, flaky, scaly skin, occurs with long-term consumption of 400 mg of kavalactones daily. The yellow skin discoloration is reversed on discontinuation of the drug. Ocular photosensitivity has also been reported. Extrapyramidal effects such as oral and lingual dyskinesia, oculogyric crisis, and exacerbations of Parkinson's disease have been reported at doses of 100 to 450 mg/day. Drowsiness, lethargy, hepatotoxicity, and visual impairment have all been documented.

Kava potentiates anticoagulants and the effects of central nervous system depressants (e.g., alcohol, barbiturates, and opiates). Patients receiving anxiolytics, hypnotics, sedatives, warfarin, or other anticoagulants should avoid using kava. Patients who do take kava should not consume alcohol.

CLINICAL CAUTION

Kava kava is contraindicated in the following:

- Pregnancy, breast-feeding
- Neonates, infants, and children
- Depression
- Persons with neurologic conditions (e.g., possible dopamine antagonism may worsen symptoms of Parkinson's disease)

PRACTICE TIPS

- Kavalactones in doses of 60 to 120 mg/day should not be prescribed for any longer than 3 months.
- Too high a dose of kava can induce temporary paralysis; it is not the most suitable local anesthetic.
- Patients receiving narcotic analgesics (e.g., codeine) may become excessively drowsy if they take kava or 5-hydroxytryptophan, valerian, or melatonin.

REFERENCES

1. *Piper methysticum* (kava kava), *Altern Med Rev* 3:458-60, 1998.
2. Keledjian J, Duffield PH, Jamieson DD, et al: Uptake into mouse brain of four compounds present in the psychoactive beverage kava, *J Pharm Sci* 77:1003-6, 1988.
3. Boonen G, Haberlein H: Influence of genuine kavapyrone enantiomers on the GABA-A binding site, *Planta Med* 64:504-6, 1998.
4. Seitz U, Schule A, Gleitz J: [3H]-monoamine uptake inhibition properties of kava pyrones, *Planta Med* 63:548-9, 1997.
5. Schirrmacher K, Busselberg D, Langosch JM, et al: Effects of (+/−)-kavain on voltage-activated inward currents of dorsal root ganglion cells from neonatal rats, *Eur Neuropsychopharmacol* 9:171-6, 1999.
6. Langosch JM, Normann C, Schirrmacher K, et al: The influence of (+/−)-kavain on population spikes and long-term potentiation in guinea pig hippocampal slices, *Comp Biochem Physiol A Mol Integr Physiol* 120:545-9, 1998.
7. Beaubrun G, Gray GE: A review of herbal medicines for psychiatric disorders, *Psychiatr Serv* 51:1130-4, 2000.
8. Pittler MH, Ernst E: Efficacy of kava extract for treating anxiety: systematic review and meta-analysis, *J Clin Psychopharmacol* 20:84-9, 2000.
9. Ernst E: The risk-benefit profile of commonly used herbal therapies: ginkgo, St. John's wort, ginseng, echinacea, saw palmetto, and kava, *Ann Intern Med* 136:42-53, 2002.
10. Cauffield JS, Forbes HJ: Dietary supplements used in the treatment of depression, anxiety, and sleep disorders, *Lippincots Prim Care Pract* 3:290-304, 1999.
11. Volz HP, Kieser M: Kava-kava extract WS 1490 versus placebo in anxiety disorders—a randomized placebo-controlled 25-week outpatient trial, *Pharmacopsychiatry* 30:1-5, 1997.
12. Malsch U, Kieser M: Efficacy of kava-kava in the treatment of non-psychotic anxiety, following pretreatment with benzodiazepines, *Psychopharmacology (Berl)* 157:277-83, 2001.
13. Attele AS, Xie J-T, Yuan C-S: Treatment of insomnia: an alternative approach, *Altern Med Rev* 5:249-59, 2000.
14. Steiner GG: The correlation between cancer incidence and kava consumption, *Hawaii Med J* 59:420-2, 2000.
15. Cupp MJ: Herbal remedies: adverse effects and drug interactions, *Am Fam Physician* 59:1239-45, 1999.

■ CHAPTER 78 ■

LICORICE (*GLYRRHIZA GLABRA*)

Licorice, which is regarded as an unsafe herb, is a popular food flavoring.

Licorice is derived from the root of *Glycyrrhiza* species (Fabaceae). Glycyrrhizic acid, an important constituent of licorice, is widely used as a sweetener in food products and chewing tobacco.

Animal experiments have demonstrated that licorice and its extracts have anti-inflammatory, antiallergic, immunomodulating, anti-ulcer, phytoestrogen, and hepatoprotective activities.[1] Licorice has traditionally been used as an expectorant and a treatment for indigestion.

MECHANISM OF ACTION

Glycyrrhizin, rich in the aqueous extract of licorice root, is a triterpenoid saponin with hepatoprotective and antiviral activity. Glycyrrhizin stimulates the adrenal glands and potentiates the anti-inflammatory effects of glucocorticoids, mimics aldosterone, increases levels of interferon, and augments natural killer cell activity. Glycyrrhetic acid, the biologically active metabolite of glycyrrhizic acid, is a 200 to 1000 times more potent inhibitor of 11-β-hydroxysteroid dehydrogenase than glycyrrhizic acid.[2] The glycyrrhizin from ingested licorice is converted by the intestinal flora and absorbed as the aglycone, glycyrrhetinic acid. Glycyrrhizin is believed to achieve at least part of its anti-inflammatory activity through inhibition of complement and the lytic pathway in which the membrane attack complex is formed.[3] Glycyrrhetinic acid is a constituent in licorice believed to relieve peptic ulcers.

Isoflavans from *Glycyrrhiza glabra* have been shown to be effective in protecting mitochondrial function from oxidative stresses.[4] Licorice inhibits low-density lipoprotein cholesterol oxidation by a mechanism involving free radical scavenging. Glabridin, the major isoflavan in licorice root, is a phytoestrogen that binds to the human estrogen receptor.[5] Animal studies have shown that glabridin has an estrogen receptor–dependent, growth-promoting effect at low concentrations (10 nmol/L-10 μmol/L) and an estrogen receptor–independent antiproliferative activity at concentrations in excess of 15 μmol/L.[6]

DOSE

Traditional doses used are 2 to 6 mL of 1:1 extract per day or 1.2 to 4.6 g of deglycyrrhizinized licorice extract British Pharmacopoeia per day. When used as a flavoring component (e.g., in gargles, cough mixtures, or lozenges), a maximum daily dose of 100 mg of glycyrrhizin is regarded as acceptable.

CLINICAL USES

Once mixed with saliva, the chewable wafer form of deglycyrrhizinated licorice relieves ulcer dyspepsia by coating the gastrointestinal lining.[7] It should be taken 30 minutes before a meal. Licorice may decrease gastric irritation by inhibiting 5-hydroxyprostaglandin dihydrogenase and D-13-prostaglandin reductase, enzymes that inactivate protective prostaglandins in gastric mucosa.[8] Patients with inflammatory bowel disease may also benefit.[7] Licorice may be used to sooth inflamed skin or a sore throat.

TOXICITY/DRUG INTERACTIONS

Licorice root can safely be used for treating duodenal and gastric ulcers, but in excess doses it can cause hypokalemia, hypertension, and heart failure.[9] In fact, licorice has been identified as an unsafe herb.[10] Consumption of 400 mg of glycyrrhizin per day causes side effects in most people. However, small but significant increases in systolic pressure have been reported in persons who consume 135 mg of glycyrrhizin daily (50 g of licorice). A "no effect" level of 12 mg of glycyrrhizic acid per day has been proposed.[11] For a person with a body weight of 60 kg, this equals 6 g of licorice a day, assuming that licorice containing 0.2% of glycyrrhizic acid is used.

Licorice may impair the effects of antihypertensive medication, and through its potassium-depleting effect, may adversely affect patients receiving cardiac glycosides and diuretics. A high potassium intake minimizes the hypertensive effects of licorice. Long-term high-dose administration of licorice extract may induce edema, hypertension, and hypokalemia; long-term lower-dose licorice consumption may induce mild hypertension. The hypertensive, hypokalemic response to licorice is dose-dependent and varies among individuals. Use of licorice (or glycyrrhizin) at doses of 100 mg or more per day for more than 4 weeks requires monitoring of potassium levels in patients receiving thiazide diuretics.[8]

Licorice potentiates the effects of oral and topical corticosteroids.[12]

CLINICAL CAUTION

Medical supervision is required if licorice is to be used for more than 4 weeks at doses of 100 mg/day or more for patients receiving digoxin, thiazide diuretics, or antihypertensive agents. Licorice increases the risk of hypokalemia with furosemide and other loop diuretics and halves the bioavailability of nitrofurantoin. It is contraindicated in persons with cholestasis, cirrhosis, hypertension, or hypokalemia.

An individual consuming a lot of licorice who has increased blood pressure and edema should be evaluated for an acquired form of apparent mineralocorticoid excess syndrome.[13] Sodium retention and potassium loss may result from suppression of the renin-angiotensin-aldosterone system caused by licorice.[8]

PRACTICE TIPS

- Licorice in high doses (5-15 g of root equivalent to 200-600 mg of glycyrrhizin) should not be taken for longer than 6 to 8 weeks without professional monitoring.
- The deglycyrrhizinated form of licorice has no side effects.
- Grapefruit juice potentiates the side effects of licorice by inhibiting renal 11-β-hydroxysteroid.
- Licorice should be avoided during pregnancy, although doses of less than 3 g/day are probably safe.
- Patients with hypertension who continue to eat licorice may reduce any untoward reactions by eating a diet rich in potassium.

REFERENCES

1. Shibata S: A drug over the millennia: pharmacognosy, chemistry, and pharmacology of licorice, *Yakugaku Zasshi* 120:849-62, 2000.
2. Ploeger B, Mensinga T, Sips A, et al: The pharmacokinetics of glycyrrhizic acid evaluated by physiologically based pharmacokinetic modeling, *Drug Metab Rev* 33:125-47, 2001.
3. Fujisawa Y, Sakamoto M, Matsushita M, et al: Glycyrrhizin inhibits the lytic pathway of complement—possible mechanism of its anti-inflammatory effect on liver cells in viral hepatitis, *Microbiol Immunol* 44:799-804, 2000.
4. Haraguchi H, Yoshida N, Ishikawa H, et al: Protection of mitochondrial functions against oxidative stresses by isoflavans from *Glycyrrhiza glabra*, *J Pharm Pharmacol* 52:219-23, 2000.
5. Tamir S, Eizenberg M, Somjen D, et al: Estrogen-like activity of glabrene and other constituents isolated from licorice root, *J Steroid Biochem Mol Biol* 78:291-8, 2001.
6. Tamir S, Eizenberg M, Somjen D, et al: Estrogenic and antiproliferative properties of glabridin from licorice in human breast cancer cells, *Cancer Res* 60:5704-9, 2000.
7. Diefendorf D, Healey J, Kalyn W, editors: *The healing power of vitamins, minerals and herbs*, Surry Hills, Australia, 2000, Readers Digest.
8. Braun L: Herb-drug interaction guide, *Aust Fam Physician* 30:259-60, 2001.
9. Craig WJ: Health-promoting properties of common herbs, *Am J Clin Nutr* 70:491S-499S, 1999.

10. Klepser TB, Klepser ME: Unsafe and potentially safe herbal therapies, *Am J Health Syst Pharm* 56:125-38, 1999.
11. van Gelderen CE, Bijlsma JA, van Dokkum W, et al: Glycyrrhizic acid: the assessment of a no effect level, *Hum Exp Toxicol* 19:434-9, 2000.
12. Fugh-Berman A: Herb-drug interactions, *Lancet* 355:134-8, 2000.
13. Olukoga A, Donaldson D: Liquorice and its health implications, *J R Soc Health* 120:83-9, 2000.

■ CHAPTER 79 ■

MAGNESIUM (MG)

Magnesium deficiency, one of the most frequent electrolyte abnormalities seen in clinical practice, is also probably the most underdiagnosed one.

Magnesium, an important intracellular cation, is present in numerous enzymatic systems and is crucial for adenosine triphosphate metabolism. It influences neuromuscular, cardiovascular, immunologic, and hormonal function. Magnesium is a smooth muscle relaxant; it dilates coronary arteries and peripheral vessels, exerts antiarrhythmic effects, may have a permissive effect on catecholamine actions, and can play a role in various thrombogenic conditions.[1]

MECHANISM OF ACTION

Magnesium is a cofactor in many enzymes, of which more than 300 are involved in food catabolism. It plays an important role in intracellular homeostasis, including activation of thiamine and, consequently, an array of crucial body functions. As an essential cofactor for adenosine 5'-phosphate production, magnesium plays a pivotal role in the breakdown of glycogen, the oxidation of fat, and the synthesis of protein. Magnesium is involved in the transmission of the second messenger system.

Magnesium regulates membrane stability. It influences various cellular functions including transport of potassium and calcium ions, cell proliferation, signal transduction, and energy metabolism. It is required for the metabolism of a number of minerals including calcium, potassium, phosphorus, zinc, copper, iron, sodium, lead, and cadmium and for the production of gastric hydrochloric acid, acetylcholine, and nitric oxide.

FOOD SOURCES

The best dietary sources of magnesium include green leafy vegetables, nuts, peas, beans, and whole grains (i.e., cereal grains) from which the germ or outer layers have not been removed. A half a cup of cooked spinach supplies 78 mg of magnesium, one fifth of the daily requirement. Hard water has more magnesium than soft water. Absorption of magnesium is reduced on a high-fat or high-fiber diet, because it is bound in the intestine by phytates and oxalates. Around one third of dietary magnesium is absorbed.

DOSE

The recommended daily allowance of magnesium is 350 mg or 150 mg/1000 kcal. Supplementation is usually in the range of 300 to 1000 mg, with a therapeutic dose range of 1000 to 1500 mg/day.[2] Suggested therapeutic doses are 400 mg daily to prevent heart disease; 400 mg twice daily to treat arrhythmia, heart failure, or asthma; 500 mg for hypertension or diabetes; and 150 mg combined with 600 mg of malic acid to treat fibromyalgia.[3] Magnesium sulfate can cause diarrhea, magnesium diglycinate is well-absorbed, and magnesium oxide is poorly absorbed. Absorption is 35% to 40%, and the body content is 25 g. Physiologic studies suggest that women with no clinical evidence of magnesium deficiency may not respond to short-term supplementation with any increases in the mass of the exchangeable magnesium body pool or in magnesium turnover rates.[4] Magnesium toxicosis is unlikely in persons with normal renal function; the supplemental dosage of magnesium is determined not only by intake but also by absorption, metabolism, and excretion.

CLINICAL USES

Magnesium sulfate (10 mg) is well-recognized as an effective laxative. In magnesium-depleted patients, both refractory hypocalcemia and hypokalemia respond to magnesium replacement. Furthermore, animal experiments have shown that magnesium supplementation, although reducing apparent calcium absorption, promotes bone formation, prevents bone resorption, and increases the dynamic strength of bone.[5] Magnesium is routinely included with calcium in osteoporosis prevention supplements. Of the total body content of magnesium, half is stored in bone. Magnesium (200 mg) in combination with vitamin B_6 (50 mg) may marginally reduce anxiety-related premenstrual symptoms.[6] Furthermore, anecdotal evidence suggests that 70% of patients seen in primary practice because of nervous system–type complaints respond to magnesium: 50% report having more energy while taking magnesium, and 38% of patients believe their musculoskeletal problems are relieved by use of this mineral. Oral administration of magnesium, 500 mg/day, has been reported to relieve exercise-induced muscle spasms within a few days,[7] but conflicting trial results for magnesium in the treatment of fibromyalgia have been reported.[8,9]

Magnesium has also been postulated to play a role in establishing a threshold for migraine attacks. Magnesium counteracts vasospasm; inhibits platelet aggregation; stabilizes cell membranes; and affects serotonin receptors, nitric oxide, and eicosanoid synthesis and release.[10,11] Furthermore, up to 50% of patients with migraine have lowered levels of ionized magnesium during an acute migraine attack.[12]

Although epidemiologic studies suggest a link between low magnesium status and diabetes mellitus and hypertension, there is little clinical evidence that magnesium supplementation can be used to improve glucose control or manage hypertension. Randomized clinical trials are urgently needed to determine whether magnesium supplementation will alter the natural history of chronic cardiovascular diseases and whether any benefits detected are limited to patients with magnesium deficiency.[13] Intravenous magnesium sulphate ($MgSO_4$) has a statistically significant, albeit clinically limited, effect on ventricular rate.[14] The effect of intravenous magnesium is not altered by any associated magnesium deficiency.

Magnesium has been used in the treatment of preeclampsia and eclampsia, certain types of ventricular tachycardia, and acute asthma in certain patients.[15,16]

TOXICITY/DRUG INTERACTIONS

Doses in excess of 500 mg/day have been associated with gastrointestinal disturbances, including diarrhea.[7] Drowsiness, lethargy, sluggishness, and stupor have also been reported. Magnesium supplementation may exacerbate cardiac and renal disease.

Many therapeutic drugs (e.g., diuretics, chemotherapeutics, immunosuppressive agents, and antibiotics) cause hypomagnesemia as a result of increased urinary loss. Magnesium can reduce the efficacy of tetracyclines.

CLINICAL CAUTION

More than half the population in developed countries may have an inadequate dietary intake.[17] Magnesium deficiency may present as psychologic changes such as apathy, depression, and anorexia and neuromuscular excitability including muscle weakness, myalgia, spasms, tremors, and arrhythmia. In severe cases, coma and convulsions may occur.

Magnesium deficiency has been postulated to be associated with disorders as diverse as cardiac disease; hypertension; preeclampsia; diabetes mellitus; depressed immunity; premenstrual syndrome; osteoporosis; mood swings; and peroxynitrite damage presenting as migraine, multiple sclerosis, glaucoma, or Alzheimer's disease.[18-20] Magnesium deficiency is a recognized risk factor for hypertension, cardiac arrhythmia, and ischemic heart disease, especially when the deficiency is associated with coronary vasospasm and night cramps. In patients with magnesium deficiency, serum magnesium level is unreliable, erythrocyte magnesium content is a better indicator, and the electrocardiogram shows lengthened QRS complexes, peaked T waves, ST depression, and a delayed QT interval.[20] Patients respond to 200 mg three times a day.

PRACTICE TIPS

- Magnesium supplements are absorbed best when taken with meals; taking magnesium supplements with meals reduces the risk of diarrhea.
- Calcium deficiency and magnesium deficiency have a similar clinical presentation; magnesium is a cofactor in calcium mobilization.
- In humans, magnesium deficiency produces a drop in the serum calcium level. When magnesium supplements are taken, an appropriate regimen includes calcium, with the ratio of calcium to magnesium being 2:1.
- Excess coffee or alcohol or profuse sweating can reduce magnesium levels.
- Correction of magnesium deficiency (400 mg daily) may reduce muscle cramps and correct a reduced pain threshold.
- A neutraceutical regimen for nocturnal cramps includes magnesium (4.5 mg/kg body weight), 2 g of calcium daily, and 300 IU of vitamin E daily.
- Persons with hypertension who have magnesium deficiency may respond to administration of 400 to 800 mg of magnesium daily.

REFERENCES

1. Iannello S, Belfiore F: Hypomagnesemia. A review of pathophysiological, clinical and therapeutical aspects, *Panminerva Med* 43:177-209, 2001.
2. Brighthope I: Nutritional medicine tables, *J Aust Coll Nutr Env Med* 17:20-5, 1998.
3. Diefendorf D, Healey J, Kalyn W, editors: *The healing power of vitamins, minerals and herbs*, Surry Hills, Australia, 2000, Readers Digest.
4. Feillet-Coudray C, Coudray C, Tressol JC, et al: Exchangeable magnesium pool masses in healthy women: effects of magnesium supplementation, *Am J Clin Nutr* 75:72-8, 2002.
5. Toba Y, Kajita Y, Masuyama R, et al: Dietary magnesium supplementation affects bone metabolism and dynamic strength of bone in ovariectomized rats, *J Nutr* 130:216-20, 2000.
6. De Souza MC, Walker AF, Robinson PA, et al: A synergistic effect of a daily supplement for 1 month of 200 mg magnesium plus 50 mg vitamin B_6 for the relief of anxiety-related premenstrual symptoms: a randomized, double-blind, crossover study, *J Womens Health Gend Based Med* 9:131-9, 2000.
7. Lukaski HC: Magnesium, zinc and chromium nutriture and physical activity, *Am J Clin Nutr* 72(suppl 2):585S-593S, 2000.
8. Russell IJ, Michalek JE, Flechas JD, et al: Treatment of fibromyalgia syndrome with Super Malic: a randomized, double blind, placebo controlled, crossover pilot study, *J Rheumatol* 22:953-8, 1995.
9. Manuel y Keenoy B, Moorkens G, et al: Magnesium status and parameters of the oxidant-antioxidant balance in patients with chronic fatigue: effects of supplementation with magnesium, *J Am Coll Nutr* 19:374-82, 2000.

10. McCarty MF: Magnesium taurate and fish oil for prevention of migraine, *Med Hypotheses* 47:461-6, 1996.
11. Gawaz M: Antithrombocytic effectiveness of magnesium, *Fortschr Med* 114: 329-32, 1996.
12. Mauskop A, Altura BM: Role of magnesium in the pathogenesis and treatment of migraine, *Clin Neurosci* 5:24-7, 1998.
13. Fox C, Ramsoomair D, Carter C: Magnesium: its proven and potential clinical significance, *South Med J* 94:1195-201, 2001.
14. Eray O, Akca S, Pekdemir M, et al: Magnesium efficacy in magnesium deficient and nondeficient patients with rapid ventricular response atrial fibrillation, *Eur J Emerg Med* 7:287-90, 2000.
15. Dacey MJ: Hypomagnesemic disorders, *Crit Care Clin* 17:155-73, viii, 2001.
16. Ramsey PS, Rouse DJ: Magnesium sulfate as a tocolytic agent, *Semin Perinatol* 25:236-47, 2001.
17. Saris NE, Mervaala E, Karppanen H, et al: Magnesium. An update on physiological, clinical and analytical aspects, *Clin Chim Acta* 294:1-26, 2000.
18. Johnson S: The multifaceted and widespread pathology of magnesium deficiency, *Med Hypotheses* 56:163-70, 2001.
19. Sanders GT, Huijgen HJ, Sanders R: Magnesium in disease: a review with special emphasis on the serum ionized magnesium, *Clin Chem Lab Med* 37:1011-33, 1999.
20. Taylor M: Nutritional management of an elderly patient—the importance of magnesium, *J Aust Coll Nutr Env Med* 18:21, 1999.

■ CHAPTER 80 ■

MANGANESE (MN)

> When trace minerals are widely dispersed in food, deficiencies are
> unlikely if a balanced varied diet is eaten.

Manganese is an important trace element that facilitates synthesis of
mucopolysaccharides, lipids, and thyroxine. It is an antioxidative transition
metal and helps prevent tissue damage caused by lipid oxidation.

MECHANISM OF ACTION

Manganese activates several enzymes, is a constituent of several metalloen-
zymes, and may play a role in calcium mobilization. As part of the enzyme
superoxide dismutase, manganese reduces the risk of exposure to free radicals. As a constituent of pyruvate carboxylase, it generates oxaloacetate, a
substrate in the tricarboxylic acid (Krebs) cycle, and may play a role in glucose homeostasis. It also activates enzymes involved in cartilage synthesis;
facilitates formation of urea; and activates various kinases, decarboxylases,
transferases, and hydroxylases.

FOOD SOURCES

Sources include nuts, fruits, and vegetables—especially hazelnuts, blackberries, pineapple, lentils, beans, and whole grains. Manganese is lost in milling
of whole grains. Absorption varies from 10% to 40%. The body content is
0.012 g.

DOSE

Body levels of manganese are controlled by biliary excretion. The recommended intake ranges from 2 to 5 mg daily; however, this may be excessive
because some consider a manganese intake of more than 10 mg per day
from food or 4.2 mg from water to be toxic. The therapeutic dose range is 2 to
50 mg/day.[1]

CLINICAL USES

Manganese is suspected to facilitate control of blood sugar in diabetes and to reduce inflammation in arthritis. Further research is required before any recommendation can be made.

As a component of superoxide dismutase, manganese may be used as a marker to help define therapeutic strategies in the clinical management of glioblastoma. Patients with glioblastomas and high levels of manganese superoxide dismutase show a median survival time of 6.11 months, whereas patients with glioblastomas and low levels of this enzyme have a median survival time of 12.17 months.[2] Glioblastomas can be divided into two distinct groups on the basis of their content of manganese superoxide dismutase.

TOXICITY/DRUG INTERACTIONS

Oral manganese is essentially nontoxic. Mild airborne manganese poisoning may impair both memory and coordination. Fatigue, weakness, anorexia, apathy, depression, and disturbed sleep have all been reported. Irritability, hallucinations, and poor coordination have been reported in persons with severe manganism.

Manganese in excess amounts can cause irreversible nervous system damage.[3] The neurologic signs of manganism resemble several clinical disorders collectively described as *extrapyramidal motor system dysfunction*, and in particular, idiopathic Parkinson's disease and dystonia.[4] Tremors are a sign of excess.

CLINICAL CAUTION

Deficiency may cause growth impairment and tendon and bone disorders in animals but is probably not a problem in humans. Aberrant manganese metabolism may be found in certain cases of multiple sclerosis and amyotrophic lateral sclerosis.

PRACTICE TIPS

• There is no reliable indicator of manganese status in adults.

REFERENCES

1. Brighthope I: Nutritional medicine tables, *J Aust Coll Nutr Env Med* 17:20-5, 1998.

2. Ria F, Landriscina M, Remiddi F, et al: The level of manganese superoxide dismutase content is an independent prognostic factor for glioblastoma. Biological mechanisms and clinical implications, *Br J Cancer* 84:529-34, 2001.
3. Lee JW: Manganese intoxication, *Arch Neurol* 57:597-9, 2000.
4. Aschner M: Manganese: brain transport and emerging research needs, *Environ Health Perspect* 108(suppl 3):429-32, 2000.

■ CHAPTER 81 ■

MEADOWSWEET (*FILIPENDULA ULMARIA L*)

> Salicyclic acid, extracted from meadowsweet, causes gastric discomfort, but decoctions of the herb can prevent acetylsalicylic acid (aspirin)–induced gastric lesions in rats.

Meadowsweet has been used as an antacid, anti-inflammatory, mild urinary antiseptic, and astringent. It has traditionally been favored for treatment of gastrointestinal tract disturbances ranging from flatulence to hyperacidity.

MECHANISM OF ACTION

Active constituents of meadowsweet include flavonoids, phenolic glycosides, and essential oils. Salicylates are found in various forms in the flowers and leaves. The herb has antioxidant, anticoagulant, and fibrinolytic activity.

DOSE

The usual daily dose of meadowsweet is 2.5 to 3.5 g of flowers, 4 to 5 g of herb, 3 to 6 mL of 1:2 liquid extract, or 7.5 to 15 mL of 1:5 tincture.[1]

CLINICAL USES

There are no clinically proven uses for meadowsweet, although one clinical trial suggests that it may be useful in the treatment of cervical dysplasia.[1]

In laboratory studies, residues from meadowsweet flowers were found to exhibit strong antioxidative properties and have been recommended as preservatives for margarine.[2]

TOXICITY/DRUG INTERACTIONS

Side effects are rare at recommended doses but include anorexia, nausea, and vomiting. Concurrent use of meadowsweet with warfarin, heparin, aspirin, or any other drug with an anticoagulant effect should be avoided.[3]

CLINICAL CAUTION

Meadowsweet is contraindicated in patients with salicylate sensitivity. Until further evidence is available, meadowsweet should not be prescribed for children or used during pregnancy.

PRACTICE TIPS

• Use of meadowsweet should be avoided by patients with asthma.

REFERENCES

1. Mills S, Bone K: *Principles and practice of phytotherapy*, Edinburgh, 2000, Churchill Livingstone.
2. Sroka Z, Cisowski W, Seredynska M, et al: Phenolic extracts from meadowsweet and hawthorn flowers have antioxidative properties, *Z Naturforsch [C]* 56:739-44, 2001.
3. Heck AM, DeWitt BA, Lukes AL: Potential interactions between alternative therapies and warfarin, *Am J Health Syst Pharm* 57:1221-7, 2000.

■ CHAPTER 82 ■

MISTLETOE (*VISCUM ALBUM*)

> The capacity of mistletoe to modulate immunity may prove to be a two-edged sword, with neoplasia sometimes being enhanced and other times being retarded.

Mistletoe (*Viscum album*) is a semi-parasitic plant of several trees (e.g., apple, oak, and pine). It is also traditionally used as a sedative and for treatment of headache, epilepsy, paralysis, hypertension, and debility. Mistletoe lectins have been shown to have cytotoxic effects on cancer cells in vitro.[1]

Mistletoe is a toxic plant and should be kept out of the reach of children.

MECHANISM OF ACTION

Mistletoe contains tyramine, a number of antioxidants, and a galactoside-specific lectin. Results of in vitro and in vivo studies suggest that this lectin has immunomodulatory capacity as reflected in upregulation of the production of proinflammatory cytokines.[2] However, the clinical outcome is unpredictable, because mistletoe lectins may stimulate growth in cell lines.

Mistletoe, like allicin from garlic, induces programmed cell death, thus arresting cellular proliferation.[3] Programmed cell death (apoptosis) is reduced in cancer and increased in neurodegenerative diseases. Soy bean, garlic, ginger, and green tea—which in epidemiologic studies have been suggested to reduce the incidence of cancer—may also do so by inducing programmed cell death.

DOSE

Mistletoe is usually taken three times daily as 3 to 6 g of dried leaves, 2 to 3 mL of 1:1 dilution of fluid extract, or 0.5 mL of 1:5 tincture.

CLINICAL USES

Total extracts of mistletoe (e.g., Iscador) have been developed to treat cancer. A prospective, long-term, epidemiologic, cohort study demonstrated that treatment with Iscador can result in a clinically relevant prolongation of survival time in patients with cancer and that Iscador appears to stimulate self-regulation.[4]

Clinical experience among patients who are seropositive for human immunodeficiency virus (HIV) also suggests that mistletoe inhibits the progression of HIV infection. One study indicated that mistletoe extract induced immunomodulation that may inhibit the progression of HIV infection and could be administered safely to HIV-positive patients.[5]

TOXICITY/DRUG INTERACTIONS

Although mistletoe is regarded as a dangerous plant, side effects are seldom reported and include dry mouth, rarely dyspepsia, gastrointestinal upset, mild drowsiness, lethargy, photosensitivity, ataxia, and seizures. Although only a few adverse reactions have been noted, cases of anaphylactic shock have been described.[6]

Mistletoe induces several isoenzymes of the hepatic cytochrome P-450 enzyme system and therefore may influence the metabolism of numerous drugs. Mistletoe decreases the efficacy of warfarin and interacts with oral contraceptives and estrogen.

CLINICAL CAUTION

Mistletoe is a uterine stimulant and should not be taken by pregnant women.

PRACTICE TIPS

• The clinical cost-benefit of using mistletoe has yet to be established.

REFERENCES

1. Primack A: Complementary/alternative therapies in the prevention and treatment of cancer. In Spencer JW, Jacobs JJ, editors: *Complementary/alternative medicine: an evidence-based approach*, St Louis, 1998, Mosby.
2. Gabius HJ: Probing the cons and pros of lectin-induced immunomodulation: case studies for the mistletoe lectin and galectin-1, *Biochimie* 83:659-66, 2001.
3. Thatte U, Bagadey S, Dahanukar S: Modulation of programmed cell death by medicinal plants, *Cell Mol Biol (Noisy-le-grand)* 46:199-214, 2000.
4. Grossarth-Maticek R, Kiene H, Baumgartner SM, et al: Use of Iscador, an extract of European mistletoe (*Viscum album*), in cancer treatment: prospective nonrandomized and randomized matched-pair studies nested within a cohort study, *Altern Ther Health Med* 7:57-66, 68-72, 74, 2001.

5. Gorter RW, van Wely M, Reif M, et al: Tolerability of an extract of European mistletoe among immunocompromised and healthy individuals, *Altern Ther Health Med* 5:37-44, 47-8, 1999.
6. Hutt N, Kopferschmitt-Kubler M, Cabalion J, et al: Anaphylactic reactions after therapeutic injection of mistletoe (*Viscum albumL.*), *Allergol Immunopathol (Madr)* 29:201-3, 2001.

■ CHAPTER 83 ■

PAU D'ARCO (*TABEBUIA* SPECIES)

> In clinical trials lapachol has been shown to have side effects, but there is no evidence that pau d'arco has similar untoward effects, since herbs and their isolated constituents may have dissimilar clinical outcomes.

Pau d'arco, or taheebo, is derived from the inner bark of a tree, *Tabebuia impetiginosa*. In Brazil, it is used as an analgesic, anti-inflammatory, antineoplastic, and diuretic. Its antimicrobial, immunostimulant, and cytotoxic properties are under investigation.

MECHANISM OF ACTION

Important active constituents in pau d'arco include the naphthoquinones (e.g., lapachol and furonaphthoquinones), anthraquinones, and benzoic acid derivatives. Quinones are important components of the electron transfer chain. Both ubiquinol, the reduced form of coenzyme Q, and menaquinone (vitamin K) have significant antioxidant properties. Menaquinone has an anticoagulant effect.

Two cyclopentene dialdehydes isolated from the bark of *T. impetiginosa* have demonstrated anti-inflammatory activity.[1] Animal experiments have shown that an aqueous extract of the inner bark of *T. avellanedae* has pain- and edema-reducing effects.[2]

The bark of pau d'arco, like the bulbs of *Allium sativum*, has an antimicrobial effect.

DOSE

The traditional daily dose of pau d'arco is 1.5 to 3.5 g or 3 to 7 mL of a 1:2 extract in 45% ethanol.

CLINICAL USES

Both the anti-inflammatory activity and free radical quenching properties of this herb may be helpful in the treatment of psoriasis. In vitro tests with β-lapachone displayed activity comparable to that of the antipsoriatic drug anthralin against the growth of a human keratinocyte cell line.[3]

The stem bark of pau d'arco has broad-spectrum antimicrobial activity against gram-positive and gram-negative bacteria and fungi.[4] Extracts produced by boiling the bark of *T. impetiginosa* were found to be active against *Staphylococcus aureus* and *Escherichia coli*.[5] Extracts of the leaves inhibit the growth of *Candida* species.

The herb may also benefit persons with impaired immunity (e.g., patients with chronic fatigue syndrome, acquired immunodeficiency syndrome, or cancer). Lapachol is considered to have antitumor activity and may be used as complementary therapy for certain malignancies.

TOXICITY/DRUG INTERACTIONS

A mild contact dermatitis has been reported. High doses may cause nausea and vomiting. Strict adherence to recommended doses is advocated to prevent potential adverse effects, with respect to both bleeding and free radical pathology.

CLINICAL CAUTION

High doses of naphthoquinones have an anticoagulant effect and may cause bleeding.

PRACTICE TIPS

- Pau d'arco should be avoided or used with great caution during pregnancy.
- Pau d'arco tea used as a lukewarm douche is reputed to restore vaginal flora and to treat vaginal candidiasis.
- Compresses soaked in pau d'arco tincture have been used to treat warts. Compresses are applied nightly until the warts disappear.
- Blood counts of patients receiving high doses of pau d'arco should be monitored.

REFERENCES

1. Koyama J, Morita I, Tagahara K, Hirai K. Cyclopentene dialdehydes from *Tabebuia impetiginosa*, *Phytochemistry* 53:869-72, 2000.
2. Miranda FG, Vilar JC, Alves IA, et al: Antinociceptive and antiedematogenic properties and acute toxicity of *Tabebuia avellanedae* Lor. Ex Griseb. Inner bark aqueous extract, *BMC Pharmacol* 1:6, 2001.

3. Muller K, Sellmer A, Wiegrebe W: Potential antipsoriatic agents: lapacho compounds as potent inhibitors of HaCaT cell growth, *J Nat Prod* 62:1134-6, 1999.
4. Binutu OA, Lajubutu BA: Antimicrobial potential of some plant species of the Bigoniaceae family, *Afr J Med Sci* 23:269-73, 1994.
5. Anesini C, Perez C: Screen of plants used in Argentine folk medicine for antimicrobial activity, *J Ethnopharmacol* 39:119-28, 1993.

▪ CHAPTER 84 ▪

PEPPERMINT (*MENTHA PIPERITA*)

Peppermint oil is used to treat functional dyspepsia but may exacerbate gastroesophageal reflux.

Peppermint (*Mentha piperita*), a naturally occurring hybrid of water mint (*M. aquatica*) and spearmint (*M. spicata*), is best known for its role as a popular flavoring agent. Its volatile oils, extracted from leaves and stems harvested just before the plant flowers, are used for medicinal purposes.

Peppermint is usually taken after a meal to relieve intestinal colic and dyspepsia. It has traditionally been used to manage bronchospasm. Peppermint is frequently included in topical applications for myalgia and neuralgia.

MECHANISM OF ACTION

Peppermint oil is rich in menthol, menthone, and menthyl acetate. The essential oil also contain flavonoids, tannins, and triterpenes. Peppermint oil is used as a spasmolytic, reducing smooth muscle contractions in diverse circumstances. It is usually taken after a meal to reduce indigestion and colonic spasms by dampening the gastrocolic reflex.[1] Peppermint oil inhibits muscle spasm initiated by serotonin and substance P. It increases the pain threshold through activation of the endogenous opiate system and may have a mild sedative effect on the central nervous system.

Menthol stimulates the secretion of digestive enzymes and bile and is a mild anesthetic. It can enhance skin penetration of other agents. Topical preparations of menthol relieve pain if they are applied early.

Peppermint oil has been found to have an antibacterial and antifungal effect.

DOSE

Plants in which the whole peppermint leaf contains at least 12 mg/kg and cut leaf contains at least 9 mg/kg essential oil are selected. Traditionally, a daily dose consists of 6 to 9 g of dried leaf, 1.5 to 4 mL of 1:2 liquid extract, 3.5 to 11 mL of 1:5 tincture, or 0.15 to 0.6 mL (3-12 drops) of essential oils.

CLINICAL USES

Clinical trials support menthol inhalation to dampen airways responsiveness in patients with asthma, peppermint oil ingestion to relieve irritable bowel syndrome and functional dyspepsia, and topical application of these extracts for headaches.[2] Use of peppermint oil to relieve abdominal discomfort is promising but inconclusive. In a prospective, randomized, double-blind, placebo-controlled, clinical study, three in four patients taking an enteric-coated peppermint oil formulation (Colpermin) three to four times daily, 15 to 30 minutes before meals for 1 month, experienced less severe abdominal pain, less abdominal distension, reduced stool frequency, fewer borborygmi, and less flatulence.[3] A randomized, double-blind, controlled trial in which children with irritable bowel syndrome were given pH-dependent, enteric-coated peppermint oil capsules also showed that three in four patients experienced less severe abdominal pain.[4] A review of clinical trials of peppermint extract as a symptomatic treatment for irritable bowel syndrome—which included eight randomized, controlled trials and five placebo-controlled, double-blind trials—indicated that although *Mentha piperita* appeared to provide symptom relief, methodological flaws associated with most studies precluded definitive judgment on the efficacy of this treatment.[5]

Peppermint oil, in combination with caraway oil, has been used with success in the treatment of functional dyspepsia. Enteric-coated capsules containing a fixed combination of 90 mg of peppermint oil and 50 mg of caraway oil have been found to reduce the intensity of pain, pressure, heaviness, and fullness in patients with dyspepsia.[6] Another study of 120 outpatients with functional dyspepsia compared this combination with cisapride (10 mg three times per day), a prokinetic agent. Comparable results were attained with both treatments in the Dyspeptic Discomfort Score regardless of the presence of *Helicobacter pylori*.[7] It is worth noting that laboratory studies have shown that the essential oils of peppermint and four of its major constituents do exhibit bactericidal activity against various organisms including *H. pylori*.[8]

As a smooth muscle relaxant, peppermint oil may also be helpful in the management of diffuse esophageal spasm, an uncommon condition that results in simultaneous esophageal contractions. A manometric study showed that peppermint oil, 5 drops in 10 mL of water, completely eliminated simultaneous esophageal contractions in all patients without lowering esophageal sphincter pressure or altering the pressure or duration of contractions in both the upper and lower esophagus.[9]

Despite the growing popularity of aromatherapy, an experimental study in humans demonstrated that the effects of essentials oils or their components, including peppermint, on alertness, as judged by motor and reaction times, are mainly psychologic.[10] In contrast, animal experiments suggest that peppermint oil may be effective for treating mental fatigue because mice respond to intraperitoneal administration of various constituents of peppermint oil with increased ambulatory activity.[11]

TOXICITY/DRUG INTERACTIONS

In general, the oils, but not the leaf, of peppermint have been associated with side effects. High doses of essential oils may cause headaches, skin rashes, bradycardia, ataxia, pyrosis, and muscle tremors. Peppermint oil should be avoided or used cautiously in patients with salicylate sensitivity or aspirin-induced asthma.

Provided that the concentration of pulegone, a constituent of peppermint oil, does not exceed 1%, it appears that peppermint oil is safe when used in cosmetic formulations.[12]

CLINICAL CAUTION

Peppermint oil is contraindicated in patients with symptoms of esophageal reflux, gall stone colic, and liver disease. Peppermint oil should not be applied to the facial area of infants and young children, since spasm of the glottis has been reported.

PRACTICE TIPS

- Peppermint tea is reputed to relieve flatulence. When tea is prepared by soaking two teaspoons of dried peppermint leaves in boiling water for 5 to 10 minutes, the cup should be covered to trap the volatile oils.
- Peppermint oil in boiling water may be inhaled to increase bronchial secretions.
- Patients should be cautioned not to use peppermint oil with a heating pad or near an open flame.

REFERENCES

1. Spirling LI, Daniels IR: Botanical perspectives on health peppermint: more than just an after-dinner mint, *J R Soc Health* 121:62-3, 2001.
2. Mills S, Bone K: *Principles and practice of phytotherapy*, Edinburgh, 2000, Churchill Livingstone.
3. Liu JH, Chen GH, Yeh HZ, et al: Enteric-coated peppermint-oil capsules in the treatment of irritable bowel syndrome: a prospective, randomized trial, *J Gastroenterol* 32:765-8, 1997.
4. Kline RM, Kline JJ, Di Palma J, et al: Enteric-coated, pH-dependent peppermint oil capsules for the treatment of irritable bowel syndrome in children, *J Pediatr* 138:125-8, 2001.
5. Pittler MH, Ernst E: Peppermint oil for irritable bowel syndrome: a critical review and metaanalysis, *Am J Gastroenterol* 93:1131-5, 1998.
6. May B, Kohler S, Schneider B: Efficacy and tolerability of a fixed combination of peppermint oil and caraway oil in patients suffering from functional dyspepsia, *Aliment Pharmacol Ther* 14:1671-7, 2000.

7. Madisch A, Heydenreich CJ, Wieland V, et al: Treatment of functional dyspepsia with a fixed peppermint oil and caraway oil combination preparation as compared to cisapride. A multicenter, reference-controlled double-blind equivalence study, *Arzneimittelforschung* 49:925-32, 1999.
8. Imai H, Osawa K, Yasuda H, et al: Inhibition by the essential oils of peppermint and spearmint of the growth of pathogenic bacteria, *Microbios* 106(suppl 1):31-9, 2001.
9. Pimentel M, Bonorris GG, Chow EJ, et al: Peppermint oil improves the manometric findings in diffuse esophageal spasm, *J Clin Gastroenterol* 33:27-31, 2001.
10. Ilmberger J, Heuberger E, Mahrhofer C, et al: The influence of essential oils on human attention. I: alertness, *Chem Senses* 26:239-45, 2001.
11. Umezu T, Sakata A, Ito H: Ambulation-promoting effect of peppermint oil and identification of its active constituents, *Pharmacol Biochem Behav* 69:383-90, 2001.
12. Nair B: Final report on the safety assessment of *Mentha piperita* (peppermint) oil, *Mentha piperita* (peppermint) leaf extract, *Mentha piperita* (peppermint) leaf, and *Mentha piperita* (peppermint) leaf water, *Int J Toxicol* 20(suppl 3):61-73, 2001.

■ CHAPTER 85 ■

PHYTOCHEMICALS (PHYTONUTRIENTS)

A diet rich in fruits and vegetables provides a health advantage beyond that attributable to energy, vitamins, and minerals.

Phytonutrients are a diverse group of chemicals that provide plants with protection against various predators and diseases. Although they are not a source of energy, minerals, or vitamins, when consumed in moderate amounts by humans, phytochemicals have a health-promoting effect.[1] Despite having no known role in nutrition, many phytochemicals possess properties that might be beneficial in preventing disease. Phytochemicals may demonstrate antioxidant, antimutagenic, antiestrogenic, anticarcinogenic, and anti-inflammatory effects. Phytosterols found in plant oils are noted for their an anti-inflammatory and immune-modulating effects, whereas phytoestrogens found in soy products are recognized for their hormonal and antioxidant effects.

MECHANISM OF ACTION

The protective effect of a phytonutrient depends on its chemistry. Phytochemicals include the phenolic compounds.[2] Phenols are ubiquitous phytonutrients found in cereals, fruits, and vegetables. They impart an astringent flavor to fresh food and can be a source of discoloration and "off flavors." Phenol is synthesized from L-tyrosine or L-phenylalanine via the shikimic pathway in plants. Enzymes for the synthesis and catabolism of phenol are not found in animal cells. Animals who eat plants accumulate phenols in their tissues. Because phenols readily coprecipitate with protein, they are readily eliminated from food during the manufacturing process.

FOOD SOURCES

Plant-derived phenols in the human diet include the following:

- Simple phenols such as hydroxybenzoic acid. Their richest sources are acidic tasting fruits. Tea, berries, a number of culinary herbs, and coffee are good sources. They have a powerful antioxidant effect.

- Phenylpropanoids such as hydroxycinnamic acid. Coffee, grains, and fruits are good sources. Ferulic acid (oryzanol), derived from rice bran oil, is a strong antioxidant, and caffeic acid has anticarcinogenic activity. Consuming moderate amounts of cinnamates may protect against a range of genotoxic substances.
- Flavonoids, three-ringed hydroxylated polyphenols. Flavonoids have an ideal chemical structure for free radical scavenging. Variations around the middle phenol ring have resulted in flavonoids being categorized into the following seven groups: flavones (e.g., luteolin and rutin), flavon-3-ols (e.g., quercetin and kaempferol), flavanon(ol)es (e.g., hesperidin and naringenin), flavan-3-ols (e.g., catechins), anthocyanins (e.g., cyanidin), chalones (e.g., phloretin), and isoflavones (e.g., genistein). Good sources of flavones are fruit skin, lemon, and onion; good sources of flavon-3-ols are black grapes, onions, and broccoli; good sources of flavanon(ol)es are citrus fruits; good sources of flavan-3-ols are red wine and tea; good sources of anthocyanins are red wine, grapes, and strawberries; good sources of chalones are apples; and good sources of isoflavones are soybeans and chickpeas (see Chapters 65 and 93). Isoflavones, indoles, isothiocyanates, and lignans all modify and dampen the effect of endogenous estrogens and may reduce the risk of cancer.
- Allylic sulfides. Garlic and onions are a good source of allylic sulfides. They raise high-density lipoprotein cholesterol levels, lower triglyceride levels, and suppress tumor growth.
- Carotenoids. Good sources are green leafy and yellow-orange vegetables. Carotenoids have an antioxidant effect.
- Monoterpenes. Rich sources are cherries and citrus fruit. Monoterpenes block certain carcinogens.
- Saponins. Rich sources are soybeans, chickpeas, nuts, oats, asparagus, and tomatoes. Saponins have a hypocholesterolemic effect and enhance immunity.

DOSE

The bioavailability in human subjects of nonnutrient plant factors is of great importance relative to their reported health-protective effects. Required intakes have not been adequately defined; however, a diet rich in fruits and vegetables is highly recommended.

CLINICAL USES

The clinical use of phytonutrients varies depending on their chemical structure. As a group, they reduce the risk of heart disease and cancer. In view of their diversity, phytonutrients may have an impact on several stages of atherosclerosis and/or carcinogenesis, for example[3]:

- Phenols, glucosinolates, and indoles, thiocyanates and isothiocyanates, and coumarins can induce a multiplicity of phase II enzymes. Phase II enzymes tend to increase the solubility of compounds and inactivate enzymes.
- Phenols and ascorbate block the formation of carcinogens such as nitrosamines.
- Flavonoids and carotenoids act as antioxidants, essentially disabling the carcinogenic potential of specific compounds.
- Carotenoids and sterols, lipid-soluble compounds, may alter membrane structure or integrity.
- Sulfur-containing compounds may suppress DNA and protein synthesis.
- Carotenoids may suppress DNA synthesis and enhance cellular differentiation.
- Phytoestrogens may compete with estradiol for estrogen receptors in a way that is generally antiproliferative.
- Different phytochemicals may influence almost every stage of carcinogenesis.

Fortunately, their overall impact appears to be to reduce the likelihood of disease.

TOXICITY/DRUG INTERACTIONS

This varies depending on the phytochemical involved.

CLINICAL CAUTION

Drug interactions with certain phytochemicals may occur.

PRACTICE TIPS

- Cruciferous vegetables should be microwaved or lightly steamed to preserve the phytonutrients.
- Chopping or crushing garlic and onions releases allyl sulfides, enhancing their biologic activity.
- Carotenoids are best absorbed when eaten in a meal containing fat or oil.
- Isoflavones and other phenolic compounds are retained in many processed foods.
- Flavonoids and monoterpenes are found in the skin and pulp of citrus fruits and in apples.

REFERENCES

1. Jacobs DR, Murtaugh MA: Its more than an apple a day: an appropriately processed plant-centered dietary pattern may be good for your health, *Am J Clin Nutr* 72:899-900, 2000.
2. Miller NJ, Rruiz-Larrea MB: Flavonoids and other plant phenols in the diet: their significance as anti-oxidants, *J Nutr Environ Med* 12:39-51, 2002.
3. Lamartiniere CA: Protection against breast cancer with genistein: a component of soy, *Am J Clin Nutr* 71(suppl 6):1705S-1707S, 2000.

■ CHAPTER 86 ■

PHYTOESTROGENS

> The clinical impact of phytoestrogens is dose-related and modified by the endogenous estrogen status of the woman; in premenopausal women, phytoestrogens suppress estrogenic stimulation, and in postmenopausal women, they stimulate estrogen receptors.

Various phytonutrients may act as phytoestrogens. Major dietary sources of phytoestrogens are soy products and flaxseed. Although exogenous estrogens derived from these and other plants are weaker than endogenous estrogens, diets rich in phytoestrogens have been shown to have clinical effects.[1]

The estrogenic potency of phytochemicals varies, depending on their source and concentration. The relative potency of phytoestrogens is also modified by their activation by intestinal bacteria and the hormonal status of the woman.

MECHANISM OF ACTION

Some phytonutrients have a hormone-modulating effect. Isoflavonoids and lignans stimulate hepatic production of sex hormone binding globulin (SHBG). SHBG binds testosterone; the amount of circulating SHBG influences the concentration of active (i.e., unbound) testosterone. Although phytoestrogens can influence the hormone status of both sexes, women are particularly affected. In menstruating women, phytoestrogens tend to depress estrogenic activity, and in postmenopausal women, the opposite is true.

Estrone, the dominant endogenous estrogen in postmenopausal women, is derived from androstenedione produced in the adrenal glands, and to a lesser extent, the ovaries. Androstenedione is converted to estrone in adipose tissue, the liver, and the kidneys. Estrone is around 12 times weaker than estradiol, the ovarian estrogen produced by menstruating women. Overall, phytoestrogens are 160 to 100,000 times weaker than estradiol.[2] In view of both the concentration and potency of estrone, phytoestrogens are of more importance as estrogen analogues in postmenopausal women.

Research has shown that herbal constituents have the capacity to compete with estradiol and progesterone, binding to intracellular receptors in intact human breast cancer cells.[3] The six most competitive estradiol-binding herbs that are commonly consumed are soy, licorice, red clover, thyme, turmeric, hops, and verbena. In vitro studies have indicated that red clover and hops show significant competitive binding to both α- and β-estrogen receptors, as does chasteberry.[4] Genistein is the most active component of red clover. The six most competitive progesterone-binding herbs and spices commonly consumed are oregano, verbena, turmeric, thyme, red clover, and damiana. In general, estradiol-binding herbal extracts are agonists, much like estradiol, whereas progesterone-binding extracts are neutral agents or antagonists.

In addition to hormonal modulation, phytoestrogens are noted for their antioxidant effect.[5] Isoflavones are well absorbed and appear to be sufficiently bioavailable to act as antioxidants in vivo. The inhibitory effect of isoflavones is further enhanced in the presence of ascorbic acid. Habitual dietary preferences also appear to influence the activation phytoestrogens. Gut bacteria remove a glycoside from isoflavone precursors to create the active isoflavones genistein, daidzein, and equol. Equol, a bacterial metabolite of daidzein, is a more potent antioxidant that daidzein. From a cardiovascular perspective, genistein appears to be the most potent antioxidant of the phytoestrogenic isoflavones, enhancing the resistance of low-density lipoproteins to oxidation.[6] However, the low reactivity of phytoestrogens with peroxyl radicals suggests that an antioxidant mechanism other than free radical scavenging reactions may account for their antioxidant effect.[7] Epidemiologic studies have shown that the intake of other flavonoids, especially quercetin, is inversely associated with mortality from ischemic heart disease. Along with their ability to alter hormone levels and their antioxidant activity, phytoestrogens may affect the development of cancer by inducing increased cellular differentiation through stabilizing protein-linked DNA strand breakage, modulating signal transduction pathways involved in cell division, inhibiting endothelial cell proliferation, impairing angiogenesis and tumor growth, and having a cytostatic effect.[8]

FOOD SOURCES

The major classes of physiologically active phytoestrogens are as follows:

- Isoflavones found in legumes, clover, alfalfa. Soybeans and soy foods contain 0.2 to 1.6 mg of isoflavones for each gram of dry weight. Soy isoflavones are 85% degraded in the intestine; differences in fecal flora determine the nature and bioavailability of isoflavones absorbed. Gut bacteria metabolize phytoestrogen precursors, producing genistein, daidzein, and equol. These active isoflavones have an estrogenic and antioxidant effect, and genistein has an antithrombotic effect by inhibiting platelet aggregation. Although all these active isoflavones do have an estrogenic effect, equol is some 1000 times and genistein 100,000 times weaker than estradiol. Isoflavones are considered in more detail in the section on soy products.

- Lignins found in whole grains and whole meal bread, rye, seeds, especially linseed (flaxseed), legumes, nuts (peanuts), fruits (e.g., pears, peaches), and vegetables (e.g., tomatoes). Lignin precursors are broken down by bowel bacteria into enterolactone and enterodiol (mammalian lignin). Whole-grain cereals are good sources of enterolactone and enterodiol. Lignans also have an antioxidant effect.
- Coumestans found in clover (5.6 mg/g dry weight), alfalfa, and soybean sprouts. Coumestans are estimated to have 30 to 100 times more estrogenic potency than the isoflavones but are 160 times less potent than estradiol. They have steroid-like activity but are not important in humans as a source of phytoestrogens (see Chapter 93).
- Phytosterols. Beta-sitosterol has estrogenic activity but is some 400 times weaker than estradiol. Because absorption is limited, dietary phytosterols have little, if any, phytoestrogenic effect in vivo (see Chapter 87).
- Triterpenoid and steroidal saponins. The structure of the saponins is similar to that of steroidal hormones. Ginseng and licorice are sources of triterpenoid saponins.
- Resorcylic acid lactones (e.g., zearalenone). Whole grains (e.g., wheat, rye, corn, oats) contain a fungus that produces the estrogenic substances zearalenol and zearalenone, which are stronger phytoestrogens than the lignin produced by the plant.

DOSE

Required intakes of phytoestrogens have not been adequately defined; however, a diet rich in fruits and vegetables is highly recommended.

CLINICAL USES

In a recent workshop, it was concluded that isoflavone-containing soy foods may have favorable effects on the cardiovascular system, but major knowledge gaps still exist regarding the effects of phytoestrogen supplements on bone disease, various cancers, menopausal symptoms, and cognitive function.[9]

Although phytoestrogens are less potent than hormone replacement therapy, they do have greater tissue selectivity and should be considered as treatment for menopausal women and men at risk of ischemic heart disease.[10] Animal experiments do suggest that dietary phytoestrogens significantly reduce aortic cholesterol content with a potency comparable to that of estrogen replacement.[11]

Epidemiologic and pathologic data suggest that thyroid cancer may well be an estrogen-dependent disease. A population-based, case-control study of thyroid cancer suggests that thyroid cancer prevention through dietary modification of phytoestrogen intake may be possible, but further research is required.[12] Further research is also required before phytoestrogens can be recommended as a hormone replacement option for patients with breast cancer.[13]

TOXICITY/DRUG INTERACTIONS

At high concentrations, phytoestrogens have been shown to inhibit DNA synthesis; whereas at lower concentrations, closer to probable levels in humans, induction of DNA has been noted.[14] Available data do not unequivocally support the beneficial effects of phytoestrogens, and, in the absence of satisfactory clinical findings, any untoward effects are cause for concern.[15] Excessive consumption should be avoided until more evidence is available.[1]

CLINICAL CAUTION

Infant soy formulas are rich in phytoestrogens. However, apart from a few women reporting slightly longer duration of menstrual bleeding and greater discomfort with menstruation, exposure to soy formula does not appear to lead to different general health or reproductive outcomes than exposure to cow's milk formula.[16]

PRACTICE TIPS

- Phytoestrogens are too weak to trigger ovulation.

REFERENCES

1. Jacobs JJ: Complementary/alternative therapies in select populations: women. In Spencer JW, Jacobs JJ, editors: *Complementary/alternative medicine: an evidence-based approach*, St Louis, 1998, Mosby.
2. Tricky R: *Women, hormones and the menstrual cycle*, Crows Nest, United Kingdom, 1998, Allen & Unwin.
3. Zava DT, Dollbaum CM, Blen M: Estrogen and progestin bioactivity of foods, herbs, and spices, *Proc Soc Exp Biol Med* 217:369-78, 1998.
4. Liu J, Burdette JE, Xu H, et al: Evaluation of estrogenic activity of plant extracts for the potential treatment of menopausal symptoms, *J Agric Food Chem* 49: 2472-9, 2001.
5. Wiseman H: The bioavailability of non-nutrient plant factors: dietary flavonoids and phyto-oestrogens, *Proc Nutr Soc* 58:139-46, 1999.
6. Ruiz-Larrea MB, Mohan AR, Paganga G, et al: Antioxidant activity of phytoestrogenic isoflavones, *Free Radic Res* 26:63-70, 1997.

7. Hwang J, Sevanian A, Hodis HN, et al: Synergistic inhibition of LDL oxidation by phytoestrogens and ascorbic acid, *Free Radic Biol Med* 29:79-89, 2000.

8. Humfrey CD: Phytoestrogens and human health effects: weighing up the current evidence, *Nat Toxins* 6:51-9, 1998.

9. Lu LJ, Tice JA, Bellino FL: Phytoestrogens and healthy aging: gaps in knowledge. A workshop report, *Menopause* 8:157-70, 2001.

10. Ariyo AA, Villablanca AC: Estrogens and lipids. Can HRT designer estrogens, and phytoestrogens reduce cardiovascular risk markers after menopause? *Postgrad Med* 111:23-30, 2002.

11. Alexandersen P, Haarbo J, Breinholt V, et al: Dietary phytoestrogens and estrogen inhibit experimental atherosclerosis, *Climacteric* 4:151-9, 2001.

12. Horn-Ross PL, Hoggatt KJ, Lee MM: Phytoestrogens and thyroid cancer risk: the San Francisco bay area thyroid cancer study, *Cancer Epidemiol Biomarkers Prev* 11:43-9, 2002.

13. This P, De La Rochefordiere A, Clough K, et al: The Breast Cancer Group of the Institut Curie. Phytoestrogens after breast cancer, *Endocr Relat Cancer* 8:129-34, 2001.

14. Wang C, Kurzer MS: Phytoestrogen concentration determines effects on DNA synthesis in human breast cancer cells, *Nutr Cancer* 28:236-47, 1997.

15. Strom BL, Schinnar R, Ziegler EE, et al: Exposure to soy-based formula in infancy and endocrinological and reproductive outcomes in young adulthood, *JAMA* 286:807-14, 2001.

16. Sirtori CR: Risks and benefits of soy phytoestrogens in cardiovascular diseases, cancer, climacteric symptoms and osteoporosis, *Drug Saf* 24:665-82, 2001.

■ CHAPTER 87 ■

PHYTOSTEROLS

The clinical impact of margarine rich in phytosterols may not be limited to reduction of blood lipid levels.

Phytosterols, or plant sterols, although structurally similar to cholesterol, are found at a concentration 800 to 1000 times lower than cholesterol in humans. Sterols and sterolins are bound to dietary fiber, making digestion difficult. About 5% of total dietary β-sitosterol is absorbed. The most common phytosterols are β-sitosterol, campesterol, and stigmasterol.

In animals, these plant sterols exhibit anti-inflammatory, antineoplastic, antipyretic, and immune-modulating activity.[1] In humans, they are used in functional foods to lower blood cholesterol levels.

MECHANISM OF ACTION

Phytosterols have diverse effects on the structure and function of membranes; they affect signal transduction pathways that regulate tumor growth and apoptosis, immune function, and cholesterol metabolism. A proprietary mixture of phytosterols seems to target specific T-helper lymphocytes, helping to normalize their function and improve T-lymphocyte and natural killer cell activity.[2] A dampening effect on overactive antibody responses and normalization of the dehydroepiandrosterone to cortisol ratio have also been reported. Furthermore, a blend of sterols and sterolins is capable of reducing the secretion of proinflammatory cytokines and tumor necrosis factor-α.[3]

The reestablishment of these physiologic parameters may benefit management of various chronic immune-mediated conditions including rheumatoid arthritis, acquired immunodeficiency syndrome, and cancer.

FOOD SOURCES

Plant oils contain the highest concentration; nuts and seeds, a moderate concentration; and fruits and vegetables, the lowest concentration of phytosterols.[4] Oranges and passion fruit are among the best fruit sources.

Peanuts and peanut products, such as peanut oil, peanut butter, and peanut flour, are good sources of phytosterols. Depending on the peanut variety, roasted peanuts may contain 61 to 114 mg of phytosterols per 100 g, and 78% to 83% of this is in the form of β-sitosterol. Unrefined peanut oil contains 207 mg of phytosterols per 100 g of oil. This value is higher than that of unrefined olive oil. Refining these oils results in reduction of phytosterol's concentration in the oil. This loss is greater in the case of olive oil than peanut oil. Further refining, such as deodorization, results in significant loss of phytosterols, but hydrogenation after refining has a minimal effect on phytosterol loss. Peanut butter, which represents 50% of the peanuts consumed in the United States, contains 144 to 157 mg of phytosterols per 100 g. Peanut flour, which is made by removing some of the oil from peanuts, contains 55 to 60 mg phytosterols per 100 g.[4]

Gamma-oryzanol, a mixture of phytosterols, is found in rice bran oil. Rice bran products are of interest as functional foods.[5]

Some margarines are a source of phytosterols. Margarine to which phytosterols have been added is marketed as a functional food for reducing cholesterol absorption. Phytosterols reduce cholesterol absorption by steric hindrance.

DOSE

The dose of phytosterols has yet to be established. Doses of 60 to 120 mg of β-sitosterol combined with 600 to 1200 μg of β-sitosterolin have been used, as have doses of 100 to 500 mg of γ-oryzanol daily. Animal fats inhibit absorption.

CLINICAL USES

Plant sterol esters reduce cholesterol absorption and lower circulating blood cholesterol concentrations when incorporated into the habitual diet. A randomized, double-blind, three-group, parallel controlled study demonstrated that incorporation of esterified plant sterols in a reduced-fat spread is a beneficial adjunct to the low-fat dietary management of hypercholesterolemia.[6] In fact, products enriched with plant sterol and stanol esters selectively lower low-density lipoprotein (LDL) cholesterol levels. In 16 recently published human studies, phytosterol therapy was accompanied by an average 10% reduction in the total cholesterol level and a 13% reduction in the LDL cholesterol level.[7] Results of another randomized, double-blind trial of two rapeseed oil–based test margarines, one with added stanols and another with added sterols, confirmed the benefit of phytosterols, demonstrating that both test margarines reduced significantly and equally total and LDL serum cholesterol concentrations, when they were consumed as part of a low-fat diet.[8] The effects were noted after several weeks of supplementation.

Phytosterols may also be of benefit in reestablishing optimal immune parameters. Epidemiologic and experimental studies suggest that dietary phytosterols may offer protection from the most common cancers in Western societies, such as colon, breast, and prostate cancer.[9] However, an epidemiologic study suggested that consuming plant sterols (285 ± 97 mg/d) from bread (38%), vegetable fats (26%), and fruits and vegetables (21%) was not associated with a lower risk of colon and rectal cancers.[10] Two clinical trials have demonstrated good responses when benign prostatic hypertrophy was treated with 60 to 130 mg β-sitosterol over a 6-month period.[1] Reviews of current research are available.[11]

TOXICITY/DRUG INTERACTIONS

Consumption appears to be safe, although one possible concern is lower concentrations of plasma carotenoids.[12] Whether this affects health over the long term or in selected patient groups is not known. A randomized, double-blind study showed that phytosterol esters were well-tolerated with no evidence of adverse effects at a daily intake of up to 9.0 g for 8 weeks.[13] All groups receiving phytosterols had significant increases in serum campesterol, but β-sitosterol levels did not differ from those of control groups. Blood concentrations of all fat-soluble vitamins and carotenoids remained within normal reference ranges. In any event, when spreads containing sterol or stanol esters are used, consumption of an additional daily serving of a carotenoid-rich vegetables or fruits (e.g., carrots, sweet potatoes, pumpkin, tomatoes, apricots, spinach, or broccoli) is recommended to maintain plasma carotenoid concentrations while significantly lowering LDL cholesterol levels.[14] Subjects ate 25 g of a fat spread containing a maximum of 2.5 g of plant stanol esters daily.

Doses of 600 mg of γ-oryzanol daily may cause a dry mouth, hot flashes, and irritability.

CLINICAL CAUTION

Phytosterols had been used for their lipid-lowering effect for many years before the immunologic impact of these phytosterols was recognized. Phytosterols may have other unexpected side effects. Rice bran oil and γ-oryzanol, with their mixture of phytosterols, have been shown in vitro and in animal models to modulate pituitary secretion, inhibit gastric acid secretion, and inhibit platelet aggregation, and have antioxidant action.[15]

PRACTICE TIPS

• Phytosterol supplements should taken on an empty stomach, one hour before meals.

REFERENCES

1. Monograph. Plant sterols and sterolins, *Altern Med Rev* 6:203-6, 2001.
2. Bouic PJ, Lamprecht JH: Plant sterols and sterolins: a review of their immune-modulating properties, *Altern Med Rev* 4:170-7, 1999.
3. Bouic PJ: Sterols/sterolins: the natural, nontoxic immuno-modulators and their role in the control of rheumatoid arthritis, *Arthritis Trust* Summer:3-6, 1998.
4. Awad AB, Chan KC, Downie AC, et al: Peanuts as a source of beta-sitosterol, a sterol with anticancer properties, *Nutr Cancer* 36:238-41, 2000.
5. Jariwalla RJ: Rice-bran products: phytonutrients with potential applications in preventive and clinical medicine, *Drugs Exp Clin Res* 27:17-26, 2001.
6. Maki KC, Davidson MH, Umporowicz DM, et al: Lipid responses to plant-sterol-enriched reduced-fat spreads incorporated into a National Cholesterol Education Program Step I diet, *Am J Clin Nutr* 74:33-43, 2001.
7. Moghadasian MH, Frohlich JJ: Effects of dietary phytosterols on cholesterol metabolism and atherosclerosis: clinical and experimental evidence, *Am J Med* 107:588-94, 1999.
8. Hallikainen MA, Sarkkinen ES, Gylling H, et al: Comparison of the effects of plant sterol ester and plant stanol ester-enriched margarines in lowering serum cholesterol concentrations in hypercholesterolaemic subjects on a low-fat diet, *Eur J Clin Nutr* 54:715-25, 2000.
9. Awad AB, Fink CS: Phytosterols as anticancer dietary components: evidence and mechanism of action, *J Nutr* 130:2127-30, 2000.
10. Normen AL, Brants HA, Voorrips LE, et al: Plant sterol intakes and colorectal cancer risk in the Netherlands Cohort Study on Diet and Cancer, *Am J Clin Nutr* 74:141-8, 2001.
11. Bouic PJ: The role of phytosterols and phytosterolins in immune modulation: a review of the past 10 years, *Curr Opin Clin Nutr Metab Care* 4:471-5, 2001.
12. Plat J, Kerckhoffs DA, Mensink RP: Therapeutic potential of plant sterols and stanols, *Curr Opin Lipidol* 11:571-6, 2000.
13. Davidson MH, Maki KC, Umporowicz DM, et al: Safety and tolerability of esterified phytosterols administered in reduced-fat spread and salad dressing to healthy adult men and women, *J Am Coll Nutr* 20:307-19, 2001
14. Noakes M, Clifton P, Ntanios F, et al: An increase in dietary carotenoids when consuming plant sterols or stanols is effective in maintaining plasma carotenoid concentrations, *Am J Clin Nutr* 75:79-86, 2002.
15. Cicero AF, Gaddi A: Rice bran oil and gamma-oryzanol in the treatment of hyperlipoproteinaemias and other conditions, *Phytother Res* 15:277-89, 2001.

CHAPTER 88

POTASSIUM (K)

Muscle weakness and cardiac arrhythmia may result from either a
deficiency or an excess of potassium.

Potassium is a major intracellular cation. Along with other electrolytes,
potassium is involved in acid-base balance, nerve conduction, and water balance. It influences smooth, striated, and cardiac muscle contraction. Potassium
helps regulate blood pressure.

MECHANISM OF ACTION

Potassium passes across cell membranes in exchange for sodium. It is a
major factor in determining intracellular fluid osmolality. It enters cells
through potassium channels. Potassium channels are multi-subunit complexes important for the differential distributions of K^+ conductance at the
cell surface, and hence, the electrical activity of cells and tissues.[1] By maintaining the resting membrane potential, potassium plays an important role
in transmission of nerve impulses, smooth and skeletal muscle contraction,
and maintenance of a normal cardiac rhythm. Potassium is involved with
insulin in the movement of blood glucose into cells. It is required for glycogen deposition in the liver and in skeletal muscle. In mitochondria, the
adenosine triphosphate–sensitive K^+ channel is important in cell signaling
pathways both for ischemic protection and for gene transcription.[2]

Changes in pH, and hence hydrogen ion concentration, affect potassium
balance.

FOOD SOURCES

Because potassium is an intracellular ion, good sources are intact cells. Foods
rich in potassium include squash, potatoes, spinach, lentils, beans, peas,
watermelon, raisins, orange juice, bananas, and cantaloupe. Animal products such and meat and milk are also good sources.

Potassium is lost when foods are boiled. Vegetables should be steamed,
and fresh whole fruits should be eaten when possible.

DOSE

An adequate daily intake of potassium is 1600 to 2000 mg or 40 to 50 mEq. The recommended daily allowance of potassium is 2 to 2.5 g, and supplementary doses range from 3 to 10 g. The body content of potassium is 180 g, and absorption is 100%.

CLINICAL USES

Potassium is prescribed for diarrhea and to replace losses resulting from use of diuretics.

Low potassium intake may play an important role in the genesis of high blood pressure. Although no consensus about the role of potassium intake in prevention or control of hypertension currently exists,[3] some studies support the protective value of a high intake of potassium. A randomized, double-blind, placebo-controlled trial showed that supplementation with 60 mmol of potassium chloride resulted in a substantial reduction (mean, 5 mm Hg) in systolic blood pressure in a population that habitually consumed a high-sodium and low-potassium diet.[4] Results from 33 randomized, controlled trials confirm that potassium supplementation is associated with a significant reduction in mean systolic (−4.44 mm Hg) and diastolic (−2.45 mm Hg) blood pressure.[5] The blood pressure effects of potassium administration appear to be enhanced when the intake of sodium is high.

TOXICITY/DRUG INTERACTIONS

Provided that renal function is normal, hyperkalemia caused by potassium supplementation is unlikely. Hyperkalemia presents as muscle weakness, confusion, anxiety, cardiac arrhythmia, or dyspnea.

Potassium may interact with various medications, particularly those used to treat hypertension and cardiac complaints. Angiotensin-converting enzyme inhibitors and nonsteroidal anti-inflammatory drugs increase the risk of hyperkalemia; whereas laxatives, steroids, and loop and thiazide diuretics increase the risk of hypokalemia.

CLINICAL CAUTION

Minor side effects of potassium deficiency include diarrhea, nausea, muscle weakness, abdominal discomfort, and flatulence. More severe deficiency may precipitate cardiac arrhythmia, mood changes, and paresis.

PRACTICE TIPS

- Patients taking certain extended-release potassium chloride tablets may notice the tablet in their stool; this is the shell of the tablet that remains after the potassium has been absorbed.
- Leg cramps that occur during exercise may be indicative of potassium deficiency.

REFERENCES

1. Deutsch C: Potassium channel ontogeny, *Annu Rev Physiol* 64:19-46, 2002.
2. Garlid KD, Paucek P: The mitochondrial potassium cycle *IUBMB Life* 52:153-8, 2001.
3. Dickey RA, Janick JJ: Lifestyle modifications in the prevention and treatment of hypertension, *Endocr Pract* 7:392-9, 2001.
4. Gu D, He J, Wu X, Duan X, et al: Effect of potassium supplementation on blood pressure in Chinese: a randomized, placebo-controlled trial, *J Hypertens* 19: 1325-31, 2001.
5. Whelton PK, He J: Potassium in preventing and treating high blood pressure, *Semin Nephrol* 19:494-9, 1999.

■ CHAPTER 89 ■

QUERCETIN

The clinical effects of quercetin and rutin are not identical; the physiologic functions of antioxidants overlap, but the precise chemical nature of any particular antioxidant modifies its potency and spectrum of activity.

Quercetin is the major bioflavonoid in the human diet. One of the most abundant of the naturally occurring flavonoids, it is frequently found in a wide variety of vegetables and herbs as rutin. Quercetin is the aglycone, or sugarless form of rutin (quercetin-3-rutoside). Quercetin is a flavon-3-ol, and rutin is a flavone. The best sources of quercetin and rutin are onions, kale, broccoli, and berries. Quercetin is found in all berries, and its concentration may reach 121 mg/kg in cranberries.[1]

Quercetin appears to have many beneficial effects on human health, including activity against cardiovascular disease, cancer, peptic ulcers, allergy, inflammation, and cataracts. Although quercetin (i.e., the aglycone form of the bioflavonoid) is touted as a dietary supplement for preventing or treating atherosclerosis, diabetes, cataracts, peptic ulceration, cancer, and prostatitis, it is rutin's ability to reduce capillary permeability that makes it recommended for treatment of varicose veins and as an adjunct to other supplements in the treatment of osteoarthritis.

MECHANISM OF ACTION

The bioflavonoids have antioxidant activity. Quercetin is directly, and rutin is rapidly, metabolized by intestinal bacteria through quercetin, to 3,4-dihydroxyphenylacetic acid, a phenolic compound with antioxidant activity. A reaction between this phenolic compound and free radical species forms phenoxy radicals that are considerably less reactive.[2] Laboratory studies have shown that dihydroquercetin was the only flavanone capable of reducing the ascorbyl radical, thus fulfilling the so-called ascorbate-protective function.[3] Quercetin is an effective protector against lipid oxidation in the cell membrane. In vitro studies have shown dietary quercetin to be capable of inhibiting peroxynitrite-induced oxidative modification of low-density lipoprotien cholesterol.[4] Such protection occurs in association with the lipophilic antioxidants lycopene, beta-carotene, and α-tocopherol present within the lipoprotein particle. Laboratory data suggest that quercetin and other antioxidants such as tea polyphenols (e.g., epigallocatechin gallate) dampen mitochondrial reactive oxygen species production.[5]

Quercetin inhibits inflammatory processes.[2,3] Several mechanisms are involved including potent antioxidant activity, membrane stabilization, inhibition of the enzyme hyaluronidase, and dampening of eicosanoid (particularly leukotriene) production. Quercetin exhibits antitumor properties through various mechanisms including immune stimulation, free radical scavenging, alteration of the mitotic cycle in tumor cells, gene expression modification, anti-angiogenesis, and/or apoptosis induction.[2,6] Quercetin influences gene expression and significantly reduces natural killer cell cytotoxicity.

However, there does appear to be conflict between in vitro and in vivo outcomes of quercetin. This may be related to a biphasic concentration effect. Although flavonoids are effective radical scavengers, the rather high redox potentials for most flavonols may explain their occasional prooxidative behavior.

DOSE

The dose of quercetin has not been established, but dietary supplements of both quercetin and rutin provide around 500 mg per dose. An oral dose of 400 to 500 mg three times per day is typically used in clinical practice; this may be reduced to 250 mg three times per day when quercetin chalcone, a water-soluble molecule, is used.[7]

The estimated average daily dietary intake of quercetin by an individual in the United States is 25 mg.[8] Most animal and human trials of oral dosages of quercetin aglycone show absorption in the vicinity of 20%. A daily dose 1500 mg is required to achieve serum quercetin concentrations consistent with anticancer activity ($\geq$10 μmol/L). Because of the poor bioavailability of quercetin, use of a water-soluble quercetin analogue, quercetin chalcone, may be prudent.[7]

CLINICAL USES

Quercetin may benefit patients with certain types of cancer. Treatment of human epidermoid cancer cells with quercetin results in strong dose-and time-dependent cell growth inhibition.[9] A combination of modified citrus pectin and quercetin chalone has been found to be effective in treating solid tumors in mice.[10]

Bioflavonoids may benefit the cardiovascular system. Epidemiologic studies suggest that the intake of flavonols and flavones is inversely associated with subsequent coronary heart disease.[11] On the other hand, rutin is believed to have beneficial effects on capillary permeability, venous insufficiency, and venous hypertension.[12,13]

Quercetin may ease discomfort. Quercetin is well tolerated and provides significant symptomatic improvement in most men with chronic pelvic pain syndrome.[14] It is effective for treatment of prostatitis in oral doses of 500 mg twice daily. Laboratory investigations suggest that it has an antimicrobial effect.[15] In vitro studies suggest that quercetin may be useful in reducing or preventing photobiologic damage caused by ultraviolet A irradiation[16] and may contribute to the reduction of copper toxic effects by chelating copper and enhancing metallothoinein induction by copper in a dose-dependent manner.[17] Other potential uses include treatment of gout through inhibition of xanthine oxidase; treatment of peptic ulcers through inhibition of lipid peroxidation of stomach cells, gastric acid secretion, and growth of *Helicobacter pylori*; and prevention of diabetic complications through inhibition of aldose reductase.

TOXICITY/DRUG INTERACTIONS

Human studies have not shown any adverse effects from taking quercetin either as a single dose of up to 4 g or after 1 month of administration of 500 mg twice daily. A single intravenous bolus of quercetin at a dose of 100 mg is also apparently well tolerated.

Quercetin inhibits sulfotransferase and modifies drug metabolism, affecting drugs such as salbutamol and acetaminophen (paracetamol) at the level of both the intestinal mucosa and liver.[18]

CLINICAL CAUTION

Many, but not all, studies have indicated that quercetin and its glycosides lack carcinogenicity.

PRACTICE TIPS

• Quercetin should be taken 20 minutes before meals.
• Quercetin is a more powerful antioxidant than vitamin E.

REFERENCES

1. Hakkinen SH, Karenlampi SO, Heinonen IM, et al: Content of the flavonols quercetin, myricetin, and kaempferol in 25 edible berries, *J Agric Food Chem* 47:2274-9, 1999.
2. Lamson DW, Brignall MS: Antioxidants and cancer III: quercetin, *Altern Med Rev* 5:196-208, 2000.

3. Bors W, Michel C, Schikora S: Interaction of flavonoids with ascorbate and determination of their univalent redox potentials: a pulse radiolysis study, *Free Radic Biol Med* 19:45-52, 1995.

4. Terao J, Yamaguchi S, Shirai M, et al: Protection by quercetin and quercetin 3-O-beta-D-glucuronide of peroxynitrite-induced antioxidant consumption in human plasma low-density lipoprotein, *Free Radic Res* 35:925-31, 2001.

5. Feng Q, Kumagai T, Torii Y, et al: Anticarcinogenic antioxidants as inhibitors against intracellular oxidative stress, *Free Radic Res* 35:779-88, 2001.

6. Kang ZC, Tsai SJ, Lee H: Quercetin inhibits benzo[a]pyrene-induced DNA adducts in human Hep G2 cells by altering cytochrome P-450 1A1 gene expression, *Nutr Cancer* 35:175-9, 1999.

7. Manach C, Regerat F, Texier O, et al: Bioavailability, metabolism and physiological impact of 4-oxo-flavonoids, *Nutr Res* 16:517-34, 1996.

8. NTP Technical Report (No. 409) on the toxicology and carcinogenesis studies of quercetin in F344/N rats. NIH Publication No. 91-3140 (1991). U.S. Department of Health and Human Services, Public Health Service, National Toxicology Program, Research Triangle Park, NC.

9. Lamson DW, Brignall MS: Natural agents in the prevention of cancer, part two: preclinical data and chemoprevention for common cancers, *Altern Med Rev* 6:167-87, 2001.

10. Bhatia N, Agarwal C, Agarwal R: Differential responses of skin cancer-chemopreventive agents silibinin, quercetin, and epigallocatechin 3-gallate on mitogenic signaling and cell cycle regulators in human epidermoid carcinoma A431 cells, *Nutr Cancer* 39:292-9, 2001.

11. Hayashi A, Gillen AC, Lott JR: Effects of daily oral administration of quercetin chalcone and modified citrus pectin, *Altern Med Rev* 5:546-52, 2000.

12. Hollman PC, Katan MB: Absorption, metabolism and health effects of dietary flavonoids in man, *Biomed Pharmacother* 51:305-10, 1997.

13. Mills S, Bone K: *Principles and practice of phytotherapy*, Edinburgh, 2000, Churchill Livingstone.

14. Shoskes DA, Zeitlin SI, Shahed A, et al: Quercetin in men with category III chronic prostatitis: a preliminary prospective, double-blind, placebo-controlled trial, *Urology* 54:960-3, 1999.

15. Gatto MT, Falcocchio S, Grippa E, et al: Antimicrobial and anti-lipase activity of quercetin and its C2-C16 3-O-acyl-esters, *Bioorg Med Chem* 10:269-72, 2002.

16. Erden Inal M, Kahraman A, Koken T: Beneficial effects of quercetin on oxidative stress induced by ultraviolet A, *Clin Exp Dermatol* 26:536-9, 2001.

17. Kuo SM, Huang CT, Blum P, et al: Quercetin cumulatively enhances copper induction of metallothionein in intestinal cells, *Biol Trace Elem Res* 84:1-10, 2001.

18. Marchetti F, De Santi C, Vietri M, et al: Differential inhibition of human liver and duodenum sulphotransferase activities by quercetin, a flavonoid present in vegetables, fruit and wine, *Xenobiotica* 31:841-7, 2001.

■ CHAPTER 90 ■

Saw Palmetto (*Serenoa repens*)

> Before prostatic hyperplasia is treated, it is good clinical practice to rule out a covert prostate malignancy.

Saw palmetto has been available for several years for the treatment of men with benign prostatic hyperplasia. Its medicinal properties are derived from the blue-black berries of the small palm tree *Serenoa repens*. The n-hexane lipidosterolic extract of the dwarf American palm is a complex mixture of various compounds that exert anti-inflammatory, spasmolytic, and some endocrine effects. It is as effective as reference medications in improving urologic symptoms and flow in patients with benign prostatic hyperplasia.

MECHANISM OF ACTION

Saw palmetto contains various lipids including phytosterols, a potent lipase, flavonoids, and polysaccharides. In vitro studies suggest that 5α-reductase inhibition, adrenergic receptor antagonism, and intraprostatic androgen receptor blockade may underlie the benefits of this herb. The lipidosterolic extract of *S. repens* appears to benefit benign prostatic hyperplasia by the following:

- Antiandrogenic effect. Androgen deprivation can reduce obstructive symptoms in prostatic hyperplasia. This is achieved through inhibition of type 1 and type 2 isoenzymes of 5α-reductase and through interference with the binding of dihydrotestosterone to cytosolic androgen receptors in prostate cells. The β-sitosterol-3 D-glucoside found in saw palmetto inhibits conversion of testosterone, by 5α-reductase, to the more active 5α-dihydrotestosterone. Dihydrotestosterone is about five times more potent than testosterone. Results from four randomized, placebo-controlled, double-blind trials, lasting 4 to 26 weeks, have shown that although β-sitosterols do not reduce prostate size, they do improve urinary symptoms and flow.[1]
- Anti-inflammatory effect. The berries inhibit cyclooxygenase and 5-lipoxygenase, and consequently, eicosanoid synthesis.

DOSE

The German Commission E suggests a dose of 320 mg (160 mg of liposterol extract twice daily).[2] The extract is 8:1 to 10:1 concentrate compared with the original dried berry. This equates to 2 to 4 g of dried whole berries each day.

Aqueous preparations should be avoided because they lack the active components of this herb.

CLINICAL USES

Saw palmetto is useful for treating obstructions to urinary flow caused by mild or moderate prostatic hypertrophy. A review of trials determined that there is good evidence for the efficacy of saw palmetto in the treatment of benign prostatic hyperplasia.[3] In controlled clinical trials of men with benign prostatic hypertrophy, oral administration of *S. repens*, 160 mg twice daily for 1 to 3 months, relieved dysuria, reduced the frequency of nocturia by 33% to 74%, and improved peak urinary flow rate by 26% to 50%.[4] A saw palmetto herbal blend was found to result in prostate epithelial contraction, and histologic studies showed that the percentage of atrophic glands increased from 25% to 41% in patients with moderate symptoms.[5] In fact, results of a large comparative trial suggest that men with moderate benign prostatic hypertrophy who received saw palmetto, 160 mg twice daily, had outcomes similar to those of men who received finasteride, 5 mg once daily for 6 months. Smaller comparative trials revealed few significant differences between *S. repens* and α-adrenergic receptor antagonists. Although placebo-controlled trials and meta-analyses suggest that saw palmetto leads to subjective and objective improvement in men with lower urinary tract symptoms, it must be noted that most studies are significantly limited by methodologic flaws, small patient numbers, and brief treatment intervals.[6] Nonetheless, a recent cost-benefit evaluation of herbal therapies indicated that saw palmetto had been shown, in short-term trials, to be efficacious in reducing the symptoms of benign prostatic hyperplasia.[7]

TOXICITY/DRUG INTERACTIONS

Saw palmetto is safe at recommended doses.[8] Although the long-term effectiveness, safety, and ability of saw palmetto to prevent complications in benign prostatic hypertrophy are not known, a review involving almost 3000 men from 18 randomized trials that lasted 4 to 48 weeks revealed that adverse effects caused by *S. repens* were mild and infrequent.[9] Saw palmetto is well tolerated; its major adverse effects are minor gastrointestinal problems such as nausea, abdominal pain, or diarrhea and headache. Taking saw palmetto with meals may eliminate any associated minor gastrointestinal problems.

A literature review to determine the possible interactions between ginkgo, St. John's wort, ginseng, garlic, echinacea, saw palmetto, and kava revealed no interactions between saw palmetto and the prescribed drugs reviewed.[10] However, concurrent use with androgens is not recommended because the effect of saw palmetto is likely to be impaired.

CLINICAL CAUTION

Patients taking saw palmetto should be monitored so that any cholestasis and/or breast enlargement can be detected early.

S. repens is a useful alternative to α-adrenergic receptor antagonists and finasteride in the treatment of men with benign prostatic hyperplasia, but because saw palmetto and finasteride have similar actions, if they are used together, they may have an exaggerated clinical effect.

PRACTICE TIPS

- Use of saw palmetto is probably most effective when the gland is only slightly enlarged.
- It is prudent to measure the level of prostate specific antigen before the herb is administered.

REFERENCES

1. Wilt T, Ishani A, MacDonald R, et al: Beta-sitosterols for benign prostatic hyperplasia, *Cochrane Database Syst Rev* 2:CD001043, 2000.
2. Blumenthal M, Busse, Goldberg, et al (eds): *The Complete German Commission E Monographs: Therapeutic Guide to Herbal Medicines*, Texas, 1999, American Botanical Council.
3. Linde K, ter Riet G, Hondras M, et al: Systematic reviews of complementary therapies—an annotated bibliography. Part 2: herbal medicine, *BMC Complement Altern Med* 1:5, 2001.
4. Plosker GL, Brogden RN: *Serenoa repens* (Permixon). A review of its pharmacology and therapeutic efficacy in benign prostatic hyperplasia, *Drugs Aging* 9:379-95, 1996.
5. Marks LS, Partin AW, Epstein JI, et al: Effects of a saw palmetto herbal blend in men with symptomatic benign prostatic hyperplasia, *J Urol* 163:1451-6, 2000.
6. Gerber GS: Saw palmetto for the treatment of men with lower urinary tract symptoms, *J Urol* 163:1408-12, 2000.
7. Ernst E: The risk-benefit profile of commonly used herbal therapies: ginkgo, St. John's wort, ginseng, echinacea, saw palmetto, and kava, *Ann Intern Med* 136: 42-53, 2002.
8. Klepser TB, Klepser ME: Unsafe and potentially safe herbal therapies, *Am J Health Syst Pharm* 56:125-38, 1999.

9. Wilt T, Ishani A, Stark G, et al: *Serenoa repens* for benign prostatic hyperplasia, *Cochrane Database Syst Rev* 2:CD001423, 2000.
10. Izzo AA, Ernst E: Interactions between herbal medicines and prescribed drugs: a systematic review, *Drugs* 61:2163-75, 2001.

CHAPTER 91

SELENIUM (SE)

Doses above the RDA of selenium (40 to 70 µg) are needed to inhibit genetic damage and cancer (>100 µg), but excessive doses of selenium may cause oxidative damage, leading to genomic instability; how much is enough?

Selenium, an essential trace element, is found in seafood, liver, lean red meat, and grains grown in selenium-rich soil. Selenium deficiency is a problem in areas of the world where the soil contains little selenium; selenium intake is on the decline in many areas (e.g., the United Kingdom). Subclinical selenium deficiency may be associated with reduced immunocompetence, depression, and reproduction problems in both males and females. There is evidence that selenium has a protective effect against some forms of cancer and that it may enhance male fertility, decrease cardiovascular disease mortality, and regulate inflammatory mediators in asthma.[1] It has also been postulated that optimal levels of selenium may be potentially useful for reducing the risk of atherosclerosis, cataracts, emphysema, inflammatory-immune disease, senile dementia, aging, and rheumatoid arthritis.

MECHANISM OF ACTION

Selenium is incorporated as selenocysteine at the active site of a wide range of selenoproteins. Selenoproteins are involved in functions as diverse as stabilizing the integrity of the sperm flagella and as essential as thyroid hormone metabolism aiding conversion of thyroxine (T_4) to the active thyroid hormone, 3,3'5-triiodothyronine (T_3). Selenium is an indispensable component of several major metabolic pathways.[2]

Selenium makes an important contribution to the anti-oxidant system. It acts as an anti-oxidant as a component of glutathione peroxidase and has a sparing effect on vitamin E. Glutathione peroxoidase prevents generation of free radicals that destroy polyunsaturated fatty acids in cell membranes. In fact, cellular and plasma glutathione peroxidase are the functional parameters used for the assessment of selenium status. Selenium enhances glucuronyl transferase activity, the enzyme required for detoxification of xenobiotic chemicals in the liver, and is involved in the degradation of intracellular peroxides and the regulation of prostaglandin synthesis.

Selenium is postulated to reduce the risk of cancer by a variety of mechanisms.[3,4] Selenium is believed to strengthen the immune system. It may also reduce the risk of cancer by enhancing stability of the genome by inhibiting carcinogen-induced covalent DNA adduct formation, retarding oxidative damage to DNA, lipids, and proteins, retarding angiogenesis, and modulating cellular events critical in cell growth inhibition. Laboratory studies, which demonstrated oxidative stress was induced by sodium selenite at high concentrations in both acute and chronic treatments of prostate cancer cells, suggested different mechanisms were involved.[5] After acute exposure to selenite, cells exhibited mitochondrial injury and cell death, mainly apoptosis. Chronic exposure selenium exerted its effects on human prostate cancer cells by altering the intracellular redox state, which subsequently blocked the cell cycle.

FOOD SOURCES

Brewers yeast, kelp, seaweed, brazil nuts, seafood (e.g. tuna, herring), garlic, milk, eggs, and kidneys are all possible sources.

DOSE

The RDA for selenium is 40 to 70 µg for healthy males and 45 to 55 µg for healthy females. The RDA for children starts at 10 µg and increases to 30 µg by the age of 10 years. The therapeutic dose range is 200 to 800 µg/day.[6] Selenium has a narrow safety margin, with clinical toxicity reported on daily doses of 1000 to 2000 µg over a month. The dose for long-term use is thought to fall between 100 to 400 µg. Extrapolation from animal experiments suggests that 400 to 700 µg/day may be required for cancer protection. Since 400 µg daily is probably the upper limit of safety, daily doses of 100 to 200 µg may be more realistic objectives for inhibiting genetic damage and cancinogenesis in humans.[7] Such recommendations are contrary to the traditional nutritional essentiality paradigm; however, as such advice is consistent with a better health outcome, it is perhaps time that the paradigm be reviewed.[8]

One of the safest selenium supplements is selenium organically bound to yeast. Yeast-based selenium is approximately 40% selenomethionine, 20% other amino acid conjugates (e.g., selenocysteine, methylselenocysteine), and 40% unidentified selenopeptides.[9] Doses of 500 to 1000 µg appear to be well tolerated. Selenite and selenate are more bioavailable than selenomethionine; however, selenomethionine appears more effective at increasing selenium status. In one animal study, co-administration of vitamin C nullified the chemopreventive effect of inorganic selenium (selenite), but not that of selenomethionine. Animal studies have confirmed that the dose and form of selenium compounds are critical factors in determining cellular responses, inorganic selenium at doses up to 10 µmol, and organic selenium compounds at doses equal to or greater than 10 μmol eliciting distinctly different cellular responses.[7] Animal studies using a variety of different tumorigenesis models have largely found that selenium has significant chemopreventive activity.

CLINICAL USES

Administration of 200 μg selenium from 0.5 g Brewer's yeast has been shown to reduce the incidence of several types of cancers in a human trial.[10] This placebo-controlled, prospective study found that, although a daily supplement of 200 μg selenium over a mean of 4.5 years showed no protective effects against the primary endpoint of squamous and basal cell carcinomas of the skin, the selenium-treated group had substantial reductions in the incidence of prostate cancer and total cancer incidence and mortality.[10] This dose is three or four times the RDA. Nonetheless, such findings are supported by epidemiologic studies, which have shown that low selenium status is associated with an increased total cancer incidence, particularly of gastrointestinal, prostate, and lung cancers.[11] Certainly, epidemiologic, laboratory, and serendipitous results of two randomized clinical trials suggest that men with high selenium and vitamin E intake have a lower risk of prostate cancer.[12] A case control study has also found that low plasma selenium is associated with a four-to five-fold increased risk of prostate cancer.[13] Because plasma selenium decreases with patient age, supplementation may be particularly beneficial to older men.

While the protective effect of selenium against cancer is fairly well documented, there is less clinical evidence to support the anti-inflammatory effect of selenium in arthritis. A recent clinical trial failed to demonstrate that selenium treatment (200 μg/day) achieved any clinical benefit in rheumatoid arthritis.[14]

Animal studies suggest other areas for investigation. It is possible that selenium deficiency and vitamin E deficiency can activate latent viruses such as herpes.[15] Animal studies have also shown that mice on either a selenium- or vitamin E–deficient diet developed myocarditis when exposed to coxsackie virus infection; those with adequate selenium or vitamin E status did not.[15] Viral-induced neuropathy was found to abate once selenium, vitamin E, carotenoid, and riboflavin blood levels were increased. It appears that a normally avirulent viral genome may become pathogenic in a nutritionally deprived host. An experimental animal study has also found that growth retardation induced by selenium deficiency is associated with impaired bone metabolism and a reduction in bone mineral density.[16]

TOXICITY/DRUG INTERACTIONS

Selenium toxicity is increased in animals with low or depleted stores of vitamin E. Chronic ingestion of more than 0.6 mg/day can cause garlic breath, paresthesias, hair loss, gastric disturbances, brittle fingernails, and dermatitis. Hepatorenal damage, nausea, a metallic taste, nervous irritability, depression, weakness, unusual fatigue, and nausea and vomiting have also been reported.

CLINICAL CAUTION

- Less than 11 µg selenium daily is thought to definitely put people at risk of selenium deficiency and genetic damage.[7] An increased risk of cancer is suspected to be associated with selenium deficiency. Clinically, findings consistent with selenium deficiency include fingernail and skin changes, cardiomyopathy, and skeletal muscle fatigue, tenderness, and weakness.
- Patients on monoamine inhibitors should avoid yeast-containing selenium products.
- Although an adequate vitamin C status is important for normal selenium metabolism, megadoses of vitamin C may decrease absorption of selenium taken as sodium selenite.[17]

PRACTICE TIPS

- Animal studies have shown selenium causes birth defects when given in large doses.
- Close monitoring of patients on selenium supplementation is necessary.
- Vitamin E 500 IU enhances the efficacy of selenium.
- Selenium and vitamin E have closely related mechanisms of action, and deficiency in one often overlaps with deficiency in the other.
- Muscular pain associated with selenium deficiency may be corrected with 200 µg daily.
- Selenium modulates T lymphocyte–mediated immune responses and stimulates peripheral lymphocytes to respond to antigens.
- Selenium 50 µg daily combined with beta-carotene 15 mg and vitamin E 20 IU may reduce the risk of cancer.
- Selenium does not protect against skin cancer, whether it be basal or squamous cell cancer.

REFERENCES

1. Brown KM, Arthur JR: Selenium, selenoproteins and human health: a review, *Public Health Nutr* 4(2B):593-9, 2001.
2. Holben DH, Smith AM: The diverse role of selenium within selenoproteins: a review, *J Am Diet Assoc* 99(7):836-43, 1999.
3. Kim YS, Milner J: Molecular targets for selenium in cancer prevention, *Nutr Cancer* 40(1):50-4, 2001.

4. Lu J, Jiang C: Antiangiogenic activity of selenium in cancer chemoprevention: metabolite-specific effects, *Nutr Cancer* 40(1):64-73, 2001.

5. Zhong W, Oberley TD: Redox-mediated effects of selenium on apoptosis and cell cycle in the LNCaP human prostate cancer cell line, *Cancer Res* 61(19):7071-8, 2001.

6. Brighthope I: Nutritional medicine tables, *J Aust Coll Nutr Env Med* 17:20-5, 1998.

7. El-Bayoumy K: The protective role of selenium on genetic damage and on cancer, *Mutat Res* 475(1-2):123-39, 2001.

8. Combs GF: Impact of selenium and cancer-prevention findings on the nutrition-health paradigm, *Nutr Cancer* 40(1):6-11, 2001.

9. Nelson MA, Porterfield BW, Jacobs ET, Clark LC: Selenium and prostate cancer prevention, *Sem Urol Oncol* 17(2):91-6, 1999.

10. Clark LC, Dalkin B, Krongrad A, et al: Decreased incidence of prostate cancer with selenium supplementation: results of a double-blind cancer prevention trial, *Br J Urol* 81(5):730-4, 1998.

11. Lamson DW, Brignall MS: Natural agents in the prevention of cancer part I: human chemoprevention trials, *Altern Med Rev* 6(1):7-19, 2001.

12. Brawley OW, Parnes H: Prostate cancer prevention trials in the USA, *Eur J Cancer* 36(10):1312-5, 2000.

13. Brooks JD, Metter EJ, Chan DW, et al: Plasma selenium level before diagnosis and the risk of prostate cancer development, *J Urol* 166(6):2034-8, 2001.

14. Peretz A, Siderova V, Neve J: Selenium supplementation in rheumatoid arthritis investigated in a double blind, placebo-controlled trial, *Scand J Rheumatol* 30(4):208-12, 2001.

15. Beck MA: Nutritionally induced oxidative stress: effect on virus disease, *Am J Clin Nutr* 71(6 Suppl):1676S-81S, 2000.

16. Moreno-Reyes R, Egrise D, Neve J, et al: Selenium deficiency-induced growth retardation is associated with an impaired bone metabolism and osteopenia, *J Bone Miner Res* 16(8):1556-63, 2001.

17. van den Brandt PA, Goldbohm RA, van't Veer P, et al: A prospective cohort study on selenium status and the risk of lung cancer, *Cancer Res* 53(20):4860-5, 1993.

■ CHAPTER 92 ■

SODIUM (NA)

> After many years of recommending that patients with hypertension reduce their salt intake, the salt hypothesis remains unproven and nothing more than a popular postulate.

Sodium, the major cation in extracellular fluid, is critical for regulation of body fluids. It influences acid-base balance, nerve function, water balance, and blood pressure. The intake of sodium tends to be much higher than the recommended allowance, and a major source is from salt added to processed food.

MECHANISM OF ACTION

Sodium is involved in the conduction of electrical impulses. Around two thirds of adenosine triphosphate (ATP) synthesized by cells is used to maintain the sodium-potassium transport system. The transporter protein ATPase requires sodium, potassium, and magnesium ions. For every ATP molecule hydrolyzed, three molecules of sodium move out of and two molecules of potassium move into the cell. This active transport system maintains an electrical potential with the inside of the cell being more negative than the outside. The excitability of nerve and muscle cells results from their ability to change this resting potential in response to electrochemical stimuli. Electrical impulses are transmitted as a result of changes in membrane permeability, movement of ions across the cell membrane, and restoration of the resting membrane potential by the ATP pump.

Sodium influences the fluid balance. It achieves fluid balance by attracting water. In contrast to the ATP-driven protein channel pump that moves sodium and potassium across the membranes of most cells, an active antiport proton pump moves sodium and hydrogen in opposite directions across cells in the small intestine and proximal renal tubular cells. Passive movement of sodium in distal renal tubular cells also influences fluid balance. Passive transport of sodium is by diffusion and electrical attraction. The epithelial sodium channel expressed in aldosterone-responsive epithelial cells of the kidney and colon plays a critical role in the control of sodium balance, blood volume, and blood pressure. Aldosterone conserves sodium by increasing activity of the sodium pump in the kidney.

FOOD SOURCES

Sodium is plentiful. It is found in fruits and vegetables, but more concentrated sources of sodium are table salt, sea salt, processed food, kelp, and celery. Hidden sources include toothpaste, certain mouthwashes, and medications (e.g., antacids, cough mixtures). The body content of sodium is 64 g and absorption is 100%.

DOSE

Current daily dietary guidelines for sodium are 2.4 g/day or 6 g of sodium chloride. This is far in excess of any physiologic need, and it is likely the harmful effects of sodium are expressed above a threshold of approximately 2.3 g (100 mmol) daily.[1]

CLINICAL USES

Sodium is prescribed for heat exhaustion. A 0.1% sodium chloride solution may be given orally. Heat cramps can be treated by taking 1 g salt hourly in large volumes of water.

Two determinants of blood pressure are circulating blood volume and vascular tone, both of which are influenced by sodium. Sodium restriction is routinely recommended for borderline and definitive cases of hypertension. However, the hypothesis that suggests higher levels of salt in the diet leads to higher levels of blood pressure and increases the risk of cardiovascular disease remains unproven.[2] In fact, the often quoted support derived from the Intersalt cross-sectional study of salt levels and blood pressures in 52 populations is based on somewhat contradictory data. Four of the populations did have low levels of salt and blood pressure, but across the other 48 populations, blood pressures went down as salt levels went up. Recent rigorous reviews of salt restriction trials in normal subjects show extremely small effects ranging from 1 to 2 mm Hg for systolic blood pressure and 0.1 to 1.0 mm Hg for diastolic pressure.[3] Furthermore, this drop in blood pressure is achieved at greater levels of sodium restriction than are consistent with recommendations for the general population. Population studies have not been able to show an association between salt intake and unfavorable health outcome. Experimental evidence suggests that the effect of a large reduction in salt intake on blood pressure is modest. Furthermore, based on population and randomized studies, the effect of an extreme salt reduction of 100 mmol on blood pressure in hypertensive persons only accounts for about one third of the effect of antihypertensive medication.[4] However, although the damaging potential of salt to the heart and kidney seems to be largely independent of the ongoing arterial pressure response, left ventricular mass is closely related to salt intake and a high salt intake induces hyperfiltration and raises glomerular pressure in the kidney. Despite sodium restriction being a popular clinical recommendation, the health consequences of sodium reduction have yet to be determined.

Salt reduction may have unfavorable effects on heart rate and serum levels of renin, aldosterone, catecholamines, and lipids. In short-term clinical studies, very low sodium intakes (<50 mmol/day) have been associated with greater values for total and low-density lipoprotein cholesterol, fasting and postglucose insulin, uric acid, and plasminogen activator inhibitor-1.[5] Short-term sodium restriction also enhances the activity of the renin-angiotensin system.[5] However, it should be noted that the long-term safety of the very low salt diets suggested by epidemiologic studies is not entirely consonant with the short-term clinical trials data in which sodium is studied as an isolated intervention.

Routinely, advocating salt restriction in the management of hypertension is being questioned.[4] Despite a potentially enormous impact if blood pressure decreased 1 to 2 mm Hg for every 75 to 100 mmol difference in sodium intake, the paucity and inconsistency of data linking sodium intake to health outcomes suggest that caution be exercised in advocating salt restriction.[6] A preferable approach would seem to be to adopt an individualized strategy. Calculation of specific individual "salt-sensitive risk profiles" based on knowledge of hypertension genes and environmental risk factors influencing the pressor response to salt is desirable.[7] The role of single-nucleotide polymorphisms in determining salt sensitivity or salt resistance in general populations requires further clarification. Genetically defined forms of a salt sensitivity and salt resistance in human monogenic diseases and in animal models have been reviewed,[8] as has the pathophysiology of essential hypertension.[9]

TOXICITY/DRUG INTERACTIONS

Dizziness, fluid retention, irritability, hypertension, and premenstrual blues may result from sodium toxicity.[10]

CLINICAL CAUTION

Persons complaining of lassitude, nausea, muscle weakness, and cramps may be sodium deficient.

PRACTICE TIPS

- Chronic diarrhea and excess sweating increase the requirement for sodium.
- Dietary sodium is associated with an obligatory calcium loss.

- Urinary sodium is an important determinant of calciuria in preadolescent and adolescent females.
- A diet rich in processed foods is likely to be high in sodium.

REFERENCES

1. Kaplan NM: The dietary guideline for sodium: should we shake it up? No, *Am J Clin Nutr* 71(5):1020-6, 2000.
2. Freedman DA, Petitti DB: Salt and blood pressure. Conventional wisdom reconsidered, *Eval Rev* 25(3):267-87, 2001.
3. Swales J: Population advice on salt restriction: the social issues, *Am J Hypertens* 13(1 Pt 1):2-7, 2000.
4. Graudal N, Galloe A: Should dietary salt restriction be a basic component of antihypertensive therapy? *Cardiovasc Drugs Ther* 14(4):381-6, 2000.
5. Egan BM, Lackland DT: Biochemical and metabolic effects of very-low-salt diets, *Am J Med Sci* 320(4):233-9, 2000.
6. Alderman MH: Salt, blood pressure, and human health, *Hypertension* 36(5):890-3, 2000.
7. Zoccali C, Mallamaci F: The salt epidemic: old and new concerns, *Nutr Metab Cardiovasc Dis* 10(3):168-71, 2000.
8. Rossier BC, Pradervand S, Schild L, Hummler E: Epithelial sodium channel and the control of sodium balance: interaction between genetic and environmental factors, *Annu Rev Physiol* 64:877-97, 2002.
9. Kurokawa K: Salt, kidney and hypertension: why and what to learn from genetic analyses? *Nephron* 89(4):369-76, 2001.
10. Brighthope I: Nutritional medicine tables, *J Aust Coll Nutr Env Med* 17:20-5, 1998.

■ CHAPTER 93 ■

SOY PRODUCTS

> The Japanese live longer and have less heart disease and breast cancer than Americans; they also eat about six times more soy products than Americans.

Soybeans, and particularly the isoflavones contained in soy, have generated interest as chemopreventive agents. Soybeans and soyfoods are, for practical purposes, the only nutritionally relevant dietary sources of isoflavones. Isoflavonoids are one of over 4,000 different polyphenolic compounds collectively called flavonoids that occur ubiquitously in foods of plant origin. The bioavailability of isoflavones has been shown to be influenced not only by their chemical form in foods, their hydrophobicity, and their susceptibility to degradation but also by the food matrix in which they are consumed and the microbial flora of the consumer.[1] In nonfermented foods, isoflavones appear as a conjugate, in fermented foods aglycones dominate.

Based on recent data of their conformational binding to estrogen receptors, soy isoflavones may be viewed as natural selective estrogen receptor modulators.[2] Genistein and daidzein, the major metabolites of soy isoflavone metabolism by bowel bacteria, are estrogen analogues.[3] Epidemiologic data indicate that women ingesting large amounts of phytoestrogens, particularly as isoflavones in soy products, have less cardiovascular disease, breast and uterine cancer, and menopausal symptoms than those eating Western diets.[4] Isoflavones are weak estrogens in that they bind to estrogen receptors, but they also have important nonhormonal properties.

While plant-derived estrogen analogs may confer significant health advantages, including cholesterol reduction, antioxidant activity, and possibly a reduced cancer risk, concern has also been raised that phytoestrogens may disrupt endocrine balance and create a major health hazard.

MECHANISM OF ACTION

Soybeans are a healthy food source rich in a number of constituents that have beneficial physiologic effects. In addition to their nutritional value, soybeans are a good source of fiber, prebiotics, and isoflavones. A number of the health benefits of soybeans have been specifically linked to one or more of these constituents.

The high fiber content of soybeans also favors a low glycemic index. Soy fiber supplements improve glucose tolerance and insulin response in subjects with glucose intolerance.

Soybeans contain oligosaccharides that function as prebiotics, promoting the growth of commensal bowel flora such as bifidobacteria. These probiotic bacteria promote bowel and cardiovascular health and may reduce the risk of colon cancer. Soy oligosaccharides, such as raffinose, stachyose, and verbascose, are fermented in the intestine to gas and short chain fatty acids. Short chain fatty acids produced by fermentation of oligosaccharides can hinder hepatic cholesterol synthesis and may lower blood cholesterol levels. In addition, soy products reduce blood cholesterol levels by the 7S globulin protein-enhancing low-density lipoprotein (LDL) receptor activity, increasing LDL degradation and, through isoflavones, offering an estrogen-mediated antioxidant effect. A randomized, double-blind, controlled trial that supplemented hypercholesterolemic postmenopausal women with soy protein containing either a low or high content of isoflavones found soy protein had a cholesterol-lowering effect regardless of the isoflavone concentration of the supplement.[5] This tends to confirm that isoflavone may not alone account for the hypocholesterolemic effects of soy.

Nonetheless, soybeans are the major dietary source of isoflavonoids; soy isoflavones are a dietary source of estrogens. Phytoestrogen derivatives bind at estrogen receptor sites and exhibit a biphasic effect on estrogen receptors, acting as an agonist at low concentrations and an antagonist at higher levels.[6] Phytoestrogens bind to β-estrogen receptors. Whereas α-estrogen receptors dominate breast, uterine, and ovarian tissue, β-estrogen receptors occur predominantly in prostate, bone, and vascular tissue. While the isoflavones in soybeans may reduce the risk of certain cancers, soybeans have other anticarcinogenic properties. In fact, multiple antineoplastic actions have been demonstrated, including protease inhibition, antimitotic effect, antiangiogenesis, inhibition of protein tyrosine kinase activity, and 5-α-reductase inhibition.[7]

In addition to having an antineoplastic, antioxidant, hypocholesterolemic, and glucose-normalizing effect, soybeans are a nutritious source of fiber, fat, protein, and even some minerals.[8]

FOOD SOURCES

Soy products are rich sources of nutrients and phytochemicals. Soy protein is a complete protein equivalent to egg albumin. Compared to other beans, soybeans are rich sources of polyunsaturated fat (20%) with a ratio of linoleic to α-linolenic acid around 7:1. Soybeans are a good source of fiber. One serving (31g/⅙ cup) of uncooked soybeans provides 5.4 g fiber, of which 2 g is soluble. They are also a good vegetable source of iron (16 mg/100 g dry wt), calcium (276 mg/100 g dry wt), and zinc (4.8 mg/100 g dry wt). Although availability varies depending on processing and phytate content, soybeans are a better source of minerals than other beans.

The concentration of soy protein is around 13 g in a cup of firm tofu, 6 g in one soy sausage, 10 to 12 g in a soy burger, 14 g in one soy protein bar, 19 g in ¼ cup of roasted soy nuts, and 10 g in an 8-ounce glass of plain soy milk.

Apart from soybeans, good sources of isoflavones are chickpeas, kidney beans, lentils, and red clover. The diverse constituents of soy, however, do provide a rationale for augmenting the diet with soy foods rather than isoflavone extracts. In fact, discrepancies in research outcomes may be related to differences in the study population, but they may also be attributable to differences in the soy supplement used.

DOSE

The dose of isoflavones has not been established. However, the minimal daily requirement appears to be about two servings (i.e., 200 g tofu, 2 cups soy milk, or 1 cup soy flour). One serving of traditional soy foods usually provides between 25 to 40 mg isoflavones. Dietary supplements usually contain 50 to100 mg of mixed isoflavones. The threshold intake of phytoestrogens necessary to have a biologic effect in humans appears to be 30 to 50 mg/day, a quantity attainable by the inclusion of modest amounts of soy in the diet.[9] However, taking soy protein (40 g/day) with 1.39 mg isoflavones per gram of protein for 6 months decreased the risk factors associated with cardiovascular disease in postmenopausal women; soy with isoflavone content of 2.25 mg or more per gram of protein was required to protect against spinal bone loss.[10] A red clover isoflavone preparation containing genistein, daidzein, formononetin, and biochanin increased the bone mineral density of the proximal radius and ulna by 4.1% over 6 months with 57 mg/day and by 3.0% with 85.5 mg/day of isoflavones.[11] The response with 28.5 mg/day of isoflavones was not significant. Spinal studies suggest that a dose threshold may be significant; the same may be true for cardiovascular health. This cross-over, randomized, controlled study that supplemented postmenopausal women with a red clover isoflavone preparation using different doses of phytoestrogens (28.5 mg, 57 mg, or 85.5 mg) each day for 6 months detected a rise in HDL cholesterol (15% to 28%) and a fall in serum apolipoprotein B (11% to 17%), unrelated to dose.[11] Such studies confirm that isoflavones are an active principle contributing to cardiovascular and skeletal health and emphasize the desirability of identifying minimal effective dose thresholds required to achieve various biologic functions.

It is also relevant that soy has been found to alter estrogen metabolism in both pre-and postmenopausal women. Consumption of 65 mg/day isoflavones by postmenopausal women was found to increase serum 2-OH:16-OH estrone ratios.[12] Urinary excretion of 2-OH estrone was increased by consumption of 158 mg/day soy isoflavones for an entire menstrual cycle in pre-menopausal women.[13] Consumption of 154 mg/day soy isoflavones for one menstrual cycle was associated with a 25% reduction in circulating 17-β-estradiol concentrations in premenopausal women.[14]

CLINICAL USES

Soy may have a cardioprotective effect. Epidemiologic and laboratory evidence has long suggested that soy foods and compounds may prevent heart disease through favorable changes to lipid profile and a possible effect on arterial compliance. While epidemiologic evidence continues to support this hypothesis,[15] clinical evidence is less clear cut. A randomized, placebo-controlled, double-blind, crossover trial of healthy postmenopausal women found taking a soybean tablet containing 80 mg/day of isoflavone for 8 weeks failed to significantly modify blood pressure, peripheral vasodilation, endothelial function, or lipoprotein levels.[16] Another randomized, controlled, double-blind trial on healthy persons over 50 years of age found those on a soy protein isolate with 40 g soy protein and 118 mg isoflavones had a mildly greater fall in both diastolic and systolic blood pressure and a significantly greater improvement in overall lipid profile than the control casein group.[17]

In addition to affecting blood pressure, soy products can improve the lipid profile. Soybeans are good source of saponins, which bind with and help excretion of cholesterol. Consumption of isoflavones as a constituent of isolated soy protein results in small but significant improvement in the lipid profile in normocholesterolemic and mildly hypercholesterolemic post-menopausal women.[18] A randomized, double-blind, crossover pilot study in elderly men consuming two soy beverages daily, each containing 20 g isolated soy protein, decreased serum cholesterol levels.[19] Replacing animal with soy protein has been shown to reduce total and LDL-cholesterol concentrations in humans. Consuming as little as 20 g soy protein daily, instead of animal protein, for 6 weeks reduced concentrations of non-HDL cholesterol and apo B by approximately 2.6% and 2.2%, respectively.[20] Soy may not only achieve more favorable lipid ratios, it may also reduce the quantity of oxidized cholesterol.

A randomized trial found consuming soy containing naturally occurring amounts of isoflavone phytoestrogens reduced lipid peroxidation in vivo and increased the resistance of LDL to oxidation.[21] This effect was dependent on the dose of isoflavones ingested. Consuming soy foods with 33 g soy protein that provided 86 mg isoflavones per 2000 kcal daily and doubling the soluble fiber intake reduced levels of circulating oxidized LDL, even in subjects taking vitamin E (400 to 800 mg/d), found no evidence of increased urinary estrogenic activity.[22] This suggests soy consumption may reduce cardiovascular disease risk without increasing the risk for hormone-dependent cancers.

In view of its estrogen analogues, soy is of potential benefit to postmenopausal woman. Although soy failed to prevent hot flashes in breast cancer survivors[23] and perimenopausal women in doses of 80.4 mg isoflavone daily,[24] a double-blind, randomized, multicenter study did find soy isoflavone extract (50 mg/day genistein and daidzein) decreased the frequency and severity of hot flushes within 2 weeks of supplementation.[25] This clinical trial is consistent with a prospective study that suggested that hot flushes were significantly inversely associated with consumption of soy products in terms of both the total amount soy product consumed and the isoflavone intake.[26] As a rule of thumb, 60 to 140 mg/day soy can be used to relieve menopausal flushes.

While uncertainty about the impact of isoflavones on flushes is perplexing, it is the potential of soy products to alter bone mass that has more profound health implications. High consumption of soy products has been shown to increase bone mass in postmenopausal women.[27] Weight and years since menopause, significant independent predictors of bone mineral density, were controlled in the study. A 24-week, double-blind trial concluded soy isoflavones (80.4 mg/day) attenuated bone loss from the lumbar spine in perimenopausal women.[28] The authors suggested isoflavones, not soy protein, exerted the effect. Preliminary human studies suggest that postmenopausal woman have an increased lumbar bone density after consuming 40 g soy protein with 2.25 mg isoflavones per gram each day for 6 months.[10] Animal studies suggest that soy is more protective of trabecular than cortical bone.[29] Several studies have also found that in comparison with animal protein, soy protein decreases calcium excretion, a result of the lower sulfur amino acid content of soy protein.[30]

Soybeans may influence hormone-dependent cancers. Early consumption of soy foods in young girls may reduce breast cancer in later life.[31,32] Consumption of an isoflavone-containing soya diet reduces levels of ovarian steroids in normal women over the entire menstrual cycle without affecting gonadotropins.[14] Although not statistically significant, men who ate tofu five times or more a week are at a lower risk of prostate cancer than those who ate it once or less a week.

TOXICITY/DRUG INTERACTIONS

Adding a soy beverage containing 20 g of protein and 38 mg of total isoflavones to their usual diet had no significant effect on the menstrual cycle, serum sex hormones, or urinary estrogen metabolite ratio in premenopausal women.[33] However, some research has shown soy isoflavones have an estrogenic effect on the normal breast. Clinical trials found consumption of 45 mg isoflavones increased the proliferation of normal breast tissue.[34,35]

Preliminary in vitro studies suggest soy may attenuate the estrogen-receptor antagonist activity of tamoxifen.[36] Isoflavones may potentiate the effect of oral contraceptives and hormone replacement therapy.

CLINICAL CAUTION

In the absence of adequate research, conservative use of soy in patients with breast cancer and other endocrine related tumors is recommended.

The validity of extrapolating reports that soy isoflavones potentially have a negative effect on cognitive function in the aged, may induce chromosomal changes in cells exposed in vitro, and could potentiate chemical carcinogens to clinical situations is questionable.[37] Nonetheless, perhaps caution should be exercised in use of these phytonutrients. This is particularly true if the clinical efficacy of soy isoflavones in reducing plasma cholesterol levels, preventing cancer in endocrine influenced tissues, and preventing or treating postmenopausal symptoms and osteoporosis is weak.

PRACTICE TIPS

- Processing does not destroy isoflavones, so canned beans remain a good source.
- It may be wise for elderly people to limit their tofu intake until further notice.
- Soaking soybeans and throwing away the water a number of times before cooking can reduce flatus resulting from gas production caused by oligosaccharide fermentation.

REFERENCES

1. Birt DF, Hendrich S, Wang W: Dietary agents in cancer prevention: flavonoids and isoflavonoids, *Pharmacol Ther* 90(2-3):157-77, 2001.
2. Setchell KD: Soy isoflavones—benefits and risks from nature's selective estrogen receptor modulators (SERMs), *J Am Coll Nutr* 20(5 Suppl):354S-62S, 2001.
3. Alhasan SA, Ensley JF, Sarkar FH: Genistein induced molecular changes in a squamous cell carcinoma of the head and neck cell line, *Int J Oncol* 16(2):333-8, 2000.
4. Lissin LW, Cooke JP: Phytoestrogens and cardiovascular health, *J Am Coll Cardiol* 35(6):1403-10, 2000.
5. Mackey R, Ekangaki A, Eden JA: The effects of soy protein in women and men with elevated plasma lipids, *Biofactors* 12(1-4):251-7, 2000.
6. Miodini P, Fioravanti L, Di Fronzo G, Cappelletti V: The two phyto-oestrogens genistein and quercetin exert different effects on oestrogen receptor function, *Br J Cancer* 80(8):1150-5, 1999.
7. Lamson DW, Brignall MS: Natural agents in the prevention of cancer, part two: preclinical data and chemoprevention for common cancers, *Altern Med Rev* 6(2):167-87, 2001.
8. Anderson JW, Smith BM, Washnock CS: Cardiovascular and renal benefits of dry beans and soybean intake, *Am J Clin Nutr* 70(3 Suppl):464S-74S, 1999.
9. Setchell KD: Phytoestrogens: the biochemistry, physiology, and implications for human health of soy isoflavones, *Am J Clin Nutr* 68(6 Suppl):1333S-46S, 1998.
10. Potter SM, Baum JA, Teng H, et al: Soy protein and isoflavones: their effects on blood lipids and bone density in postmenopausal women, *Am J Clin Nutr* 68(6 Suppl):1375S-9S, 1998.

11. Clifton-Bligh PB, Baber RJ, Fulcher GR, et al: The effect of isoflavones extracted from red clover (Rimostil) on lipid and bone metabolism, *Menopause* 8(4):259-65, 2001.

12. Xu X, Duncan AM, Wangen KE, Kurzer MS: Soy consumption alters endogenous estrogen metabolism in postmenopausal women, *Cancer Epidemiol Biomark Prev* 9(8):781-6, 2000.

13. Lu LJ, Cree M, Josyula S, et al: Increased urinary excretion of 2-hydroxyestrone but not 16-alpha-hydroxyestrone in premenopausal women during a soya diet containing isoflavones, *Cancer Res* 60(5):1299-305, 2000.

14. Lu LJ, Anderson KE, Grady JJ, et al: Decreased ovarian hormones during a soya diet: implications for breast cancer prevention, *Cancer Res* 60(15):4112-21, 2000.

15. Goodman-Gruen D, Kritz-Silverstein D: Usual dietary isoflavone intake is associated with cardiovascular disease risk factors in postmenopausal women, *J Nutr* 131(4):1202-6, 2001.

16. Simons LA, von Konigsmark M, Simons J, Celermajer DS: Phytoestrogens do not influence lipoprotein levels or endothelial function in healthy, postmenopausal women, *Am J Cardiol* 85(11):1297-301, 2000.

17. Teede HJ, Dalais FS, Kotsopoulos D, et al: Dietary soy has both beneficial and potentially adverse cardiovascular effects: a placebo-controlled study in men and postmenopausal women, *J Clin Endocrinol Metab* 86(7):3053-60, 2001.

18. Wangen KE, Duncan AM, Xu X, Kurzer MS: Soy isoflavones improve plasma lipids in normocholesterolemic and mildly hypercholesterolemic postmenopausal women, *Am J Clin Nutr* 73(2):225-31, 2001.

19. Urban D, Irwin W, Kirk M, et al: The effect of isolated soy protein on plasma biomarkers in elderly men with elevated serum prostate specific antigen, *J Urol* 165(1):294-300, 2001.

20. Teixeira SR, Potter SM, Weigel R, et al: Effects of feeding 4 levels of soy protein for 3 and 6 wk on blood lipids and apolipoproteins in moderately hypercholesterolemic men, *Am J Clin Nutr* 71(5):1077-84, 2000.

21. Wiseman H, O'Reilly JD, Adlercreutz H, et al: Isoflavone phytoestrogens consumed in soy decrease F(2)-isoprostane concentrations and increase resistance of low-density lipoprotein to oxidation in humans, *Am J Clin Nutr* 72(2):395-400, 2000.

22. Jenkins DJ, Kendall CW, Garsetti M, et al: Effect of soy protein foods on low-density lipoprotein oxidation and ex vivo sex hormone receptor activity a controlled crossover trial, *Metabolism* 49(4):537-43, 2000.

23. Quella SK, Loprinzi CL, Barton DL, et al: Evaluation of soy phytoestrogens for the treatment of hot flashes in breast cancer survivors: A North Central Cancer Treatment Group Trial, *J Clin Oncol* 18(5):1068-74, 2000.

24. St Germain A, Peterson CT, Robinson JG, Alekel DL: Isoflavone-rich or isoflavone-poor soy protein does not reduce menopausal symptoms during 24 weeks of treatment, *Menopause* 8(1):17-26, 2001.

25. Upmalis DH, Lobo R, Bradley L, et al: Vasomotor symptom relief by soy isoflavone extract tablets in postmenopausal women: a multicenter, double-blind, randomized, placebo-controlled study, *Menopause* 7(4):236-42, 2000.

26. Nagata C, Takatsuka N, Kawakami N, Shimizu H: Soy product intake and hot flashes in Japanese women: results from a community-based prospective study, *Am J Epidemiol* 153(8):790-3, 2001.

27. Somekawa Y, Chiguchi M, Ishibashi T, Aso T: Soy intake related to menopausal symptoms, serum lipids, and bone mineral density in postmenopausal Japanese women, *Obstet Gynecol* 97(1):109-15, 2001.
28. Alekel DL, Germain AS, Peterson CT, et al: Isoflavone-rich soy protein isolate attenuates bone loss in the lumbar spine of perimenopausal women, *Am J Clin Nutr* 72(3):844-52, 2000.
29. Messina MJ: Legumes and soybeans: overview of their nutritional profiles and health effects, *Am J Clin Nutr* 70(3 Suppl):439S-50S, 1999.
30. Messina M, Messina V: Soyfoods, soybean isoflavones, and bone health: a brief overview, *J Ren Nutr* 10(2):63-8, 2000.
31. Brown NM, Lamartiniere CA: Xenoestrogens alter mammary gland differentiation and cell proliferation in the rat, *Environ Health Perspect* 16:708-13, 1995.
32. Lamartiniere CA, Moore JB, Brown NM, et al: Genistein suppresses mammary cancer in rats, *Carcinogenesis* 16(11):2833-40, 1995.
33. Martini MC, Dancisak BB, Haggans CJ, et al: Effects of soy intake on sex hormone metabolism in premenopausal women, *Nutr Cancer* 34(2):133-9, 1999.
34. Hargreaves DF, Potten CS, Harding C, et al: Two-week dietary soy supplementation has an estrogenic effect on normal premenopausal breast, *J Clin Endocrinol Metab* 84(11):4017-24, 1999.
35. McMichael-Phillips DF, Harding C, Morton M, et al: Effects of soy-protein supplementation on epithelial proliferation in the histologically normal human breast, *Am J Clin Nutr* 68(6 Suppl):1431S-6S, 1998.
36. Schwartz JA, Liu G, Brooks SC: Genistein-mediated attenuation of tamoxifen-induced antagonism from estrogen receptor-regulated genes, *Biochem Biophys Res Comm* 253(1):38-43, 1998.
37. Sirtori CR: Risks and benefits of soy phytoestrogens in cardiovascular diseases, cancer, climacteric symptoms and osteoporosis, *Drug Saf* 24(9):665-82, 2001.

■ CHAPTER 94 ■

ST. JOHN'S WORT (*HYPERICUM PERFORATUM*)

> Herbs are natural but not necessarily without untoward effects; in fact, patients on St. John's wort are advised not to discontinue this drug without professional supervision.

St. John's wort is a perennial shrub that bears yellow flowers. It is regarded as an important natural antidepressant. Traditionally, this herb is also considered to have antiviral, anti-inflammatory, and analgesic activity.

MECHANISM OF ACTION

Hypericum perforatum contains numerous biologically active constituents such as naphthodianthrones, including hypericin and its derivatives, hyperforin, flavonoids (hyperoside, rutin, quercetin, etc.), catechin, epicatechin, procyanidin B_2, amino acid derivatives (melatonin, GABA), and essential oils. It is thought that St. John's wort may be effective through cumulative activity on a number of neurotransmitters and steroid hormones. It is not yet known definitively which constituents are responsible for *Hypericum*'s antidepressant effects, but there is a positive correlation between the hyperforin concentration and the antidepressant efficacy of this herb.[1]

Hypericum's antidepressant effect may be achieved by the following:

- Inhibiting serotonin, dopamine, norepinephrine, GABA, and L-glutamate reuptake. Hypericin extract appears to inhibit serotonin uptake by postsynaptic receptors and increase synaptic dopamine concentration.
- Inhibition of monoamine oxidase. However, this is only achieved at doses exceeding those typically found in commercially available extracts. Quercetin and xanthones in the roots and leaves may inhibit monoamine oxidase.

Since *Hypericum* extracts have only weak activity in assays related to mechanisms of the synthetic antidepressants, it has been postulated that the clinical efficacy of St. John's wort could be attributable to the combined contribution of several mechanisms, each one too weak by itself to account for the overall effect.[2] St. John's wort has also been shown to inhibit free radical production in both cell-free and human vascular tissue.[3]

DOSE

In clinical trials, typical dosages of standardized *Hypericum* extracts range from 300 mg of 0.3% hypericin liquid tincture taken three times daily for mild to moderate depression to 600 mg solid extract taken three times daily for more severe depression.[4] Traditionally the following doses have been used:

• 2 to 5 g dried herb each day or equivalent to 1.0 to 2.7 mg of total hypericin.
• 2 to 3 standardized hypericin tablets per day (1.5 g with 0.9 mg hypericin).
• Liquid extract 3 to 6 ml of 1:2 liquid extract or 7.5 to 15 ml of 1:5 tincture daily.

As a dietary supplement, St. John's wort is currently largely unregulated, but the Food and Drug Administration is reviewing plans to tighten this regulatory oversight.[5]

CLINICAL USES

Reviews of clinical trials consistently conclude that St. John's wort is more effective than placebo in the short-term treatment of mild to moderate depression.[6-8] In a double-blind, placebo-controlled trial, 105 mildly depressed subjects were given a standardized extract of St. John's wort at a dose of 300 mg three times daily.[9] Significant improvements, using the Hamilton Depression Scale, were noted with respect to depressive mood, sleep, and anxiety. A randomized, placebo-controlled, crossover study of 72 patients with major depression also found significant improvement in depression within the first 2 weeks of the trial in patients taking 300 mg three times daily of a standardized *Hypericum* extract.[10] A study of 209 severely depressed patients comparing *Hypericum* standardized extract, 600 mg tid, with imipramine, 50 mg tid, found similarly positive results in both groups, except that the *Hypericum* group experienced significantly fewer side effects (34.6% versus 81.4%).[11] Although controlled studies are needed to determine the long-term efficacy of *Hypericum* in mild to moderate depression, in view of its favorable side effect profile, *Hypericum* offers a realistic alternative to other antidepressants.[8]

A small study has also detected a significant reduction in the Hamilton Depression Scale scores of patients with seasonal affective disorder treated with 300 mg tid standardized *Hypericum* extract, regardless of light exposure.[12] The psychologic symptoms of menopause may also respond to this herb.

Results from an open trial of 450 mg of 0.3% hypericin, a psychoactive compound in *Hypericum*, given twice daily suggest patients with obsessive-compulsive neurosis may benefit.[13]

In addition to a beneficial effect on psychologic problems, *Hypericum* extracts have been reported to demonstrate the following[12]:

- In vitro antiviral effects. Hypericin may improve CD4/CD8 ratios in HIV/AIDS patients. Hypericin is active against enveloped viruses (e.g., herpes and parainfluenza).
- Enhanced wound healing. This is due in part to its antimicrobial effects. Topical *Hypericum* ointment heals burns faster and prevents keloid formation. *Hypericum* infusion, prepared by packing *Hypericum* flowers and leaves into a jar and covering them with olive or safflower oil, is traditionally used to speed the healing of burns and wounds. The jar is placed in the sun and shaken daily. The oil is poured off after 2 to 3 weeks and can be used in wound dressings and as a massage oil. The red-pigmented oil can stain clothing.

Traditionally, *Hypericum* is believed to have anti-inflammatory and analgesic properties.

TOXICITY/DRUG INTERACTIONS

The incidence of adverse events in those treated with St. John's wort is between 1% and 3%, some 10 times less than that with synthetic antidepressants. Although St. John's wort causes fewer side effects than other antidepressants, further trials are still needed to establish its long-term efficacy and safety.[8] Despite St. John's wort being generally regarded as a safe herb, side effects such as gastrointestinal tract disturbances, allergic reactions, fatigue, dizziness, confusion, dry mouth, or photosensitivity have been reported in up to 1 in 40 persons.[14] Furthermore, serious concerns exist about its interactions with several conventional drugs.[15,16] Medication dosages of other drugs (e.g., digoxin, warfarin) may need to be adjusted in patients treated with *Hypericum*.

Hypericum may alter the efficacy of various drugs by modifying their metabolism through induction of several isoenzymes of the hepatic cytochrome P_{450} enzyme system. Recent analysis of over 100 studies confirmed therapeutic preparations of *Hypericum* extract had a potentially significant pharmacologic effect on depression but cautioned that little information existed regarding the safety of *Hypericum*, including potential herb-drug interactions.[17] Furthermore, a single-blind, placebo-controlled, parallel study found that *Hypericum* extract LI160 (900 mg/day) reduced the requirement for digoxin; the effect became increasingly pronounced until the tenth day of combined therapy.[18] Care should also be exercised when the drug is used in patients taking oral contraceptives, theophylline, and warfarin. Since *Hypericum* may inhibit monoamine oxidase, its use with pseudoephedrine and ephedrine should be avoided.

Women using oral contraception should be warned that the effectiveness of this contraceptive method may be modified by this herb.[19]

The threshold dose for an increased risk of photosensitization, the most common side effect, is about 2 to 4 g/day of a usual commercial extract (5 to 10 mg hypericin).[20] One should avoid using this herb for patients with known photosensitivity.

CLINICAL CAUTION

Caution should be exercised when using *Hypericum* in the following:

- Fair-skinned individuals. Photosensitivity presents as pruritus and erythema 1 day after exposure to sunlight. After oral consumption of *Hypericum* 600 mg three times daily, one must reduce tanning time by 21%.[21]
- Persons taking medication such as warfarin, oral contraceptives/estrogen, and digoxin. Dosages may require adjustment (e.g., *Hypericum* may lower digoxin levels by 25%).[22]
- Patients taking tricyclic antidepressants or monoamine oxidase inhibitors. Avoid using this herb in patients on medications that affect neurotransmitters.

PRACTICE TIPS

- At least 4 weeks of therapy is required before clinical relief of depression should be expected.
- If a significant response to depression is not detectable within 4 to 6 weeks, treatment with *Hypericum* should be discontinued.
- Avoid excess exposure to sunlight if taking high doses (2.7 mg or more per day of total hypericin).
- If switching from a selective serotonin uptake inhibitor to St. John's wort, allow a washout period of 2 weeks between medications.

REFERENCES

1. Laakmann G, Schule C, Baghai T, Kieser M: St. John's wort in mild to moderate depression: the relevance of hyperforin for the clinical efficacy, *Pharmacopsychiatry* 31(Suppl 1):S54-9, 1998.
2. Bennett DA, Phun L, Polk JF, et al: Neuropharmacology of St. John's wort (hypericum), *Ann Pharmacother* 32(11):1201-8, 1998.
3. Hunt EJ, Lester CE, Lester EA, Tackett RL: Effect of St. John's wort on free radical production, *Life Sci* 69(2):181-90, 2001.
4. Miller AL: St. John's wort (Hypericum perforatum): clinical effects on depression and other conditions, *Alt Med Rev* 3(1):18-26, 1998.

5. Gaster B, Holroyd J: St. John's wort for depression: a systematic review, *Arch Intern Med* 160(2):152-6, 2000.
6. Stevinson C, Ernst E: Hypericum for depression. An update of the clinical evidence, *Eur Neuropsychopharmacol* 9(6):501-5, 1999.
7. Nathan P: The experimental and clinical pharmacology of St. John's wort (Hypericum perforatum L.), *Mol Psychiatry* 4(4):333-8, 1999.
8. Linde K, ter Riet G, Hondras M, et al: Systematic reviews of complementary therapies—an annotated bibliography. Part 2: Herbal medicine, *BMC Comp Alter Med* 1(1):5, 2001.
9. Sommer H, Harrer G: Placebo-controlled double blind study examining the effectiveness of an Hypericum preparation in 105 mildly depressed patients, *J Geriatr Psychiatry Neurol* 7(Suppl 1):S9-11, 1994.
10. Hansgen KD, Vesper J, Ploch M: Multicenter double-blind study examining the antidepressant effectiveness of the Hypericum extract LI 160, *J Geriatr Psychiatry Neurol* 7(Suppl 1):S15-8, 1994.
11. Vorbach EU, Arnoldt KH, Hubner WD: Efficacy and tolerability of St. John's wort extract LI 160 versus imipramine in patients with severe depressive episodes according to ICD-10, *Pharmacopsychiatry* 30(Suppl 2):S81-5, 1997.
12. Hypericum, *Altern Med Rev* 4(3):190-2, 1999.
13. Taylor LH, Kobak KA: An open-label trial of St. John's wort (Hypericum perforatum) in obsessive-compulsive disorder, *J Clin Psychiatry* 61(8):575-8, 2000.
14. Cupp MJ: Herbal remedies: adverse effects and drug interactions, *Am Fam Physician* 59(5):1239-45, 1999.
15. Ernst E: The risk-benefit profile of commonly used herbal therapies: ginkgo, St. John's wort, ginseng, echinacea, saw palmetto, and kava, *Ann Intern Med* 136(1):42-53, 2002.
16. Izzo AA, Ernst E: Interactions between herbal medicines and prescribed drugs: a systematic review, *Drugs* 61(15):2163-75, 2001.
17. Greeson JM, Sanford B, Monti DA: St. John's wort (Hypericum perforatum): a review of the current pharmacological, toxicological, and clinical literature, *Psychopharmacology* 153(4):402-14, 2001.
18. Johne A, Brockmoller J, Bauer S, et al: Pharmacokinetic interaction of digoxin with an herbal extract from St. John's wort (Hypericum perforatum), *Clin Pharmacol Ther* 66(4):338-45, 1999.
19. Preboth M: Safety and efficacy of St. John's wort, *Am Fam Physician* 64:692-3, 2001.
20. Schulz V: Incidence and clinical relevance of the interactions and side effects of Hypericum preparations, *Phytomedicine* 8(2):152-60, 2001.
21. Brockmoller J, Reum T, Bauer S, et al: Hypericin and pseudohypericin: pharmacokinetics and effects on photosensitivity in humans, *Pharmacopsychiatry* 30(Suppl 2):S94-101, 1997.
22. Morelli V, Zoorob RJ: Alternative therapies: Part I. Depression, diabetes, obesity, *Am Fam Physician* 62(5):1051-60, 2000.

▪ CHAPTER 95 ▪

STINGING NETTLE (*URTICA DIOICA*)

> Nettle causes discomfort in hypersensitive patients but provides pain relief in others.

Anecdotal evidence suggests that nettle may have an analgesic effect. The leaf is used in the treatment of musculoskeletal complaints while the root is used for the symptomatic treatment of benign prostatic hyperplasia. Taken with lots of water, nettle has also been used as for urinary irrigation in urolithiasis (gravel). Nettle is reputed to have diuretic and antihistaminic properties.

MECHANISM OF ACTION

The fresh stinging hairs on the leaves of nettle contain histamine, serotonin, and acetylcholine. Nettle leaf, which contains flavonols, glycosides, sterols, and silicon, has been found to have an anti-inflammatory effect and an inhibitory effect on cytokines.[1] In a whole blood culture system, a nettle extract inhibited lipopolysaccaride and stimulated monocyte cytokine expression, indicating an immunomodulating effect.[2] It appears that the effective ingredient of nettle leaf extract may act by mediating a switch in T helper cell–derived cytokine patterns. Stinging nettle leaf extract may inhibit the inflammatory cascade in autoimmune diseases like rheumatoid arthritis.

Nettle root inhibits cellular proliferation in benign prostatic hyperplasia. The root is rich in sterols and sterolglycosides, phenylpropanes, and coumarins. In vitro, it has been found to inhibit cellular proliferation of prostate cells and impair the activity of sex hormone–binding globulin. Testosterone is largely bound to sex hormone–binding globulin; free testosterone exerts biologil effects.

Nettle may also act as a diuretic.[3]

DOSE

Traditionally, the daily dose *Urtica dioica* has been 8 to 12 g dried herb, 3 to 6 ml of 1:2 liquid extract or 7 to 14 ml of 1:5 leaf tincture, and 4 to 6 g dried root or 4 to 9 ml of 1:2 nettle root liquid extract.

CLINICAL USES

There is clinical evidence to support the use of nettle leaf in osteoarthritis and allergic rhinitis and the use of nettle root to relieve urologic symptoms in benign prostatic hyperplasia.[4]

Extracts from the fruits of saw palmetto and the roots of nettle are popular, safe, and effective options in benign prostatic hyperplasia.[5] Doses of 600 to 1200 mg daily of nettle root extract (5:1) or 3 to 6 g of nettle root over 3 or more weeks reduce frequency and improve urine flow in patients with benign prostatic hyperplasia. A clinical trial found that a combination of nettle and saw palmetto achieved an efficacy equivalent to finasteride in the management of benign prostatic hyperplasia.[6] The herbal preparation was better tolerated. Experiments have shown that a 20% methanolic extract of stinging nettle roots has an antiproliferative effect on human prostatic epithelial, but not stromal, cells.[7]

Stinging nettle leaf extracts are registered in Germany for use as adjuvant therapy of rheumatic diseases. Self-selected patients with joint pain using the nettle sting reported benefit with no observed side effects except a transient urticarial rash.[8]

After 1 week's treatment with nettle, a randomized, controlled, double-blind, crossover study concluded that patients with osteoarthritic pain at the base of the thumb or index finger had significantly less pain and disability.[9] Patients with arthritis require an extract equivalent to 9 g/day of nettle leaf.

Doses of 250 mg of standardized nettle extract taken three times daily may benefit allergic patients. Nettle relieves hay fever controlling watery eyes and nasal congestion. A randomized, double-blind study using 300 mg/day of freeze-dried *Urtica dioica* in the treatment of allergic rhinitis found more than half the study patients regarded it as helpful.[10] The benefits may be attributable to histamine acting as an autocoid or local hormone to modulate the immune response.

TOXICITY/DRUG INTERACTIONS

Nettle is a safe herb except for the occasional case of contact allergy. Ingestion of nettle root may occasionally cause mild gastrointestinal tract problems. *Urtica dioica* is contraindicated in persons who are allergic to nettle stings.

CLINICAL CAUTION

Concurrent use of nettle and diuretics increases the risk of dehydration and hypokalemia.

PRACTICE TIP

• Drinking 1 cup of hot nettle tea made from a teaspoon of dried herb may act as a diuretic, increasing urine flow.

REFERENCES

1. Ernst E, Chrubasik S: Phyto-anti-inflammatories. A systematic review of randomized, placebo-controlled, double-blind trials, *Rheum Dis Clin North Am* 26(1):13-27, vii, 2000.
2. Klingelhoefer S, Obertreis B, Quast S, Behnke B: Antirheumatic effect of IDS 23, a stinging nettle leaf extract, on in vitro expression of T helper cytokines, J *Rheumatol* 26(12):2517-22, 1999
3. Diefendorf D, Healey J, Kalyn W (ed): The healing power of vitamins, minerals and herbs, Surry Hills, Australia, 2000, Readers Digest.
4. Mills S, Bone K: Principles and practice of phytotherapy Edinburgh, 2000, Churchill Livingstone.
5. Koch E: Extracts from fruits of saw palmetto (Sabal serrulata) and roots of stinging nettle (Urtica dioica): viable alternatives in the medical treatment of benign prostatic hyperplasia and associated lower urinary tracts symptoms, *Planta Med* 67(6):489-500, 2001.
6. Sokeland J: Combined sabal and urtica extract compared with finasteride in men with benign prostatic hyperplasia: analysis of prostate volume and therapeutic outcome, *BJU Int* 86(4):439-42, 2000.
7. Konrad L, Muller HH, Lenz C, et al: Antiproliferative effect on human prostate cancer cells by a stinging nettle root (Urtica dioica) extract, *Planta Med* 66(1): 44-7, 2000.
8. Randall C, Meethan K, Randall H, Dobbs F: Nettle sting of Urtica dioica for joint pain–an exploratory study of this complementary therapy, *Complement Ther Med* 7(3):126-31, 1999.
9. Randall C, Randall H, Dobbs F, et al: Randomized controlled trial of nettle sting for treatment of base-of-thumb pain, *J R Soc Med* 93(6):305-9, 2000.
10. Mittman P: Randomized, double blind study of freeze dried urtica dioica in the treatment of allergic rhinitis, *Planta Med* 56(1):44-7, 1990.

■ CHAPTER 96 ■

TURMERIC (*CURCUMA LONGA*)

> Dose may be critical; curcumin enhances healing of peptic ulcers at one dose, at another it may be ulcerogenic.

Turmeric, also known as Indian saffron, is a member of the ginger family. It is popular as a cooking spice and has long been regarded as an aromatic digestive stimulant. It has anti-inflammatory, antioxidant, and topical antimicrobial properties.

MECHANISM OF ACTION

The active ingredient in turmeric is curcumin. The anti-inflammatory effect of curcumin is mediated by inhibition of neutrophil function and modification of eicosanoid synthesis. Curcumin inhibits leukotriene and, to a lesser extent, cyclooxygenase production. Its antiplatelet activity is mediated both by inhibiting arachidonic acid's incorporation into and release from platelets and by selective inhibition of thromboxane.

Turmeric has antioxidant activity. Animal and in vitro studies have shown that curcumin prevents lipid oxidation and counteracts increases in blood and hepatic cholesterol in animals on cholesterol rich diets.

In vitro and in vivo studies show curcuminoids act as biologic response modifiers, resulting in significant increases in CD4 and CD8 counts. The essential oil also has antihistaminic properties.

DOSE

An adult maintenance dose of 100 mg may be increased to therapeutic levels of up to 1500 mg, depending on the condition being treated.

CLINICAL USES

Clinically, curcumin may be used for its anti-inflammatory, antioxidant, or antimicrobial and nematocidal activities.[1] Curcumin has been used with some success in the short-term treatment of rheumatoid arthritis (120 mg/day), as a hypolipdemic agent (50 g/day), and in the treatment of flatulence (2 g/day).[2] Curcumin also has an antispasmodic effect.

Curcumin's major anti-inflammatory impact is largely mediated by modifying leukotriene production. The anti-inflammatory effect of turmeric (400 mg) appears to be enhanced if used with bromelain (500 mg) three times a day. Despite lacking an analgesic and antipyetic effect, turmeric, because of its anti-inflammatory action, may be useful in treating rheumatoid arthritis.[3] Its anti-inflammatory effect may also contribute to its beneficial effect in the management of peptic ulcers. Two capsules filled with turmeric (300 mg each) taken five times daily, 30 to 60 minutes before meals, at 16:00 hours and at bedtime, achieved ulcer healing in 48% of cases after 4 weeks of treatment and in 76% of patients after 12 weeks.[4] Further research is required.

Animal experiments suggest curcumin has the potential to become a therapeutic anticancer agent. It significantly inhibits prostate cancer growth and may have the capacity to prevent progression of this cancer to its hormone refractory state.[5] Curcumin, like other plant-derived phenolics, decreases tumor formation in mice.[6] Plant-derived phenolic compounds manifest many beneficial effects and can potentially inhibit several stages of carcinogenesis in vivo.

TOXICITY/DRUG INTERACTIONS

Curcumin is safe in recommended doses. A few patients may have an allergic response. An ulcerogenic effect is possible when it is used in doses high enough to achieve an anti-inflammatory effects nearly equivalent to NSAIDs.

CLINICAL CAUTION

Avoid curcumin or use with caution in patients with symptomatic gallstones. Curcumin has a choleritic effect. It is contraindicated during pregnancy and the periconceptual period. Persons taking antiplatelet or anticoagulant therapy should avoid high doses of curcumin.

PRACTICE TIPS

- Persons with hyperlipidemia may benefit from 1 teaspoon of curcumin in water before the main meal.

REFERENCES

1. Araujo CC, Leon LL: Biological activities of Curcuma longa L, *Mem Inst Oswaldo Cruz* 96(5):723-8, 2001.

2. Mills S, Bone K: *Principles and practice of phytotherapy*, Edinburgh, 2000,Churchill Livingstone.
3. Pinn G: Herbal therapy in rheumatology, *Aust Fam Phys* 30:878-83, 2001.
4. Prucksunand C, Indrasukhsri B, Leethochawalit M, Hungspreugs K: Phase II clinical trial on effect of the long turmeric (Curcuma longa Linn) on healing of peptic ulcer, *Southeast Asian J Trop Med Public Health* 32(1):208-15, 2001.
5. Dorai T, Cao YC, Dorai B, et al: Therapeutic potential of curcumin in human prostate cancer. III. Curcumin inhibits proliferation, induces apoptosis, and inhibits angiogenesis of LNCaP prostate cancer cells in vivo, *Prostate* 47(4): 293-303, 2001
6. Mahmoud NN, Carothers AM, Grunberger D, et al: Plant phenolics decrease intestinal tumors in an animal model of familial adenomatous polyposis, *Carcinogenesis* 21(5):921-7, 2000.

■ CHAPTER 97 ■

VALERIAN (VALERIANA OFFICINALIS)

Valerian is a useful sedative in most people but some find it stimulating.

The rootstock of valerian has been shown to have sleep-inducing, anxiolytic, and tranquilizing effects in animal studies and clinical trials.[1] It is widely used as a hypnotic and daytime sedative and is recommended for the treatment of patients with mild psychophysiologic insomnia.

The U.S. Food and Drug Administration regards valerian as a generally safe herb. Although valerian extracts have been demonstrated to cause both CNS depression and muscle relaxation,[1] the primary active ingredient of valerian has yet to be identified.

MECHANISM OF ACTION

Valerian contains valepotriates, valerenic acid, and unidentified aqueous constituents that contribute to the sedative properties of valerian. The proportion of these constituents can vary greatly between and within species. Investigations have shown that valerian extracts affect GABA(A) receptors and can also interact at other presynaptic components of GABAergic neurons.[2] Sedation may result from an interaction of valerian constituents with central GABA(A) receptors. Valerenic acid has been shown to inhibit enzyme-induced breakdown of GABA in the brain, resulting in sedation.

DOSE

Placebo-controlled trials show that 400 to 900 mg of valerian extract at bedtime improves sleep quality, decreases sleep latency, reduces the number of night awakenings, and improves insomnia.[1] The usual dose range prescribed is 3 to 9 grams of dried root or rhizome daily, 2 to 6 ml of 1:2 liquid extract, or 5 to 15 ml of 1:5 tincture daily.

CLINICAL USES

Valerian is used as an anxiolytic, a mild sedative-hypnotic, and deserves consideration as an adjunct in depression. Seven days on a standard dose of valerian reduced physiologic reactivity, as measured by systolic blood pressure, to psychologically stressful laboratory situations in healthy volunteers.[3] At least two of three patients in an open trial taking 1 to 3 capsules of valerian root (470 mg) reported at least moderate sleep improvement.[4]

There is even some clinical evidence that valerian is a useful hypnotic and may alleviate symptoms of benzodiazepine withdrawal. Although valerian has been shown to decrease sleep latency and nocturnal awakenings and improve subjective sleep quality, placebo effects were marked in some studies, and in some cases the beneficial effects are not seen until after 2 to 4 weeks of therapy.[5] This may partially explain why a review of randomized, placebo-controlled, double-blind trials of the effect of valerian on insomnia was inconclusive.[5] Certainly, a randomized, double-blind, placebo-controlled, cross-over study that found no effect after a single dose of valerian showed a significant increase in sleep efficiency after multiple-dose treatment over 14 days.[6]

In comparison with placebo, slow-wave sleep latency is reduced after administration of valerian. The authors concluded that treatment with an herbal extract of *Radix valerianae* demonstrated positive effects on sleep structure and sleep perception.[6] When 500 mg of valerian extract was combined with 120 mg of hop extract, declines in the sleep latency and the wake time were noted after 2 weeks.[7] Sleep stage 1 was reduced and slow-wave sleep increased. Patients judged themselves more refreshed in the morning and no adverse events were observed.

TOXICITY/DRUG INTERACTIONS

Valerian is generally regarded as a safe herb.[8] A randomized, controlled, double-blind trial found a single evening dose of native valerian root extract (600 mg LI 156) did not impair the reaction abilities, concentration, and coordination the following morning.[9] Similar results were reported after treatment over a 2-week period. Another study over 6 weeks using 600 mg daily of valerian found the majority of patients reported no side effects and of those that did, the most prevalent untoward effect was vivid dreams.[10] However, patients using large doses over several years may experience serious withdrawal symptoms following abrupt discontinuation.[1]

Valerian may enhance the sedative effects of α- and/or β-blockers, analgesics, anesthetics, and tricyclic antidepressants. Persons using hypnotic or sedative drugs who take valerian may experience excessive drowsiness. Valerian may negate the therapeutic effects of warfarin, monoamine oxidase inhibitors, and phenytoin. There are also concerns about carcinogenicity.

CLINICAL CAUTION

Valerian overdose may cause blurred vision, headaches, arrhythmia, restlessness, and nausea.

PRACTICE TIPS

- Individuals who find valerian stimulating should avoid its use.
- In some individuals valerian causes drowsiness.
- Valerian preparations have a disagreeable odor.

REFERENCES

1. Attele AS, Xie J-T, Yuan C-S: Treatment of insomnia: an alternative approach, *Altern Med Rev* 5(3):249-59, 2000.
2. Ortiz JG, Nieves-Natal J, Chavez P: Effects of *Valeriana officinalis* extracts on [3H]flunitrazepam binding, synaptosomal [3H]GABA uptake, and hippocampal [3H]GABA release, *Neurochem Res* 24(11):1373-8, 1999.
3. Cropley M, Cave Z, Ellis J, Middleton RW: Effect of kava and valerian on human physiological and psychological responses to mental stress assessed under laboratory conditions, *Phytother Res* 16(1):23-7, 2002.
4. Dominguez RA, Bravo-Valverde RL, Kaplowitz BR, Cott JM: Valerian as a hypnotic for Hispanic patients, *Cultur Divers Ethnic Minor Psychol* 6(1):84-92, 2000.
5. Beaubrun G, Gray GE: A review of herbal medicines for psychiatric disorders, *Psychiatr Serv* 51(9):1130-4, 2000.
6. Stevinson C, Ernst E: Valerian for insomnia: a systematic review of randomized clinical trials, *Sleep Med* 1(2):91-9, 2000.
7. Donath F, Quispe S, Diefenbach K, et al: Critical evaluation of the effect of valerian extract on sleep structure and sleep quality, *Pharmacopsychiatry* 33(2):47-53, 2000.
8. Klepser TB, Klepser ME: Unsafe and potentially safe herbal therapies, *Am J Health Syst Pharm* 56(2):125-38; quiz 139-41, 1999.
9. Kuhlmann J, Berger W, Podzuweit H, Schmidt U: The influence of valerian treatment on "reaction time, alertness and concentration" in volunteers, *Pharmacopsychiatry* 32(6):235-41, 1999.
10. Wheatley D: Kava and valerian in the treatment of stress-induced insomnia, *Phytother Res* 5(6):549-51, 2001.

▪ CHAPTER 98 ▪

Vitamin A

> Ingesting excess amounts of preformed vitamin A is hazardous, but consuming vast quantities of carotenoids, the precursors of vitamin A, is safe and may even be beneficial.

Vitamin A is required for normal vision and plays an important role in immune competence at the level of both the superficial barrier (i.e., skin and mucous membranes) and the immune system.

Vitamin A comes in two distinct forms, retinol (the animal form) and β-carotene (the plant form). Retinol is the major transport and storage form of vitamin A. Retinol-binding protein transports vitamin A from the liver to the rest of the body. Vitamin A reserves may be depleted in 3 to 12 months.

Vitamin A is involved in production of visual purple, mucopolysaccharide synthesis, maintenance of epithelial tissue, and regulation of genes. It can influence reproduction, growth, and carcinogenesis.

MECHANISM OF ACTION

Retinols, the animal form of vitamin A, are fat soluble and active in the human body in three different configurations. Retinol, the alcohol form, can be reversibly oxidized to retinal, the aldehyde form, which can be irreversibly converted to retinoic acid. All-trans retinoic acid, 9-cis retinoic acid, and 13-cis retinoic acid are isomers that are interconverted in humans and that may be less hepatotoxic than retinol. Each form of vitamin A has its own receptor protein.

The retinal form of vitamin A is required for vision. On exposure to light, trans-retinal is converted to cis-retinal. Opsin releases this retinal isomer, changing the configuration of the visual pigment. The change in shape of visual pigment (i.e., rhodopsin in the rods and iodopsin in the cones) initiates transmission of impulses to the cerebral cortex.

Retinoic acid is the form of vitamin A necessary for the normal growth and differentiation of epithelial tissue.[1] It binds with nuclear receptor sites. The effects of vitamin A on cellular differentiation are mediated by two separate classes of nuclear receptors, retinoic acid receptors (α, β, and γ) and the retinoid X receptors (α, β, and γ). Retinoid receptors modify the effects of many compounds, including prostaglandins, vitamin D, and steroid and thyroid hormones.[2]

Vitamin A is required for both innate and specific immunity. Vitamin A deficiency impairs innate immunity by impeding normal regeneration of mucosal barriers damaged by infection and by diminishing the function of neutrophils, macrophages, and natural killer cells. Studies in animal models and cell lines show that vitamin A and related retinoids play a major role in immunity, including expression of mucins and keratins, lymphopoiesis, apoptosis, cytokine expression, and production of antibody.[3] Retinoids also modify the function of neutrophils, natural killer cells, monocytes or macrophages, T lymphocytes, and B lymphocytes.[3] Vitamin A is required for adaptive immunity and plays a role in the development of both T-helper (Th) cells and B cells. In particular, vitamin A deficiency diminishes antibody-mediated responses directed by Th2 cells, although some aspects of Th1-mediated immunity are also diminished.[4]

Retinoids play an important role in regulating the growth and differentiation of cells, including premalignant and malignant cells, especially epithelial cells. At the molecular level, aberrant expression and function of nuclear retinoid receptors have been found in various types of cancer, including premalignant lesions. Aberrations in retinoid signaling are early events in carcinogenesis.

FOOD SOURCES

Vitamin A is obtained from the diet in the form of retinyl esters, which are subsequently de-esterified to retinol. About half of the vitamin A activity is derived from animal and half from plant sources. Preformed vitamin A (retinol) is present in liver, fatty fish, dairy products, and fortified margarine. Inclusion of fortified dairy products in the diet may be a practical, sustainable, and cost-effective approach for improving vitamin intake and status in the elderly.[5] Although plants do not contain vitamin A, they are an important source of carotenoids. Six apricots daily can provide the RDA of RE as well as 6 grams of fiber for just over 100 calories.

A proportion of dietary carotenoids are converted to retinol in the intestine and liver. Refer to Chapter 54 for more information about these vitamin A precursors.

DOSE

It has been suggested that for optimal health, the daily intake of vitamin A is around 1.5 to 3 mg or 0.005 to 0.01 µmol of preformed vitamin A.[6] Although the system of international units has officially been discontinued, it continues to be widely used, especially on supplement labels. The conversion is 1 IU equates to 0.3 µg retinal equivalents (RE), 0.3 µg retinol, 0.3 µg retinol acetate, 0.4 µg retinol propionate, or 0.5 µg retinol palmitate.[7] The daily adult male requirement is 1000 retinol equivalents (RE) consumed as 3330 international units (IU) of retinol or 5000 IU as a combination of retinol and β-carotene. The daily requirement for adult females is 800 RE as 2665 IU of retinol or 4000 IU as a combination of retinol and β-carotene. Traditionally, 1 RE was equated to 6 µg or 10 IU of β-carotene. However, recent studies have shown that the basis for describing vitamin A activity of carotenoids overestimates the bioavailability of provitamin A carotenoids and their bio-conversion to retinol (vitamin A). Instead of 6 µg from a mixed diet, 21 µg of β-carotene are required to provide 1 µg of retinol or 1 RE of vitamin A.[8] The therapeutic dose range of vitamin A is 10,000 to 500,000 IU/day.[9]

CLINICAL USES

Excessively dry eyes may be a sign of hypovitaminosis A, especially in individuals with malabsorption. Xerophthalmia results from keratinization of the cornea. It may be exacerbated in patients with zinc deficiency. Vitamin A is indisputably effective for xerophthalmia. An oral dose of 7500 to 15,000 RE/day (25,000 to 50,000 IU/day) is recommended.

An intake of at least 3 mg vitamin A, along with 130 mg vitamin C and 67 mg vitamin E or more daily, is thought to possibly reduce the risk of cancer.[6] A population-based case control of colorectal adenoma suggested that the risk of developing colorectal adenomas is reduced in those with high vitamin A levels but unrelated to serum vitamin C and E and carotene levels.[10] Despite this and other promising epidemiologic studies, human studies using vitamin A or retinoids as chemopreventive agents have been largely disappointing.[11] This may to some extent be explained by the relationship between vitamin A and the carotenoids. Beta-carotene has distinct immunologic effects. It affects the number of NK and T helper cells and enhances macrophage function independently of vitamin A. Supplementation of elderly adults with 30 to 60 mg β-carotene for 2 months increased white cells, particularly NK and lymphocytes with interleukin-2 receptors.

Unlike vitamin A, β-carotene can reduce lipid peroxidation and modulate enzymatic activity of lipoxygenases. However, the immunologic impact of vitamin A is not solely attributable to its carotene precursor. Animal studies do suggest vitamin A and retinoids regulate epithelial cell differentiation and maintenance and inhibit tumor angiogenesis.[12]

Animal research has demonstrated that retinoids have a chemopreventive effect in many types of cancer, and in vitro research has identified a number of promising mechanisms of action. Vitamin A decreases serum insulin-like growth factor-1, inhibits 5-α-reductase (the enzyme that catalyzes formation of dihydrotestosterone), and up-regulates transforming growth factor-β.[13] Animal and epidemiologic studies also suggest a lower dietary vitamin A intake increases the risk of cancer, while retinoids at pharmacologic doses exhibit various cancer protective effects.[14] Retinoids may suppress transformation of cells in vitro, reduce premalignant human epithelial lesions, and prevent recurrence of primary epithelial malignancies.[14] A combination of retinoids with vitamin D analogs have been found to have synergistic inhibitory effects on tumor cell proliferation and on the angiogenic capability of malignancies.[15] Small doses of both agents applied simultaneously are efficacious.

Vitamin A has a number of other promising and interesting clinical applications. Retinoids protect gastric mucosa against the ulcerogenic effects of indomethacin treatment without any inhibition of gastric acid secretion.[16] This effect was noted both in healthy persons and in patients with peptic ulcers. cAMP is the intracellular signal involved in the protection of gastric mucosa induced by retinoids and in the development of gastric mucosal damage produced by chemicals (e.g., ethanol, HCl). Vitamin A protects gastric mucosa by mechanism unrelated to prostaglandins, the target of NSAIDs.

Correction of UV-induced vitamin A deficiency deserves investigation as a strategy for the prevention of skin cancer and aging. Current data suggest dermal vitamin A is a direct target of both UVB and UVA and participates in an adaptive response to UV exposure.[17] Human epidermis contains vitamin A, the enzymes responsible for its metabolism toward either storage or activation, the binding proteins for its protection and specific transport, and the nuclear receptors involved in vitamin A-induced gene-activity modulation. This system may be drastically altered upon ultraviolet light exposure because vitamin A absorbs in the UVB range.

There is a potential for therapeutic supplements of vitamin A in children with insulin-dependent diabetes mellitus to reduce or prevent atherogenic risk. A case-control study found children with poor metabolic control of their type 1 diabetes mellitus were at greater risk of atherosclerosis and relative vitamin A deficiency than those with good metabolic control of their illness.[18] Relationships between retinol and retinol-binding protein and atherogenic indicators were detected.

With new, more effective, and less toxic retinoids being developed, there are great expectations for the use of these derivatives, alone or in combination with other drugs. With new delivery systems being developed, it is hoped vitamin A may provide therapeutic solutions to conditions as diverse as benign proliferative skin diseases, such as psoriasis and skin cancer.[19]

TOXICITY/DRUG INTERACTIONS

Vitamin A supplementation requires careful monitoring. The relative severity of side effects varies widely between patients and, apart from skeletal and skin changes, most signs and symptoms disappear within 7 days.

Side effects are more likely to occur in adults taking 7500 RE/day for 8 months or more or taking a stat dose of 450,000 RE. Pregnant women should avoid daily doses of 1800 RE and over.

Acute toxicity, which occurs around 660,000 IU/day, presents with headache, nausea, ataxia, depression, bleeding gums, confusion, dizziness or drowsiness, and diplopia.

Chronic toxicity in adults (25,000 to 50,000 IU/day) presents with hypercalcemia, skin desquamation, hair loss, hepatosplenomegaly, and rheumatologic complications including hyperostoses, arthralgia and myalgia, and teratogenic abnormalities. Hypervitaminosis A is sometimes associated with abnormalities of calcium metabolism and bone mineral status, and a recent study found a negative association between reported dietary vitamin A intake and bone mineral density. A prospective study with 18 years of follow-up suggested long-term intake of a diet high in retinol may promote the development of osteoporotic hip fractures in women.[20] However, although the prevalences of high fasting serum retinyl esters concentration and low bone mineral density were both substantial in the NHANES III, there were no significant associations between fasting serum retinyl esters and any measure of bone mineral status.[21]

Children are at increased risk of chronic toxicity when taking 5400 RE to 15,000 RE for several months or of developing acute symptoms when taking 22,500 RE to 105,100 RE stat. In children, chronic toxicity (20,000 IU/day) may present raised intracranial pressure and vomiting. Acute toxicity in children presents blurred vision, headache, and vomiting.[22]

Vitamin A participates in a number of nutrient-nutrient interactions. While large doses of vitamin K may impair absorption of vitamin A, hypervitaminosis A causes hypoprothrombinemia, which can be corrected with vitamin K. Vitamin C may reduce the toxic effects of hypervitaminosis A. Vitamin E may enhance the therapeutic efficacy of vitamin A by protecting against the oxidative destruction of this vitamin. Zinc deficiency impairs vitamin A function, limiting the bioavailability of this vitamin. A randomized, double-blind, placebo-controlled, intervention trial found combined zinc and vitamin A supplementation improved vitamin A nutriture in vitamin A-deficient children.[22]

CLINICAL CAUTIONS

Impaired dark adaptation (night blindness) is an indication of marginal vitamin A deficiency. Vitamin A deficiency also leads to drying of the conjunctiva and mucous membranes; a rough dry skin with follicular hyperkeratosis is common.

PRACTICE TIPS

- Vitamin A supplementation during pregnancy can cause birth defects or growth retardation in the fetus.
- The risk of cataracts is reduced in persons eating a diet rich in RE.

- Chronic vitamin A overdose should be excluded in patients with bone or joint pain, convulsions, photosensitivity, polyuria, excessive fatigue, and dry cracked skin or lips.

REFERENCES

1. Hansen LA, Sigman CC, Andreola F, et al: Retinoids in chemoprevention and differentiation therapy, *Carcinogenesis* 21(7):1271-9, 2000.
2. Singh DK, Lippman SM: Cancer chemoprevention part 1: retinoids and carotenoids and other classic antioxidants, *Oncology* 12(11):1643-58, 1998.
3. Semba RD: Vitamin A and immunity to viral, bacterial and protozoan infections, *Proc Nutr Soc* 58(3):719-27, 1999.
4. Stephensen CB: Vitamin A, infection, and immune function, *Annu Rev Nutr* 21:167-92, 2001.
5. Herrero C, Granado F, Blanco I, Olmedilla B: Vitamin A and E content in dairy products: their contribution to the recommended dietary allowances (RDA) for elderly people, *J Nutr Health Aging* 6(1):57-9, 2002.
6. Gey KF: Vitamins E plus C and interacting conutrients required for optimal health. A critical and constructive review of epidemiology and supplementation data regarding cardiovascular disease and cancer, *Biofactors* 7(1-2):113-74, 1998.
7. Mason P: *Dietary supplements*, Bath, UK, 2001, Pharmaceutical Press.
8. West CE: Meeting requirements for vitamin A, *Nutr Rev* 58(11):341-5, 2000.
9. Brighthope I: Nutritional medicine tables, *J Aust Coll Nutr Env Med* 17:20-5, 1998.
10. Breuer-Katschinski B, Nemes K, Marr A, et al: Relation of serum antioxidant vitamins to the risk of colorectal adenoma, *Digestion* 63(1):43-8, 2001.
11. Lamson DW, Brignall MS: Natural agents in the prevention of cancer part I: human chemoprevention trials, *Altern Med Rev* 6(1):7-19, 2001.
12. Primack A: Complementary/alternative therapies in the prevention and treatment of cancer. In Spencer JW, Jacobs JJ: *Complementary/alternative medicine: an evidence-based approach*, St Louis, 1998, Mosby.
13. Whelan P: Retinoids in chemoprevention, *Eur Urol* 35(5-6):424-8, 1999.
14. Sun SY, Lotan R: Retinoids and their receptors in cancer development and chemoprevention, *Crit Rev Oncol Hematol* 41(1):41-55, 2002.
15. Majewski S, Kutner A, Jablonska S: Vitamin D analogs in cutaneous malignancies, *Curr Pharm Des* 6(7):829-38, 2000.
16. Mozsik G, Bodis B, Figler M, et al: Mechanisms of action of retinoids in gastrointestinal mucosal protection in animals, human healthy subjects and patients, *Life Sci* 69(25-26):3103-12, 2001.
17. Saurat JH: Skin, sun, and vitamin A: from aging to cancer, *J Dermatol* 28(11):595-8, 2001.
18. Baena RM, Campoy C, Bayes R, et al: Vitamin A, retinol binding protein and lipids in type 1 diabetes mellitus, *Eur J Clin Nutr* 56(1):44-50, 2002.
19. Zouboulis CC: Retinoids-which dermatological indications will benefit in the near future? *Skin Pharmacol Appl Skin Physiol* 14(5):303-15, 2001.
20. Feskanich D, Singh V, Willett WC, Colditz GA: Vitamin A intake and hip fractures among postmenopausal women, *JAMA* 287(1):47-54, 2002.

21. Ballew C, Galuska D, Gillespie C: High serum retinyl esters are not associated with reduced bone mineral density in the Third National Health And Nutrition Examination Survey, 1988-1994, *J Bone Miner Res* 16(12):2306-12, 2001.

22. Rahman MM, Wahed MA, Fuchs GJ, et al: Synergistic effect of zinc and vitamin A on the biochemical indexes of vitamin A nutrition in children, *Am J Clin Nutr* 75(1):92-8, 2002.

■ CHAPTER 99 ■

VITAMIN B_1 (THIAMIN)

> Adding bicarbonate to green vegetables to retain their color after cooking results in substantial loss of thiamin; this vitamin is unstable in an alkaline environment.

This water-soluble B vitamin is essential for converting carbohydrate into energy. Thiamin is important in nerve transmission. It works synergistically with other vitamins of the B complex, particularly riboflavin (B_2) and niacin (B_3).

MECHANISM OF ACTION

Frequently found in its coenzyme form of thiamin pyrophosphate, this vitamin is largely concerned with decarboxylation of α-ketoacids (e.g., pyruvate) involved in energy production and transketolation of intermediates in the pentose phosphate pathway of carbohydrate metabolism. It is required for oxidation of alcohol. Alcoholics are at particular risk of thiamin deficiency.

Thiamin is required for synthesis of acetylcholine and is important for neural transmission.

FOOD SOURCES

Thiamin is found in various foods, including cereals (whole grain and enriched), peas, beans, nuts, and meats (especially pork and beef). Some thiamin in foods is lost with cooking.

Thiamin is best taken with meals, since it is better absorbed in an acidic environment.

DOSE

Requirements for thiamin depend on energy intake. The RDA is 1.2 mg for men and 1.1 mg for women. The EAR is 1.0 mg/day for men and 0.9 mg/day for women. During pregnancy and lactation, the EAR 1.2 mg/day and RDA 1.4 mg/day. For children, the RDA increases gradually from 0.3 mg/day until it reaches the adult dose. The therapeutic dose range is 10 to 1000 mg/day by injection.[1] The UL has not been established.

Alcoholics require 150 mg of vitamin B_1 daily.

CLINICAL USES

The use of vitamin B_1 is recognized for treatment of beriberi, a condition resulting from thiamin deficiency. Treatment in adults is 5 to 10 mg of vitamin B_1 three times a day; in children, the dose is 10 mg/day. Severe thiamin deficiency may cause depression, memory problems, weakness, dyspnea, and tachycardia. Early signs of beriberi that are often missed include anorexia, constipation, muscle weakness, paresthesia, and pedal edema. Numbness and tingling attributable to peripheral neuropathy can be relieved by 10 mg vitamin B_1 daily.

Wet beriberi presents with cardiac failure. Thiamin deficiency impairs cellular metabolism in all tissues. In the heart, this results in impaired contractile strength; in the blood vessels, this results in vasodilatation. The cardiac failure of wet beriberi results from a combination of reduced venous return and impaired cardiac muscle contractility compromising cardiac output. Dry beriberi presents with neurologic problems. Persistent thiamin deficiency in dry beriberi may cause Korsakoff's psychosis and Wernicke's encephalopathy. Acute Wernicke-Korsakoff syndrome, a form of amnesia caused by brain damage occurring in long-term alcoholics, is normally reversible with thiamin but may proceed to profound dementia.[2]

A review of clinical trials concluded that while magnesium was promising, 100 mg vitamin B_1 daily was an effective treatment for dysmenorrhea.[3]

A 500-mg dose of vitamin B_1 in the morning may be helpful for depression.

TOXICITY/DRUG INTERACTIONS

Oral thiamin is nontoxic. Allergic reactions may rarely occur. Lasix increases urinary excretion of thiamin, and supplementation with 200 mg of thiamin daily may benefit cardiac failure patients on this drug.

CLINIC CAUTION

Thiamin deficiency is associated with apathy, insomnia, and fatigue. Early signs of beriberi are often missed. Biochemical changes precede clinical signs. Erythrocyte transketolase activity in excess of 1.25 indicates deficiency, as does an erythrocyte thiamin concentration of less than 70 nmol/L.

PRACTICE TIPS

- Thiamin may serve as an insect repellant.
- Older people are often mildly deficient and benefit from 10 mg daily.

REFERENCES

1. Brighthope I: Nutritional medicine tables, *J Aust Coll Nutr Env Med* 17:20-5, 1998.
2. Rodriguez-Martin JL, Qizilbash N, Lopez-Arrieta JM: Thiamine for Alzheimer's disease (Cochrane Review), *Cochrane Database Syst Rev* 2:CD001498, 2001.
3. Wilson ML, Murphy PA: Herbal and dietary therapies for primary and secondary dysmenorrhoea (Cochrane Review), *Cochrane Database Syst Rev* 3:CD002124, 2001.

■ CHAPTER 100 ■

VITAMIN B$_2$ (RIBOFLAVIN)

A relative deficiency of vitamin B$_2$ can result from excess supplementation with vitamin B$_6$; deficiency or excess of one B vitamin can precipitate a metabolic imbalance with other members of the B group.

Riboflavin is a water-soluble vitamin of the B group that is important in energy metabolism. Riboflavin is sensitive to light but largely heat resistant. Since riboflavin is sensitive to light, it is lost when milk is stored in glass bottles, hence the trend to opaque containers.

MECHANISM OF ACTION

The major form of riboflavin is as a part of the coenzymes flavin mononucleotide (FMN) and flavin-adenine dinucleotide (FAD). In these forms, riboflavin acts as a catalyst for redox reactions in a large number of energy-producing pathways, including oxidation of glucose, certain amino acids, and fatty acids. It is also involved in the conversion of pyridoxine to its active co-enzyme and is required for tryptophan metabolism.

FOOD SOURCES

This soluble B vitamin is found naturally in many foods, including milk and dairy products, fish, meats (especially liver and kidney), green leafy vegetables, and whole grains and is added to fortified cereal and breads. Riboflavin is better absorbed from animal sources than vegetable sources.

DOSE

The RDA of vitamin B$_2$ is 1.3 mg/day for men and 1.1 mg/day for women. The EAR is 1.1 mg/day for men and 0.9 mg/day for women. For pregnancy, the RDA is 1.4 mg/day and the EAR 1.2 mg/day. For lactation, the RDA is 1.6 mg/day and EAR is 1.3 mg/day. By 3 years of age, children require 0.8 mg/day; this gradually increases to adult levels by 11 years of age. The usual therapeutic dose range is 12 to 200 mg/day; rarely 5000 mg/day is required.[1] The UL has not been determined.

CLINICAL USES

In later stages, riboflavin deficiency is associated with cheilosis, angular stomatitis, glossitis, and normochromic normocytic anemia. Erythrocyte flavin values below 270 nmol/L (10 µg/100 ml) indicate deficiency. Riboflavin deficiency is corrected by taking 5 to 30 mg of vitamin B_2 in divided doses for several days followed by 1 to 4 mg/day.

Vitamin B_2 may be helpful for migraine prophylaxis. A daily dose of 400 mg over 3 months is suggested. A randomized trial of 3 months duration found more than half of the migraine subjects responded favorably to this dose.[2] Since beta-blockers and riboflavin act on two distinct pathophysiologic mechanisms, combining both treatments might enhance their efficacy without increasing central nervous system side effects.[3] A combination product containing magnesium, riboflavin, and feverfew is another option for headache management.[4]

Riboflavin supplementation exerts a weak protective effect on cortical cataract formation.[5] However, although 25 mg a day may protect against cataracts, it has been suggested that high doses may exacerbate existing cataracts.[6]

TOXICITY/DRUG INTERACTIONS

Riboflavin does not cause any side effects. Supplementation with boron and/or vitamin B_6 may cause a relative riboflavin deficiency. Excessive or prolonged use of alcohol, barbiturates, oral contraceptives, phenothiazines, and probenecid may induce a riboflavin deficiency.

CLINICAL CAUTION

Usually associated with other nutrient deficiencies, riboflavin deficiency presents early with a sore throat, pharyngeal redness, and photosensitive, itching, and burning eyes.

PRACTICE TIPS

- Persons taking large doses of riboflavin should be warned to expect yellow discoloration of their urine.
- Consider adding vitamin B complex when supplementing single members of the B group.

REFERENCES

1. Brighthope I: Nutritional medicine tables, *J Aust Coll Nutr Env Med* 17:20-5, 1998.
2. Schoenen J, Jacquy J, Lenaerts M: Effectiveness of high-dose riboflavin in migraine prophylaxis. A randomized controlled trial, *Neurology* 50(2):466-70, 1998.
3. Sandor PS, Afra J, Ambrosini A, Schoenen J: Prophylactic treatment of migraine with beta-blockers and riboflavin: differential effects on the intensity dependence of auditory evoked cortical potentials, *Headache* 40(1):30-5, 2000.
4. Mauskop A: Alternative therapies in headache. Is there a role? *Med Clin North Am* 85(4):1077-84, 2001.
5. Kuzniarz M, Mitchell P, Cumming RG, Flood VM: Use of vitamin supplements and cataract: the Blue Mountains Eye Study, *Am J Ophthalmol* 132(1):19-26, 2001.
6. Diefendorf D, Healey J, Kalyn W, editors: *The healing power of vitamins, minerals and herbs*, Surry Hills, Australia, 2000, Readers Digest.

▪ CHAPTER 101 ▪

VITAMIN B₃ (NIACIN)

> Niacinamide and nicotinic acid do not have identical therapeutic or side effects; it may be important to specify the chemical nature of a supplement prescribed.

Vitamin B_3 is found in two forms, the niacin, or nicotinic acid, and niacinamide, or nicotinamide, forms. The clinical effects of these two forms are not identical. Niacin lowers blood lipids and aggravates asthma; niacinamide does not. Niacin is a precursor to glucose tolerance factor while niacinamide is not.

Deficiency of vitamin B_3 is associated with pellagra.

MECHANISM OF ACTION

The nicotinamide component of the coenzyme nicotinamide adenine dinucleotide (NAD) and nicotinamide adenine dinucleotide phosphate (NADP) acts as a hydride ion acceptor or donor in numerous redox reactions. NAD is important in intracellular respiration and as a codehydrogenase for oxidation of energy sources (e.g., alcohol, lactate, pyruvate, α-hydroxybutyrate). In addition to its role in electron transfer, NAD is important for DNA repair and calcium mobilization.

NADP(H) is essential for the cytochrome P450 detoxification system. It very effectively inactivates singlet oxygen and is involved in reductive biosynthesis of fat and steroids. It also acts as a codehydrogenase in the glucose phosphate shunt.

In pharmacologic doses, nicotinic acid causes peripheral vasodilation and inhibits synthesis of very-low-density lipoproteins, the precursors of LDL cholesterol.

FOOD SOURCES

Niacin is found in fish, eggs, whole grains, liver, meat, and legumes. Alkali treatment of grain increases the bioavailability of niacin. In addition to dietary niacin, humans convert tryptophan to niacin, with 60 mg of tryptophan being converted to 1 mg of vitamin B_3. The conversion of tryptophan to niacin requires an adequate supply of vitamin B_6, riboflavin (B_2), and iron.

DOSE

Niacin intake can be measured as the preformed vitamin or can take into consideration the diet's content of tryptophan, in which case the required intake is measured in terms of niacin equivalents (NE). The RDA for niacin is 7 mg/1000 kcal or 13 to 18 mg RDA with a world range of 9 to 24 mg. The RDA for men is 16 mg/day NE and for women, 14 NE. The EAR is 12 mg/day NE for men and 11 NE for women. By 3 years of age, children require 9 mg/day. The RDA for pregnancy is 18 mg/day NE and for lactation, 17 mg/day NE. For pregnancy, the EAR is 14 mg/day NE and for lactation, 13 mg/day NE. The therapeutic dose range is 20 to 10,000 mg/day.[1] A more conservative supplemental dose range is 13 to 300 mg. The UL for adults is 35 mg/day of niacin; this is reduced to 30 mg/day of niacin for pregnant women and teenagers. Requirements are increased by a high-carbohydrate diet.

CLINICAL USES

Pellagra, the result of severe vitamin B_3 deficiency, presents with diarrhea, dermatitis, and dementia. The dermatitis is most noted in sun-exposed areas, with forearms, hands, and neck developing a crazy-paving appearance. The dementia is associated with confusion, hallucinations, and seizures. Up to 500 mg/day of oral niacin may be required, depending on the severity of the deficiency.

When treating hyperlipidemia, niacin, not niacinamide, is required.[2] At a dose of 1.5 to 3.0 grams/day, niacin effectively blocks adipose tissue lipolysis, inhibits synthesis and secretion of VLDL by the liver, lowers lipoprotein(a), and increases HDL. Up to 90% of patients respond when higher doses are used. A maximum daily dose of 6 grams may be given, provided an immediate-release preparation is prescribed. Dose levels of 2 grams daily are recommended if a sustained-release preparation is available. It is good practice to start on 100 mg niacin tid and gradually increase the dose to 500 mg tid or qid. Up to a 25% reduction in total cholesterol is possible. A statin-niacin regimen is regarded as safe and effective in managing dyslipidemias in most patients at risk for cardiovascular events who respond poorly to either agent used alone.[3] At around 3000 mg/day, niacin achieves a significant increase in HDL, a decrease in LDL cholesterol and triglycerides, and only a modest increase in blood glucose levels (0.3 to 0.4 mmol/L) with no change in HbA. Although current guidelines do not recommend use of niacin in patients with diabetes because of concerns about adverse effects on glycemic control, niacin may be useful in type 2 diabetics.[4] Niacinamide may relieve symptoms of hypoglycemia, but it fails to lower blood lipids.

Vitamin B$_3$ can be used to enhance perfusion. Even though flushing provides only a temporary therapeutic benefit, vitamin B$_3$ may be used to relieve chilblains and muscle cramps caused by impaired perfusion in peripheral vascular disease. Doses of 100 to 300 mg/day are recommended. The dose of niacin is increased to 500 mg tid for treating Raynaud's disease. Perfusion is even more effectively improved with a combined approach using α-tocopherol-nicotinate 200 mg tid. In addition to its hypolipidemic and flushing effects, niacin significantly decreases fibrinogen. In view of both its lipid and anticoagulant effects, 100 to 150 mg of niacin given orally three to five times per day deserves serious consideration in the treatment of peripheral vascular disease.[5]

Vitamin B$_3$ may promote psychologic health. As part of a B complex, 50 mg niacin is used to treat depression and anxiety.[6] Higher doses of niacinamide (500 to 1000 mg tid) may be helpful for anxiety and/or depression in persons with sugar intolerance. A 500-mg dose of vitamin B$_3$ taken an hour before bedtime is recommended for insomnia.[6] The hypothesis is that vitamin B$_3$ saturation will encourage diversion of tryptophan to serotonin production. Niacinamide in dosages of 3 grams daily has been used in schizophrenia.

Niacinamide has also been reported to increase joint mobility and function and decrease joint stiffness, deformity, swelling, and pain.[7] A daily dose of 1000 mg has been suggested for arthritis.[6]

TOXICITY/DRUG INTERACTIONS

Niacinamide is nontoxic in recommended therapeutic doses. However, nausea, vomiting, and hepatotoxicity have been reported at doses of 3 grams/day. High doses may also cause diarrhea, dizziness, blurred vision, arrhythmia, arthralgia, and myalgia. At a dose of 3 grams/day, niacinamide impairs glycemic control. Asthma is not triggered by niacinamide.

The spectrum of toxicity from least to most toxic is niacinamide, niacin, and sustained-release niacin preparations. Nausea and hepatotoxicity are especially marked with slow-release forms of niacin. Niacin toxicity starts at 100 mg and completely overlaps the therapeutic dose. Nausea, vomiting, and hepatotoxicity have been reported at doses of 1.5 grams/day for niacin. Asthma, aggravated by histamine release, may be caused by niacin. The vasodilatory effect of niacin (at dosages of 100 to 200 mg), when not used to increase perfusion, is regarded as a side effect. Flushing presents with a burning tingling sensation, pruritus, and reddening of the face, arms, and chest. Headaches may occur. Flushing appears to be more closely related to a continuous rise in plasma niacin than to the absolute dose. Niacin-induced flushing usually occurs within 15 to 30 minutes and may be reduced by taking niacin with meals, avoiding hot drinks, and taking 300 mg of aspirin 30 minutes before the niacin dose. In doses of 100 to 500 mg tid, other adverse effects of niacin are hyperglycemia, hyperuricemia, and raised liver enzymes. Monitoring of liver function is recommended at doses over 250 mg/day.

Isoniazid increases the requirement for niacin. Other interactions include alcohol, aspirin, nitroglycerine, warfarin, and cholesterol-lowering medications. The risk of myopathy is increased when niacin and HMG-CoA reductase inhibitors are combined.

Niacin competes with uric acid for excretion and may precipitate gout in susceptible persons. Patients with gout, peptic ulceration, or liver disease should avoid niacin supplementation.

CLINICAL CAUTION

Early signs of deficiency include anorexia, weight loss, stomach problems, skin problems, burning sensations, sores in the mouth, anemia, and mental problems such as anxiety, tension, and depression. Early evidence of deficiency is urinary excretion of less than 5.8 μmol/day of N^1-methyl-nicotinamide.

PRACTICE TIPS

- Patients starting on niacin may experience dizziness on getting up quickly; this usually is resolved within 14 days.
- Although niacinamide raises liver enzymes, it does not produce the other adverse effects of niacin, making it a safer but less effective drug.
- Use of niacin to reduce blood lipids should only be undertaken under medical supervision.
- Although results are unproven, 50 to 100 mg niacin may reduce symptoms of tinnitus.
- Dysmenorrhea may respond to starting 100 mg niacin bd 7 to 10 days before menstruation and every 3 hours during cramps. Rutin 60 mg and vitamin C 300 mg enhance the spasmolytic effect.

REFERENCES

1. Brighthope I: Nutritional medicine tables, *J Aust Coll Nutr Env Med* 17:20-5, 1998.
2. Wang W, Basinger A, Neese RA, et al: Effect of nicotinic acid administration on hepatic very low density lipoprotein-triglyceride production, *Am J Physiol Endocrinol Metab* 280(3):E540-7, 2001.
3. Taher TH, Dzavik V, Reteff EM, et al: Tolerability of statin-fibrate and statin-niacin combination therapy in dyslipidemic patients at high risk for cardiovascular events, *Am J Cardiol* 89(4):390-4, 2002.
4. Elam MB, Hunninghake DB, Davis KB, et al: Effect of niacin on lipid and lipoprotein levels and glycemic control in patients with diabetes and peripheral

arterial disease: the ADMIT study: a randomized trial. Arterial Disease Multiple Intervention Trial, *JAMA* 284(10):1263-70, 2000.

5. Chesney CM, Elam MB, Herd JA, et al: Effect of niacin, warfarin, and antioxidant therapy on coagulation parameters in patients with peripheral arterial disease in the arterial disease multiple intervention trial, *Am Heart J* 140(4):631-6, 2000.

6. Diefendorf D, Healey J, Kalyn W, editors: *The healing power of vitamins, minerals and herbs*, Surry Hills, Australia, 2000, Readers Digest.

7. Hoffer A: Treatment of arthritis by niacin and nicotinamide, *Can Med Assoc J* 81:235, 1959.

▪ CHAPTER 102 ▪

VITAMIN B₅ (PANTOTHENIC ACID)

> Adequate amounts and an acceptable ratio of all vitamins of the B group are required for optimal function.

Panothenic acid is a B group vitamin required for catabolism of carbohydrates, proteins, and fats. Its name is derived from the Greek word *pantos*, meaning everywhere. It is involved in many metabolic reactions and has been used to promote a healthy nervous system. Vitamin B₅ is routinely included in antistress vitamin B complex formulations.

Pantothenic acid may be helpful in conditions such as migraine, chronic fatigue syndrome, and allergy.

MECHANISM OF ACTION

Pantothenic acid is a component of coenzyme A, a cofactor and acyl group carrier for many metabolic reactions. As a component of acetyl CoA and succinyl CoA, pantothenic acid plays a central role in the tricarboxylic acid cycle and in the synthesis of fatty acids, including membrane phospholipids. Pantothenic acid derivatives have a hypolipidemic effect in mice with induced hypothalamic obesity.[1] The mechanism could be related to a reduced resistance to insulin and activation of lipolysis in serum and adipose tissue.

Pantothenic acid is important for synthesis of steroids, amino acids, neurotransmitters, and vitamins A and D.

FOOD SOURCES

Pantothenic acid is widely distributed in foods. Peas and beans (except green beans), lean meat, poultry, fish, and whole grain cereals are all good sources. Cooked liver and sunflower seeds are excellent sources as well.

Little pantothenic acid is lost from foods with ordinary cooking; however, refining of grains results in substantial losses. Freezing, thawing, and canning cause depletion of this vitamin. Pantothenic acid is synthesized by intestinal bacteria.

DOSE

Lack of pantothenic acid is so rare that there is no RDA or RNI for this vitamin. Although biochemical indices of adequate pantothenate nutrition and a satisfactory estimate of requirements may be lacking,[2] the AI of pantothenic acid for adults is 5 mg/day and increased to 6 mg/day in pregnancy and to 7 mg/day during lactation. The UL has not been set. The therapeutic dose range is 50 to 2000 g/day.[3]

CLINICAL USES

Pantothenic acid is not the focus of recent clinical trials. However, a double-blind study found pantothenic acid, in a dose of 900 mg daily, reduced LDL and elevated HDL cholesterol in certain types of hyperlipidemia.[4] Some two decades ago, a double-blind, placebo-controlled trial found arthritis patients taking 500 to 2000 mg calcium pantothenate daily reported significant pain relief.[5] Those with rheumatoid arthritis also reported less morning stiffness and disability.

Laboratory studies suggest that higher quantities of pantothenate are locally required to enhance wound healing. Calcium D-pantothenate was found to accelerate the wound-healing process by increasing the number of migrating cells, their distance, and hence their speed in cell cultures.[6] In addition, cell division was increased and protein synthesis changed. The clinical usefulness of this observation has yet to be established.

TOXICITY/DRUG INTERACTIONS

No toxicity has been reported. Alcohol and oral contraceptives may increase the requirement for pantothenic acid. Biotin deficiency may be aggravated by pantothenic acid deficiency.[7]

CLINICAL CAUTION

Pantothenic acid deficiency may present with irritability and restlessness, fatigue, apathy, sleep disturbance, gastrointestinal upsets, and motor and sensory neurologic changes (e.g., burning feet). However, before diagnosing a vitamin B_5 deficiency, one must confirm that the patient is either on a semisynthetic diet devoid of pantothenic acid or consuming pantothenic acid antagonists.

PRACTICE TIPS

- No clinical problems have been found to be caused by a lack of pantothenic acid alone.
- Research is too limited to recommend use of pantothenic acid.

REFERENCES

1. Naruta E, Buko V: Hypolipidemic effect of pantothenic acid derivatives in mice with hypothalamic obesity induced by aurothioglucose, *Exp Toxicol Pathol* 53(5):393-8, 2001.
2. Bender DA: Optimum nutrition: thiamin, biotin and pantothenate, *Proc Nutr Soc* 58(2):427-33, 1999.
3. Brighthope I: Nutritional medicine tables, *J Aust Coll Nutr Env Med* 17:20-5, 1998.
4. Gaddi A, Descovich GC, Noseda G, et al: Controlled evaluation of pantethine, a natural hypolipidemic compound, in patients with different forms of hyperlipoproteinemia, *Atherosclerosis* 50(1):73-83, 1984.
5. Calcium pantothenate in arthritic conditions. A report from the General Practitioner Research Group, *Practitioner* 224(1340):208-11, 1980.
6. Weimann BI, Hermann D: Studies on wound healing: effects of calcium D-pantothenate on the migration, proliferation and protein synthesis of human dermal fibroblasts in culture, *Int J Vitam Nutr Res* 69(2):113-9, 1999.
7. Ramakrishna T: Vitamins and brain development, *Physiol Res* 48(3):175-87, 1999.

■ CHAPTER 103 ■

VITAMIN B$_6$

Peripheral neuropathy, a manifestation of vitamin B$_6$ deficiency, can be precipitated by megadose supplementation.

Vitamin B$_6$ is found in six forms—pyridoxine, pyridoxal, pyridoxamine, and their respective 5′-phosphates. The pyridoxine, pyridoxal, and pyridoxamine derivatives are oxidized to pyridoxal, which is rapidly phosphorylated in the liver. Formation of the metabolically active form of vitamin B$_6$, pyridoxal-5-phosphate, requires vitamin B$_2$ and magnesium. Pyridoxal-5-phosphate is the most direct clinically relevant measure of vitamin B$_6$ status.

Vitamin B$_6$ is necessary for metabolism of proteins, carbohydrates, and fats. It is involved in amino group transfer and protein synthesis, heme biosynthesis, synthesis of essential fatty acids, glycogen breakdown, and synthesis of neurotransmitters including dopamine, serotonin, γ-aminobutyric acid (GABA), histamine, adrenalin, noradrenalin, and taurine. It is also involved in the transulfuration pathway of homocysteine to cysteine. Its participation in many vital metabolic pathways has created potential interest in its use in the management of diverse conditions ranging from carpal tunnel syndrome and diabetic neuropathy, through premenstrual syndrome and morning sickness, to cardiovascular disease and asthma.

MECHANISM OF ACTION

The metabolically active coenzyme form of vitamin B$_6$, pyridoxal 5′-phosphate, is a cofactor for over 100 enzymes. Pyridoxal 5′-phosphate–dependent enzymes are involved in the following[1]:

- Decarboxylation of amino acids to yield amines, many of which are important neurotransmitters and hormones.
- Transamination of amino acids to keto acids, which are then oxidized and used as metabolic fuel.
- Phosphorolytic cleavage of glycogen (from liver and muscle) to glucose-1-phosphate.
- Formation of α-aminolevulinic acid, a precursor to heme.
- Decarboxylation of phosphatidylserine to phosphatidylethanolamine in phospholipid synthesis.

• As a co-factor in a variety of reactions involving side-chain cleavage, including cystathionine synthase and cystathionase.

Pyridoxamine is a potent inhibitor of both advanced glycation end products and advanced lipid peroxidation formation. It may prove useful for limiting chemical modification of tissue proteins and associated pathology of aging and chronic diseases, including diabetes and atherosclerosis.[2]

Vitamin B_6 enhances immune responsiveness.

FOOD SOURCES

Vitamin B_6 is found in various foods, including brewer's yeast, liver, oatmeal, cereals, legumes, egg yolk, soybeans, avocado, walnuts, and whole grain cereals. Half of the vitamin B_6 content of food is lost during processing. Although some forms of vitamin B_6 are lost from food during ordinary cooking, pyridoxine is unaffected.

DOSE

While the RDA for adults is set at 1.0 mg/1000 kcal or 1.5 to 4 mg/day, requirements may be higher in persons on very-high-protein diets. The typical therapeutic dose is 50 to 200 mg/day, but the therapeutic dose range is 10 to 1000 mg/day.[3] The UL for adults is 100 mg/day as pyridoxine. A useful conversion is

dietary B_6 equivalents (mg) = food B_6 (mg) + (1.27 × mg synthetic B_6)

Plasma pyridoxal-5-phosphate reflects tissue stores and is the best single indicator of vitamin B_6 status. Plasma pyridoxal-5-phosphate levels of 10 nmol/L are suboptimal. The plasma level of B_6 reflects intake, while red cell transaminase enzyme reactivation reflects function and tissue status. Urinary xanthurenic acid excretion is tested after a tryptophan load.

CLINICAL USES

Although somewhat controversial, there is some scientific support for use of this vitamin in various conditions.

Vitamin B_6 can modify homocysteine levels. Homocysteine has toxic effects on vascular endothelial cells, and plasma pyridoxal-5-phosphate levels below 20 nmol/L are found in 10% of patients with coronary artery disease but only 2% of controls.[4] Moderately elevated plasma homocysteine levels were halved in persons supplemented with 1 mg/day folic acid, 0.05 mg/day vitamin B_{12}, and 10 mg/day vitamin B_6.[5] A randomized, double-blind, placebo-controlled trial found low-dose vitamin B$_6$ (1.6 mg/day) supplementation reduced fasting total homocysteine concentrations in healthy elderly persons who were made replete with folate (400 µg/day for 6 weeks prior to the study) and riboflavin (1.6 mg/day for 18 weeks prior to the study).[6] Furthermore, a prospective study concluded that an intake of folate and vitamin B$_6$ above the current recommended dietary allowance may be important in the primary prevention of coronary heart disease among women.[4] However, another study found that, while daily treatment with 15 mg folic acid and 600 mg pyridoxine significantly lowered plasma total homocysteine, it did not improve any of the associated coagulation and hemostasis cardiovascular risk factors in type 2 diabetics mellitus with hyperhomocysteinemia.[7] Nonetheless, a clinical study of consecutive type 2 diabetics did conclude homocysteine was independently associated with the prevalence of diabetic neuropathy.[8] Homocysteine values are inversely related to vitamin levels.

The nutritional status of vitamin B$_6$ also has a significant and selective modulatory impact on central production of both serotonin and GABA, neurotransmitters that control depression, pain perception, and anxiety. Pooled data of nine trials suggest doses of pyridoxine up to 100 mg/day are likely to be of benefit in treating premenstrual symptoms, including premenstrual depression.[9] Similarly, 100 to 200 mg pyridoxine daily for at least 12 weeks may prove beneficial in treating carpal tunnel syndrome, given its ability to alter pain perception and increase the pain threshold.[10] A review of clinical trials, however, did conclude that the evidence for the use of pyridoxine as the sole treatment of carpal tunnel syndrome is weak.[11] It has also been reported that 20 mg vitamin B$_6$ daily may improve memory in the healthy elderly.[12]

Other possible indications for vitamin B$_6$ are morning sickness and sideroblastic anemia. A double-blind trial using pyridoxine (25 mg every 8 hours for 3 days) in the treatment of morning sickness resulted in a significant reduction in vomiting and an improvement in nausea in those who initially reported severe nausea.[13] Pyridoxal-5-phosphate is necessary for the activation of glycine in the initial stages of heme production. From a therapeutic point of view, pyridoxal-5-phosphate should be tried in all cases of symptomatic primary sideroblastic anemia that have shown no response to pyridoxine.

TOXICITY/DRUG INTERACTIONS

Vitamin B$_6$ toxicity manifests as sensory peripheral neuritis. Potentially toxic levels in adults can result either from prolonged daily intake of vitamin B$_6$ in excess of 100 mg or consumption of 2 g/day over a shorter period. Chronic pyridoxine intake may cause sensory neuropathy by exceeding the liver's ability to phosphorylate pyridoxine to the active coenzyme pyridoxal phosphate. The resultant high pyridoxal level may be either be directly neu-rotoxic or cause toxicity through competition with pyridoxal binding sites. This problem can be avoided by supplementing with pyridoxal phosphate.[14] In reality, most reported cases of neuropathy associated with pyridoxine supplementation have involved doses of at least 500 mg/day for 2 years or more.[15] In fact, it has been suggested that it takes doses in excess of 1000 mg/day for long periods to cause a reversible neuropathy.[3]

Pyridoxine will reduce the efficacy of levodopa in controlling parkinson-ian symptoms, the magnitude of the effect proportional to the dose of pyri-doxine. In doses of 25 mg/day, vitamin B_6 antagonizes the effect of levodopa. Other antiparkinsonian drugs, benserazide and carbidopa, cause vitamin B_6 depletion by forming hydrazones.

Estrogen is suspected to induce vitamin B_6 deficiency or depletion. There have been many reports of abnormal tryptophan metabolism in women tak-ing either oral contraceptive or menopausal hormone replacement therapy.[1] High-dose oral contraceptive use slightly decreases plasma pyridoxal phos-phate. This probably reflects hormonal stimulation of tryptophan catabolism rather than a deficiency of vitamin B_6 per se. The antituberculosis drug iso-niazid can also result in a functional vitamin B_6 deficiency.

Vitamin B_6 enhances absorption of zinc picolinate, and vitamin C defi-ciency may increase vitamin B_6 excretion.

CLINICAL CAUTION

Early evidence of vitamin B_6 deficiency presents with insomnia, irritability, depression, and, later, confusion. Seborrheic dermatitis, neuropathy, epilep-tiform convulsions, microcytic anemia, and glossitis have been reported. Chronic deficiency may lead to hyperoxaluria and an increased risk of kid-ney stones.

PRACTICE TIPS

- Infants receiving unfortified formulas, such as evaporated milk, may need additional pyridoxine.
- The risk of developing sensory neuropathy decreases rapidly at doses under 1 g/day.
- Vitamin B_6 supplementation can cause a relative deficiency of vitamin B_2.
- Pregnant women, women taking oral contraceptives, and alcoholics are at increased risk of vitamin B_6 deficiency
- Vitamin B_6 deficiency impairs both humoral and cell-mediated immune responses.

REFERENCES

1. Bender D: Non-nutritional uses of vitamin B$_6$, *Br J Nutr* 81(1):7-20, 1999.
2. Onorato JM, Jenkins AJ, Thorpe SR, Baynes JW: Pyridoxamine, an inhibitor of advanced glycation reactions, also inhibits advanced lipoxidation reactions. Mechanism of action of pyridoxamine, *J Biol Chem* 275(28):21177-84, 2000.
3. Brighthope I: Nutritional medicine tables, *J Aust Coll Nutr Env Med* 17:20-5, 1998.
4. Rimm EB, Willett WC, Hu FB, et al: Folate and vitamin B$_6$ from diet and supplements in relation to risk of coronary heart disease among women, *JAMA* 279(5):359-64, 1998.
5. Ubbink JB, van der Merwe A, Vermaak WJ, Delport R: Hyperhomocysteinemia and the response of vitamin supplementation, *Clinical Invest* 71(12):993-8, 1993.
6. McKinley MC, McNulty H, McPartlin J, et al: Low-dose vitamin B$_6$ effectively lowers fasting plasma homocysteine in healthy elderly persons who are folate and riboflavin replete, *Am J Clin Nutr* 73(4):759-64, 2001.
7. Baliga BS, Reynolds T, Fink LM, Fonseca VA: Hyperhomocysteinemia in type 2 diabetes mellitus: cardiovascular risk factors and effect of treatment with folic acid and pyridoxine, *Endocrinol Pract* 6(6):435-41, 2000.
8. Ambrosch A, Dierkes J, Lobmann R, et al: Relation between homocysteinaemia and diabetic neuropathy in patients with Type 2 diabetes mellitus, *Diabet Med* 18(3):185-92, 2001.
9. Wyatt KM, Dimmock PW, Jones PW, et al: Efficacy of vitamin B$_6$ in the treatment of premenstrual syndrome: systematic review, *BMJ* 318(7195):1375-81, 1999.
10. Jacobson MD, Plancher KD, Kleinman WB: Vitamin B$_6$ (pyridoxine) therapy for carpal tunnel syndrome, *Hand Clin* 12(2):253-7, 1996.
11. Vitamin B$_6$ (pyridoxine and pyridoxal 5'-phosphate)—monograph, *Altern Med Rev* 6(1):87-92, 2001.
12. Riggs KM, Spiro A, Tucker K, Rush D: Relations of vitamin B$_{12}$, vitamin B$_6$, folate, and homocysteine to cognitive performance in the Normative Aging Study, *Am J Clin Nutr* 63(3):306-14, 1996.
13. Sahakian V, Rouse D, Sipes S, et al: Vitamin B$_6$ is effective therapy for nausea and vomiting of pregnancy: a randomized, double-blind placebo-controlled study, *Obstet Gynecol* 78(1):33-6, 1991.
14. Werbach MR: *Textbook of nutritional medicine*, Tarzana, CA, 1999, Third Line Press.
15. Bendich A, Cohen M: Vitamin B$_6$ safety issues, *Ann N Y Acad Sci* 585:321-30, 1990.

■ CHAPTER 104 ■

VITAMIN B$_{12}$ (COBALAMIN)

Vegans are at risk of vitamin B$_{12}$ deficiency; this vitamin only occurs naturally in animal products.

Cyanocobalamin and hydroxycobalamin are manmade forms of vitamin B$_{12}$. Vitamin B$_{12}$ is essential for myelination of nerves, hematopoiesis, and synthesis of nucleic acids. It is intimately involved in folate metabolism.

The requirement for vitamin B$_{12}$ is increased in pregnancy, celiac disease, and gastrointestinal disorders involving intrinsic factor production in the stomach or absorption in the ileum, as in pernicious anemia. Vitamin B$_{12}$ deficiency is also reported to be a risk factor for heart disease, stroke, Alzheimer's disease, and accelerated aging.

MECHANISM OF ACTION

Vitamin B$_{12}$ is implicated in methyl biosynthesis and methyl group transfer. The active form of vitamin B$_{12}$ is methylcobalamin. Along with folic acid, pyridoxine, and riboflavin, vitamin B$_{12}$ is a source of coenzymes that participate in one carbon metabolism. A carbon unit from serine or glycine is transferred to tetrahydrofolate to form methylene-tetrahydrofolate. This is used as such for the synthesis of thymidine, which is incorporated into DNA, for the oxidation to formyl-tetrahydrofolate, or for the reduction to methyl-tetrahydrofolate. Formyl-tetrahydrofolate is used for the synthesis of purines, the building blocks nucleic acids. Methyl-tetrahydrofolate is used to methylate homocysteine to form methionine, a reaction catalyzed by a B$_{12}$-containing methyltransferase. Homocysteine is a product of methionine metabolism and a precursor of methionine synthesis. Elevated plasma homocysteine is a risk factor for cardiovascular disease, stroke, thrombosis and is associated with loss of neurocognitive function as in Alzheimer's disease.[1] These associations may be due to a neurotoxic effect of homocysteine and/or to decreased availability of S-adenosylmethionine, resulting in hypomethylation in brain tissue. Hypomethylation is thought to exacerbate a depressive tendency in people. Much of the methionine that is formed is converted to S-adenosylmethionine, a universal donor of methyl groups.

Vitamin B$_{12}$ is also a coenzyme for conversion of methylmalonyl-CoA to succinyl-CoA, an intermediate in the tricarboxylic acid cycle.

FOOD SOURCES

Dietary sources of vitamin B_{12} include shellfish, organ meats (e.g., liver, kidney), meat, fermented cheeses, milk, and egg yolk. It is not found in any vegetables. Vegetarians can obtain vitamin B_{12} from yeast grown on a special B_{12}-enriched medium. Spirulina contains vitamin B_{12} in a nonphysiologic form. Intestinal bacteria synthesizes vitamin B_{12}, but B_{12} produced in the colon is not absorbed. Absorption occurs in the ileum. Active absorption of vitamin B_{12} requires intrinsic factor, a glycoprotein secreted by gastric parietal cells. The elderly and vegans are at particular risk of vitamin B_{12} deficiency. Absorption also occurs by passive diffusion.

About 30% of B_{12} is lost during cooking.

DOSE

The RDA for vitamin B_{12} is 2.4 µg/day for adults and increases to 2.6 µg/day during pregnancy and 2.8 µg/day during lactation. The RDA is 0.7 µg/day by the age of 3 years, and gradually increases to the adult level by the teens. The EAR is 2 µg/day for adults, increasing to 2.2 µg/day during pregnancy and 2.4 µg/day during lactation. The UL has not been set at this time. Supplemental doses range from 5 to 50 µg/day, although a therapeutic dose range of 10 to 5000 µg/day has been suggested.[2]

Serum B_{12} levels should exceed 120 pmol/L (170 pg/ml), although values at this level do not exclude deficiency. Serum B_{12} levels reflect intake. Serum homocysteine is raised in vitamin B_{12} deficiency.

CLINICAL USES

It is recommended that persons over 50 years of age take vitamin B_{12} supplementation. The prevalence of vitamin B_{12} deficiency, which is higher than previously reported, increases with age, especially in persons over 65 years.[3] Absorption requires the presence of both intrinsic factor and adequate gastric acid. Since many elderly people have a degree of atrophic gastritis, it has been suggested they meet their daily vitamin B_{12} requirements from fortified food or supplements rather than relying entirely on natural sources. There are a number of reasons, including cardiovascular health, to support a food fortification policy based on vitamin B_{12} and folic acid.[4,5]

Vitamin B_{12} deficiency results in pernicious anemia. Early evidence of deficiency is fatigue, weakness, lack of appetite, and glossitis. Progression to pernicious anemia results in hematologic and neurologic changes. Subacute combined degeneration of the spinal cord presents with paresthesia, sensory loss, and ataxia. Major changes include sensory disturbances with tingling and numbness that is worst in the lower limbs, loss of vibration sense, an abnormal gait, and cognitive changes, including poor concentration, memory impairment, and frank dementia. Visual changes, impaired bladder and bowel control, and impotence have also been reported. The onset is insidious. The hematologic changes of megaloblastic anemia are indistinguishable from folic acid deficiency. While folate supplementation will normalize the blood picture, neurologic damage progresses and the patient develops overt subacute combined degeneration of the spinal cord. Ideally, intervention with vitamin B$_{12}$ occurs early while the condition is reversible.

An accepted regime for treating vitamin B$_{12}$ deficiency is to initially administer 1000 μg of vitamin B$_{12}$ intramuscularly each week.[6] The patient usually responds rapidly, and the dose is then decreased to 1000 μg each month for as long as needed. Patients with overt atrophic gastritis require regular injections to avoid vitamin B$_{12}$ deficiency. Strict vegetarians who fail to take vitamin B$_{12}$ supplements are similarly at risk of neurologic disorders. In these cases, oral supplementation suffices.

Vitamin B$_{12}$ has long been used as a panacea for vague illnesses. An informal study found that a substantial proportion of patients with normal serum B$_{12}$ concentrations did indeed feel better following injections of hydroxycobalamin, but not following injections of sterile water.[7] Open trials reported the maximum feeling of well-being was achieved using dosages ranging from 3000 μg four times weekly to 9000 μg/day.

Although a longitudinal, multicenter study of an elderly population found no significant correlations between mental health and vitamin B$_{12}$ or folate,[8] there is a persistent belief that vitamin B$_{12}$ may affect mental alertness. A study of vegans did suggest that cobalamin deficiency, in the absence of hematologic signs, may lead to impaired cognitive performance in adolescents.[9] Vitamin B$_{12}$ deficiency is frequently associated with Alzheimer's disease,[3] and a combination of vitamin B$_{12}$ and bright light therapy has been shown to improve the daytime vigilance level of early Alzheimer-type dementia patients.[10] A pilot study found methylcobalamin had a positive psychotropic alerting effect modulating the sleep-wake cycle toward sleep reduction.[11] Vitamin B$_{12}$ may indeed exert a direct influence on melatonin, a hormone involved in the regulation of the sleep-wake cycle. However, a double-blind study found 3 mg methylcobalamin administered over 4 weeks was not an effective treatment for sleep-wake rhythm disorders.[12] Nonetheless, a later double-blind study using a larger dose detected slight and inconsistent improvement.[13] Methylcobalamin appears to have low therapeutic potency and may possibly boost other treatment methods for this disorders.

Vitamin B$_{12}$ has a number of other potential uses. A randomized, prospective clinical trial concluded that a vitamin B$_{12}$ cream containing avocado oil had considerable potential as a well-tolerated, long-term, topical therapy of psoriasis.[14] Open trials involving patients with vertebral pain syndromes, degenerative neuropathies, and cancer reported excellent pain relief with injections of 5000 to 10,000 μg/day.

Further investigation into a role for vitamin B$_{12}$ in treatment of multiple sclerosis and prevention of ischemic heart disease also deserves consideration.

TOXICITY/DRUG INTERACTIONS

Vitamin B_{12} is nontoxic, but it may occasionally cause diarrhea and pruritus. High doses may exacerbate acne. Of more concern is that high doses of folic acid may mask a vitamin B_{12} deficiency.

Absorption of vitamin B_{12} may be impaired by drugs that reduce hydrochloric acid secretion (e.g., ranitidine). Alcohol, antibiotics, colchicine, methyldopa, and metformin are among the drugs that reduce absorption of this vitamin.

CLINICAL CAUTION

Early evidence of deficiency is tiredness, weakness, lack of appetite, and glossitis. Treatment of pernicious anemia with folic acid improves the blood picture but neural damage progresses.

PRACTICE TIPS

- Liver stores last 3 to 5 years and therefore deficiency only becomes evident after some years of inadequate intake or absorption.
- Vitamin B_{12} appears to exert a substantial analgesic effect at pharmacologic dosages.
- Avoid taking vitamin C within 1 hour of taking oral vitamin B_{12}.

REFERENCES

1. Selhub J: Folate, vitamin B_{12} and vitamin B_6 and one carbon metabolism, *J Nutr Health Aging* 6(1):39-42, 2002.
2. Brighthope I: Nutritional medicine tables, *J Aust Coll Nutr Env Med* 17:20-5, 1998.
3. Wynn M, Wynn A: The danger of B_{12} deficiency in the elderly, *Nutr Health* 12(4):215-26, 1998.
4. Quinlivan EP, McPartlin J, McNulty H, et al: Importance of both folic acid and vitamin B_{12} in reduction of risk of vascular disease, *Lancet* 359(9302):227-8, 2002.
5. SoRelle R: Fortification of food with vitamin B_{12} in addition to folic acid might reduce cardiovascular disease risk, *Circulation* 105(4):E9070, 2002.
6. Werbach MR: Nutritional strategies for treating chronic fatigue syndrome, *Altern Med Rev* 5(2):93-108, 2000.
7. Newbold HL: Vitamin B_{12}: placebo or neglected therapeutic tool? *Med Hypotheses* 28(3):155-64, 1989.
8. Eussen S, Ferry M, Hininger I, et al: Five year changes in mental health and associations with vitamin B_{12}/folate status of elderly Europeans, *J Nutr Health Aging* 6(1):43-50, 2002.

9. Louwman MW, van Dusseldorp M, van de Vijver FJ, et al: Signs of impaired cognitive function in adolescents with marginal cobalamin status, *Am J Clin Nutr* 72(3):762-9, 2000.

10. Ito T, Yamadera H, Ito R, et al: Effects of vitamin B$_{12}$ and bright light on cognitive and sleep-wake rhythm in Alzheimer-type dementia, *Psychiatry Clin Neurosci* 55(3):281-2, 2001.

11. Mayer G, Kroger M, Meier-Ewert K: Effects of vitamin B$_{12}$ on performance and circadian rhythm in normal subjects, *Neuropsychopharmacology* 15(5):456-64, 1996.

12. Okawa M, Takahashi K, Egashira K, et al: Vitamin B$_{12}$ treatment for delayed sleep phase syndrome: a multi-center double-blind study, *Psychiatry Clin Neurosci* 51(5):275-9, 1997.

13. Takahashi K, Okawa M, Matsumoto M, et al: Double-blind test on the efficacy of methylcobalamin on sleep-wake rhythm disorders, *Psychiatry Clin Neurosci* 53(2):211-3, 1999.

14. Stucker M, Memmel U, Hoffmann M, et al: Vitamin B$_{12}$ cream containing avocado oil in the therapy of plaque psoriasis, *Dermatology* 203(2):141-7, 2001.

■ CHAPTER 105 ■

VITAMIN C (ASCORBATE)

Current thinking suggests doubling the RDA for vitamin C to around 100 mg daily, yet it is used therapeutically in doses of up to 100 g/day, and 10 g/day is not unusual.

The cost and safety profile of vitamin C favors its empiric use in recommended doses. It is under investigation for its potential use in the prevention and treatment of a myriad of conditions including cardiovascular disease, cancer, and infections including coryza and oxidative stress.

MECHANISM OF ACTION

Ascorbate is well recognized to benefit wound healing.[1] In fact, an animal study confirmed that those receiving the higher dose of vitamin C demonstrated greater wound integrity than those receiving a more moderate dose of the vitamin.[2] Vitamin C stimulates procollagen, enhances collagen synthesis, increases alkaline phosphatase activity, and helps maintain the intercellular matrix. Vitamin C, in addition to being involved in the transport of nutrients such as iron, copper, and folic acid, reduces redox active transition metal ions in the active sites of specific biosynthetic enzymes. In fact, much of the interest in vitamin C has focused on its antioxidant role.

Vitamin C is a major antioxidant defense in the aqueous phase and for transfer of radicals from the lipid to aqueous phase.[3] Vitamin C spares vitamin E. Vitamin C is water soluble and can directly react with superoxide, hydroxyl radicals, and singlet oxygen.[4] The ability of vitamin C to scavenge reactive oxygen and nitrogen species may enable it to prevent oxidative damage to important biologic macromolecules such as DNA, lipids, and proteins. However, vitamin C does show both reducing and oxidizing activities, depending on the environment.[5] At lower concentrations, ascorbic acid displays an antioxidant property, preventing spontaneous, stress, or antitumor agent-induced apoptosis. Higher concentrations of vitamin C induce apoptotic cell death in various tumor cell lines, possibly via its pro-oxidant action.

Vitamin C supplementation bolsters the immune responses. Normal volunteers supplemented with 1 to 3 g/day vitamin C showed increased neutrophil motility and chemotaxis, immunoglobulin levels, and lymphocyte blastogenesis in response to mitogens.[6] In addition to modifying the immunologic activity of leukocytes, vitamin C enhances production of interferon and modulates inflammation.

The biochemical activity of vitamin C has recently been reviewed.[7]

FOOD SOURCES

Vitamin C is found in various foods including peppers, black currants, citrus fruits (oranges, lemons, grapefruit), green vegetables (peppers, broccoli, cabbage), tomatoes, rosehips, and potatoes. It is best to eat fresh fruits and vegetables, since losses of up to 90% have been reported with cooking and canning. For example, exposure to air, drying, salting, or cooking (especially in copper pots), mincing of fresh vegetables, or mashing potatoes reduces the vitamin C content of foods. Freezing does not usually cause loss of vitamin C unless foods are stored for a very long time. Vitamin C loss is decreased by using very little water for cooking and by microwaving.

The bioavailability of ascorbic acid is enhanced in citrus extract.[8]

DOSE

The RDA for ascorbic acid for infants is 30 mg, for children 45 mg, and for teenagers and adults 50 to 75 mg. The RDA increases to at least 70 mg during pregnancy and 90 mg during lactation. It has been postulated that the minimal daily requirement of vitamin C to allow 3% utilization and maintain a body pool of 1500 mg is 45 mg. Signs of scurvy appear when the body pool level of vitamin C reaches 300 mg, blood levels fall to 1 mg and under, and leukocyte levels fall to 70 mg/L. A daily intake of 45 mg is anticipated to prevent deficiency; it is unlikely to provide efficient protection as an antioxidant. In fact, it is well recognized that smokers require at least an additional 40 mg/day vitamin C above the RDA.[9] Even this level may well fail to be protective.

A daily intake of 150 to 200 mg vitamin C provides health benefits beyond that offered by the RDA. More recently, the RDA for vitamin C for adult nonsmokers has been raised to 60 mg/day, based on a mean requirement of 46 mg/day to prevent scurvy. However, biochemical, clinical, and epidemiologic evidence suggests an intake of 90 to 100 mg/day vitamin C is required for optimum reduction of chronic disease risk in nonsmokers, suggesting a new RDA of 120 mg/day vitamin C would be more appropriate.[10] Gey[3] concurs; he suggests a dietary intake of 22 mg/day plus supplementation with 130 mg/day vitamin C comes closer to what may be an optimal dose for wellness.

An adequate intake is estimated to be 200 mg/day or five servings of fruit and vegetables.[11] More recently, five portions of fruits and vegetables or 1 to 2 cups of black, green, or oolong tea have been reported as roughly equivalent to the total in vitro radical scavenging capacity of 400 mg vitamin C.[12] Bioavailability may alter in vivo efficacy. The antioxidant capacity of vitamin

C does not increase linearly with its serum concentration, and efficiency for scavenging free radicals declines as the concentration of ascorbate increases. Nonetheless, the optimal intake may be around 150 mg/day.

An even higher dose is required in smokers to compensate for their exposure to free radicals in cigarette smoke. A randomized, double-blind, placebo-controlled trial found 2 months of daily supplementation with 500 mg of vitamin C decreased smoking-related lipid peroxidation markers of oxidative stress in humans with a high, but not a low, BMI.[13] There was no indication that an antioxidant combination was more effective than vitamin C alone.

There appears to be a good correlation between serum levels and dietary intake of vitamin C up to 300 mg/day. At a blood level of 2 mg/L or more, the renal threshold for vitamin C is 14 mg/L. While the clinical importance of precise vitamin C blood levels is difficult to interpret, 2 mg/L is considered acceptable, as are leukocyte ascorbate levels of greater than 150 mg/L. Plasma ascorbate levels reflects recent diet while leukocyte vitamin C levels provide an indication of chronic depletion.

CLINICAL USES

The earliest symptom of scurvy, occurring only after many weeks of deficient vitamin C intake, is fatigue. The most common cutaneous findings are follicular hyperkeratosis, perifollicular hemorrhages, ecchymoses, xerosis, leg edema, poor wound healing, and bent or coiled body hairs. Gum abnormalities include gingival swelling, purplish discoloration, and hemorrhages. Back and joint pain, probably due to hemorrhage, is common, as is anemia. Leukopenia may be encountered as may syncope and sudden death. Treatment with vitamin C results in rapid, often dramatic, improvement.[14] Adults require 500 mg/day, children 100 to 300 mg/day, for at least 2 weeks.

Vitamin C in excess of the RDA appears to have beneficial effects; in fact, a daily intake of vitamin C in doses of at least the following[9,15]:

- 200 mg improves sperm quality 15%, while 1000 mg achieves a 40% improvement.
- 178 mg increases the forced expiratory volume.
- 50 mg at meals more than doubles nonheme iron absorption.
- 300 mg reduces the risk of cataract.
- 217 mg reduces the risk of heart disease.
- 225 mg reduces the risk of certain cancers.
- 1 g/day, over 4 to 6 weeks, is helpful for multiple episodes of furunculosis associated with neutrophil dysfunction.[16]
- 2 g hourly may help to control acute vital illness (e.g., colds and flu).
- 1 g hourly enhances healing in acute physical stress (e.g., burns, wounds).
- 5 to 10 g/day may aid degenerative low back pain.
- 5 to 10 g/day may be beneficial for chronic illness.

- 10 to 30 g/day assists persons with chronic fatigue syndrome.
- 3 to 10 g/day reduces chemical hypersensitivity and allergy.
- 5 g/day may alleviate mild anxiety.
- 5 to 10 g/day may be helpful for moderate anxiety, depression, insomnia, and confusion.
- 4 to 12 g acidifies urine. Vitamin C is beneficial in treatment and prevention of urinary tract infection. Laboratory studies suggest that acidification of nitrite generated by bacteria in urine results in the formation of nitric oxide and other reactive nitrogen oxides, which are toxic to a variety of microorganisms including *Escherichia coli, Pseudomonas aeruginosa,* and *Staphylococcus saprophyticus.*[17]
- 10 to 60 g/day may be used for severe depression and psychosis.
- 10 to 100 g/day may assist drug and alcohol withdrawal.
- Intravenous administration of sodium ascorbate is recommended for doses over 10 g/day.

The potential for vitamin C to enhance cardiovascular and musculoskeletal health, prevent and treat viral infections, and prevent cancer deserves special mention. Vitamin C is one of a very few intervention options that may raise HDL cholesterol levels. For each 1 mg/dl increase in serum ascorbic acid level, a 2 mg/dl increase in HDL-C level in women with total serum cholesterol levels of 200 mg/dl or more has been noted.[18] Another study confirmed 1000 mg vitamin C lowered LDL and raised HDL in a randomized, controlled, crossover trial.[19] On the other hand, an 8-month randomized, double-blinded, placebo-controlled trial of vitamin C supplementation (1 g/day) observed no overall effect on plasma concentrations of HDL, LDL, or total cholesterol, apolipoprotein (apo) B, or triglyceride.[20] The authors did not rule out the possibility that vitamin C supplementation might increase HDL cholesterol or apo A-I concentrations among individuals with lower plasma vitamin C levels.

It has been suggested that the potential for ascorbate to protect against atherosclerosis through inhibition of LDL oxidation, vascular endothelial dysfunction, and leukocyte adhesion to endothelium should not be ignored.[21] Such antioxidant protection may be particularly important for nonsmokers exposed to smoke-filled environments. In nonsmoking subjects, even a short period of passive smoking reduces serum antioxidant defense and accelerates lipid peroxidation, leading to accumulation of their low-density lipoprotein cholesterol in cultured human macrophages. Researchers found that, although 3 g of vitamin C did not influence the plasma antioxidant defense or the resistance of LDL to oxidation in normal air, it did prevent the smoke-induced decrease in plasma antioxidant defenses, the reduced resistance of LDL to oxidation, and the accelerated formation of serum thiobarbituric acid reactive substances in blood samples 1½ hours after passive smoking had been initiated.[22]

On the other hand, a double-masked, placebo-controlled, randomized, clinical trial found long-term oral supplementation of clinically healthy hypercholesterolemic men with 500 mg of slow-release ascorbate daily failed to lower lipid peroxidation in vivo, whereas 200 mg/day of D-α-tocopherol acetate did.[23] Subjects entering the study had both normal vitamin C and E levels. Despite failure of vitamin C to lower peroxidation levels in this study, in view of the potential for vitamin C to prevent the pro-oxidant activity of vitamin E, it remains likely that an optimum vitamin C intake or body status may help protect against atherosclerosis and its clinical sequelae.[21]

Vitamin C enhances musculoskeletal health. A population-based sample of postmenopausal women found taking both estrogen and vitamin C resulted in a significantly higher bone mineral density level.[24] Vitamin C is a marker for osteoblast formation. Vitamin C may also modify the impact of exercise. A double-blind, crossover study found supplementation of normal volunteers with 1 g vitamin C three times daily reduced delayed-onset muscle soreness following strenuous exercise.[25]

Vitamin C may protect against cancer. A number of mechanisms are postulated, including the following[26]:

- Antioxidant activity at both the level of initiation and promotion of carcinogenesis. Its direct in vitro cytotoxicity to certain cancer cell lines, however, is probably the result of hydrogen peroxide production within the cell.
- Preventing production of mutagenic nitrosamines. Conversion of nitrites to nitrous oxide by gastric bacteria predisposes to production of mutagenic nitrosamines through interaction of dietary amines with dietary nitrates. Vitamin C reduces such conversion.
- Stimulation of the immune system.
- An effect on liver enzymes responsible for detoxification and transformation of carcinogens.

Epidemiologic evidence supports a protective role for vitamin C against cancer. However, its efficacy does vary depending on the malignancy involved. Vitamin C appears to be particularly effective with respect to non-hormone-dependent cancers such as those of the lung and stomach.[27] Vitamin C intake has been shown to have an inverse relationship with gastric cancer. Recent follow-up studies on high-risk populations suggest that ascorbic acid, the reduced form of vitamin C, protects against gastric cancer. The mechanism underlying this protective effect requires further clarification. *H. pylori* is a significant risk factor for gastric cancer,[28] and the in vivo effect of vitamin C on this organism is dubious at best. Laboratory studies have found that, while vitamin C may inhibit the growth of gastric cancer cells and alter *H. pylori*-induced cell cycle events at concentrations comparable with those in gastric juice, it has no effect on *H. pylori* growth or pathogenicity.[29] Furthermore, the in vitro inhibitory effect of vitamin C on gastric cancer cells was lost at vitamin C concentrations found in patients with *H. pylori* infection.[29]

Vitamin C may offer a degree of chemoprotection against colon cancer. Three out of four intervention trials have found a significant benefit from vitamin C supplementation (3 to 4 g/day), often along with other interventions, in the treatment of patients with colonic polyps. While the data are not unanimous, there is evidence to support the possibility that oral vitamin C can help reduce the area, proliferation, and recurrence of precancerous colonic lesions.[30]

No consistent benefits have emerged from epidemiologic studies between dietary vitamin C intake and prostate or breast cancer risk; however, in view of persuasive retrospective studies, a beneficial effect from vitamin C should not be entirely discounted.[30] Retrospective dietary data has suggested that each 300 mg of dietary vitamin C intake is associated with roughly a 30% decrease in breast cancer risk. Yet, when the same research group analyzed prospective dietary studies, no association was detected between dietary vitamin C and breast cancer risk. Furthermore, another prospective trial found no relationship between plasma levels of ascorbate and risk of breast cancer in the subsequent 5 years. More investigations are required.

Controversy regarding the potential of vitamin C to prevent the common cold persists. A test population reported that vitamin C reduced flu and cold symptoms by 85%.[31] The symptoms of study subjects were monitored while they were treated with hourly doses of 1000 mg of vitamin C for the first 6 hours and then three times daily thereafter. The potential benefits of intervening with vitamin C in viral infections remains of interest (see case study in Chapter 1).

TOXICITY/DRUG INTERACTIONS

Vitamin C is safe at levels of supplementation up to 600 mg/day, and in fact higher levels up to 2000 mg/day are generally regarded as devoid of risk.[32] Although more than 1 g/day may cause an osmotic diarrhea, headache, fatigue, or insomnia in some people, toxicity is rare in doses of less than 5 g/day.[33]

High doses of vitamin C have long been suspected to increase the risk of urolithiasis. Oxalate is an excretory product of ascorbic acid. Concerns that vitamin C supplementation may cause oxalate stones is unfounded, since vitamin C intake above that which maintains a plasma level of 10 mg/L is excreted unchanged. Oxalate excretion does not increase with dietary vitamin C intake in a dose-response relationship.[34] Furthermore, no association between serum ascorbic acid level and prevalence of kidney stones has been detected.[35] However, large doses of ascorbic acid, but not ascorbate, may lower urinary pH and enhance excretion of alkaline drugs and resorption of acidic medications.

Other theoretical concerns linked with large doses of vitamin C include decreased serum vitamin B_{12} levels and increased iron absorption. Neither of these seems a realistic clinical problem. Iron overload is unlikely, since ascorbate does not affect iron absorption in iron-replete individuals,[11] and no association between serum ascorbic acid levels and decreased serum vitamin B_{12} levels has been detected.[35]

Ironically, lower doses of vitamin C may be risky in particular circumstances. Vitamin C may distort screening tests. Vitamin C in doses as low as 250 mg impairs screening for colon cancer, giving false-negative results on the guaiac stool occult blood test.[36] It may also interfere with diabetes control, giving false positives for glucosuria using cupric sulfate, as in the Clinitest, and false negatives using glucose oxidase, as with Clinistix. Ascorbic acid increases urinary excretion of uric acid and could obscure the diagnosis of gout. Doses in excess of 1 gram may be required.

A remaining and emerging concern is the possibility that vitamin C could have a pro-oxidant effect.[37] Vitamin C can serve as a pro-oxidant through formation of ascorbyl radical. It is also known this radical is quenched by vitamin E to yield the tocopherol radical, which in turn is reduced by the conversion of glutathione. The biologic relevance of any interaction of vitamin C with free, catalytically active metal ions that contribute to oxidative damage is also uncertain. While such reactions may occur in vitro, their occurrence in vivo is disputed. In vitro studies suggest daily supplementation with 500 mg of vitamin C may have an oxidant effect on certain DNA base oxidation.[38] However, such findings may be an experimental artifact.[39] A review of studies that investigated the role of vitamin C, in both the presence and absence of metal ions, in oxidative DNA, lipid, and protein damage found rather compelling evidence for antioxidant protection of lipids by vitamin C in biologic fluids, animals, and humans.[40] This protective effect was present both with and without iron cosupplementation. Data from animal studies consistently shows an antioxidant role of vitamin C.[40] In humans, cosupplementation with iron (14 mg/day) and vitamin C at either 60 or 260 mg/day for 12 weeks produced modest beneficial effects on LDL oxidation and platelet function, with no evidence for pro-oxidant effects.[41] In fact, plasma α-tocopherol concentrations were significantly increased after 6 weeks. Another human experiment confirmed ascorbic acid had an antioxidant effect. In doses up to 5000 mg, vitamin C neither induced mutagenic lesions nor had negative effects on natural killer cell activity, apoptosis, or the cell cycle.[42] Drug interactions include aspirin-promoting excretion of vitamin C, indomethacin decreasing vitamin C absorption, and the anticoagulant efficacy of warfarin being impaired by megadose vitamin C supplementation. Megadoses of vitamin C (1 g/day) increase serum levels of estrogen in women taking oral contraceptives or hormone replacement therapy.

Hypertensive patients taking calcium channel blockers may need to avoid grapefruit as a source of vitamin C since grapefruit contains naringin, a compound that impairs intestinal metabolism of these drugs.

CLINICAL CAUTION

Abrupt discontinuation of megadose vitamin C may result in rebound scurvy, a problem which may be encountered in neonates born to mothers on megadose supplementation. Selecting an appropriate dose of vitamin C remains problematic. Results of a depletion-repletion study with healthy young women using vitamin C doses of 30 to 2500 mg/day found doses above 100 mg were beyond the linear portion of a sigmoid curve, plasma and circulating cells were saturated at 400 mg/day, and urinary elimination of higher doses was noted.[43] This study also found biomarkers of endogenous oxidant stress were unchanged by vitamin C at all doses, suggesting this vitamin does not alter endogenous lipid peroxidation in healthy young women.

In persons with a glucose-6-phosphate dehydrogenase deficiency, high-dose vitamin C may trigger hemolytic anemia.

PRACTICE TIPS

- In persons with recurrent infections due to primary defects of phagocytic function, vitamin C is considered to be the specific therapy.
- Persons taking 400 mg/day vitamin C reported feeling less fatigued than those on 100 mg/day or less.
- For a cold or flu, take 5 to 10 g/day vitamin C immediately when symptoms present and continue every 2 to 4 hours until symptoms cease or a loose stool is passed.
- Megadose dose vitamin C therapy implies 10 g/day or more, a prophylactic dose of vitamin C is over 1 g/day, usually between 2 and 8 g/day, and optimal health may require an intake of around 150 to 200 mg/day.
- Ascorbic acid appears to exert a substantial analgesic effect at pharmacologic dosages.
- Megadoses of vitamin C (10 to 50 g/day) may reduce moderately severe pain while 1 g/day reduces delayed onset muscle soreness following strenuous exercise.
- Infants receiving unfortified formulas may develop a deficiency of vitamin C.
- Habitual chewing of ascorbic acid products may increase the risk of dental caries.

REFERENCES

1. Gross RL: The effect of ascorbate on wound healing, *Int Ophthalmol Clin* 40(4): 51-7, 2000.
2. Silverstein RJ, Landsman AS: The effects of a moderate and high dose of vitamin C on wound healing in a controlled guinea pig model, *J Foot Ankle Surg* 38(5):333-8, 1999.
3. Gey KF: Vitamins E plus C and interacting conutrients required for optimal health. A critical and constructive review of epidemiology and supplementation data regarding cardiovascular disease and cancer, *Biofactors* 7(1-2):113-74, 1998.
4. Clarkson PM, Thompson HS: Antioxidants: what role do they play in physical activity and health? *Am J Clin Nutr* 72(2 Suppl):637S-46S, 2000.

5. Sakagami H, Satoh K, Hakeda Y, Kumegawa M: Apoptosis-inducing activity of vitamin C and vitamin K, *Cell Mol Biol* (Noisy-le-grand) 46(1):129-43, 2000.

6. Werbach MR: Nutritional strategies for treating chronic fatigue syndrome, *Altern Med Rev* 5(2):93-108, 2000.

7. Arrigoni O, De Tullio MC: Ascorbic acid: much more than just an antioxidant, *Biochim Biophys Acta* 1569(1-3):1-9, 2002.

8. Vinson JA, Bose P: Comparative bioavailability of to humans of ascorbic acid alone or in citrus extract, *Am J Clin Nutr* 48(3):601-4, 1988.

9. Weber P, Bendich A, Schalch W: Vitamin C and human health—a review of recent data relevant to human requirements, *Int J Vit Nutr Res* 66(1):19-30, 1996.

10. Carr AC, Frei B: Toward a new recommended dietary allowance for vitamin C based on antioxidant and health effects in humans, *Am J Clin Nutr* 69(6):1086-107, 1999.

11. Levine M, Rumsey SC, Daruwala R, et al: Criteria and recommendations for vitamin C intake, *JAMA* 281(15):1415-23, 1999.

12. du Toit R, Volsteedt Y, Apostolides Z: Comparison of the antioxidant content of fruits, vegetables and teas measured as vitamin C equivalents, *Toxicology* 166(1-2):63-9, 2001.

13. Dietrich M, Block G, Hudes M, et al: Antioxidant supplementation decreases lipid peroxidation biomarker F(2)-isoprostanes in plasma of smokers, *Cancer Epidemiol Biomarkers Prev* 11(1):7-13, 2002.

14. Hirschmann JV, Raugi GJ: Adult scurvy, *J Am Acad Dermatol* 41(6):895-906, 1999.

15. Brighthope I: Nutritional medicine tables, *J Aust Coll Nutr Env Med* 17:20-5, 1998.

16. Levy R, Shriker O, Porath A, et al: Vitamin C for the treatment of recurrent furunculosis in patients with impaired neutrophil functions, *J Infect Dis* 173(6):1502-5, 1996.

17. Carlsson S, Wiklund NP, Engstrand L, et al: Effects of pH, nitrite, and ascorbic acid on nonenzymatic nitric oxide generation and bacterial growth in urine, *Nitric Oxide* 5(6):580-6, 2001.

18. Simon JA, Hudes ES: Relation of serum ascorbic acid to serum lipids and lipoproteins in US adults, *J Am Coll Nutr* 17(3):250-5, 1998.

19. Gatto LM, Hallen GK, Brown AJ, Samman S: Ascorbic acid induces a favorable lipoprotein profile in women, *J Am Coll Nutr* 15(2):154-8, 1996.

20. Jacques PF, Sulsky SI, Perrone GE, et al: Effect of vitamin C supplementation on lipoprotein cholesterol, apolipoprotein, and triglyceride concentrations, *Ann Epidemiol* 5(1):52-9, 1995.

21. Carr AC, Zhu BZ, Frei B: Potential antiatherogenic mechanisms of ascorbate (vitamin C) and alpha-tocopherol (vitamin E), *Circ Res* 87(5):349-54, 2000.

22. Valkonen MM, Kuusi T: Vitamin C prevents the acute atherogenic effects of passive smoking, *Free Radic Biol Med* 28(3):428-36, 2000.

23. Kaikkonen J, Porkkala-Sarataho E, Morrow JD, et al: Supplementation with vitamin E but not with vitamin C lowers lipid peroxidation in vivo in mildly hypercholesterolemic men, *Free Radic Res* 35(6):967-78, 2001.

24. Morton DJ, Barrett-Connor EL, Schneider DL: Vitamin C supplement use and bone mineral density in postmenopausal women, *J Bone Miner Res* 16(1):135-40, 2001.

25. Kaminski M, Boal R: An effect of ascorbic acid on delayed-onset muscle soreness, *Pain* 50(3):317-21, 1992.

26. van Poppel G, van den Berg H: Vitamins and cancer, *Cancer Letters* 114(1-2): 195-202, 1997.

27. Block G: Vitamin C and cancer prevention: the epidemiological evidence, *Am J Clin Nutr* 53(1 Suppl):270S-82S, 1991.

28. Feiz HR, Mobarhan S: Does vitamin C intake slow the progression of gastric cancer in Helicobacter pylori-infected populations? *Nutr Rev* 60(1):34-6, 2002.

29. Zhang ZW, Abdullahi M, Farthing MJ: Effect of physiological concentrations of vitamin C on gastric cancer cells and Helicobacter pylori, *Gut* 50(2):165-9, 2002.

30. Lamson DW, Brignall MS: Natural agents in the prevention of cancer, part two: preclinical data and chemoprevention for common cancers, *Altern Med Rev* 6(2):167-87, 2001.

31. Gorton HC, Jarvis K: The effectiveness of vitamin C in preventing and relieving the symptoms of virus-induced respiratory infections, *J Manipulative Physiol Ther* 22(8):530-3, 1999.

32. Diplock AT, Charleux JL, Crozier-Willi G, et al: Functional food science and defence against reactive oxidative species, *Br J Nutr* 80(Suppl 1):S77-112, 1998.

33. Pearce KA, Boosalis MG, Yeager B: Update on vitamin supplements for the prevention of coronary disease and stroke, *Am Fam Physician* 62(6):1359-66, 2000.

34. Garewal HS, Diplock AT: How safe are antioxidant vitamins? *Drug Safety* 13(1):8-14, 1995.

35. Simon JA, Hudes ES: Relation of serum ascorbic acid to serum vitamin B12, serum ferritin, and kidney stones in US adults, *Arch Intern Med* 159(6):619-24.

36. Primack A: Complementary/alternative therapies in the prevention and treatment of cancer. In Spencer JW, Jacobs JJ: Complementary/alternative medicine: an evidence-based approach, St Louis, 1999, Mosby.

37. Halliwell B: Vitamin C: antioxidant or pro-oxidant in vivo? *Free Radic Res* 25(5):439-54, 1996.

38. Podmore ID, Griffiths HR, Herbert KE, et al: Vitamin C exhibits pro-oxidant properties, *Nature* 392:559, 1998.

39. Bland JS: The pro-oxidant and antioxidant effects of vitamin C, *Altern Med Rev* 3(3):170, 1998.

40. Carr A, Frei B: Does vitamin C act as a pro-oxidant under physiological conditions? *FASEB J* 13(9):1007-24, 1999.

41. Yang M, Collis CS, Kelly M, et al: Do iron and vitamin C co-supplementation influence platelet function or LDL oxidizability in healthy volunteers? *Eur J Clin Nutr* 53(5):367-74, 1999.

42. Vojdani A, Bazargan M, Vojdani E, Wright J: New evidence for antioxidant properties of vitamin C, *Cancer Detect Prev* 24(6):508-23, 2000.

43. Levine M, Wang Y, Padayatty SJ, Morrow J: A new recommended dietary allowance of vitamin C for healthy young women, *Proc Natl Acad Sci USA* 98(17):9842-6, 2001.

■ CHAPTER 106 ■

VITAMIN D

> Calcitriol, a vitamin D analogue, reduces bone loss in postmenopausal women; natural vitamin D does not.

There are different forms of active vitamin D. Vitamin D_2 (ergocalciferol) is from plants, while vitamin D_3 (cholecalciferol) is of animal origin. Ergocalciferol is the form of vitamin D used in vitamin supplements.

Vitamin D is found naturally in fish and fish-liver oils but can also be obtained from vitamin D–fortified foods, such as milk and margarine. Cooking does not affect the vitamin D in foods. Vitamin D is synthesized in the skin on exposure to sunlight. This fat-soluble vitamin is excreted in the bile.

Vitamin D is an important hormone with diverse physiologic roles, including an effect on bone health, blood pressure regulation, and tumor suppression.[1] It is suspected to have a role in prevention of osteoporosis, hypertension, and certain cancers.

MECHANISM OF ACTION

Vitamin D is the key regulator of calcium and phosphate metabolism. The overall effect of vitamin D is to increase plasma calcium levels. Active vitamin D increases and normalizes serum calcium by increasing intestinal calcium absorption through stimulating synthesis of calcium-binding protein in intestinal epithelial cells, enhancing resorption of calcium from urine and accelerating calcium resorption from bone. Bone is the body store from which calcium is drawn to restore normal serum and interstitial fluid levels.

The liver produces 7-dehydrocholesterol, which, on exposure to sunlight, is converted to vitamin D_3 (cholecalciferol) in the skin. Previtamin D_3 then returns to liver where, along with dietary vitamin D, it is converted to 25-hydroxycholecalciferol, the storage form of the partially activated hormone. Measurement of plasma 25-hydroxycholecalciferol may be used as an indication of body vitamin D stores. Activation of 25-hydroxycholecalciferol in the kidney by 1-α-hydroxylase to 1,25 dihydroxycholecalciferol produces a fully active hormone.[2] Synthesis, largely regulated by circulating levels of 1,25 dihydroxycholecalciferol, is increased by parathyroid hormone and hypocalcemia. Parathyroid hormone speeds up conversion of

25-hydroxycholecalciferol to 1,25-dihydroxycholecalciferol. Calcitonin slows activation of vitamin D. A second metabolite—24,25 dihydroxycholecalciferol—produced in the kidney, may also contribute to the biologic activity of this vitamin.

Vitamin D increases intestinal absorption of calcium and phosphorus, initiates bone calcification, activates alkaline phosphatase, and contributes to maintaining serum calcium and phosphorus levels. Bone mineral tends to solubilize when serum calcium-phosphate concentration drops. The rate of deposition of calcium hydroxyphosphate in bone depends on both the concentration of calcium and phosphorus ions in the immediate region of bone. Calcitriol (1,25 dihdyroxy vitamin D), the active form of vitamin D, promotes bone resorption by the following[3]:

- Promoting differentiation of monocytes into macrophages that fuse to form multinuclear giant cells. These multinuclear giant cells stimulate osteoclastic bone resorption.
- Acting on T lymphocytes, producing various lymphokines including osteoclast-activating factor, a potent bone resorbing agent.
- Inhibiting collage synthesis by osteoblasts.
- Cultured chondrocytes converting vitamin D to its active form (24,25-$[OH]_2$-D).

Vitamin D appears to be important in regulation of cellular growth and differentiation. It has a role in the differentiation of keratocytes and monocytes into macrophages. Cells expressing vitamin D receptors have also been found in human tumor lines, including breast, prostate, and colon.[4] Calcitriol up-regulates androgen receptors in human prostate cancer cells. A number of vitamin D analogs exhibit potent antiproliferative activity on prostate cancer cells.[5]

Recent developments have identified a gene that determines vitamin D receptors on cells. It is anticipated that in the future, a blood test will become available to detect this marker; early recognition of persons at genetic risk may facilitate prevention of osteoporosis in the elderly.

FOOD SOURCES

An important source of vitamin D is cutaneous synthesis on sun exposure. Ten minutes of sun exposure produces roughly the RDA for vitamin D or the amount derived from eating 70 g of sardines or 22 g of herring. The benefits of sun exposure are neutralized by sunscreen. Sunscreen SP 8+ thickly applied every few hours prevents cutaneous production of cholecalciferol. To protect against skin cancer, it is desirable to select a sunscreen SP 15+. Fortunately, dietary sources of vitamin D can obviate the need for skin synthesis of this vitamin.

Cod liver oil and fatty fish (e.g. herring, kipper, mackerel, and salmon) are all good dietary sources of vitamin D.

DOSE

Most humans can meet their daily requirement by being exposed to sunlight for 5 to 10 minutes a day on 4 or 5 days of the week. The RDA of vitamin D_3 is around 200 to 400 IU or 5 to 10 µg. Recent recommendations urge higher doses for the entire population to prevent osteoporotic fractures.[1] Certainly, a randomized study of postmenopausal Dutch women concluded supplementation with more than 400 IU vitamin D_3 daily is indicated to prevent a winter decline in 25(OH)D and to control serum parathyroid hormone levels.[6] Current opinion is that to ensure adequate calcium absorption, a daily intake of 400 to 600 IU of vitamin D is recommended, either through sun exposure, diet, or supplementation.[7] The therapeutic dose range is 400 to 1000 IU/day.[8]

Conversions are 1 µg 25-hydroxyvitamin D = 80 IU, while 1 µg 1,25-dihydroxyvitamin D = 200 IU.

CLINICAL USES

Appropriate doses of daily vitamin D supplementation vary with the underlying problem. Correction of vitamin D deficiency in hypertensive patients requires 1000 to 2000 IU, osteomalacia is treated with 5000 IU vitamin D_2, hypoparathyroidism requires 25,000 to 200,000 IU of ergocalciferol, and postmenopausal osteoporosis requires 1000 to 10,000 IU. Calcitriol, the active form of vitamin D_3, is routinely used in postmenopausal osteoporosis. It increases calcium absorption and may have a weak action on bone. However, reviews of randomized or quasi-randomized trials using vitamin D or a vitamin D analogue, either alone or in combination with calcium supplementation, concluded that uncertainty remains about the efficacy of regimens that include vitamin D or its analogues in fracture prevention in involutional and postmenopausal osteoporosis.[9] What is clear is that vitamin D_3 without calcium cosupplementation is not associated with any reduction in the incidence of hip or other nonvertebral fractures.

Simultaneously, calcium supplementation is obligatory. Administration of vitamin D_3 plus calcium to frail, elderly people is associated with a reduction in hip fractures; calcitriol is effective in reducing the incidence of vertebral deformity. Similarly, a randomized trial found 400 IU vitamin D_3 per day improved bone mineral density of the femoral neck in postmenopausal women who also consumed around 1000 mg/day of dietary calcium.[10] A randomized, prospective 2-year clinical trial concluded a combination of 1-α-hydroxyvitamin D_3 with hormone replacement therapy was superior to hormone replacement alone for the preservation of bone mineral density in postmenopausal women taking calcium supplementation.[11]

The efficacy of calcitriol remains unproven as a single agent for the treatment of osteoporosis in men. After 2 years, a randomized, double-masked, double placebo-controlled trial of calcitriol (0.25 µg twice daily) or calcium (500 mg twice daily) found the number of men with vertebral fractures was similar in both groups.[12]

The benefit of vitamin D and calcium supplementation is not limited to bone. Oral bone and tooth loss correlate with bone loss at nonoral sites. A 3-year, randomized, placebo-controlled trial found vitamin D supplementation and calcium, 1000 mg/day or more, aimed at preventing osteoporosis had a beneficial effect on tooth retention.[13]

Epidemiologic studies suggest suboptimal vitamin D levels increase the risk of common tumors. In fact, epidemiologic studies suggest an association between colon, breast, and prostate cancer and low vitamin D intake and/or serum levels. Whether this association results from a cause-effect relationship or merely reflects a correlation remains disputed; whether vitamin D supplementation will be preventive remains a conundrum.

Nonetheless, vitamin D has been shown to reduce the proliferation of many tumor cell lines in vitro, including breast, prostate, and colon. It has been shown to cause G1 cell cycle arrest in prostate cancer cells, prolong survival time in breast cancer models, and inhibit the development of colon tumors in animals. Animal studies have found that vitamin D reduces tumor secretion of type IV collagenases and, consequently, the number of metastases. It may also partially inhibit angiogenesis. Synthetic vitamin D analogues have been shown to inhibit metastasis. Six out of seven men with recurrent prostate cancer treated with between 0.5 and 2.5 µg of oral calcitriol at bedtime had significant slowing of the rate of increase of prostate specific antigen (PSA) compared to pretreatment levels.[14] Hypercalcemia was a dose-limiting side effect.

In another preliminary study, 44% of patients with hormone-refractory advanced prostate cancer and bone metastases were found to have low serum concentrations of vitamin D.[15] In this trial, supplementation with 2000 IU vitamin D_2 was associated with reduced bone pain and an improved quality of life from baseline. Another pilot study suggested that 20 or 40 µg daily of 25-hydroxyvitamin D_3 orally for 6 weeks reduced the presence of immune suppressive CD34(+) cells and improved the immune competence of patients with head and neck squamous cell carcinoma.[16] The CD34(+) cells suppress autologous T-cell functions. 1-α,25-dihydroxyvitamin D_3 drives the differentiation of CD34(+). Inadequate vitamin D_3 and calcium intake may play a contributory role in the pathogenesis and progression of hypertension. A study using dual-energy x-ray absorptiometry suggested that high blood pressure might be associated with reduced bone mineral density in females with hypertension.[17] However, given the inverse association between calcium intake from dairy products and blood pressure, vitamin D intake per se may have no significant effect on blood pressure.[18] Nonetheless, short-term supplementation with 1200 mg calcium plus 800 IU vitamin D_3 was more effective in reducing systolic blood pressure in elderly women than calcium alone.[19]

TOXICITY/DRUG INTERACTIONS

Although supplementation with vitamin D is likely to be safe up to levels approaching 10,000 IU/day,[20] a prolonged daily intake of 5000 to 10,000 IU is potentially toxic. In view of the overlap between the therapeutic and toxic dose range, it is probably wise to limit long-term supplementation to 500 to 2000 IU daily. Problems are more likely to occur in adults taking 20,000 to 80,000 IU/day or more for several weeks or months. Early symptoms of overdose are bone pain, constipation in younger people and diarrhea in adults, drowsiness, a dry mouth, anorexia, a persistent headache, polyuria, polydipsia, muscle pain, and unusual tiredness. Weakness, irritability, anorexia, and gastrointestinal and urinary symptoms are all attributable to hypercalcemia induced by excess vitamin D. Late evidence of overdose are metastatic calcification, cloudy urine, pruritus, drowsiness, increased light sensitivity, and weight loss. Late symptoms of severe overdose are hypertension, arrhythmia, fever, and abdominal pain.

Vitamin D enhances the risk of side effects in persons taking thiazide diuretics, calcium, or magnesium supplements. Hypercalcemia associated with vitamin D supplementation may potentiate arrhythmia in persons on digoxin. Vitamin D supplementation may be necessary in patients on long-term anticonvulsant therapy. Cholestyramine and mineral oil reduce intestinal absorption.

CLINICAL CAUTION

Progressive loss of bone density and persistent bone pain in adults are suggestive of osteomalacia, a deficiency of vitamin D. Bone alkaline phosphatase is raised with low or normal serum calcium and phosphate and high or normal parathyroid hormone levels. Skeletal deformity may result from increased osteoid formation with inadequate bone mineralization and pseudofractures. Generalized musculoskeletal symptoms are encountered.

In children, vitamin D deficiency presents as rickets with epiphyseal enlargement and skeletal deformity caused by inadequate skeletal calcification causing weak bones (e.g., bowed legs), rheumatic pains, and exhaustion.

PRACTICE TIPS

- Use of sunscreen and the change in the zenith angle of the sun can dramatically reduce the cutaneous production of vitamin D_3.
- To achieve equivalent vitamin D synthesis on sun exposure, dark-skinned persons need to be exposed around six times longer than fair-skinned individuals.

- Vegetarians need to ensure adequate sun exposure and consumption of fortified foods (e.g., margarine) to achieve an adequate level of vitamin D.
- Excess intake of vitamin D should be avoided since this can result in soft tissue (e.g., the kidney or blood vessels) calcification.
- One must take care when prescribing calcium and/or magnesium in patients taking vitamin D supplements.

REFERENCES

1. Fuller KE, Casparian JM: Vitamin D: balancing cutaneous and systemic considerations, *South Med J* 94(1):58-64, 2001.
2. Wikvall K: Cytochrome P450 enzymes in the bioactivation of vitamin D to its hormonal form (Review), *Int J Mol Med* 7(2):201-9, 2001.
3. Gaby AR: Natural treatments for osteoarthritis, *Alt Med Rev* 4(5):330-41, 1999.
4. Lamson DW, Brignall MS: Natural agents in the prevention of cancer, part two: preclinical data and chemoprevention for common cancers, *Alt Med Rev* 6(2):167-87, 2001.
5. Zhao XY, Feldman D: The role of vitamin D in prostate cancer, *Steroids* 66(3-5):293-300, 2001.
6. Schaafsma A, Muskiet FA, Storm H, et al: Vitamin D(3) and vitamin K(1) supplementation of Dutch postmenopausal women with normal and low bone mineral densities: effects on serum 25-hydroxyvitamin D and carboxylated osteocalcin, *Eur J Clin Nutr* 54(8):626-31, 2000.
7. The role of calcium in peri- and postmenopausal women: consensus opinion of The North American Menopause Society, Menopause 8(2):84-95, 2001.
8. Brighthope I: Nutritional medicine tables, *J Aust Coll Nutr Env Med* 17:20-5, 1998.
9. Gillespie WJ, Avenell A, Henry DA, et al: Vitamin D and vitamin D analogues for preventing fractures associated with involutional and post-menopausal osteoporosis (Cochrane Review), *Cochrane Database Syst Rev* 1:CD000227, 2001.
10. Ooms ME, Roos JC, Bezemer PD, et al: Prevention of bone loss by vitamin D supplementation in elderly women: a randomized double-blind trial, *J Clin Endocrinol Metab* 80(4):1052-8, 1995.
11. Chen M, Chow SN: Additive effect of alfacalcidol on bone mineral density of the lumbar spine in Taiwanese postmenopausal women treated with hormone replacement therapy and calcium supplementation: a randomized 2-year study, *Clin Endocrinol (Oxf)* 55(2):253-8, 2001.
12. Ebeling PR, Wark JD, Yeung S, et al: Effects of calcitriol or calcium on bone mineral density, bone turnover, and fractures in men with primary osteoporosis: a two-year randomized, double blind, double placebo study, *J Clin Endocrinol Metab* 86(9):4098-103, 2001.
13. Krall EA, Wehler C, Garcia RI, et al: Calcium and vitamin D supplements reduce tooth loss in the elderly, *Am J Med* 111(6):452-6, 2001.
14. Gross C, Stamey T, Hancock S, Feldman D: Treatment of early recurrent prostate cancer with 1, 25-dihydroxyvitamin D_3 (calcitriol), *J Urol* 159(6):2035-9, 1998.

15. Van Veldhuizen PJ, Taylor SA, Williamson S, Drees BM: Treatment of vitamin D deficiency in patients with metastatic prostate cancer may improve bone pain and muscle strength, *J Urol* 163(1):187-90, 2000.

16. Lathers DM, Clark JI, Achille NJ, Young MR: Phase IB study of 25-hydroxyvitamin D(3) treatment to diminish suppressor cells in head and neck cancer patients, *Hum Immunol* 62(11):1282-93, 2001.

17. Tsuda K, Nishio I, Masuyama Y: Bone mineral density in women with essential hypertension, *Am J Hypertens* 14(7 Pt 1):704-7, 2001.

18. Jorde R, Bonaa KH: Calcium from dairy products, vitamin D intake, and blood pressure: the Tromso Study, *Am J Clin Nutr* 71(6):1530-5, 2000.

19. Pfeifer M, Begerow B, Minne HW, et al: Effects of a short-term vitamin D(3) and calcium supplementation on blood pressure and parathyroid hormone levels in elderly women, *J Clin Endocrinol Metab* 86(4):1633-7, 2001.

20. Vieth R: Vitamin D supplementation, 25-hydroxyvitamin D concentrations, and safety, *Am J Clin Nutr* 69(5):842-56, 1999.

■ CHAPTER 107 ■

VITAMIN E

Although epidemiologic evidence suggests taking at least 100 IU of vitamin E supplementation for 2 years or more lowers the risk of coronary artery disease (CAD), no association between CAD and vitamin E intake from food has been identified.

Economists estimate a savings of $5 to $6 billion annually could be achieved if all adults over the age of 50 years took at least 100 IU vitamin E daily.[1] Vitamin E is a lipid-soluble micronutrient containing eight active, naturally occurring plant constituents—tocopherols and tocotrienols. Different forms of vitamin E have overlapping and discrete biologic activities. Dietary tocotrienols are less important physiologically than the tocopherols. Although the antioxidant activity of tocotrienols is higher than that of tocopherols, tocotrienols have a lower bioavailability after oral ingestion. α-Tocopherol is more biologically active than its β-, γ-, and δ-tocopherol isomers. Various studies suggest that, after normal gastrointestinal absorption of dietary vitamin E, specific mechanisms favor the preferential accumulation of α-tocopherol in the human body. Vitamin E is found in a variety of foods, including seeds and grains.

Vitamin E functions as an antioxidant, enhances vitamin A utilization, and, at high doses, inhibits platelet aggregation. Some studies suggest vitamin E may have, among others, a protective effect against cardiovascular disease, certain cancers, diabetes, and cataracts. Total serum cholesterol and triglycerides are highly correlated with serum α- and γ-tocopherol concentrations.[2]

MECHANISM OF ACTION

Vitamin E has important antioxidant and cell signaling functions. Tocopherols and tocotrienols are part of an interlinking set of antioxidant cycles forming an antioxidant network. Vitamin E protects against lipid peroxidation by acting directly on a number of oxygen radicals including singlet oxygen, lipid peroxide products, and the superoxide radical to form the relatively harmless tocopherol radical.[3] However, α-tocopherol can act as either an antioxidant to inhibit or as a pro-oxidant to facilitate lipid peroxidation of LDL. It has been suggested that vitamin E may only be effective in combination with vitamin C as the pro-oxidant activity of α-tocopherol is prevented by ascorbate acting as a co-antioxidant.[4] Vitamin E can also work in conjunction with selenium, a co-factor for glutathione peroxidase, and various enzymes such as superoxide dismutase and catalase.

α-Tocopherol increasingly appears to play a critical role in influencing the key steps in the atherosclerotic process through its ability to modulate platelet aggregation, inhibit vascular endothelial dysfunction, and inhibit the activity of protein kinase C, a key player in many signal transduction pathways.[5] Vitamin E potentially retards atherosclerosis through its antioxidant effect on LDL, its protection of nitric oxide and endothelial cell dependent vasoactivity, its inhibition of smooth muscle cell proliferation, its inhibition of adhesion to vascular endothelium of monocytes, platelets, and other cells, and its alterations to eicosanoid production by neutrophils and monocytes.[6] It may protect against the progression of atherosclerosis through its anti-inflammatory effect. In doses of 1200 IU daily, vitamin E decreases release of reactive oxygen species and reduces lipid oxidation, it reduces cytokines such as interleukin-1ss (IL-1ss) and tumor necrosis factor-alpha (TNF-α), and decreases adhesion of monocytes to human endothelium.[7] Vitamin E, by inhibiting the activation of protein kinase C and nuclear factor-kappa B (NF-kappa B), prevents leukocyte-endothelial cell adhesion by inhibiting signal transduction involved in the surface expression of adhesion molecules of leukocytes and endothelial cells.[8] Endothelial-dependent vasodilation has also been shown to improve with vitamin E supplementation.[9]

The form of vitamin E influences its biologic function with α-tocopherol being the more important chain breaking antioxidant for inhibiting lipid peroxidation while γ-tocopherol is a more effective trap for lipophilic electrophiles such as reactive nitrogen oxide species.[10] Both α- and γ-tocopherol inhibit protein kinase C activity and therefore can hinder smooth muscle cell proliferation, but only γ-tocopherol and its water-soluble metabolite inhibits cyclo-oxygenase-2(COX-2) activity in intact cells and blocks prostaglandin E2 synthesis in lipopolysaccharide stimulated macrophages and interleukin 1β activated epithelial cells. The γ-tocopherol form of vitamin E is a more effective anti-inflammatory and a better quencher of reactive nitrogen oxide species generated in chronic inflammation. γ-Tocopherol has properties not shared by α-tocopherol.

Tocotrienols have beneficial effects in cardiovascular diseases both by inhibiting LDL oxidation and by down-regulating 3-hydroxyl-3-methylglutaryl-coenzyme A (HMG CoA) reductase, a key enzyme of the mevalonate pathway.[11] Tocotrienols penetrate rapidly through skin and efficiently combat oxidative stress induced by UV or ozone. Important novel anti-proliferative and neuroprotective effects of tocotrienols, which may be independent of their antioxidant activity, have also been described.[11]

FOOD SOURCES

Wheat germ oil, vegetable oils or their seeds (e.g. sunflower, avocados, sweet potato), and nuts (e.g. hazelnuts, almonds, peanuts) are particularly rich sources of vitamin E. Substantial quantities of vitamin E may be lost during storage, processing, and cooking. A control study on healthy volunteers confirmed that the plasma concentration of vitamin E and plasma antioxidant activity in response to oral supplementation of vitamin E are markedly affected by food intake.[12] However, dietary vitamin E appears to be a poor predictor of plasma levels of vitamin E.[13] Furthermore, while increasing dietary vitamin E intake can increase plasma α-tocopherol levels, the extent of dietary modification required to achieve potentially cardioprotective levels of plasma α-tocopherol is difficult in practice.[14] Supplementation may be necessary. As vitamin E is lipophilic, and its absorption is expected to be increased by food, vitamin E should be taken with meals. The most prevalent form of vitamin E in plant seeds and their products is γ-tocopherol, yet α-tocopherol is the form usually supplied in supplements. Furthermore, although α-tocopherol is preferentially accumulated, γ-tocopherol has properties not shared by α-tocopherol.

DOSE

The RDA for vitamin E is expressed in either mg or units. Although the system of International Units for vitamin E has been officially discontinued for several decades, in practice, both systems continue to be used and dietary supplements tend to favor use of the discontinued system. As shown in Table 107-1, the advantage of the unit system is that the dose can be readily modified to whichever particular tocopherol supplement the clinician is using.[15]

Depending on the source, the RDI of vitamin E varies from 12-30 IU each day. The Food and Nutrition Board of the Institute of Medicine recently published a new daily dietary reference intake of 15 mg (35 mol) vitamin E for adults. This increased RDA has been variously supported and criticized.[16,17] In any event, the tolerable upper intake level of vitamin E supplementation is reported to be 1000 mg (1100 IU) daily.

Although careful dietary selection exceeds the RDA and may achieve intake levels of 60 IU of vitamin E, it fails to reach the minimal therapeutic dose of 100 IU per day,[18] the 200 IU a day that may be optimal for the immune status of the elderly, or the 400-800 IU needed each day to reduce the risk of cardiovascular disease.[19] It has even been suggested that certain

TABLE 107-1 ■ Vitamin E Activity

PREPARATION	SOURCE	ACTIVITY	UNITS
1 mg d-alpha tocopherol	Natural	100%	0.67
1 mg d-alpha tocopherol acetate	Natural	91%	0.73
1 mg d-alpha tocopherol succinate	Natural	81%	0.83
1 mg dl-alpha tocopherol	Synthetic	74%	0.9
1 mg dl-alpha tocopherol acetate	Synthetic	67%	1.0
1 mg dl-alpha tocopherol succinate	Synthetic	60%	1.12

groups, in addition to a including 5-8 servings of fruit and vegetables in their daily diet, should take a daily supplement of 200 IU vitamin E.[19] Certainly, vitamin E intake from supplements, along with body mass index, are the major independent predictors of serum tocopherol levels in women; dietary factors only play a small role.[2] Vitamin E supplementation is not free of pitfalls. Synthetic vitamin E is a mixture of isomers. It contains 8 isomers, only one of which has the RRR configuration of natural vitamin E. Although the relative potency in humans is unproven, in animals the potency of natural versus synthetic vitamin E is 1.36.[20] Compared to the natural stereoisomer, RRR-alpha-tocopheryl acetate, synthetic vitamin E is an equimolar mixture of eight stereoisomers.[21]

The different tocol and tocotrienol derivatives α, β, δ, and γ have varied and specific roles with diverse tissue affinities.[22] For example, studies suggest that despite α-tocopherol's action as an antioxidant, γ-tocopherol is required to effectively remove the peroxynitrite-derived nitrating species.[23] As large doses of dietary α-tocopherol displace γ-tocopherol in plasma and other tissues and may block this action, the current wisdom of vitamin E supplementation with primarily α-tocopherol may require review. Furthermore, variations in the biologic activity of various homologous probably reflect the ease with which each attaches to the lipid membrane. The biologic activity of d-α-tocopherol is 1.49 IU/mg; in contrast, d-γ-tocopherol has a lower biologic activity of 0.15 IU/mg. Clearly, the potency of vitamin E depends on its form.

α-Tocopherol is used as the standard for calculating the vitamin E content of food. One mg of natural vitamin E, the RRR-α-tocopherol form, provides 1.49 IU of δ-α-tocopherol, while 1 mg of synthetic vitamin E, the all-rac-α-tocopherol form, provides 1.10 IU of dl-alpha-tocopherol. Natural vitamin E is more potent with 1000 mg of natural vitamin E providing 1500 IU, but 1000 mg of synthetic vitamin E only providing 1100 IU. The therapeutic dose range varies from 100 to 2000 IU per day.[24]

Increased dietary consumption of unsaturated fat may require an increased intake of vitamin E, a major fat-soluble antioxidant. An increased vitamin E intake of 0.4 mg for each gram of linoleic acid and of 3-4 mg for each gram of eicosapentaenoic and docosahexaenolic acids may be prudent. It is generally accepted that the requirement for vitamin E increases as the concentration of polyunsaturated fatty acids in the diet increases. However, a cross over trial found that 400 mg α-tocopheryl acetate failed to alter the small, but statistically significant, increase in oxidative stress reflected in plasma TBARS concentration after consuming fish oil with 2.5 g EPA and 1.8 g DHA daily.[10] Nonetheless, for persons on a diet rich in polyunsaturated fat, it may be premature to cease vitamin E supplementation. A useful formula is to take 0.25 (5PUFA kcal + g PUFAs) IU vitamin E. Otherwise, supplement 0.4 mg of vitamin E for each gram of linoleic acid and 3-4 mg for each gram of EPA or DHA. Infants receiving a formula high in polyunsaturated fatty acids should be supplemented with 15 -25 IU vitamin E daily or be given 7 IU vitamin E per 32 ounces of formula.

Store vitamin E supplements away from heat, direct light, and damp areas.

CLINICAL USES

For optimal health, a daily intake around 25-67 mg or 0.06-0.16 mmol vitamin E is suggested.[25] To avoid oxidative stress, vitamin C should also be increased so that a ratio of at least 1.3 to 1.5 is maintained. In addition to epidemiologic studies that suggest a benefit for high intakes of α-tocopherol, studies of supplementation in humans have clearly shown that α-tocopherol decreases lipid peroxidation, platelet aggregation, and functions as a potent anti-inflammatory agent.[26] Vitamin E supplementation improves the immune system and offers some protection against cardiovascular disease and certain cancers.[6] In all cases, doses are quoted in the units of the reference source. Various studies suggest clinical uses of vitamin E in daily doses of the following[27]:

- 50-1500 mg to prevent cardiovascular disease.
- 400 IU to reduce the risk of cataracts.
- 20 mg for cancer prevention, increased to 50 mg daily to reduce the risk of prostate cancer in smokers. Data from a study on volunteers suggested that smoking increased the disappearance of vitamin E from the plasma.[28]
- 800 IU in two doses of 400 IU to reverse leukoplakia or dysplasia.
- 1600 IU for 8-12 weeks to alleviate symptoms of tardive dyskinesia. Antipsychotic (neuroleptic) medication, used to treat people with chronic mental illnesses, is associated with a wide range of adverse effects, including movement disorders such as tardive dyskinesia. Small trials of uncertain quality indicate that vitamin E protects against deterioration of tardive dyskinesia, but there is no evidence that vitamin E improves symptoms.[29]
- 900 mg to reduce oxidative stress.
- 900 mg to enhance insulin action in type 1 diabetes.
- 60 mg in two doses of 30 mg daily to improve immune function. Immune function in the elderly improves on 800 IU/day.[30]

A literature search conducted from 1966 through March 1999 identified several epidemiologic studies that have demonstrated positive relationships between vitamin E intake and the prevention of atherosclerotic heart disease.[31] Positive outcomes included a 77% reduction in nonfatal myocardial infarction, but no corresponding reduction in mortality. Two prospective cohort studies suggested persons taking 100-250 IU of vitamin E a day were least likely to have a major coronary event and patients with atherosclerosis on 400-800 IU of vitamin E daily were least likely to have a clinical cardiac event.[32] Results from such studies, however, are inconsistent. In fact, although basic science and animal studies have generally supported the hypothesis that vitamin E may slow the progression of atherosclerosis and observational studies, primarily assessing patients without established coronary heart disease, have largely supported a protective role of vitamin E, early primary and secondary prevention clinical trials have essentially failed to show a significant benefit from vitamin E.[33] For example, a study using carotid ultrasound to evaluate atheroscleotic changes that demonstrated benefit from angiotensin-converting enzyme (ACE) inhibitor, ramipril, failed to show any change with 400 IU of natural vitamin E.[34] One explanation for such failure may relate to the dose and isomers used. Vitamin E in doses under 50 IU/day are clinically ineffective, doses over 100 IU/day may prevent or slow progression of coronary disease, while doses of over 1300 IU daily may be needed to reduce the chance of restenosis.[31]

The dose of vitamin E does indeed appear critical to its physiologic impact. While doses of 400 IU α-tocopherol daily have a significant protective effect on LDL oxidation,[35] at doses of 1200 IU/day, LDL oxidation is significantly greater than with 400 IU/day.[36] In vitro studies suggest that normal plasma levels of vitamin E enhance lipoxygenation of arachidonic acid and higher concentrations have a suppressive effect.[17] Daily doses of vitamin E in excess of 800 IU may adversely affect platelet function and 1200 IU per day may interfere with the function of vitamin K and granulocyte responses.[37] Daily doses of vitamin E up to 800 IU may enhance, while doses in excess of 800 IU may suppress immunity. Although there currently may be insufficient evidence to recommend routine use of vitamin E for the prevention of coronary artery disease or stroke, some consider daily doses of 100-800 IU vitamin E useful for secondary prevention.[37]

In addition to potentially benefiting persons with cardio- and cerebrovascular disease, vitamin E may assist those with peripheral vascular disease. Vitamin E is helpful for secondary prevention of intermittent claudication, providing most benefit to those with the poorest collateral circulation and pedal blood flow.[6] It may be necessary to continue therapy for 12-18 months before benefits are noted. Doses vary for 400-1200 mg/day. However, it should be noted that a review of clinical trials using vitamin E concluded there was insufficient evidence to determine whether vitamin E is an effective treatment for intermittent claudication.[38]

Life-long supplementation of patients with type 1 diabetes may deserve consideration. A double-blind study found an intake of 250 IU (168 mg) of RRR-α-tocopherol tds reduced lipoprotein peroxidation in patients with type 1 diabetes.[39] Increased vitamin E intake has also been associated with enhanced glucose tolerance and insulin action.[40] Type 2 diabetes is associated with increased free radical production, lipid peroxidation, and reduced plasma vitamin E levels. Variations of insulin sensitivity are related to the long-chain polyunsaturated fatty acid content of the phospholipid membrane of skeletal muscle. Pharmacologic doses of vitamin E and C increase insulin-stimulated cellular uptake of glucose.

Other potential uses for vitamin E involve inclusion as part of a larger nutritional protocol to prevent cancer. Vitamin E inclusive protocols significantly reduce the incidence of prostate, bladder, and stomach cancers, and prevent recurrences of colonic adenomas.[41] Mechanisms whereby vitamin E may impair carcinogenesis range from stimulation of wild-type p53 tumor suppressor gene, through down-regulation of mutant p53, activation of heat shock proteins, and an anti-angiogenic effect mediated by blockage of transforming growth factor-alpha (TGF-α).[42]

TOXICITY/DRUG INTERACTIONS

The cost and safety profile of vitamin E favors empiric use in recommended doses.[17] Within a therapeutic range of 200-1600 α-tocopherol equivalents, animal experiments have shown that vitamin E is not mutagenic, teratogenic or carcinogenic. Vitamin E, regarded as safe at levels up to 800 IU/day, is probably safe at 1600 IU/day. Although side effects may be expected to begin at doses of around 1500 IU/day,[6] even doses of 3200 mg/day have been shown to be without any consistent risk.[43] Nonetheless, some persons consuming vitamin E in doses greater than 400 IU daily over prolonged periods may experience blurred vision, diarrhea, dizziness, headache, nausea or stomach cramps, unusual tiredness, or weakness.

Vitamin E decreases platelet adhesion and, at levels above 400 IU daily, may increase clotting times.[44] Oral intake of high levels of vitamin E can exacerbate the blood coagulation defect of vitamin K deficiency caused by malabsorption or anticoagulant therapy.[45] Provided the prothrombin time or international normalized ratio is tested on starting a new drug and repeated within 7 to 14 days of taking vitamin E, it is safe to use in combination with anticoagulants. Vitamin E, by antagonizing vitamin K and inhibiting prothrombin production, may increase risk of hemorrhagic strokes.[46]

Vitamin E has a number of nutrient-nutreint and nutrient-drug interactions. Vitamin E supplementation may impair the hematologic response to iron and should be avoided in iron deficiency anemia. Large doses of iron or copper may increase the requirement for vitamin E, while zinc deficiency reduces vitamin E plasma levels. The tocopherol radical can interact with vitamin C to restore tocopherol. Vitamin C has a sparing effect on vitamin E, and moderate doses of vitamin E have a sparing effect on vitamin A. On the other hand, large doses of vitamin E may deplete vitamin A and increase the requirement for vitamin K.

Vitamin E may enhance the anti-inflammatory effect of aspirin and decrease the dose of anticoagulant, insulin, and digoxin required. Plasma levels of vitamin E may be reduced by anti-convulsants, oral contraceptives, sucralfate, colestyramine, and/or liquid paraffin.[15]

CLINICAL CAUTION

An intake of 4 mg daily may result in a critically low plasma vitamin E level of 20-25 umol/L; 30 umol/L is desirable. In reality, clinical deficiency is rare, except in persons with fat malabsorption. Symptoms suggestive of vitamin E deficiency include arreflexia, psychologic syndromes, cognitive dysfunction, nystagmus, ataxia, muscle weakness, and sensory loss in the arms or legs.[47] Menopausal symptoms, fatigue, restlessness, and insomnia may also result from deficiency.

PRACTICE TIPS

- To prevent deficiency, consider supplements of 10 mg (16.7 IU) and 8 mg (13 IU) alpha-TE (alpha tocopherol equivalents) for adult males and females, respectively.
- Most studies suggest therapeutic effects of vitamin E are more likely when intake exceeds 100 IU per day, possibility 200-400 IU per day.
- Combined daily supplementation of vitamin E (200 mg) with vitamin C (1000 mg) enhances immunity more than either vitamin alone.
- The γ-tocopherol form of vitamin E is indicated to reduce chronic inflammation, including atherosclerosis.[48]
- Supplementation with α-tocopherol decreases tissue levels of γ-tocopherol while supplementation with γ-tocopherol increases tissue levels of both α- and γ-tocopherol.
- At levels of 300-1000 IU, vitamin E appears free of side effects.
- Different antioxidants appear to act synergistically, so supplementation with vitamin E might be more effective if combined with other micronutrients.
- Supplementing selenium may minimize the effect of deficiency of vitamin E.
- Muscle cramping may be eased by vitamin E (500 IU daily).
- Dysmenorrhea may respond to 250 IU alpha-tocopherol bd starting 10 days pre-menstrually and continuing for 14 days.

REFERENCES

1. Bendich A, Mallick R, Leader S: Potential health economic benefits of vitamin supplementation, *West J Med* 166(5):306-12, 1997.
2. White E, Kristal AR, Shikany JM, et al: Correlates of serum alpha- and gamma-tocopherol in the Women's Health Initiative, *Ann Epidemiol* 11(2):136-44, 2001.
3. Clarkson PM, Thompson HS: Antioxidants: what role do they play in physical activity and health? *Am J Clin Nutr* 72(2 Suppl):637S-46S, 2000.
4. Carr AC, Zhu BZ, Frei B: Potential antiatherogenic mechanisms of ascorbate (vitamin C) and alpha-tocopherol (vitamin E), *Circ Res* 87(5):349-54, 2000.
5. Traber MG: Does vitamin E decrease heart attack risk? summary and implications with respect to dietary recommendations, *J Nutr* 131(2):395S-7S, 2001.
6. Pryor WA: Vitamin E and heart disease: basic science to clinical intervention trials, *Free Radic Biol Med* 28(1):141-64, 2000.
7. Jialal I, Devaraj S, Kaul N: The effect of alpha-tocopherol on monocyte proatherogenic activity, *J Nutr* 131(2):389S-94S, 2001.

8. Yoshikawa T, Yoshida N: Vitamin E and leukocyte-endothelial cell interactions, *Antioxid Redox Signal* 2(4):821-5, 2000.

9. Brown AA, Hu FB: Dietary modulation of endothelial function: implications for cardiovascular disease, *Am J Clin Nutr* 73(4):673-86, 2001.

10. Wander RC, Du SH: Oxidation of plasma proteins is not increased after supplementation with eicosapentaenoic and docosahexaenoic acids, *Am J Clin Nutr* 72(3):731-7, 2000.

11. Packer L, Weber SU, Rimbach G: Molecular aspects of alpha-tocotrienol antioxidant action and cell signaling, *J Nutr* 131(2):369S-73S, 2001.

12. Iuliano L, Micheletta F, Maranghi M, et al: Bioavailability of vitamin E as function of food intake in healthy subjects: effects on plasma peroxide-scavenging activity and cholesterol-oxidation products, *Arterioscler Thromb Vasc Biol* 21(10):E34-7, 2001.

13. Mahabir S, Coit D, Liebes L, et al: Randomized, placebo-controlled trial of dietary supplementation of alpha-tocopherol on mutagen sensitivity levels in melanoma patients: a pilot trial, *Melanoma Res* 12(1):83-90, 2002.

14. McGavin JK, Mann JI, Skeaff CM, Chisholm A: Comparison of a vitamin E-rich diet and supplemental vitamin E on measures of vitamin E status and lipoprotein profile, *Eur J Clin Nutr* 55(7):555-61, 2001.

15. Mason P: *Dietary supplements*, Bath, UK, 2001, Pharmaceutical Press.

16. Horwitt MK: Critique of the requirement for vitamin E, *Am J Clin Nutr* 73(6):1003-5, 2001.

17. Traber MG: Vitamin E: too much or not enough? *Am J Clin Nutr* 73(6):997-8, 2001.

18. Pearce KA, Boosalis MG, Yeager B: Update on vitamin supplements for the prevention of coronary disease and stroke, *Am Fam Physician* 62(6):1359-66, 2000.

19. Meydani M: Effect of functional food ingredients: vitamin E modulation of cardiovascular diseases and immune status in the elderly, *Am J Clin Nutr* 71(6 Suppl):1665S-8S, 2000.

20. Kayden HJ, Wisniewski T: On the biological activity of vitamin E, *Am J Clin Nutr* 72(1):201-3, 2000.

21. Traber MG: Utilization of vitamin E, *Biofactors* 10(2-3):115-20, 1999.

22. Wheatley C: Vitamin trials and cancer: what went wrong? *J Nutr Env Med* 8:277-88, 1998.

23. Christen S, Woodall AA, Shigenaga MK, et al: Gamma-tocopherol traps mutagenic electrophiles such as NO(X) and complements alpha-tocopherol: physiological implications, *Proc Natl Acad Sci U S A* 94(7):3217-22, 1997.

24. Brighthope I: Nutritional medicine tables, *J Aust Coll Nutr Env Med* 17:20-5, 1998.

25. Gey KF: Vitamins E plus C and interacting conutrients required for optimal health. A critical and constructive review of epidemiology and supplementation data regarding cardiovascular disease and cancer, *Biofactors* 7(1-2):113-74, 1998.

26. Jialal I, Traber M, Devaraj S: Is there a vitamin E paradox? *Curr Opin Lipidol* 12(1):49-53, 2001.

27. Brighthope I: Nutritional medicine—Its presence and power, *J Aust Coll Nutr Env Med* 17:5-18, 1998.

28. Traber MG, Winklhofer-Roob BM, Roob JM, et al: Vitamin E kinetics in smokers and nonsmokers, *Free Radic Biol Med* 31(11):1368-74, 2001.

29. Soares KV, McGrath JJ: Vitamin E for neuroleptic-induced tardive dyskinesia (Cochrane Review), *Cochrane Database Syst Rev* 4:CD000209, 2001.
30. Meydani M, Meisler J: A closer look at vitamin E: can this antioxidant prevent chronic disease, *Postgrad Med* 102(2):199-207, 1997.
31. Swain RA, Kaplan-Machlis B: Therapeutic uses of vitamin E in prevention of atherosclerosis, *Altern Med Rev* 4(6):414-23, 1999.
32. Haskell WL, Luskin FM, Maaarvasti FF: Complementary/alternative therapies in general medicine: cardiovascular disease. In Spencer JW, Jacobs JJ: *Complementary/alternative medicine: an evidence-based approach*, St Louis, 1999, Mosby.
33. Pruthi S, Allison TG, Hensrud DD: Vitamin E supplementation in the prevention of coronary heart disease, *Mayo Clin Proc* 76(11):1131-6, 2001.
34. Lonn E: Modifying the natural history of atherosclerosis: the SECURE trial, *Int J Clin Pract Suppl* Jan(117):13-8, 2001.
35. Jialal I, Fuller CJ, Huet BA: The effect of alpha-tocopherol supplementation on LDL oxidation. A dose-response study, *Arterioscler Thromb Vasc Biol* 15(2):190-8, 1995.
36. Fuller CJ, Huet BA, Jialal I: Effects of increasing doses of alpha-tocopherol in providing protection of low-density lipoprotein from oxidation, *Am J Cardiol* 81(2):231-3, 1998.
37. Goetzl EJ: Vitamin E modulates lipoxygenation of arachidonic acid in leukocytes, *Nature* 288:183-5, 1980.
38. Kleijnen J, Mackerras D: Vitamin E for intermittent claudication, *Cochrane Database Syst Rev* 2:CD000987, 2000.
39. Engelen W, Keenoy BM, Vertommen J, De Leeuw I: Effects of long-term supplementation with moderate pharmacologic doses of vitamin E are saturable and reversible in patients with type 1 diabetes, *Am J Clin Nutr* 72(5):1142-9, 2000.
40. Evans WJ: Vitamin E, vitamin C, and exercise, *Am J Clin Nutr* 72(2 Suppl): 647S-52S, 2000.
41. Lamson DW, Brignall MS: Natural agents in the prevention of cancer part I: human chemoprevention trials, *Altern Med Rev* 6(1):7-19, 2001.
42. Shklar G, Oh SK: Experimental basis for cancer prevention by vitamin E, *Cancer Invest* 18(3):214-22, 2000.
43. Diplock AT, Charleux JL, Crozier-Willi G, et al: Functional food science and defence against reactive oxidative species, *Br J Nutr* 80(Suppl 1):S77-112, 1998.
44. Kim JM, White RH: Effect of vitamin E on the anticoagulant response of warfarin, *Am J Cardiol* 77(7):545-6, 1996.
45. Kappus H, Diplock AT: Tolerance and safety of vitamin E: a toxicological position report, *Free Radic Biol Med* 13(1):55-74, 1992.
46. Primack A: Complementary/Alternative therapies in the prevention and treatment of cancer. In Spencer JW, Jacobs JJ: *Complementary/alternative medicine: an evidence-based approach*, St Louis, 1999, Mosby.
47. Tanyel MC, Mancano LD: Neurologic findings in vitamin E deficiency, *Am Fam Physician* 55(1):197-201, 1997.
48. Jiang Q, Christen S, Shigenaga MK, Ames BN: γ-tocopherol, the major form of vitamin E in the US diet deserves more attention, *Am J Clin Nutr* 74(6):714-22, 2001.

CHAPTER 108

VITAMIN K

Patients on anticoagulants who take large doses of vitamin E require increased vitamin K; those not on anticoagulants do not.

Vitamin K is a fat-soluble vitamin obtained from bacteria in the bowel and from dietary sources such as liver, leafy green vegetables, and milk. Dietary vitamin K includes phylloquinone (vitamin K_1) and menaquinone (vitamin K_2).

Vitamin K is a trace nutrient necessary for the synthesis of four plasma clotting factors, two anticlotting factors (protein C and protein S), and the synthesis of two bone proteins (osteocalcin and matrix Gla-protein).[1] Although vitamin K has long been recognized as important for blood coagulation, its contribution to skeletal health has only recently been appreciated.

MECHANISM OF ACTION

Vitamin K is essential for normal coagulation. It is required for the hepatic synthesis of clotting factors VII, IX, X, and prothrombin. Vitamin K is not only involved in the synthesis of clotting factors but it also contributes to the synthesis of proteins that prevent clotting.

Protein S is a vitamin K-dependent protein with anticoagulant properties. Case series have reported reduced plasma concentrations of protein S in patients with arterial thromboses, and other studies have reported increased levels in patients with coronary heart disease. A prospective survey found a one standard deviation increase in free protein S was associated with a hazard risk of 1.15 for coronary heart disease.[2] The association of free protein S with risk of coronary heart disease may reflect the effects of plaque-destabilizing inflammatory activity on protein S levels. Matrix Gla-protein also requires vitamin K for its synthesis in the smooth muscle cells of healthy vessel walls. Matrix Gla-protein is a strong inhibitor of vascular calcification, and its mRNA transcription is substantially upregulated in atherosclerotic lesions.

In addition to its effect on coagulation and the vasculature, vitamin K_1 has a potentially important role in cell signaling.[3] Vitamin K_1-dependent proteins have been identified as specific ligands for the receptor tyrosine kinases that can stimulate cell replication and transformation and participate in cell survival. Growing evidence suggests that most normal and tumor cells possess an active K_1-dependent gamma-carboxylation mechanism necessary for the production of gamma-carboxyglutamic acid-containing proteins. Gamma-carboxyglutamic acid residues in proteins facilitate calcium-dependent protein/phospholipid interaction. These observations provide an explanation for the rigid control of vitamin K_1 levels in the mammalian fetus and its minimal hepatic stores in the adult.

Recent studies suggest that vitamin K could affect bone quality. Vitamin K_2 is used in the treatment of osteoporosis, and laboratory studies suggest that vitamin K_2 inhibits apoptotic cell death of osteoblasts and maintains the number of osteoblasts.[4] Both vitamin K_2 and vitamin K_3 induce apoptosis of various cultured cells including osteoclasts and osteoblasts, by elevating peroxide and superoxide radicals.[5] Osteocalcin metabolism has been implicated in the pathogenesis of osteoporosis through a mechanism that may be linked to suboptimal vitamin K status resulting in undercarboxylation of its glutamic acid residues. A prospective study found low vitamin K intakes were associated with an increased incidence of hip fractures in elderly men and women; however, neither low vitamin K intake nor E4 allele status, postulated to affect vitamin K transport, was associated with low bone mineral density.[6] Vitamin K appears to reduce vertebral and hip fractures without increasing bone mass in patients with osteoporosis. Results of a preliminary study examining serum bone markers and ultrasound velocity support the hypothesis that carboxylation of osteocalcin is related to bone quality.[7]

FOOD SOURCES

Bacterial intestinal flora is an important source. Weight for weight, kale, spinach, soybeans, broccoli, and cabbage are the best sources. One hundred grams of kale have 700 µg of vitamin K, compared with the 100 µg found in 100 g of cabbage. Other sources include liver, leafy green vegetables, tomatoes, and lean meat.

DOSE

The current recommended dietary allowance (RDA) for vitamin K is 70 µg/day in men and 60 µg/day in women younger than 25 years, and 80 µg/day in men and 65 µg/day in women 25 years and older. The therapeutic dose range is 30 to 100 µg/day.[8] However, the amount of vitamin K required for hepatic synthesis of clotting factors is lower than that required for the more recently recognized roles of vitamin K in bone metabolism and vascular biology. The RDA for vitamin K may need revision.

CLINICAL USES

Neonates are at risk of hemorrhagic disease of the newborn. This can be prevented by an injection of vitamin K to enable them to synthesize coagulation factors while their intestine is being colonized by bacteria capable of vitamin K synthesis. One dose of vitamin K (1 mg imi) reduces clinical bleeding at 1 to 7 days, including bleeding after circumcision, and improves biochemical indices of coagulation status in neonates.[9] Injecting women with vitamin K before delivery is less successful. A review of clinical trials concluded that vitamin K administered to women before the birth failed to significantly prevent periventricular hemorrhages in preterm infants.[10]

Oral vitamin K also improves coagulation indices. A multicenter, double-blind, placebo-controlled, randomized trial found low dose oral vitamin K more effective than placebo in restoring blood coagulation to the therapeutic range in overanticoagulated patients receiving warfarin.[11]

Vitamin K may emerge as an intervention to prevent clinically overt osteoporosis. Results from a 24-month randomized, open study of osteoporotic patients suggested that vitamin K_2 (45 mg daily) effectively prevented the occurrence of new fractures, despite any increase in lumbar bone mineral density being detected.[12] Vitamin K_2 treatment enhances gamma-carboxylation of the osteocalcin molecule. A randomized study of postmenopausal women found that daily supplementation with 80 µg vitamin K_1 seemed necessary to reach premenopausal percentage carboxylated osteocalcin levels.[13] A stimulatory effect of calcium and/or vitamin D on the proportion of carboxylated osteocalcin could not be excluded. Furthermore, heparin inhibits lipoprotein-mediated carriage of vitamin K and possibly other lipids to bone and may explain heparin-induced osteoporosis.[14]

TOXICITY AND DRUG INTERACTIONS

Antibiotics alter bowel flora and may increase requirements for vitamin K by eliminating the bacterial bowel source of this vitamin. Vitamin K reduces the efficacy of anticoagulants.

A constant dietary intake of vitamin K that meets current dietary recommendations of 65 to 80 µg/day is the most acceptable practice for patients on warfarin therapy.[15] Dietary vitamin K may lead to diet-warfarin interaction. In addition to patients on warfarin being wary of green leafy vegetables and certain plant oils, they may also need to avoid prepared foods containing these plant oils, ranging from baked goods to margarine and salad dressings. Patients on anticoagulants should be encouraged to maintain consistency in their vitamin K intake and should strive to meet the RDA for vitamin K.[16,17] On average, to maintain a steady state, the warfarin dose required decreases by 11% per decade of age.

Absorption of vitamin K, like other fat-soluble vitamins, may be impaired by liquid paraffin, cholestyramine, or sucralfate.

CLINICAL CAUTION

In view of the role of vitamin K in bone and vascular metabolism, higher levels of vitamin K may be required than was previously thought. In fact, it is possible that the population may be mildly deficient in vitamin K and in older adults, this may contribute to increased bone fracture risk, arterial calcification, and cardiovascular disease.[6] Undercarboxylation of matrix Gla-protein may be a risk factor for vascular calcification and the present RDA values are possibly too low to ensure full carboxylation of matrix Gla-protein.

PRACTICE TIPS

- Patients on warfarin should take care not to alter their dietary intake of leafy green vegetables or liver.
- Vitamin K administration favors coagulation, increasing coagulation factors more than anticlotting factors.
- Although natural vitamin K is nontoxic, synthetic vitamin K can cause liver damage.

REFERENCES

1. Shirakawa Y, Shirahata A, Fukuda M: Differences in reactivity to vitamin K administration of the vitamin K-dependent procoagulant factors, protein C and S, and osteocalcin, *Semin Thromb Hemost* 26:119-262, 2000.
2. Rudnicka AR, Miller GJ, Nelson T, et al: An association between plasma free protein s concentration and risk of coronary heart disease in middle-aged men, *Thromb Res* 101(2):1-11, 2001.
3. Saxena SP, Israels ED, Israels LG: Novel vitamin K-dependent pathways regulating cell survival, *Apoposis* 6(1-2):57-68, 2001.
4. Urayama S, Kawakami A, Nakashima T, et al: Effect of vitamin K_2 on osteoblast apoptosis: vitamin K_2 inhibits apoptotic cell death of human osteoblasts induced by Fas, proteasome inhibitor, etoposide, and starosporine, *J Lab Clin Med* 136: 181-93, 2000.
5. Sakagami H, Satoh K, Hakeda Y, et al: Apoptosis-inducing activity of vitamin C and vitamin K, *Cell Mol Biol* 46:129-43, 2000.
6. Booth SL, Tucker KL, Chen H, et al: Dietary vitamin K intakes are associated with hip fracture but not with bone mineral density in elderly men and women, *Am J Clin Nutr* 71:1201-8, 2000.
7. Sugiyama T, Kawai S: Carboxylation of osteocalcin may be related to bone quality: a possible mechanism of bone fracture prevention by vitamin K, *J Bone Miner Metab* 19:146-9, 2001.

8. Brighthope I: Nutritional medicine tables, *J Aust Coll Nutr Env Med* 17:20-5, 1998.
9. Puckett RM, Offringa M: Prophylactic vitamin K for vitamin K deficiency bleeding in neonates (Cochrane Review), *Cochrane Database Syst Rev* 4:CD002776, 2000.
10. Crowther CA, Henderson-Smart DJ: Vitamin K prior to preterm birth for preventing neonatal periventricular haemorrhage, *Cochrane Database Syst Rev* 1:CD000229, 2001.
11. Crowther MA, Julian J, McCarty D, et al: Treatment of warfarin-associated coagulopathy with oral vitamin K: a randomised controlled trial, *Lancet* 356:1551-3, 2000.
12. Shiraki M, Shiraki Y, Aoki C, et ai: Vitamin K_2 (menatetrenone) effectively prevents fractures and sustains lumbar bone mineral density in osteoporosis, *J Bone Miner Res* 15:515-21, 2000.
13. Schaafsma A, Muskiet FA, Storm H, et al: Vitamin D_3 and vitamin K_1 supplementation of Dutch postmenopausal women with normal and low bone mineral densities: effects on serum 25-hydroxyvitamin D and carboxylated osteocalcin, *Eur J Clin Nutr* 54:626-3, 2000.
14. Newman P, Bonello F, Wierzbicki AS, et al: The uptake of lipoprotein-borne phylloquinone (vitamin K_1) by osteoblasts and osteoblast-like cells: role of heparan sulfate proteoglycans and apolipoprotein E, *J Bone Miner Res* 17:426-33, 2002.
15. Booth SL, Centurelli MA: Vitamin K: a practical guide to the dietary management of patients on warfarin, *Nutr Rev* 57(9 Pt 1):288-96, 1999.
16. Hylek EM: Oral anticoagulants. Pharmacologic issues for use in the elderly, *Clin Geriatr Med* 17:1-13, 2001.
17. Vermeer C, Schurgers LJ: A comprehensive review of vitamin K and vitamin K antagonists, *Hematol Oncol Clin North Am* 14:339-53, 2000.

CHAPTER 109

WITCH HAZEL (*HAMAMELIS VIRGINIANA L*)

> Popular remedies may enjoy better scientific validation at the level of the laboratory (i.e., *in vitro*) than suggested by the results of clinical trials.

The leaves and bark of this shrub are a popular remedy for minimizing bruising and reducing painful swelling. It has traditionally been used to treat hemorrhoids, varicose veins, bruises, and minor skin damage. There are also claims it may provide protection against ultraviolet (UV) radiation. Witch hazel is available over-the-counter and is used as an astringent for relief of minor skin or anorectal irritation.

MECHANISM OF ACTION

Hamamelis contains a mixture of tannins including hamamelitannin, catechins, gallotannins, and procyanidins; it also includes essential oils and flavonoids. The tannins exert an antiinflammatory effect. A number of the tannins are potent inhibitors of 5-lipoxygenase and consequently leukotriene production. Laboratory studies found hamamelitannin inhibited the tumor necrosis factor (TNF)-mediated endothelial cell death without altering the TNF-induced upregulation of endothelial adhesiveness.[1] This anti-TNF activity may explain the traditional selection of this herb for antihemorrhagic purposes. *Hamamelis* demonstrates vasoconstriction in animal experiments. The procyanidins inhibit lyso-PAF: acetyl-CoA acetyltransferase and therefore platelet activating factor (PAF) and have been shown to strongly increase the proliferation but not the differentiation of cultured human keratinocytes.[2] An *in vivo* experiment found transepidermal water loss and erythema formation may be reduced, suggesting that this extract may soothe irritated skin.

A crude hydroalcoholic extract from *Hamamelis virginiana* bark has been shown to have significant antiviral activity against herpes simplex virus type 1 (HSV-1), as well as radical scavenging properties.[3] Other laboratory studies confirm that *Hamamelis* has strong radical scavenging activity, protecting cell damage induced by active oxygen species.[4] Consequently, witch hazel may have potential as an antiaging or antiwrinkle potion for the skin.[4]

DOSE

Traditional use includes 2 g three times a day (tds) of the dried leaf and bark, 7 to 14 ml daily of 1:2 liquid leaf extract, or 0.1 to 1 g in suppositories applied tds. *Hamamelis* water may be used for topical application.

CLINICAL USES

Clinical trials support topical use of witch hazel for hemorrhoids and varicose veins.[5,6] It is used in combination with goldenseal for the treatment of varicose veins. It is also used to treat mild skin inflammation[5] and may be included in suntan lotions. A double-blind, randomized trial lasting 14 days in patients with moderately severe atopic eczema found cream with 5.35-g *hamamelis* distillate, the corresponding drug-free vehicle, and 0.5% hydrocortisone cream all significantly reduced itching, erythema, and scaling after 1 week.[7] However, *hamamelis* distillate was no more effective than the base preparation and neither were as effective as hydrocortisone. On the other hand, a study using healthy volunteers found the antiinflammatory action of aftersun lotion with 10% *hamamelis* superior to a number of other aftersun formulations.[8]

TOXICITY AND DRUG INTERACTIONS

Hamamelis is safe for long-term external application. Although no significant side effects are anticipated, ingestion of witch hazel may cause gastric irritation in susceptible individuals.

Tannins may impair absorption of minerals and B vitamins.

CLINICAL CAUTION

Avoid long-term oral ingestion in view of the tannin concentration.

PRACTICE TIPS

• Tannins should be avoided in patients with constipation.

REFERENCES

1. Habtemariam S: Hamamelitannin from *Hamamelis virginiana* inhibits the tumour necrosis factor-alpha (TNF)-induced endothelial cell death in vitro, *Toxicon* 40(1):83-8, 2002.

2. Deters A, Dauer A, Schnetz E, et al: High molecular compounds (polysaccharides and proanthocyanidins) from *Hamamelis virginiana* bark: influence on human skin keratinocyte proliferation and differentiation and influence on irritated skin, *Phytochemistry* 58:949-58, 2001.
3. Erdelmeier CA, Cinatl J Jr, Rabenau H, et al: Antiviral and antiphlogistic activities of *Hamamelis virginiana* bark, *Planta Med* 62:241-5, 1996.
4. Masaki H, Sakaki S, Atsumi T, et al: Active-oxygen scavenging activity of plant extracts, *Biol Pharm Bull* 18:162-6, 1995.
5. Mills S, Bone K: *Principles and practice of phytotherapy*, Edinburgh, 2000, Churchill Livingstone.
6. MacKay D: Hemorrhoids and varicose veins: a review of treatment options, *Altern Med Rev* 6(2):126-40, 2001.
7. Korting HC, Schafer-Korting M, Klovekorn W, et al: Comparative efficacy of hamamelis distillate and hydrocortisone cream in atopic eczema, *Eur J Clin Pharmacol* 48:461-5, 1995.
8. Hughes-Formella BJ, Bohnsack K, Rippke F, et al: Anti-inflammatory effect of hamamelis lotion in a UVB erythema test, *Dermatology* 196:316-22, 1998.

■ CHAPTER 110 ■

ZINC (ZN)

Iron and/or folic acid may reduce zinc absorption; zinc deficiency may cause intrauterine growth retardation and congenital abnormalities, yet it is common practice to encourage pregnant women to take iron and folic acid supplements.

The food guide pyramid does not provide guidelines leading to an adequate zinc intake. More than 60% of persons of 20 years and older in the United States do not consume the recommended dietary allowance (RDA) for zinc. Zinc deficiency is even more prevalent in areas where the population subsists on cereals. Furthermore, apparently healthy persons may function better with zinc supplementation. When normal volunteers with no evidence of zinc deficiency were supplemented with 135 mg of zinc daily for 15 days, they developed increased isokinetic strength and isometric endurance in their leg muscles.[1]

Zinc deficiency can cause immunodepression and produce muscle pain and fatigue. It is required for deoxyribonucleic acid (DNA) synthesis, cell division, and protein synthesis. Conditions for which zinc may offer a therapeutic benefit range from anorexia nervosa, wound healing, coryza, and acquired immunodeficiency syndrome (AIDS) to benign prostatic hyperplasia. Both prostatic fluid and the pancreas have a high concentration of zinc.

MECHANISM OF ACTION

Approximately 300 enzymes are known to require zinc for their activities. Zinc is a metalloenzyme activator. It is associated with a number of dehydrogenase enzymes (e.g., alcohol dehydrogenase, retinol dehydrogenase). As part of carbonic anhydrase, it is involved in the interconversion of carbon dioxide and contributes to acid-base balance in red cells. Zinc functions with cytosol superoxide dismutase inactivating free radicals; it is a free radical quencher. It is associated with nucleic acid metabolism and control of gene transcription. It is associated with the synthesis of proteins, the stabilization of cell membranes, and the function of receptor molecules.

Zinc plays a particularly important role in immunity.[2] Mouse models demonstrate that 30 days of suboptimal intake of zinc leads to a 30% to 80%

loss in immune defense capacity, whereas short periods of zinc supplementation substantially improve immune defense in individuals with diverse diseases.[3] Immune integrity is tightly linked to zinc status. Zinc deficiency affects leukocyte functions, impairing phagocytosis; however, its impact is most marked on the specific immune system. Zinc deficiency rapidly diminishes antibody- and cell-mediated responses in both humans and animals.[3]

Lymphopenia and thymic atrophy, the early hallmarks of zinc deficiency, are due to high losses of precursor T and B cells in the bone marrow. Zinc deficiency adversely affects lymphocyte proliferation and decreases interleukin-2 production by helper T lymphocytes. Glucocorticoid-mediated apoptosis induced by zinc deficiency causes downregulation of lymphopoiesis and ensures that the lymphopenia persists. Consequently, impaired immune function resulting from dietary zinc deficiency is characterized in part by a reduction in the number of lymphocytes and depressed cell-mediated (i.e., T lymphocyte) immune function.

Research suggests deficiencies of zinc and other essential nutrients such as methionine; cysteine; arginine; vitamins A, B, C, and E; and selenium promote the proliferation of Th2 cells at the expense of Th1 cells.[2] It has been postulated that a zinc deficiency can lead to premature transition from efficient Th1-dependent cellular immune functions to Th2-dependent humoral immune functions. On the other hand, adequate Zn^{2+} and nitrogen oxide prevents a shift of the Th1/Th2 balance toward Th2. Under Th2, levels of interleukin-4 (II-4), II-6, II-10, leukotriene B_4 (LTB_4), and prostaglandin E_2 (PGE_2) are raised, whereas levels of II-2, Zn^{2+}, and nitrogen oxide, amongst others, are lowered. Nitrogen oxide appears to be able to liberate Zn^{2+} from metallothionein, an intracellular storage molecule for metal ions. Zinc ions (Zn^{2+}) and nitrogen oxide, together with glutathione (GSH) and its oxidized form, GSSG, help to regulate immune responses to antigens.

In view of the impact that zinc deficiency has on cell-mediated immunity, it is not surprising that zinc deficiency may promote cancer. Under the influence of Th1 cells, zinc inhibits the growth of tumors by activating the endogenous tumor-suppressor endostatin, which inhibits angiogenesis.[2] It also reduces resistance to viral diseases. Viruses like human immunodeficiency virus 1 (HIV-1) multiply in Th2 cells but rarely, if ever, in Th1 cells. Furthermore, dysregulation of the Th1/Th2 balance is also believed responsible for autoimmune disorders such as diabetes mellitus. On the other hand, zinc supplementation may help to prevent diabetic complications through its intracellular activation of the enzyme sorbitol dehydrogenase.

Animal studies suggest even a marginal zinc deficiency could affect leptin secretion and serum leptin concentrations.[4] Impaired leptin secretion caused by zinc deficiency is postulated to contribute to hypogonadism observed in zinc deficiency.

FOOD SOURCES

Zinc is found in lean red meats, seafood (especially herring and oysters), yeast, pumpkin seeds, nuts, whole grains, leafy green vegetables, and legumes. Two steamed oysters provide more than the RDA of zinc.

Losses occur on refining flour and freezing foods treated with ethylenediaminetetraacetic acid (EDTA). Foods stored in uncoated tin cans may reduce the amount of zinc available for absorption from that food.

Zinc is best absorbed from animal products. In fact, meat increases zinc retention from conventional diets. Absorption from lean beef is 50%, compared with vegetable sources or whole meal bread, in which it drops to 15%. Phosphorus-containing foods such as milk or poultry, whole grains, and fiber-rich foods impair zinc absorption. Calcium increases the binding of zinc by phytate. Copper, iron, phytate, and oxalate also all interfere with zinc absorption.

The body content of zinc is 2 g.

DOSE

The RDA varies but a ballpark figure is 15 mg for males and 12 mg for females or 8 mg/1000 kcal. To correct zinc deficiency 220 mg three times daily (tds) plus 2 mg copper daily has been suggested.[1] The therapeutic dose range is 20 to 100 mg daily.[3]

Zinc sulphate is readily absorbed and zinc citrate is well absorbed. Zinc supplements are most effective if they are taken at least 1 hour before or 2 hours after meals.

Assays of zinc in granulocytes and lymphocytes provide better diagnostic criteria for marginal zinc deficiency than plasma zinc. Plasma zinc levels reflect intake; white cell zinc reflects cellular storage. When used, serum zinc should be measured in the fasting state and interpreted in conjunction with albumin. A low albumin depresses serum zinc and vice versa.

CLINICAL USES

Various studies suggest zinc supplementation of 45 to 100 mg daily promotes weight gain in anorexic females. Zinc deficiency, in addition to lethargy and retarded mentation, causes anorexia and reduced taste sensation. In fact, zinc supplementation may achieve a weight gain of 0.7 kg/month and improved taste sensation, appetite, and mood in anorexia nervosa.[6] Although it is known that persons with anorexia nervosa who are zinc deficient respond well to zinc supplementation, it remains unclear whether zinc deficiency is a cause or a consequence of the condition.

Zinc has also long been linked with wound healing. However, analysis of randomized, controlled trials comparing oral zinc sulphate with placebo or no treatment in patients with arterial or venous leg ulcers concluded there was no evidence that zinc sulphate increased ulcer healing.[7] Nonetheless, there was some evidence that oral zinc might have a beneficial effect on healing of venous ulcers in people with a low serum zinc level at baseline.

The impact of zinc on the common cold remains controversial but promising. A randomized, double-blind, placebo-controlled, clinical trial found treatment of the common cold with zinc gluconate lozenges significantly reduced the duration of cold symptoms.[8] Patients received zinc-containing lozenges or placebo lozenges every 2 hours while symptomatic. The median time to complete resolution of cold symptoms was 4.4 days in the zinc group, compared with 7.6 days in the placebo group. The mechanism of action of zinc in treating the common cold remains unknown. More recently, clinical trials with zinc gluconate (13.3 mg) reduced the median duration of illness by 1 day in the experimental, but not natural, colds study group.[9] Experimental subjects were symptomatic for 2.5 days in contrast to the 3.5 days reported by recipients of the placebo. Common adverse effects include unpleasant taste, mouth irritation, and nausea.[10] Trials of zinc lozenges continue to have mixed results.[11]

Both excessive and inadequate zinc levels can impair immune function.[12] Zinc deficiency in childhood is associated with reduced immunocompetence and increased infectious disease morbidity, whereas zinc supplementation in infants that are small for their gestational age can reduce mortality attributable to infectious disease.[13] A review of epidemiologic studies concluded zinc supplementation reduced the incidence and severity of diarrheal diseases and the occurrence of pneumonia and enabled greater increments in height in children with poor dietary zinc intake and/or bioavailability.[14] Animal studies suggest that adding zinc to oral replacement solutions may improve the physiologic status of the small intestine and potentially reduce the risks of recurrent diarrhea episodes.[15] Zinc, which inhibits the activity of prostatic 5-alpha-reductase, has been indeed been found to inhibit the growth of prostate cancer cell lines in vitro.[16] Zinc, in view of its impact on cell-mediated immune function, may yet emerge as a therapeutic aid in cancer and AIDS patients.

Certainly, there is little doubt that any zinc deficiency should be corrected. In fact, routine zinc supplementation may deserve consideration in certain population groups. Dietary supplementation with the RDA of zinc for between 1 and 2 months decreased the incidence of infection and increased the survival rate following infection in older adults.[17] Data support use in older adults of a daily multivitamin or trace-mineral supplement that includes zinc (elemental zinc, at least 20 mg daily), selenium (100 µg/day), and additional vitamin E, to achieve a daily dosage of 200 mg.[18]

TOXICITY AND DRUG INTERACTIONS

Acute zinc toxicity, induced by a single dose of 1.0 g or daily doses of 200 mg or more, presents with fever, nausea, vomiting, diarrhea, and abdominal pain. Some patients experience dizziness and muscular incoordination.

In doses in excess of 150 mg daily, zinc supplementation may cause reduced high-density lipoprotein (HDL) cholesterol levels,[19] precipitate gastric erosions, and depress immune function. Chronic zinc supplementation in excess of 50 mg/day can induce copper deficiency in humans.[20] Animal studies found that, although iron did not significantly inhibit zinc at a Fe/Zn ratio below 2:1, at higher ratios, zinc uptake and net absorption decreased significantly.[21] Between 2:1 and 5:1, a dose-dependent inhibition of zinc absorption occurred and reached a plateau beyond this ratio. In iron-deficient animals, zinc absorption only reached a plateau at a ratio of 7.5:1.

Zinc may reduce the effectiveness of therapies that rely on dopamine receptor antagonists[22] and reduce absorption of penicillamine, folic acid, and tetracyclines. The reverse is also true for the latter. Tetracyclines, copper, iron, and zinc supplements should consequently be taken at least 2 hours apart to maximize the full benefit from each supplement.

Immunostimulants such as zinc should not be given with immunosuppressants (e.g., corticosteroids and cyclosporine). Zinc interacts with vitamin A and can contribute to night blindness.

CLINICAL CAUTION

In animals, zinc deficiency manifests as stunted growth, impaired fetal development, infertility, skin rash, and anorexia. In humans, early evidence of zinc deficiency is anorexia, anosmia, and impaired taste (hypogeusia and dysgeusia). Dietary zinc deprivation causes brain dysfunctions such as learning impairment, enhanced susceptibility to epileptic seizures, and olfactory dysfunction.[23] Zinc homeostasis in the brain is closely related to neuronal activity. A clinical assessment of zinc status relies on taste. Persons with good zinc status experience a strong unpleasant taste immediately on taking a swig of the zinc tally solution. Those with a marginally adequate zinc status report a definite taste almost immediately. In contrast, moderately zinc-deficient persons report no specific taste after 10 seconds of holding the solution in their mouth; those mildly deficient report no immediate taste, but a furry, dry mineral taste develops.

Mild to moderate zinc deficiency presents with cold extremities, slow wound healing, male hypogonadism, and slow mentation. Severe zinc deficiency is associated with skin disorders, white spots on nails, alopecia, weight loss, psychiatric disorders, and intercurrent infection. Impaired immunity leads to lymphopenia and reduced T-cell function. Deficiency during growth periods results in growth failure and predisposes to congenital abnormalities. Acrodermatitis enteropathica, a genetic disorder, is fatal if the severe zinc deficiency is not controlled.

PRACTICE TIPS

- Because zinc is required for nucleic acid and protein synthesis, in cases of zinc deficiency, the cells with most rapid turnover are likely to be the first to demonstrate abnormalities (e.g., red blood cells, intestinal epithelium).
- Zinc chloride, zinc gluconate, and zinc sulfate may be used to inhibit copper absorption and as a nutritional supplement.
- When taking zinc supplements over periods exceeding 4 weeks, take a 2-mg copper supplement each day.
- Supplementation with 1500-mg calcium lowers zinc retention; supplementation with 500-mg calcium does not.
- Persons sucking zinc lozenges for colds and flu every 2 to 4 hours should avoid exceeding a daily intake of 150 mg.

REFERENCES

1. Werbach MR: Nutritional strategies for treating chronic fatigue syndrome, *Altern Med Rev* 5(2):93-108, 2000.
2. Sprietsma JE: Modern diets and diseases: NO-zinc balance. Under Th1, zinc and nitrogen monoxide (NO) collectively protect against viruses, AIDS, autoimmunity, diabetes, allergies, asthma, infectious diseases, atherosclerosis and cancer, *Med Hypotheses* 53(1):6-16, 1999.
3. Fraker PJ, King LE, Laakko T, et al: The dynamic link between the integrity of the immune system and zinc status, *J Nutr* 130(5S Suppl):1399S-406S, 2000.
4. Ott ES, Shay NF: Zinc deficiency reduces leptin gene expression and leptin secretion in rat adipocytes, *Exp Biol Med* (Maywood) 226:841-6, 2001.
5. Brighthope I: Nutritional medicine tables, *J Aust Coll Nutr Env Med* 17:20-5, 1998.
6. Brighthope I: Nutritional medicine—its presence and power, *J Aust Coll Nutr Env Med* 17:5-18, 1998.
7. Wilkinson EA, Hawke CI: Oral zinc for arterial and venous leg ulcers, *Cochrane Database Syst Rev* 2:CD001273, 2000.
8. Zinc lozenges reduce the duration of common cold symptoms, *Nutr Rev* 55(3):82-5, 1997.
9. Turner RB, Cetnarowski WE: Effect of treatment with zinc gluconate or zinc acetate on experimental and natural colds, *Clin Infect Dis* 31:1202-8, 2000.
10. Garland ML, Hagmeyer KO: The role of zinc lozenges in treatment of the common cold, *Ann Pharmacother* 32(1):63-9, 1998.
11. Turner RB, Schaffner W, Young MG: Will anything work for the common cold? *Patient Care* Nov:15-24, 2000.
12. Rink L, Gabriel P: Extracellular and immunological actions of zinc, *Biometals* 14:367-83, 2001.

13. Sazawal S, Black RE, Menon VP, et al: Zinc supplementation in infants born small for gestational age reduces mortality: a prospective, randomized, controlled trial, *Pediatrics* 108:1280-6, 2001.
14. Duggan C, Fawzi W: Micronutrients and child health: studies in international nutrition and HIV infection, *Nutr Rev* 59:358-69, Nov 2001.
15. Altaf W, Perveen S, Rehman KU, et al: Zinc supplementation in oral rehydration solutions: experimental assessment and mechanisms of action, *J Am Coll Nutr* 21(1):26-32, 2002.
16. Liang JY, Liu YY, Zou J, et al: Inhibitory effect of zinc on human prostatic carcinoma cell growth, *Prostate* 40:200-7, 1999.
17. Mocchegiani E, Muzzioli M, Giacconi R: Zinc and immunoresistance to infection in aging: new biological tools, *Trends Pharmacol Sci* 21(6):205-8, 2000.
18. High KP: Nutritional strategies to boost immunity and prevent infection in elderly individuals, *Clin Infect Dis* 33:1892-900, 2001.
19. Lukaski HC: Magnesium, zinc and chromium nutriture and physical activity, *Am J Clin Nutr* 72(2 Suppl):585S-93S, 2000.
20. Fischer PW, Giroux A, L'Abbe MR: Effect of zinc supplementation on copper status in adult man, *Am J Clin Nutr* 40:743-6, 1984.
21. Peres JM, Bureau F, Neuville D, et al: Inhibition of zinc absorption by iron depends on their ratio, *J Trace Elem Med Biol* 15:237-41, 2001.
22. Schetz JA, Chu A, Sibley DR: Zinc modulates antagonist interactions with D2-like dopamine receptors through distinct molecular mechanisms, *J Pharmacol Exp Ther* 289:956-64, 1999.
23. Takeda A: Zinc homeostasis and functions of zinc in the brain, *Biometals* 14:343-51, 2001.

APPENDICES

■ APPENDIX A ■

DEFINITIONS AND SOURCES OF DOSE INFORMATION[1,2]

adequate intake (AI): Recommended daily intake value based on the observed or experimentally determined approximations of nutrient intake of one or more groups of healthy people. AI is used as a guide to desirable intake levels of nutrients for which the recommended daily allowance cannot be determined.

estimated average requirement (EAR): Daily nutrient intake estimated to meet the requirements of half of the healthy individuals in a group; used as a guideline for assessing the likelihood of deficiency in individuals or groups.

recommended daily allowance (RDA): Average daily intake required to meet the nutrient requirements of 97% to 98% of healthy individuals; used as a target in planning dietary intake for individuals or populations.

tolerable upper limit (UL): Highest level of intake likely to pose no health risk to almost everybody. As dose increases, the risk of adverse effects increases. UL is used as a guide for selecting upper limits of nutrient intake in planning a diet to avoid the possibility of overconsumption.

Although there are no recommended daily allowances for herbs, guidelines for their clinical use as suggested in this text are derived from reputable sources[3-6] (see Table A-1). The concept of dried herb equivalent may be used as a guideline, with the product ratio expressing the weight of original dried herb starting material to the volume or weight of the finished product.

TABLE A-1 ■ Herbal Preparation

DRIED HERB	EXTRACT (DRIED HERB:WT/VOL EXTRACT)
1 g	2 mL of 1:2 liquid or 3 mL of 1:3 liquid
1 g	250 mg of 4:1 extract
1 g	200 mg of a 5:1 spray dried powder

Dried herb equivalent: 1 g = 2 mL of 1:2 liquid or 5 mL of 1:5 liquid.

REFERENCES

1. Subcommittee on Upper Reference Levels of Nutrients, Food and Nutrition Board, Institute of Medicine: *Dietary reference intakes for thiamin, riboflavin, niacin, vitamin B_6, folate, vitamin B_{12}, pantothenic acid, biotin, and choline/a report of the Standing Committee on the Scientific Evaluation of Dietary Reference Intakes and its Panel on Folate, Other B Vitamins, and Choline*, Washington, D.C., 2000, National Academy Press.
2. US Pharmacopeia, www.usp.org.
3. Blumenthal M, Klein J, Rister R, et al: *The complete German commission E monographs: therapeutic guide to herbal medicines*, Austin, TX, 1998, American Botanical Council.
4. *Physician's desk reference (PDR) for herbal medicines*, ed 2, New Jersey, 2000, Medical Economies Company. 1998.
5. Mills S, Bone K: *Principles and practice of phytotherapy*, Edinburgh, 2000, Churchill Livingstone.
6. Kiefer D, Shah S, Gardiner P, et al: Finding information on herbal therapy: a guide to useful sources for clinicians, *Altern Ther Health Med* 7:74-8, 2001.

■ APPENDIX B ■

ABBREVIATIONS

AA: arachidonic acid
ACTH: adrenocoticotrophic hormone
ADP: adenosine diphosphate
AI: adequate intake (estimate of requirement, used when unable to determine recommended daily allowance)
ATP: adenosine triphosphate
CRH: corticotrophin releasing factor/hormone
DHA: docosahexaenoic acid
DSHEA: Dietary Supplement Health and Education Act (United States)
EAR: estimated average requirement (minimal amount required by one in two persons)
EPA: eicosapentaenoic acid
EPO: evening primrose oil
FAD: flavin adenine dinucleotide
FDA: Food and Drug Administration (United States)
FEV_1: forced expiratory volume in 1 second
FMN: flavin mononucleotide
GABA: γ-aminobutyric acid
GLA: γ-linolenic acid
GRAS: generally recognized as safe (United States)
GSL: General Sales List (United Kingdom)
HDL: high-density lipoprotein cholesterol (protective factor, coronary heart disease)
HPA: hypothalamic-pituitary-adrenocorticol (axis)
IHD: ischemic heart disease
IL: interleukin, biochemical messenger of leukocyte
IU: international unit
LDL: low-density lipoprotein cholesterol (a risk factor for coronary heart disease)
LT: leukotriene
NAD: nicotine-adenine dinucleotide
NADH: reduced form of NAD
NK: natural killer
NSAIDs: Nonsteroidal anti-inflammatory drugs
n-3: omega-3 series polyunsaturated fatty acids
n-6: omega-6 series polyunsaturated fatty acids
PG: prostaglandin
PUFA: polyunsaturated fatty acid

RDA: Recommended daily allowances (average amount needed for most people)

RE: retinol equivalent

TCA: tricarboxylic acid cycle/citric acid cycle/Krebs cycle

TGA: Therapeutic Goods Administration

TNF-α: tumor necrosis factor alpha

UL: tolerable upper limit (total long-term safe daily diet + supplement intake)

INDEX